Public Health Nutrition

The Nutrition Society Textbook Series

Now widely adopted in courses throughout the world, the prestigious Nutrition Society Textbook Series provides students with both specific scientific information and appropriate context.

These groundbreaking titles:

- Provide students with the required scientific basics of nutrition in the context of a systems and health approach

- Enable teachers and students to explore the core principles of nutrition, to apply these throughout their training, and to foster critical thinking at all times
- Are fully peer reviewed, to ensure completeness and clarity of content, as well as to ensure that each book takes a global perspective.

Nutrition Research Methodologies
Edited by Lovegrove, Hodson, Sharma & Lanham-New
March 2015
ISBN: 978-1-118-55467-8

Clinical Nutrition, 2nd Edition
Edited by Elia, Ljungqvist, Stratton & Lanham-New
January 2013
ISBN: 978-1-4051-6810-6

Sport and Exercise Nutrition
Edited by Lanham-New, Stear, Shirreffs & Collins
October 2011
ISBN: 978-1-4443-3468-5

Nutrition and Metabolism, 2nd Edition
Edited by Lanham-New, MacDonald & Roche
November 2010
ISBN: 978-1-4051-6808-3

Introduction to Human Nutrition, 2nd Edition
Edited by Gibney, Lanham-New, Cassidy & Vorster
March 2009
ISBN: 978-1-4051-6807-6

Public Health Nutrition

Second Edition

Edited on behalf of The Nutrition Society by

Professor Judith L Buttriss
Director General, British Nutrition Foundation

Dr Ailsa A Welch
Reader in Nutritional Epidemiology, University of East Anglia

Dr John M Kearney
Lecturer, Epidemiology, Dublin Institute of Technology

Editor-in-Chief

Professor Susan A Lanham-New
Head of the Department of Nutritional Sciences, University of Surrey

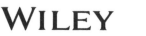

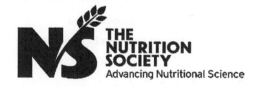

Library of Congress Cataloging-in-Publication Data

Names: Buttriss, Judith L, editor. | Welch, Ailsa A, editor. | Kearney, John M.,
 editor. | Lanham-New, Susan A, Editor-in-Chief. | The Nutrition Society (Great
 Britain), Issuing Body.
Title: Public Health Nutrition / edited on behalf of The Nutrition Society by
 Judith L. Buttriss, Ailsa A. Welch, John M. Kearney, Susan A. Lanham-New.
Other titles: Public Health Nutrition (The Nutrition Society (Great Britain))
Description: Second edition. | Chichester, West Sussex, UK ; Ames, Iowa, USA
 : John Wiley & Sons, Inc., 2017. | Includes bibliographical references and
 index.
Identifiers: LCCN 2016056644| ISBN 9781118660973 (paper) | ISBN 9781118660935
 (Adobe PDF) | ISBN 9781118660966 (epub)
Subjects: | MESH: Nutritional Physiological Phenomena | Dietetics | Public
 Health
Classification: LCC RA645.N87 | NLM QU 145 | DDC 616.3/9—dc23 LC record
available at https://lccn.loc.gov/2016056644

A catalogue record for this book is available from the British Library.

Wiley also publishes its books in a variety of electronic formats. Some content that appears in print may not be available in electronic books.

Cover image: © skystardream/iStockphoto

Set in 9.5/11pt MinionPro-Regular by Thomson Digital, Noida, India

10 9 8 7 6 5 4 3 2 1

Contents

Contributors

Professor Peter J Aggett
Lancaster University
UK

Dr Sarah C Bath
University of Surrey
UK

Bridget Benelam
British Nutrition Foundation
UK

Dr Francesco Branca
World Health Organization
Switzerland

Professor Eric J Brunner
University College London
UK

Dr Thomas Burgoine
University of Cambridge
UK

Professor Judith L Buttriss
British Nutrition Foundation
UK

Professor Janet E Cade
University of Leeds
UK

Dr U. Ruth Charrondiere
Food and Agriculture Organization of the United Nations
Italy

Dr Clare A Corish
University College Dublin
Ireland

Dr Andrea L Darling
University of Surrey
UK

Johanna T Dwyer
Tufts University
USA

Professor Ulf Ekelund
Norwegian School of Sport Sciences (NIH)
Norway

Professor Basma Ellahi
University of Chester
UK

Professor Paul Elliott
Imperial College London
UK

Cassandra H Ellis
The Nutrition Society
UK

Dr Charlotte EL Evans
University of Leeds
UK

Paul Finglas
Institute of Food Research
UK

Dr Emma Foster
Newcastle University
UK

Professor Kenneth R. Fox
University of Bristol
UK

Dr Christine Furber
The University of Manchester
UK

Jenny Gillespie
NHS Tayside
UK

Dr Bjørge H Hansen
Norwegian School of Sport Sciences (NIH)
Norway

Dr Richard PG Hayhoe
University of East Anglia
UK

Dr Anja Heilmann
University College London
UK

Dr Jayne Hutchinson
University of Leeds
UK

Elizabeth J Johnson
Tufts University
USA

Ashley T LaBrier
Tufts University
USA

Dr Amelia A Lake
Durham University
UK

Professor Susan A Lanham-New
University of Surrey
UK

Professor Alison M Lennox
University of Surrey
UK

Professor H David McCarthy
London Metropolitan University
UK

Professor Helene McNulty
Ulster University
UK

Dr Tracey A Mills
The University of Manchester
UK

Dr Emily Mohn
Tufts University
USA

Dr Farah Naja
American University of Beirut
Lebanon

Dr Lara Nasreddine
American University of Beirut
Lebanon

Dr Anne P Nugent
University College Dublin
Ireland

Dr Marga Ocke
National Institute for Public Health and the Environment
Netherlands

Dr Linda M Oude Griep
Imperial College London
UK

Jenny Plumb
Institute of Food Research
UK

Professor Margaret P Rayman
University of Surrey
UK

Mark Roe
Institute of Food Research
UK

Professor Peter J Rogers
University of Bristol
UK

Professor Tom Sanders
Kings College London
UK

Dr Paul A Sharp
Kings College London
UK

Dr Debbie M Smith
The University of Manchester
UK

Dr Sara Stanner
British Nutrition Foundation
UK

Dr Laura Stewart
NHS Tayside
UK

Professor Janice L Thompson
University of Birmingham
UK

Professor Tim G Townshend
Newcastle University
UK

Professor Richard G Watt
University College London
UK

Dr Elisabeth Weichselbaum
Nutrition Science and Consultancy
New Zealand

Dr Ailsa A Welch
University of East Anglia
UK

Dr Louise R Wilson
University of Surrey
UK

Professor Martin Wiseman
World Cancer Research Fund & University of Southampton
UK

Taryn Young
NHS Tayside
UK

As Patron of the British Nutrition Foundation I am pleased to contribute the Foreword for this comprehensive new edition of a popular textbook on Public Health Nutrition. Much has changed in the world of nutrition since the first edition was published in 2004, especially through confusing headlines and specialist research that seemed to contradict each other. The aim of the editorial team for the second edition, led by Professor Judith Buttriss from the British Nutrition Foundation, has been to bring the book up to date and, at the same time, to meet the requirements of students of nutrition and practitioners, as well as try to balance all that information. The book provides the reader with a comprehensive series of chapters in five themed sections, covering basic principles through to practical application of public health nutrition in local, national and international settings, and its translation into policy.

The Nutrition Society textbook series, first established by Professor Michael Gibney in 1998 and now under the direction of the second Editor-in-Chief, Professor Susan Lanham-New, continues to be an extraordinarily successful venture for the Society. This series of human nutrition textbooks is designed for use worldwide and this has been achieved by translating the series into many different languages including Spanish, Greek and Portuguese. The popularity of the textbooks is a tribute to the quality of the authorship and the value placed on them, both in the UK and Worldwide, as a core educational tool. I am sure this textbook will make a very valuable contribution to the Nutrition debate. Perhaps I might suggest a strapline: all things in moderation!

Preface

I am absolutely delighted in my capacity as Editor-in-Chief (E-i-C) of the Nutrition Society (NS) Textbook Series to introduce the Second Edition of *Public Health Nutrition*. So much planning and hard work has gone into producing this Second Edition, following a most successful production of *Public Health Nutrition* First Edition. We owe a great deal of thanks to Professor Barrie Margetts, Professor Lenore Arab and Dr John Kearney for their original work on this important book in the NS Textbook Series.

Public Health Nutrition 2nd Edition (PHN2e) has been led superbly by Professor Judith Buttriss (Director General, British Nutrition Foundation) as Senior Editor of the book, and her Editorial Team in the name of Dr Ailsa Welch (University of East Anglia) and Dr John Kearney (Dublin Institute of Technology). They have meticulously planned out the details of the chapters and managed to secure the world-leaders in the field to contribute key chapters. Professor Buttriss is a most inspirational leader, and the team have complemented one another admirably with their expertise and knowledge in the field, as well as providing great continuity from the First Edition. How indebted we are to all the contributors for making the book such a comprehensive review and we are absolutely thrilled, as Professor Buttriss outlines in her Introductory Chapter, to have so many global experts who have written chapters to make PHN2e a complete review of this key area.

PHN2e is intended for those with an interest in nutritional science whether they are nutritionists, food scientists, dietitians, medics, nursing staff or other allied health professionals. We hope that both undergraduate and postgraduate students will find the book of great help with their respective studies and that the book will really put public health nutrition as a *discipline* into context.

PHN2e comprises of a total 29 chapters; commencing with a detailed overview of the book structure and then a focus of five sections; namely: 1) Public Health Nutrition Tools; 2) Current State of Evidence; 3) Diet and Disease; 4) Environmental Factors and 5) Public Health Nutrition Strategies and Approaches, with each chapter providing a key summary of the take home messages.

We are extremely honoured and most sincerely grateful that the Foreword for PHE2e has been written by Her Royal Highness The Princess Royal, who has a great depth of knowledge in the field and who speaks with authority on key issues in Public health Nutrition. It gives us great confidence in this textbook to have such a Royal seal of approval.

The first and second textbooks in the Series: *Introduction to Human Nutrition* (IHN) and *Nutrition & Metabolism* (N&M), are now out in 2nd Edition and sales continue to go extremely well, with third editions now fully under-preparation. Sales of Professor Marinos Elia *et al*'s *Clinical Nutrition* 2nd Edition (CN2e - fourth textbook) continue to sell apace and our fifth textbook in the Series, *Sport and Exercise Nutrition* 1st Edition (SEN1e) has surpassed all expectations. Our sixth textbook, *Nutrition Research Methodology* 1st Edition (NRM1e) led by Professor Julie Lovegrove *et al* provides great complementarity to PHN2e, and the Series, and is proving to be an excellent textbook in its own right.

We are most grateful to the following individuals for their support and most generous Forewords in SEN1e, CN2e and NRM1e respectively; namely - Professor Richard Budgett OBE, Chief Medical Officer for the London 2012 Olympic and Paralympic Games and now Medical and Scientific Director at the International Olympic Committee (IOC) based in Lausanne, Switzerland; Dame Sally Davies, Chief Medical Officer (CMO) for England, and the UK Government's Principal Medical Adviser; Professor Lord John Krebs, Principal, Jesus College, University of Oxford and our first Chairman of the UK Food Standards Agency.

The Society is most grateful to the textbook publishers, Wiley-Blackwell for their continued help with the production of the textbook and in particular, James Watson, Jennifer Seward and Francesca Giovannetti. We would also like to thank Garima Singh from Thomson Digital for her great help with PHN2e finalisation. In addition, I would like to acknowledge formally my great personal appreciation to Professor G.Q. Max Lu AO, FRSC, FIChemE, Vice-Chancellor of the University of Surrey, and Professor David Blackbourn FRSB, Head of the School of Bioscience and Medicine, University of Surrey, for their respective great encouragement of the nutritional sciences field in general, and the Textbook Series production in particular.

Sincerest appreciation indeed to the Nutrition Society past-Presidents, Professor Sean J.J. Strain OBE (Ulster University) and Professor Catherine Geissler (King's College London) and current-President, Professor Philip Calder (University of Southampton) for their belief in the Textbook Series. With special thanks to past-Honorary Publications Officer, Professor David Bender (University College London), and present-Honorary Publications Officer Professor Paul

Trayhurn (University of Liverpool) for being such tremendous sounding boards for the Textbook Series. I am hugely grateful for their wise counsel. And finally a very big thank you indeed to Cassandra Ellis, Assistant Editor, NS Textbook Series, for her incredibly important contribution to the development of the Series.

Finally, as I always write and absolutely do not forget (ever!), the Series is indebted to the forward thinking focus that Professor Michael Gibney (University College Dublin) had at that time of the Textbook Series development. It remains such a tremendous privilege for me to continue to follow in his footsteps as the second E-i-C.

I really hope that you will find the textbook a great resource of information and inspiration . . . please enjoy, and with so many grateful thanks to all those who made it happen!

With my warmest of wishes indeed

Professor Susan A Lanham-New RNutr, FAfN FRSB
E-i-C, Nutrition Society Textbook Series and
Head, Department of Nutritional Sciences
School of Biosciences and Medicine,
Faculty of Health and Medical Sciences
University of Surrey

Introduction

Much has changed in the 12 years since the launch of the first edition of *Public Health Nutrition*. With an explosion of research in this area, changes in nutrition policy and food-related legislation, and shifts in population health, dietary patterns and the food supply, the second edition represents a complete rewrite. We are honoured to have so many global experts in public health nutrition (PHN) contributing to make this textbook a comprehensive review.

To ensure the second edition reflects the most recent knowledge and research, and meets the requirements of students and practitioners alike, an expert advisory group was consulted throughout the planning process. The group members, representing research, teaching and PHN practice, were asked to comment on the content and structure of the new edition, and to provide guidance on what they were looking for in a PHN resource.

The textbook not only introduces PHN concepts, it is also intended to support learning for students and to be a practical guide for health professionals and those working within public health. More generally, feedback highlighted the benefit of including case studies to illustrate the practical application of the evidence and how this translates to policy. Case studies have therefore been included throughout to support the evidence and to offer practical advice for those working within PHN.

The clear message throughout consultation was the importance of structure and flow through the textbook. To ensure a clear, concise structure, the 29 chapters have been divided into clearly defined sections covering five key areas of PHN.

Part One outlines PHN assessment tools. This provides an introduction to concepts in PHN, followed by an overview of dietary assessment methodology, anthropometry and physical activity measures, with a focus on contemporary measures using new technology as well as traditional methods. This part then outlines the importance of food composition data in nutrition research, food safety and food security, and discusses dietary guidelines.

Part Two moves on to considering the application of PHN tools in a review of the current evidence. It begins by outlining dietary patterns and how they are defined before discussing vitamins and minerals that are of particular concern due to prevalent deficiency. This part also examines nutrition through the lifecycle, from pre-conception to old age, considering the public health challenges and risk factors at each phase.

Part Three reviews the relationship between diet and disease. Beginning with the risks of obesity in pregnancy and childhood, chapters that follow discuss some of the comorbidities of obesity, cardiovascular disease and type 2 diabetes. The relationship between diet and cancer is also examined, with consideration to both the protective and the carcinogenic roles of dietary factors. The PHN challenges associated with bone and dental health are also reviewed, and the relationship between diet and mental health and cognitive function is explored.

Part Four looks at the impact of environmental factors on public health, starting with consideration of the effects that obesogenic environments have on diets and health. Also explored is how aspects such as advertising, health promotion, food reformulation and food legislation can affect dietary behaviours.

Finally, Part Five outlines current public health strategies, policies and approaches. It begins broadly with a global perspective, before considering community strategies and engagement, how these strategies can be used to influence behaviour change, and the importance of culturally sensitive interventions and policies. The final chapters provides an evaluation of current policies and interventions and the social determinants of diet and health.

Judith L Buttriss

About the Companion Website

This book is accompanied by a companion website:

www.wiley.com/go/buttriss/publichealth

The website includes:

- Multiple choice questions
- Short answer questions
- Essay titles
- Further readings

Part One

Public Health Nutrition Tools

1
Introduction to Public Health Nutrition

Martin Wiseman

Key messages

- Nutrition is fundamental for life and health. The term 'nutrition' encompasses both biological and sociological aspects of how cells, tissues and organisms access the substrates and cofactors that are necessary for normal conception, growth, development and ageing.
- Public health nutrition refers to nutritional aspects of public health, which is the science and art of promoting and protecting health and well-being, preventing ill health and prolonging life through the organised efforts of society.
- The historical focus of public health nutrition has been on undernutrition, which is still a major problem across all levels of development. In less economically developed countries, it most commonly manifest as deficiencies of micronutrients as well as wasting and stunting (acute and chronic malnutrition) in childhood. In economically developed countries undernutrition is a common feature of ageing, though nutrition-related chronic non-communicable diseases such as obesity, type 2 diabetes, cardiovascular disease and several common cancers predominate. Increasingly, as less economically developed countries undergo nutritional transition, they are experiencing a rising burden of these diseases, so that these are now the major nutrition-related disease burden globally.

- The characterisation of human nutrient requirements is a fundamental activity for public health nutrition, and their application in clinical or public health settings requires training and experience that marks professional nutritional practice.
- Effective public health nutrition requires three discrete functions
  - the acquisition, synthesis and dissemination of knowledge relating nutrition to health and disease;
  - surveillance programmes to detect potential nutritional problems across the life course among the population, and to monitor change;
  - evidence-informed policy development, implementation and evaluation.
- Public health nutrition policy relies on ensuring that people have the necessary information to make healthy choices around food and physical activity, as well as on ensuring that the environment in which they live is conducive to making those healthy choices. Policy makers need to balance the evidence for health need against economic and other socio-political factors in determining what action to take.

1.1 Public health and nutrition

Nutrition lies at the heart of health. Human life – from conception or even before, through fetal and childhood growth, development and maturation, to adult life and old age – creates a demand for energy and nutrients, and relies on their adequate provision, and on the body's metabolic capability to transform these substrates and cofactors into the multitude of chemicals needed by cells for normal structure and function, driven by their genetic endowment. Nutrition is the process by which cells, tissues, organs, people and populations achieve this.

Poor nutrition leads to poor health; and poor health also often leads to poor nutrition.

Public health refers to those aspects of health that affect the population as a whole, their study and the services that aim to deliver it. Public health nutrition is where these two concerns – population health and nutrition – interact or overlap.

Public health is defined as 'The science and art of promoting and protecting health and well-being, preventing ill health and prolonging life through the organised efforts of society'.

Public Health Nutrition, Second Edition. Edited by Judith L Buttriss, Ailsa A Welch, John M Kearney and Susan A Lanham-New.
© 2018 by The Nutrition Society. Published 2018 by John Wiley & Sons, Ltd.
Companion website: www.wiley.com/go/buttriss/publichealth

It is worth elaborating on that concise definition, first to note the implicit recognition that the evidence (science) underpinning actions to promote or protect health may often be incomplete, and that professional judgement (art) is needed to interpret and apply it. This is no different in concept from the application of science in clinical care, where the demand for evidence-based practice exposes gaps in knowledge of how to manage the very variable presentations of individual patients, but does not paralyse clinical action. Second, it is important that prolongation of life is linked with the promotion of health and prevention of ill health, in order to avoid prolonged disability with ageing. The aim is to shorten the period of ill health (compression of morbidity) before death in old age. Third, public health needs to be organised. It is not a default, as can be seen in the many parts of the world where effective public health structures and systems do not exist, and where infant and maternal mortality are high, expectation of life is low, and infectious and increasingly non-communicable diseases are common, as was the case in now economically developed countries in the past. Finally, the responsibility to make efforts falls not only to the small group of people who are professionals in public health, but to society as a whole. This recognises that the determinants of health in populations have little to do with the health care system (which deals with the problems of failed health), and are mostly related to the wider environmental conditions in which people are conceived, born, grow, live, work and age. Public health is about creating environments that are conducive to health, and public health nutrition is about creating environments that are conducive to healthy nutrition.

1.2 History of nutrition in public health

The ancients regarded food and medicine as related aspects, and since the demonstration in the 18th century by James Lind that lime juice was effective in curing and preventing scurvy (even though the finding was initially ignored and later had to be rediscovered), it has been clear that the provision of appropriate quality and quantity of food is essential in securing people's health.

The importance of food for growth, development and health was apparent despite lack of knowledge of the biological processes involved. This ignorance of the detail of the body's nutritional demands and how different foods and diets can meet them meant that it was difficult to derive rational nutrition policies.

The UK offers a good illustration. In the UK during the First World War, disruption to food imports from abroad had a major impact on the food supply (see Table 1.1), but there was insufficient understanding of

Table 1.1 When food imports were seriously disrupted in the First World War (WW1), limited nutrition knowledge meant that a coherent food policy was not possible and the food supply was adversely affected. In contrast, despite similar disruption to food imports in the Second World War (WW2), the application of the new nutritional science into effective policy ensured that the food supply was maintained and equitably distributed to secure the health of the population.

	WW1	WW2
Milk	−26%	+28%
Eggs	−40%	−6%
Meat	−27%	−21%
Vegetables	−9%	+34%

Source: Magee (1946). Reproduced with permission of BMJ Publishing Ltd.

the nutritional consequences for a coherent political response to be mounted.

Subsequently, the British population experienced food shortages, and malnutrition was a major problem. After the establishment of the Ministry of Health in 1919, food and nutrition were early targets for a more systematic approach to policy. In 1921 the Ministry published a report on 'Diet in Relation to Normal Nutrition' that identified the importance of so-called 'protective foods' – green leafy vegetables, milk and eggs – for healthy growth in children. This period coincided with the explosion of nutrition research into the accessory food factors (vitamins, minerals and trace elements) and the biological mechanisms for their effects – a discipline which spawned the new word 'biochemistry'. By the time of the Second World War, when there was a similar disruption as in the first war to the food imports on which the British food supply depended, nutritional science had progressed sufficiently for the Government to base its food policy on sound science. This policy, which involved public education with enhanced local food production and controls on the equitable distribution of food, led to quite different effects on the food supply (see Table 1.1), and its success to the British Ministries of Food and Health later receiving the prestigious Lasker Award for public health.

This period set the foundations for the essential elements of food and nutrition policy into the future. The key aspects are

- a transparent mechanism for the provision of scientific nutrition advice to government;
- reliable means for monitoring diet and nutrition status among the population;
- effective means of developing and evaluating policies to assure the quality and quantity of the food supply, and the nutritional health of the population.

The most prominent aspect of nutritional advice was the establishment by groups of experts of so-called recommended daily (or dietary) allowances. These set the amounts of essential nutrients needed to be consumed by populations to minimise risk of deficiencies, based on the growing science. These reports, published in the UK in the same series as the 1921 report for the Ministry of Health, have now been supplanted in most countries, following the UK 1991 report on dietary reference values, by attempts to describe the estimated range of dietary requirements for different nutrients among populations, including the balance of macronutrients considered desirable to reduce risk of chronic disease.

The establishment in Britain in 1940 of the National Food Survey was the forerunner of a systematic programme of diet and nutrition surveys which characterise the food and drink consumption of the population from childhood to old age, as well as their nutrition status in terms of anthropometry and biochemical measurements of blood and urine, and relevant physiological measures such as blood pressure. Such food and health monitoring systems play an essential role in the detection of nutritional problems in the population, tracking their development, and evaluating the effectiveness of policies to address them.

The success of the wartime food policy in the UK may in part be ascribed to the possibility of applying stringent controls and restrictions on the national diet due to the national emergency, as well as the coincidentally high levels of physical activity that were prevalent at the time. However, such restrictive approaches, though effective, are unlikely to find favour beyond the stringent circumstances of such an emergency, and a critical issue for policy makers is to find effective means of promoting healthy nutrition without inappropriate interference with people's freedom to choose how they live. This dilemma has been addressed by various commentators, including the Nuffield Council on Bioethics.

1.3 Nutrition and public health in different parts of the world

For the majority of the 20th century, nutrition policy in industrialised countries was directed to the elimination of classic micronutrient deficiency diseases such as scurvy and rickets, which were major scourges in particular among the least affluent in society. In less economically developed countries, gross malnutrition with wasting and stunting of children, and high levels of maternal and child mortality, as well as specific nutrient deficiencies, remain common, mirroring the situation of the previous century in industrialised countries.

During the latter part of the 20th century and in the 21st century, the prominence in economically developed countries of deficiency diseases diminished with better access for all to a wide variety of foods, and effective food fortification policies. However, this was replaced by a growing burden of chronic non-communicable disease, at first cardiovascular disease, but increasingly cancers, obesity and diabetes. At the same time, some micronutrient deficiencies – in particular rickets – began to re-emerge, while undernutrition in the ageing population has become an important concern, sometimes simply due to poor dietary intake (with low lean mass and activity levels), and sometimes consequent to disease.

In less economically developed countries, the problems of malnutrition with stunting and wasting continue to dominate, but as the populations undergo an economic transition from rural to more urbanised ways of life, they also undergo a nutrition transition so that rates of obesity, and other chronic non-communicable diseases, are also rising, creating the so-called double burden (of over– and undernutrition). In places such as Thailand and Chile, which have had tangible success in reducing undernutrition, this has been at the cost of a rise in prevalence of overweight and obesity.

Clearly, malnutrition in all its forms affects all parts of the globe, though its segmentation within society varies.

1.4 Current role of nutrition in public health

Socio-demographic changes are affecting many parts of the globe. In most countries people are living longer, while economic development is also driving increased urbanisation, with rapid and profound changes in ways of life. In more affluent countries, average smoking rates are declining, while prevalence of overweight and obesity are increasing, and levels of physical activity have fallen. Traditional diets are being replaced by typical 'westernised' patterns, with more processed foods including fats, oils, refined starches and sugars, higher salt intake and a greater reliance on foods from animal as opposed to plant sources.

In less economically developed countries there is a rising burden of cardiovascular disease, and increasingly also the cancers more typical of affluent nations – breast, colorectal and prostate – related to nutritional factors, in place of the cancers caused by infections – liver, stomach and cervix. Lung cancer remains a scourge – though mostly of men – as smoking rates have not declined as in more affluent countries, and indeed are still rising in some.

In more affluent nations, rates of cardiovascular disease are declining, so that with increasing age the major non-communicable disease group is predicted to be cancers, many of which are related to dietary patterns, body fatness and physical activity levels.

Meanwhile malnutrition – stunting and wasting in children, short stature in adulthood, as well as specific micronutrient deficiencies – remains prevalent, often within the same communities as increasing overweight and obesity. Even in richer countries, where food security is less of a problem, micronutrient deficiencies such as rickets remain persistent in vulnerable groups, and are possibly increasing.

1.5 Nutrition through the life course

Nutritional problems have always been recognised at all stages of the life course. Maternal overweight or obesity, or underweight, are known to influence the outcome of pregnancy both for the mother and the infant. Low birth weight remains a problem among low-income countries, and nutritional factors are key. Poor growth with wasting and stunting are classic nutritional problems of undernutrition, which remain prevalent in low income countries, while increasingly in high income countries obesity is becoming a serious problem in childhood. One consequence of the nutrition transition is the development of a cohort of people of short stature from undernutrition in childhood, but who then become overweight or obese; this combination carries enhanced risk for nutrition-related problems, in particular for maternal and fetal outcomes in pregnancy. Adolescence is a period of rapid growth and development, with increased demands for energy and nutrients, and so is a period of vulnerability to any constraint on supply, and this can be compounded by early pregnancy, which drives competing demands between mother and fetus. Micronutrient deficiencies remain prevalent where food supply is monotonous and insecure, emphasising the need for dietary diversity, while adult obesity with its attendant co-morbidities of diabetes, cardiovascular disease and some cancers is a major problem for high-income countries and increasingly so for middle– and even low-income countries. Undernutrition is also becoming an important cause of morbidity and mortality among older people.

There is growing recognition of the impact of nutrition not only in the immediate context, but as a determinant of future health. Non-communicable chronic diseases such as obesity, diabetes, cardiovascular disease and cancers result from the interaction of people's current exposures – their diet, activity levels and nutritional state – with their susceptibility. Susceptibility is partly determined by genetic endowment; however, it is now clear that early life events (in particular constraint of growth due to imbalance between the amount or quality of the demands for energy or nutrients, and their supply,

from conception to adulthood) can have a profound impact on later risk of these conditions.

1.6 Principles of public health nutrition

Effective public health nutrition requires three discrete functions

- the acquisition, synthesis and dissemination of knowledge relating nutrition to health and disease;
- surveillance programmes to detect potential nutritional problems across the life course among the population, and to monitor change;
- evidence-informed   policy   development   and implementation.

The primary prevention of disease relies on the identification of the causes of disease, so that they may be addressed. The identification of infectious causes has led to the development of vaccination and antibiotics, and of means to control their vectors, such as the mosquito for malaria. The identification of a deficiency of the essential nutrients allowed for dietary approaches to their prevention, and policies such as food fortification. For nutrition-related chronic non-communicable diseases, with multiple causes and highly variable susceptibility in the population, not only is the identification and characterisation of the pathways of causation complex, but equally the appropriate medical, public health or political response is often difficult to agree. Nevertheless, an analogous approach to these problems allows an open dialogue on how to address them.

It is essential that any approach relies on the whole body of scientific evidence. As in all health practice, this may be epidemiological information, clinical trial data or laboratory evidence, or less reliable forms. In clinical medicine, randomised controlled trials (RCTs) are rightly regarded as superior to other forms of investigation because of their ability to test relevant hypotheses with a robust design and avoid the problems of confounding that arise in epidemiological studies. However, for primary prevention of chronic non-communicable disease that manifests in adulthood but has roots in early life, and where the impact of environmental exposures takes decades, it is less clear that RCTs have net overall advantage. While well-designed and –executed RCTs have strong internal validity (they give a correct answer to the hypothesis tested), they often lack external validity (that is, they cannot test the right hypothesis) perhaps because they are not conducted in an appropriate population or use atypical exposures. For primary prevention, intelligent interrogation of the whole body of evidence is required to infer causation from observed associations. This can be aided by using accepted frameworks such as that derived by Bradford Hill. Such synthetic approaches to the evidence can identify preferred patterns of diet or lifestyle likely to reduce disease and promote health.

Once such patterns are identified, it is important to explore to what extent they are present in the population, and in potentially vulnerable subgroups. For this reason, proactive nutritional surveillance of the population is a necessary component of rational public health nutrition. Such monitoring surveys may identify the prevalence of disease risk factors in the population such as obesity or physical inactivity, or of biological factors such as high blood pressure or disordered blood lipids. They also allow the impact of policy to be evaluated.

Vulnerable subgroups may be defined in several ways. They are often defined in terms of age, sex, ethnicity or socio-economic state. However, it is equally possible to conceive vulnerability from a biological perspective. Diet and health surveys allow the distribution of relevant variables (such as risk factors or markers of nutritional status) within the population to be calculated. Though one aim of policy is to shift the whole distribution of risk in a population in a beneficial direction, interest – aided by newer technologies – is increasingly being paid to exploring the variability itself. Such variability reflects individual characteristics that determine susceptibility (e.g. to disease), and characterising the risks of individuals *within* the population and their determinants (as well as the determinants of differential risk *between* populations, which may be different) is an increasing focus of attention. For example, fortification of staple foods with folic acid has been proposed (and in some countries implemented) to ensure adequate intake in women who become pregnant to reduce the risk of neural tube defects in their offspring. However, there are concerns that such broad exposure to fortified foods might lead to excessive intakes among those who already have high intakes, emphasising the need to consider the shape of the distribution of intake, and not only the average.

Finally, effective public health action requires the development of policies based on the evidence. Though seemingly obvious, much nutrition policy may nevertheless be based on preconceptions or ideological preferences. Because the evidence for effectiveness of policy is difficult to obtain by conventional medical models of investigation, policy needs first to identify the nutritional problems that need addressing; to develop policies based on the best evidence available (even if incomplete) and implement them in a way that can be evaluated to allow the policy to be continuously improved (that is, to develop evidence from the evaluation of policies in action). Because policy often involves politics, and the

solution needs to embrace not only the health aspects but also socio-political considerations, tensions may arise in identifying the appropriate intervention or its degree. This aspect has been addressed by the Nuffield Council on Bioethics, which developed a 'ladder' of different degrees of intervention as a framework for consideration (Figure 1.1). While this ladder offers a valuable framework, it is predicated on relatively simple, single actions. This limits its practical use in public health, which has the characteristics of a complex system. Failure to recognise the inherent complexity in the determinants of people's behaviour may in part be responsible for the relatively modest effects observed from many more linear interventions, as well as unwillingness to adopt policies that are more restrictive.

The question arises as to who should take action. The definition of public health draws attention to the need for organised efforts of society. While it falls clearly to the health professions and politicians to take the lead in the organisation of society's efforts, it is clear that the roots of environmental exposures linked to health or disease fall far outside the ambit of health practice. The complex environmental determinants of people's behaviour are formed by the cumulated actions of all sectors of society, many of whom have no sense of their role or responsibility in public health. Yet, it is only by engaging with all sectors, and creating a synergy of action, that the environment will become conducive to the promotion of healthy long life for all. Much public health policy is driven by professional and other sectors, attempting to impose top-down change on people, while examples of success are often characterised by a groundswell of demand form the grassroots (bottom-up). Finding ways to engage with people through their own communities, and manage the interface between them (us) and more powerful sectors, is critical for lasting and substantive success.

1.7 Conclusions

Public health nutrition, like other health professions, relies on the application of incomplete evidence in biological, psychological and sociological spheres. It requires the engagement of parts of society that are outside traditional health sectors, and the capacity to identify, collect, synthesise and disseminate relevant information, and to use it effectively to influence important players from the public to politicians. Public health nutritionists have a lead responsibility in organising the efforts of all parts of society to create an environment conducive to good nutrition and health.

The range of options available to government and policy makers can be thought of as a ladder of interventions with progressive steps from individual freedom and responsibility, towards state intervention as one moves up the ladder. In considering which 'rung' is appropriate for a particular public health goal, the benefits to individuals and society should be weighed against the erosion of individual freedom. Economic costs and benefits would need be taken into account alongside health and societal benefits. The ladder of possible policy action is as follows:

Eliminate choice. Regulate in such a way as to entirely eliminate choice, for example through compulsory isolation of patients with infectious diseases.

Restrict choice. Regulate in such a way as to restrict the options available to people with the aim of protecting them, for example removing unhealthy ingredients from foods, or unhealthy foods from shops or restaurants.

Guide choice through disincentives. Fiscal and other disincentives can be put in place to influence people not to pursue certain activities, for example through taxes on cigarettes, or by discouraging the use of cars in inner cities through charging schemes or limitations of parking spaces.

Guide choices through incentives. Regulations can be offered that guide choices by fiscal and other incentives, for example offering tax-breaks for the purchase of bicycles that are used as a means of travelling to work.

Guide choices through changing the default policy. For example, in a restaurant, instead of providing chips as a standard side dish (with healthier options available), menus could be changed to provide a more healthy option as standard (with chips as an option available).

Enable choice. Enable individuals to change their behaviours, for example by offering participation in an NHS 'stop smoking' programme, building cycle lanes, or providing free fruit in schools.

Provide information. Inform and educate the public, for example as part of campaigns to encourage people to walk more or eat five portions of fruit and vegetables per day.

Do nothing or simply monitor the current situation.

Figure 1.1 The intervention ladder. Source: Nuffield Council on Bioethics (2007). Reproduced with permission of Nuffield Council on Bioethics.

References

Magee, H.E. (1946) Application of nutrition to public health: some lessons of the war. *British Medical Journal*, 1, 475–482.

Nuffield Council on Bioethics (2007) *Public Health: Ethical Issues.* Cambridge Publishers Ltd, Cambridge. http://nuffieldbioethics. org/wp-content/uploads/2014/07/Public-health-ethical-issues. pdf (accessed 23 November 2016).

2
Concepts and Definitions Used in Public Health Nutrition

Eric J Brunner and Ailsa A Welch

Key messages

- The main concepts and definitions used in public health are outlined.
- The nature of the evidence required to make decisions for public health nutrition is described, including issues of study design and interpretation.
- The issues of measurement error in the evidence that supports public health nutrition are discussed.
- The social determinants of diet and health are discussed.

2.1 Introduction

Public health nutrition has been defined as the science and art of preventing disease and promoting positive health by means of good nutrition. Public health nutrition, like medicine, is grounded in scientific knowledge, which is applied to a range of health-related problems and ambitions. Public health nutrition differs from clinical medicine, and clinical nutrition, in that its target is the group rather than the individual. This distinction is clear if we think about obesity: a clinical nutritionist would seek to help an individual obese child to lose weight, while a public health nutritionist would tend to work with groups of children either to lose weight or perhaps better to reduce the chance that any of them become obese. Public health nutrition is interdisciplinary in nature. The scope of knowledge and skills is wide (see Box 2.1 for examples) because the range of problems that public health nutrition can tackle is wide.

Nutritional epidemiology provides the evidence for policy and action in public health nutrition. The science base of public health nutrition continues to develop and expand, and workers in the field consider that the evidence we have now is incomplete. This situation is not an excuse for inaction, because there are many obvious problems of under- and overnutrition across the planet that need to be solved urgently. The reality is

complicated. First, we cannot always wait for faultless evidence before calling for action. Second, public health is only one voice among many that strive to influence dietary habits. Powerful stakeholders produce a food environment with high availability of low-cost, energy-dense but nutrient-poor food and drink products. Third, socioeconomic inequalities in health – deprivation and disadvantage linked to poorer health right across the social hierarchy – are generated in part by social differences in dietary patterns which are themselves shaped by market forces. (In this context, the wider environment and dietary patterns are covered in more detail in Chapters 9 and 24.)

The imperfections in our understanding of the links between diet, disease and health mean that it is important for public health nutritionists to be aware of the methods and challenges in the research: how we know what we know and what produces the evidence to support their beliefs and practice. The vital topics of the nature of evidence and what counts as weak or strong evidence, the design of studies, and the important problem of measurement error (a defining characteristic of nutrition research) are outlined briefly in Sections 2.2, 2.3 and 2.4. Section 2.6 highlights a key distinction between risk assessment and risk management. Section 2.7 presents an outline of this social determinants perspective, and makes the case for its relevance to public health nutrition.

Public Health Nutrition, Second Edition. Edited by Judith L Buttriss, Ailsa A Welch, John M Kearney and Susan A Lanham-New.
© 2018 by The Nutrition Society. Published 2018 by John Wiley & Sons, Ltd.
Companion website: www.wiley.com/go/buttriss/publichealth

2.2 Nature of evidence

Two types of evidence provide direct support for rational practice in public health nutrition. The first answers the question, 'What is going wrong?' (That is, what the problem is and what the causes of that problem are.) The second answers the question, 'How can I best intervene?' The first type of evidence tells us about the contribution of nutritional factors for causation of diseases of public health importance; for example, that a high habitual intake of saturated fatty acids increases the risk of heart attack. Such evidence generally applies to everyone, across time and place. Because of the widespread significance of nutritional effects on health it is important to make the distinction between claims which are supported by scientific studies and those based merely on enthusiasm or vested interests (Box 2.2). Such knowledge needs to be placed in a context: in the population of interest, what proportions of children and adults have high (or low) intakes? The second type of evidence helps us to identify effective ways to reduce the problem. There are often a number of different modes of intervention that could be employed. A medical model

might involve dietary advice to adults when they visit their doctor. A social marketing model might involve an advertising campaign. A fiscal model might centre on a tax on saturated fat. Some interventions may work well in one country and badly in another. Some interventions may be introduced in one year and scrapped the next, as was the case with the fat tax in Denmark in 2011 (Bodker *et al.*, 2015).

2.3 Methods and study design

It is clear that a wide spectrum of research methods sits behind the different strands of evidence. Details of the types of study design available and of their advantages and disadvantages are given in Table 2.1.

Nutritional epidemiology is the science providing the basic knowledge about the dietary causes of disease. Studies are typically large, with hundreds or thousands of participants followed for a decade or more. Such necessarily expensive longitudinal cohort studies observe the real world as opposed to laboratory-based phenomena, with the aim of testing hypotheses about diet, health and disease. The principle is simple. Individuals are ranked according to their baseline intake of the food or nutrient of interest. The hypothesis is tested by examining the strength of the association between the level of dietary exposure and the health outcome of interest. If there is an association, the rate of disease occurrence will change as intake increases. The design, execution and analysis of such studies is challenging. The challenges include measurement of complex dietary behaviour, recruitment of a large sample of study participants and their retention until sufficient outcomes (e.g. deaths, cases of disease) have occurred, and separating out the effects of numerous dietary and non-dietary exposures once the data have been collected.

At this point we must note that 'association is not the same as cause'. Observational studies suffer from a specific conceptual weakness. Exposure status, which is to say levels of dietary intakes, is self-selected. Because unhealthy (or healthy) behaviours tend to cluster in the same individual, it may be difficult to know which aspects of dietary and non-dietary behaviour are exerting causal effects, even if there is supporting evidence from laboratory or animal studies about the biological plausibility of the causal effect in question. This is the problem of confounding: the confusion of the effect of one exposure with that of one or more other exposures on the disease outcome of interest.

A confounder is a 'third' factor such as age (where exposure and outcome are the first and second factors) which is associated with the exposure and also is a risk factor for the outcome. For instance, if the question of

Table 2.1 Types of study design that provide supporting evidence for public health nutrition and their advantages and disadvantages.

Study design	Name/ alternative name	Description	Advantages	Disadvantages
Intervention study	Randomised controlled trial/ clinical trial	Comparison of event rates, behaviour and risk factor changes in individuals or groups of people exposed to an intervention (e.g. dietary advice) with a control or comparison group	Low probability of selection bias, recall bias, confounding Pilot policy change by comparing effect of new and old policies Demonstrate effectiveness	Risks of bias due to loss to follow up High time and cost requirements Educational and behavioural interventions are difficult to conceal. Resulting 'contamination' distorts observed effect sizes
Cohort study	Prospective study Follow-up study Longitudinal study	Measurement of exposures (e.g. dietary intake) with follow up over time for incident events/risk factor status Studies relationships between exposures and outcomes	Prospective study avoids recall bias Can study multiple exposures Obtain direct measures of incident disease/outcomes Observe time sequences and relationships Control for possible multiple confounders	Risks of bias due to loss to follow up High time and cost requirements Requires large sample size Difficult to eliminate confounding between correlated exposures (e.g. nutrient intakes)
Cross-sectional study	Health survey	Measurement of exposures, risk factors and disease prevalence at one point in time Studies relationships (associations) between exposures and outcomes	Low probability of selection bias, recall bias Study multiple exposures and outcomes Can control for possible multiple confounders	Requires large sample sizes Temporality of associations is not known Cannot measure incidence
Case–control study	Case–reference	Comparison of group of identified cases with a group of healthy controls. Exposure is measured retrospectively Compares level of past exposure (e.g. diet) in cases and controls	Smaller sample size than cohort study Low time and cost requirements Prospective case–control studies are possible	High probability of selection bias, recall bias, confounding. Potentially low reliability of findings Temporality of associations often not known Can only test one outcome
Ecological study	Correlational	Investigates the relationship between exposure and disease in grouped data (e.g. regions, countries)	Low time and cost requirements High potential for investigating causes of rare diseases	Inaccuracy of data Ecological fallacy: confounding cannot be controlled

Source: adapted from Bonita et al. (2006) and Thiese (2014).

interest was to understand whether increasing body mass index (BMI) is a risk factor for the onset of type 2 diabetes, age needs to be taken into account, either by analysing the effect of BMI in age groups or by statistical adjustment for age. This is important for the two reasons stated at the beginning of this paragraph. First, age and BMI are associated, such that BMI tends to increase with age, and second age and onset of type 2 diabetes are associated, such that its incidence increases with age. The design of studies and procedures in statistical analysis can take into account the problem of confounding, which in this example involves disentangling the effects of age and BMI. Confounding is an important problem in

nutritional epidemiology because diet is a complicated and multifactorial exposure or, more accurately, set of exposures. In recognition, there has been a shift away from studies of the health effects of individual foods and nutrients towards identifying dietary patterns (such as the Mediterranean diet), and examining how a healthy diet may promote health.

Trials have the potential to generate stronger evidence with minimal or no confounding, since confounding is controlled for in the study design. A trial, randomised controlled trial or intervention study differs from an observational study in that the researcher seeks to compare two or more groups that differ as a result of deliberate action rather than natural or observed variation. The researcher uses randomisation to allocate individuals to the intervention and control groups in the reasonable expectation that all confounder levels will be the same in the two groups. Then, if the condition of the two groups differs at the end of the trial, it can only be the result of the intervention. Unfortunately, randomised controlled trials using foods or whole diet as intervention are rare because they are impractical, particularly if the health outcome is chronic disease such as heart disease or cancer, when the trial would need to continue for perhaps 20 years. From an ethical standpoint, it is not possible to feed people with suspected disease-causing nutrients. With the exception of health-promoting nutrients such as vitamins, therefore, we can only test diet–disease hypotheses in observational and prospective cohort studies.

2.4 Measurement error and bias

Measurement error is an important issue in large-scale nutrition research, which often depends on self-reported dietary data. Whether a study seeks to describe the occurrence of a nutritional problem or to analyse the dietary causes of disease, there are always problems of measurement. Measurement error can be defined as the difference between the measured exposure, such as the usual dietary intake of fat, and the true exposure.

Error may be either systematic or random. Random error occurs with all measurements and is generally regarded as being caused by chance (Figure 2.1). Random error causes imprecision, or noise, in the estimate of food intake in a group of people, and can be reduced by increasing the number of observations or by improving quality control procedures when making measurements. Systematic error (or bias) is error that occurs in a consistent direction and reduces the accuracy of a measurement. Systematic error, unlike random error, is not smaller in larger studies. The consequences of measurement error are a loss of accuracy and precision, terms which have a specific meaning in scientific method. Accuracy is the degree of closeness of the measurement to its true value (see Figure 2.1a and b). Precision refers to the ability to measure without random error and means that measurements have high repeatability. Intuitively, we can predict that accurate and precise measurements of dietary intake will produce more valid results, and vice versa.

Measurement errors may arise for many reasons. There may be a flaw in the design of the measurement instrument or it may be poorly calibrated. Errors will be introduced by researchers who do not follow standard operating procedures during data collection and during

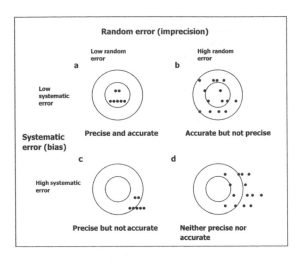

Figure 2.1 Representation of the effects of random and systematic error on measurements: (a) measurements that are both accurate and precise; (b) accurate measurements free of systematic error but affected by random error; (c) measures free of random error but affected by systematic error (inaccurate but precise); (d) measures that include both systematic and random error (inaccurate and imprecise). *Source*: Adapted from Gerstman (2003).

processing of the raw data. Characteristics of the study participant, such as their degree of obesity and level of health consciousness, are sources of error when dietary assessment is based on self-report. Food tables, from which nutrient intakes are derived, are approximate. Techniques to estimate or reduce the effects of measurement error are available, but often not employed. Validation techniques have been used to estimate dietary measurement error by using biological measures such as 24-h urinary excretion of nitrogen (to estimate protein intake), potassium or sucrose, or circulating concentrations of vitamins C and E, carotenoids or retinol, or fatty acids, but biomarkers are only available for a limited set of nutrients.

In contrast to validation, which attempts to identify the type and scale of measurement error, calibration techniques adjust for systematic over– or underestimation of dietary intakes between studies and populations. An example is the calibration of dietary intakes using a method considered more accurate than the main method when estimating the association between disease risk and dietary intake. The EPIC-Europe Study (European Prospective Investigations into Cancer and Nutrition Study) utilised a calibration method by incorporating data from a standardised computer-based 24-h recall to make an improved estimate of the association between diet, estimated using a food frequency questionnaire, and risk of colorectal cancer in 10 European countries (Norat *et al.*, 2005). Another example is the biomarker-calibrated association between carotenoid intake and incidence of cataracts, which utilised a biomarker in addition to the dietary estimate of carotenoids (Freedman *et al.*, 2011). Addition of the biomarker strengthened the association between carotenoids and incidence of cataract formation.

Dietary intake is generally measured by some form of diary or questionnaire. The weighed intake method, which requires the study participant to weigh and record every item of food eaten for several days, is considered to be one of the most accurate methods. This activity is a burden and it is not surprising that many studies adopt simpler and easier methods to measure dietary intake, such as a food frequency questionnaire asking respondents to estimate how often, on average, they eat a given food over a year. These methods are less burdensome than a food diary, but the trade-off is likely to be increased measurement error.

Measurement errors have important impacts on the interpretation of dietary studies. When the aim is to understand the true association between diet and a disease outcome, the accuracy and precision of the study measures must be carefully considered in order to evaluate the extent to which the observed association between dietary intake and disease outcome is valid (Schatzkin and Kipnis, 2004). The fundamental objective in nutritional epidemiology is often to classify the dietary intake of each participant in a study, so that the group can be ordered correctly (ranked) according to their level of intake. As the degree of measurement error increases, misclassification increases, and the observed association between dietary intake and disease will increasingly be distorted.

Specific forms of bias can occur when measuring dietary intake. Reporting bias, or social desirability bias, occurs when respondents report what they think is an acceptable level of intake; for example, reporting less alcohol or higher fruit and vegetable consumption than is actually the case. This common behaviour leads to misreporting (under- or overreporting) of nutrient and energy intake. It is known that underreporting of energy intake increases with increasing BMI (Bingham *et al.*, 1997; Brunner *et al.*, 2001). As a result, contradictory findings may emerge, such that obese people appear to have lower energy intake than thinner or normal weight people. Misreporting is common. It is linked not only with higher BMI, but other variables such as socioeconomic status. Researchers have tried to reduce this source of bias by excluding the data from individuals who under- or overreported the most, but such an approach is no longer recommended because it introduces further bias, known as selection bias, which distorts estimates of the quantities or relationships of interest (Stubbs *et al.*, 2002).

Recall bias is another type of reporting bias, known for producing spurious findings in case–control studies of chronic diseases such as cancer. Recall bias leads to systematic differences in recall due to current or prior events or experiences. Although it may be convenient to measure past diet at the time of onset of a disease in a study of disease causation, there is a risk that recall of behaviours including diet (perhaps two decades earlier) will be influenced by knowing the diagnosis, while recall bias in the control or comparison group might be quite different. The net result is that the risk factors identified in such retrospective studies may reflect current popular attitudes to diet and health as much if not more than the actual past differences in diet between cases and controls. A further problem with recall of past diet is that current diet has been found to influence recall of past diet to a large extent (Willett, 2013).

Publication bias undermines the validity of many fields of science, and is the consequence of selective publication of positive results. In some cases, the body of evidence on a topic, particularly when financial interests are involved, may need to be examined carefully to check that it is valid. How best to support weight loss in overweight and obese people is an issue of great significance at present. A recent trial found that significant weight loss was eight times more likely after 6 months with behavioural counselling in a supportive group than with self-motivation alone (Johnston *et al.*, 2013) Such an effect may be valid and generally applicable; however, Weight Watchers International paid for the study and presumably did so because it wished to generate evidence for commercial advantage. In such situations, it is reasonable to consider whether results may need to be replicated by an independent research group, without commercial involvement.

Research in the field of nutrition is influenced by various parts of the food and dieting industry. Beyond potential publication bias, it is appropriate to ask whether certain research topics are neglected because the industry is rich, whereas public research funds are scarce. As a result, research on benefits and harms and the effectiveness of different interventions to achieve behaviour change is lacking (Kivimaki *et al.*, 2015). Those working in health care and public health who are required to develop health interventions or policy should be aware of the types of potential bias that may have occurred in shaping the body of evidence when making their decisions.

2.5 Interpretation of study design and hierarchy of the evidence

Many factors may influence the validity of a study. If the body of evidence supporting a policy action in public

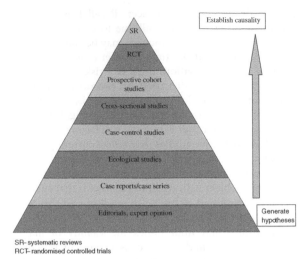

SR- systematic reviews
RCT- randomised controlled trials

Figure 2.2 Hierarchy of epidemiological study design for establishing causality. SR: systematic review; RCT: randomised controlled trial.

health nutrition is based mainly on weak study designs, then the policy decision is open to challenge. The 'hierarchy of evidence' shown in Figure 2.2 is a general guide to the strength and quality of findings according to the design of the study. Designs located higher up the pyramid will tend to provide more solid evidence than those nearer the base. Public health practitioners need to be aware of this hierarchy and the advantages and disadvantages of the different study designs detailed in Table 2.1. Systematic reviews, which are literature reviews that collect and critically analyse multiple research studies or papers according to a predetermined protocol, are considered the optimal type of evidence for making decisions in public health nutrition. Randomised controlled trials are considered to be the type of study design that is best to infer causation. However, designing randomised controlled trials in nutrition can be difficult. A randomised trial is practical for testing the effectiveness of a drug in acute disease; for example, an antibiotic in patients with blood poisoning. Demonstrating that one dietary pattern is superior to another in preventing heart attacks is a more challenging task altogether.

When interpreting the results of studies associating diet with health or disease outcomes it is important to understand the size or scale of the effects that are found and to interpret them in relation to a number of factors, including study design (McLeod *et al.*, 2016). It is often the case that the size of a relationship will be small. If the study is large, the associations will be statistically significant, and vice versa. In this context, it is important to consider whether the scale or size of the effect of the relationship found has clinical and/or public health relevance (McLeod *et al.*, 2016).

2.6 Risk assessment versus risk management

Risk assessment in public health characterises the nature and size of the health risks associated with particular exposures. Risk assessment by means of surveys and clinical screening provides the motivation for public health nutritionists to act. The next step is risk management, involving intervention rather than observation. Risk management refers to the planning and implementation of actions to reduce or eliminate risk. What we need to know here is how best to achieve the change in dietary intake that is wanted. If we can put together strong evidence on the links between diet and health, along with strong evidence on the effectiveness and cost-effectiveness of interventions to change the target population's diet, then we have a formula for positive change. See Figure 2.3.

Risk assessment is a fundamental activity in public health that helps to identify priorities for action, or risk management. Examples of sources of population surveillance information available for the UK are shown in Box 2.3 These surveys provide data for trends in food consumption, obesity and other health-related factors. Such information is usually broken down into demographic groups including sex, age group, region and socioeconomic position. At present, there is widespread concern about the high prevalence of obesity in the UK and other countries. In just 30 years, adult obesity prevalence has risen threefold in England, from about 8% in the early 1980s to 25% in 2011. The challenge of epidemic obesity is that effective solutions are hard to find either for prevention or treatment.

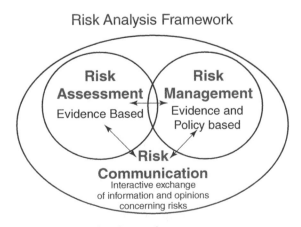

Figure 2.3 Risk analysis framework.

Box 2.3 Examples of sources of data for risk assessment

UK National Diet and Nutrition Survey. This is a continuous cross-sectional survey, designed to assess the diet, nutrient intake and nutritional status of the general population aged 18 months upwards living in private households in the UK (https://www.gov .uk/government/collections/national-diet-and-nutrition-survey).

Health Survey for England. This is a series of annual surveys designed to measure health and health-related behaviours (including some aspects of nutrition) in adults and children (http://data.gov.uk/dataset/health_survey_for_england).

Family Food Survey. This is part of the Living Costs and Food Survey: "Living Costs and Food Module of the Integrated Household Survey". This collects information on spending patterns and the cost of living that reflects household budgets.

Information about spending patterns for the consumer price indices, and about food consumption and nutrition, is provided with details on purchased quantities, expenditure and nutrient intakes derived from both household and eating-out food and drink. The survey has been ongoing (with modifications) since 1940 (https://www.gov.uk/government/collections/family-food-statistics).

Individual-level risk assessment should lead to some form of risk management if there is a problem, according to the principles of screening (Harris *et al.*, 2011). Screening is considered unethical if nothing can be done to ameliorate the problem that has been identified. If this logic is extended from screened individuals to surveyed populations, risk management should be based on evidence that a particular intervention is effective. Dietary advice given to adults who do not have disease is potentially an important means by which to promote health, but do we know that it works? The *Cochrane Database of Systematic Reviews* is an online collection of reviews of effectiveness of health care and public health interventions (http://www.thecochranelibrary.com/). One of the Cochrane reviews summarises the evidence from randomised controlled trials on this question. This systematic review shows that dietary advice given to healthy people is modestly effective, leading to reductions in total and low-density lipoprotein cholesterol of 0.15 mmol/L and systolic blood pressure of 2.6 mmHg. The changes, when sustained during adult life, translate into estimated 11% reduction in major coronary events and 19% in strokes. The evidence suggests that diet is a safe and effective alternative to long-term statin and blood pressure lowering treatment among healthy people at low risk of heart disease. In contrast, it is not certain that benefits exceed harms in this low-risk group in those who elect for drug-based risk factor lowering. This example of risk assessment indicates that risk management by dietary advice may be an effective alternative to drug treatment in individuals at low risk of heart disease.

2.7 Social determinants of diet and health

Diet explains part of variation in health between individuals and between populations. Within populations, epidemiologists study differences in health between groups defined by demographic factors such as age. Socioeconomic position has emerged as an important and potentially modifiable determinant of health. The link between lower social status and health has behavioural dimensions, including smoking and diet (Stringhini *et al.*, 2010). A public health view on this is to understand that the social pattern of behaviour has its origins in culture, early life and the transmission of risk across generations (Giesinger *et al.*, 2014). Such observations are significant to public health policy for two reasons. First, health differences or inequalities invariably favour rich and wealthy groups and disadvantage poor groups, producing a stepwise social gradient in health. Second, the social gradient in health can in principle be reduced by policy that helps to equalise access to the goods and services that determine health across social groups.

One of these services is health care, and in the UK there has been a system of universal free access for more than 60 years, based on the principle of fairness (equity). The research shows that, after taking health care need into account, access is indeed generally equitable. Despite equity in health care, health inequalities persist in the UK. This situation illustrates the importance of considering living conditions, including those which influence our diet, to understand the reasons for health inequalities, and then to take effective action to promote public health and reduce health inequality.

This view of public health is different from the approach that concentrates on the individual and their risk factor status. Isolated cases of vitamin C deficiency can be managed by doctors, but if a survey of adults on a low income finds that more than one-third of respondents have depleted or deficient plasma vitamin C levels, then we need to look beyond low fruit and vegetable intake as the explanation. It may come as a surprise that a UK survey, carried out in 2003–2005, produced precisely these findings (Mosdol *et al.*, 2008). The public health approach is to ask what 'upstream' factors, such as price and availability, produce such a widespread problem, with a view to prevention rather than cure.

The environmental factors which influence diet are depicted in the conceptual model (Figure 2.4), which serves as a framework for thinking about nutrition in a social determinants perspective. There are four levels: (1) the inner, individual level (white) of food and nutrient intakes, immersed in and influenced by three sets of factors; (2) the 'micro' or local food environment (pale

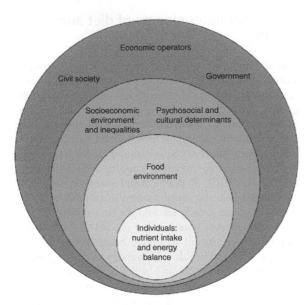

Figure 2.4 Social determinants of diet. Four levels: individual (white); micro (local; pale grey); meso (social; mid grey); macro (national/international; dark grey). *Source*: adapted from a conceptual framework developed by the Prevention of Obesity in Europe (EURO-PREVOB) consortium (2007–2010), http://prevob.lshtm.ac.uk/.

grey) of retailers, caterers and advertising images; (3) the 'meso' or sociocultural factors (mid grey), including norms about food preferences and the salience of healthy eating in family and social networks; and (4) 'macro' national and international factors (dark grey), such as taxation, regulation, food production together with public discussion about food issues. The model is simplistic and it is a generalisation. It omits much important specificity, such as climate, that would need to be added to a case study for every food or food group. The social determinants of diet model is intended to act as a pointer to the levers of change. We hope the reader will consider how far removed it is from the older theories and practices of education and behaviour change which have dominated the field of public health nutrition for many years. (See also Chapter 24 on the wider environment.) The present unsatisfactory state of nutrition-linked public health suggests we do need to find a wider range of effective ways to promote health by means of good nutrition.

2.8 Conclusion

In this chapter we have summarised the concepts and the nature of the evidence, particularly for nutritional epidemiology, when used in public health nutrition, and while we recognise the many imperfections inherent in this process, we reiterate the importance of diet and nutrition-related activities to improve the health of populations.

References

Bingham, S.A., Gill, C., Welch, A. *et al.* (1997) Validation of dietary assessment methods in the UK arm of EPIC using weighed records, and 24-hour urinary nitrogen and potassium and serum vitamin C and carotenoids as biomarkers. *International Journal of Epidemiology*, **26** (Suppl 1), S137–S151.

Bodker, M., Pisinger, C., Toft, U. and Jorgensen, T. (2015) The rise and fall of the world's first fat tax. *Health Policy*, **119**, 737–742.

Bonita, R., Beaglehole, R. and Kjellstrom, T. (2006) *Basic Epidemiology*, 2nd edn. WHO Press, Geneva.

Brunner, E., Stallone, D., Juneja, M. *et al.* (2001) Dietary assessment in Whitehall II: comparison of 7 d diet diary and food-frequency questionnaire and validity against biomarkers. *British Journal of Nutrition*, **86**, 405–414.

Freedman, L.S., Midthune, D., Carroll, R.J. *et al.* (2011) Using regression calibration equations that combine self-reported intake and biomarker measures to obtain unbiased estimates and more powerful tests of dietary associations. *American Journal of Epidemiology*, **174**, 1238–1245.

Gerstman, B. (2003) *Epidemiology Kept Simple: An Introduction to Traditional and Modern Epidemiology*. John Wiley & Sons Inc., Hoboken, NJ.

Giesinger, I., Goldblatt, P., Howden-Chapman, P. *et al.* (2014) Association of socioeconomic position with smoking and mortality: the contribution of early life circumstances in the 1946 birth cohort. *Journal of Epidemiology and Community Health*, **68**, 275–279.

Harris, R., Sawaya, G.F., Moyer, V.A. and Calonge, N. (2011) Reconsidering the criteria for evaluating proposed screening programs: reflections from 4 current and former members of the U. S. Preventive Services Task Force. *Epidemiologic Reviews*, **33**, 20–35.

Johnston, C.A., Rost, S., Miller-Kovach, K. *et al.* (2013) A randomized controlled trial of a community-based behavioral counseling program. *The American Journal of Medicine*, **126**, 1143. e19–1143.e24.

Kivimaki, M., Vineis, P. and Brunner, E.J. (2015) How can we reduce the global burden of disease? *The Lancet*, **386**, 2235–2237.

McLeod, L.D., Cappelleri, J.C. and Hays, R.D. (2016) Best (but oft-forgotten) practices: expressing and interpreting associations and effect sizes in clinical outcome assessments. *American Journal of Clinical Nutrition*, **103**, 685–693.

Mosdol, A., Erens, B. and Brunner, E. J. (2008) Estimated prevalence and predictors of vitamin C deficiency within UK's low-income population. *Journal of Public Health*, **30**, 456–460.

Norat, T., Bingham, S., Ferrari, P. *et al.* (2005) Meat, fish, and colorectal cancer risk: the European Prospective Investigation into cancer and nutrition. *Journal of the National Cancer Institute*, **97**, 906–916.

Offit, P. (2013) The vitamin myth. *The Atlantic*, July 19. http://www.theatlantic.com/health/archive/2013/07/the-vitamin-myth-why-we-think-we-need-supplements/277947/ (accessed November 24 2016).

Schatzkin, A. and Kipnis, V. (2004) Could exposure assessment problems give us wrong answers to nutrition and cancer questions? *Journal of the National Cancer Institute*, **96**, 1564–1565.

Stringhini, S., Sabia, S., Shipley, M. *et al.* (2010) Association of socioeconomic position with health behaviors and mortality. *JAMA*, **303**, 1159–1166.

Stubbs, J., O'Reilly, L., Fuller, Z. *et al.* (2002) Detecting and modelling mis-reporting of food intake in adults. https://www.

researchgate.net/profile/James_Stubbs3/publication/265671753_Detecting_and_Modelling_Mis-Reporting_of_Food_Intake_in_Adults/links/55b61f9e08aec0e5f436de73.pdf (accessed 4 January 2017).

Thiese, M.S. (2014) Observational and interventional study design types; an overview. *Biochemia Medica*, **2**, 199–210.

Willett, W. (2013) *Nutritional Epidemiology*, 3rd edn. Oxford University Press, Oxford.

3
Assessment of Dietary Habits

Marga Ocke and Emma Foster

Key messages

- Different types of dietary assessment methods exist to estimate food consumption of individuals. Four main traditional types are food records, 24-h dietary recalls, dietary history and food frequency questionnaires (FFQs).
- Biomarkers of intake are biochemical indicators measured in biological specimens that are associated with dietary intake. Recovery biomarkers provide an estimate of absolute intake levels and predictive biomarkers show a dose relationship with intake levels. Concentration and replacement biomarkers cannot be translated into absolute levels of intake, but the biomarker concentrations do correlate with intakes of corresponding food components.
- Food records and 24-h dietary recalls repeated on non-consecutive days can be used to estimate the distribution of usual intake for a population by analytically estimating and removing the effects of within-person variation in the observed intake. FFQs are used to collect data on food intake over a longer time period and can be used to rank individuals according to intake.
- Young children up till the age of 7 years have insufficient abilities to cooperate in dietary assessment procedures. Parents are reliable reporters of children's food intake at home, but not for out-of-

home consumption. From the age of 8 years onwards there is a rapid increase in the ability to self-report food consumption.
- Four types of measurement error exist: random within-person error, systematic within-person error, random between-person error and systematic between-person error. A validation study provides insight into the type and size of measurement error.
- Dietary assessment methods which rely on self-reporting of food intakes are prone to bias. Types of bias include recruitment bias (recruiting a sample which is not representative of the general population), low energy reporting, changes to intake to facilitate recording and social desirability bias (reporting food intakes which the individual perceives to be more socially acceptable than their true intake).
- Dietary assessment with new technologies potentially offers advantages, such as increased participation rates, reduced participant burden, reduced cost and improved consistency of data coding. In addition, technology offers the opportunity to collect rich contextual information. Feasibility and validity studies are needed to establish whether the potential advantages are achieved and to check the impact on the quality of the dietary data.

3.1 Introduction

Assessment of dietary habits is a challenge. A range of different types of dietary assessment methods exist for estimating food consumption of individuals. There is no perfect method; and no best method for all purposes. In Section 3.2 we describe the different types of dietary assessment methods with focus on new developments, uses, and strengths and weaknesses. An overview can be found in Table 3.1. Then in Section 3.3 we describe some selective issues that are applicable to many or all dietary assessment methods, like portion size assessment, nutrient calculations and measurement error.

The information provided should help researchers to select the method appropriate for the purpose and target population of a specific study.

3.2 Dietary assessment methods

Dietary records

In the dietary record method, the subject is asked to record all food and beverages immediately before or after they are consumed. The food diary in which the recording is done can be open, semi-open or closed. A closed form is a precoded list of all of the commonly eaten foods

Public Health Nutrition, Second Edition. Edited by Judith L Buttriss, Ailsa A Welch, John M Kearney and Susan A Lanham-New.
© 2018 by The Nutrition Society. Published 2018 by John Wiley & Sons, Ltd.
Companion website: www.wiley.com/go/buttriss/publichealth

Table 3.1 Different methods of dietary assessment.

Method	Description	Advantages	Disadvantages
Dietary records	Respondents keep records of all food and drink they consume. Amounts of foods may be weighed or estimated using portion size assessment aids. An interview may be conducted at the end of the recording period to check for completeness of information.	Does not rely on memory. Can provide accurate information on foods and drinks consumed during the reporting period.	Respondents must be literate and have some level of food knowledge. High burden on respondents may lead to response bias and changes to diet to facilitate recording. May result in underestimation of intakes due to underreporting or undereating.
Variations: Image-capture-based records	Mobile phones or digital cameras are used to capture images of all food and drink consumed.	May be more engaging and less burdensome for the participant.	Risk of blurred or incomplete images. Foods may be difficult to identify from images or obscured by other foods.
24-h dietary recall	Trained interviewers take the respondents through the previous day or 24 h asking them to recall all foods and drinks they consumed.	Does not require respondent to be literate. Low respondent burden.	One day may not be representative of usual intake. Relies on memory.
Variations: Multiple-pass 24-h recall	The respondent is taken through their day's food intake in several stages, gathering information on foods and amounts consumed and checking for forgotten items.	Multiple passes aid memory.	Interviews may be long, increasing the burden on the respondent.
Computer-administered 24-h recall		Convenient for the respondent. Automation of coding. Reduced cost. Increased consistency.	Automation of interview results in loss of flexibility. Respondents must be computer literate and have access to the internet.
Dietary history	Interviewer asks about usual daily intake, followed by a cross-check with food list and 3-day food record.	Allows estimation of habitual food intake. Respondent literacy not required.	Requires highly skilled interviewer. Estimating usual intake is a complex cognitive task, and so respondent burden may be high.
Variations: Computer-based diet history		Improved consistency of interview and coding.	Most still require interviewer due to the complexity of the method.
Food frequency questionnaire (FFQ)	Preprinted list of foods where respondent is asked to report usual frequency of consumption. Sometimes questions on usual amounts consumed are included.	Allows estimation of usual food intake of a group or ranking of individuals. Low burden and low cost. Can be administered by post.	Relies on memory. Estimating usual intake is a complex cognitive task. Absolute level of individual intake not well estimated. Longer food lists may lead to overestimation.
Variations: Computer-administered FFQ		System can check for completeness of answers and implausible amounts. System can provide assistance; for example, audio help.	
Biomarkers for intake	Biochemical indicators which are associated with dietary intake.	Objective measure of intake of certain nutrients or foods. Independent of biases associated with self-reported intake.	Only available for a limited range of foods and nutrients. Expensive. The need for samples of blood, urine or saliva may reduce participation rates.

(continued)

Table 3.1 (*Continued*)

Method	Description	Advantages	Disadvantages
Observation	Researchers observe participants and record their food and drink intake.	Can provide very accurate information on food and drinks consumed. Low respondent burden.	Resource intensive and so costly. Participant may change their behaviour due to being observed. Practical only in institutional settings and small-scale studies.
Variations: Automatic image-capture methods	Wearable cameras are set to capture images at set intervals.	Low respondent burden. Reduced likelihood of changes to intake.	Not all eating occasions may be captured. Risk of data loss. Privacy issues.

in units of specified portion size. A semi-open form may be meal based and prestructured with many foods and amount options listed, but including sufficient space for other foods. Portion size estimation can either be through weighing (weighed food record) or estimated using standard units, household measures or food photographs (estimated food record). The quality of the food recording can be improved by training the respondents to record the level of detail needed to describe adequately the foods and amounts consumed, and by checking the completed food record in detail with the participant during an interview.

Traditionally, the dietary recording is done in a paper diary; however, various alternative procedures are currently available and being developed. Selective examples include the following.

NutriNet-Santé is an online dietary record for use with adults (Hercberg *et al.*, 2010). It is a meal-based record, whereby participants log on and record all foods and drinks consumed for each eating occasion (breakfast, lunch, dinner and others) along with portion size estimates using food photographs.

Images of food taken using Sensecam or on a smartphone have been used to record food intake paired with: a traditional food diary, automated recognition of food type and portion size, or food identification and estimation of portion size by a trained dietitian (e.g. O'Loughlin *et al.*, 2013). The use of such technology may result in improved consistency between respondents: in a food diary one person may write 'Pie', whilst another may write 'Mr Kipling Apple Pie'. This variation in detail is removed by the use of images. There is, however, the risk that images may be blurred or data lost due to limited storage capacity. Automated recognition of food type and portion size is currently limited, in that foods need to be individually served in clear containers for this to be possible, and it does not work well for mixed dishes or layered foods. Nevertheless, this is an exciting possibility for the future.

Uses

Food recording on two or more non-consecutive days provides data on within– and between-individual variation, which allows for the estimation of the distribution of usual intake for a population. Multiple days of recording may allow individuals to be classified according to their usual intakes. The number of days needed to record food intake depends on the aim of the survey and the within-individual variation in intakes of the nutrients of interest.

Children <10 years old are unlikely to supply adequate records. However, dietary records may be completed by someone other than the subject; for example, the parent or caregiver. The food record is often used for national food consumption surveys, particularly in children. In Europe it is the method recommended by the European Food Safety Authority (EFSA) for the youngest age group (<10 years) (EFSA, 2009).

Strengths and weaknesses

A food record does not depend on memory. Thus, it has the potential to be very accurate, particularly if amounts are weighed. However, the usual eating pattern may be influenced by the recording process. In general, respondents must be literate and highly cooperative. This requirement may lead to response bias as a result of overrepresentation of more highly educated individuals interested in diet and health. Keeping a food record, especially a weighed food record, is a considerable respondent burden. Nowadays, no more than three or four consecutive days' food recording are recommended because of respondent fatigue. Intakes obtained through food records tend to be underestimated because of underreporting and or undereating.

Twenty-four-hour dietary recall

The principle of a 24-h dietary recall is that a participant recalls actual food and beverage consumption for the past

24 h or the preceding day. Most commonly, the recalled day is defined as from when the respondent gets up one day until the respondent gets up the next day, but variations to this exist. Variations in timeframe are also in use; for example, a 48-h dietary recall.

The 24-h recall is often structured in multiple steps or passes with specific probes to help the respondent to remember all foods consumed throughout the day. Food quantities are usually assessed by use of household measures, food models or photographs. It is advised that no prior notification is given to the participant about whether or when they will be interviewed about their food intake. Although notification could help the memory of some subjects, others might change their usual diet for the occasion.

The diet recall was traditionally conducted as a personal interview with open forms, precoded questionnaires or tape recorders, but computer-assisted interviews have become common; for example, AMPM (Conway et al., 2004) and GloboDiet (Slimani et al., 2011). With computer-assisted personal interviewing (CAPI) the interviewer is guided by automatic response routing to ask tailored questions and prompts for specific foods. The system thus helps to ensure completeness and consistency across interviewers. There are automated links to food lookup tables and data quality checks. The systematic questions can result in the interview duration being longer, as there may be more steps to identifying or describing a food. There is also some loss of flexibility for the interviewer to respond appropriately to an individual participant's answers.

More recently, online self-administered 24-h diet recalls have been developed; for example, ASA24 (Kirkpatrick et al., 2014). The computer acts as the interviewer and all foods are automatically coded so the cost of data collection is significantly reduced. Many of these systems include automated prompts for items commonly consumed together and checks for missing drinks or long time gaps where no foods are reported. They have the advantage that data collection can be at a time and location convenient to the respondent. They do, however, require subjects to be computer literate and to have access to the internet. There may also be some loss of flexibility. Interviewers can tailor their questions to the level of food knowledge of their respondent and use more descriptive questions about colour, texture and taste to elucidate details of the types of foods consumed, whereas a preprogrammed computer system cannot.

Uses

The 24-h dietary recall is appropriate for describing the mean intake of a group. Two or more non-consecutive days provide data on within- and between-individual variation, which allows for the estimation of the

distribution of usual intake for a population. The repeated 24-h dietary recall is often used for national food consumption surveys; in Europe it is the recommended method by EFSA for that purpose in adults (EFSA, 2009).

Because the recall method depends on the subject's ability to remember and adequately describe their diet, this method is not suitable for children younger than around 7 years (without help of a caregiver) and persons with impaired short-term memory. The prevalence of impaired short-term memory increases above the age of 75 years.

Strengths and weaknesses
Strengths are that the administration time can be short, and the respondent burden is relatively small. In the case of interviewer administration, literacy is not required. Weaknesses are that a respondent's recall depends on short-term memory, and it is known that omission and intrusions occur; portion size is difficult to remember and might be misestimated; and intakes tend to be underreported.

Dietary history

The dietary history assesses an individual's total daily food intake and usual meal pattern over a longer period of time (e.g. the past month or year). In 1947, Burke developed the dietary history technique in three parts: (1) an interview about the subject's usual daily pattern of food intake with quantities specified in household measures, (2) a cross-check using a detailed list of foods and (3) a food diary in which the subject recorded food intake for 3 days. Today, the diet history is applied in many ways. Usual portion sizes are estimated with standard household measures, food pictures and standard units and may be checked by weighing.

A number of computerised/online versions of the diet history have been developed; for example, DISHES98 (Mensink et al., 2001). However, with the exception of an audio-guided self-administered diet history questionnaire developed by Slattery et al. (2008), these still require a dietitian or nutritionist to be present to assist the respondent due to the complexity of the method. In the case of interviews, highly trained nutritionists with well-developed social skills are required to conduct the interview, and the interview is very liable to evoke socially desirable answers.

Uses
The dietary history is used for assessment of usual meal patterns and details of food intake of an individual. A short version of this method with a limited checklist of foods is often used in the clinical setting for diagnosis and

as a basis for therapeutic dietary guidelines. Respondent literacy is not required for an interviewer-administered dietary history. The method is not suitable for children under the age of 10, who are likely to lack the cognitive skills required to average their usual dietary intake over a long period of time.

Strengths and weaknesses

The dietary history method allows assessment of intake over a longer time period. In the case of a cross-check dietary history, the different checks likely improve quality of the dietary data obtained. Respondents are asked to make many judgments about the usual food intake and the amounts of those foods, and the recall period is difficult to conceptualise and remember accurately. This is particularly the case for participants with an irregular dietary pattern. Reports covering a longer period may be influenced by present consumption. The respondent burden and requirements might lead to response bias as a result of overrepresentation of more highly educated individuals interested in diet and health.

Food frequency questionnaires

The FFQ is a preprinted list of foods on which subjects are asked to estimate the frequency and very often also the amount of habitual consumption during a specified period. FFQs vary in the foods listed, length of the reference period, response intervals for specifying frequency of use, procedure for estimating portion size (pictures, household measures, units) and manner of administration. The most optimal food list depends on the research questions and study population. The development of the FFQ is crucial for its quality and may take a lot of time when an evaluation is included.

Traditionally, FFQs were self-administered on paper, but interviewer administration is also done. Nowadays, online FFQs are common. Web-based questionnaires have the advantage that they can easily give cognitive support; a number of systems include audio-help, touch screen functionality or options for the questions to be 'read out'. The data accuracy and completeness can also be improved by having checks for implausible entries and systems to prevent respondents skipping questions.

Uses

The first FFQs were developed for large epidemiological studies; for instance, on the relation between diet and chronic disease.

The food frequency method estimates the usual food (group) intake of an individual. Individuals can be ranked according to nutrient intake, but the absolute level of intake is often not estimated well.

Strengths and weaknesses

A self-administered questionnaire may require little time to complete and to code; the response burden is generally low and response rates, therefore, are relatively high. The method can be automated easily and is not very costly. Weaknesses of this method include that memory of food use in the past is required and that the respondent's burden is governed by number and complexity of foods listed and quantification procedure. The listing of foods may be incomplete or missing details. Longer food lists and longer reference periods often lead to overestimation of intake. Because of these problems, relationships in epidemiological studies may be attenuated, obscuring relationships that might exist.

Biomarkers of intake

Biomarkers of intake are biochemical indicators measured in biological specimens (e.g. urine, blood (fractions)) that are associated with dietary intake. Dietary biomarkers can be divided into several classes; that is, recovery biomarkers, predictive biomarkers, concentration biomarkers and replacement biomarkers (Jenab et al., 2009). Recovery biomarkers provide an estimate of absolute intake levels, and predictive biomarkers show a dose relationship with intake levels. Whereas concentration and replacement biomarkers cannot be translated into absolute levels of intake, the biomarker concentrations do correlate with intakes of corresponding food components. There are only a few recovery biomarkers available. Examples are urinary nitrogen, sodium and potassium, and doubly labelled water. Vitamin and mineral levels in blood fall in the class of concentration biomarkers.

New dietary biomarkers are emerging through biomarker discovery strategies using non-targeted metabolomics. These recent techniques of metabolite profiling or fingerprinting allow for simultaneous monitoring of multiple and dynamic components of biological fluids. This may provide metabolic signals indicative of food intake. Samples of urine from short-term food intervention studies or from cohort studies in which participants consumed a freely chosen diet can be analysed through numerous analytical platforms, followed by multivariate data analysis. Biomarkers discovered in this way are generally indicators for intake of very specific foods, like salmon and raspberries (Lloyd et al., 2011).

Uses

Biomarkers for intake are often used as an objective reference measure to validate other dietary assessment methods. Sometimes biomarkers are used as a (better) substitute for dietary assessment. For example, accurate assessment of total sodium intake using self-reported methods is very difficult because people cannot quantify discretionary salt well, and because sodium contents in foods differ largely between brands, whereas food composition tables are usually not brand specific. In addition, the use of biomarkers in combination with other dietary assessment methods is increasingly recommended (see Section 3.2: 'Combined methods').

Strengths and weaknesses

The main strength of dietary biomarkers is that they are objective measures and are independent of all the biases and errors associated with self-reported dietary assessment. Weaknesses are that they are available only for a limited number of nutrients and foods. Genetic variation and other factors may influence nutrient metabolism and may affect the utility of a dietary biomarker to properly reflect dietary exposures. Biomarkers can tell us about the intake of specific nutrients or foods but cannot provide detailed information on the rich variety of foods and nutrients which make up an individual's total dietary intake. The requirement to collect blood and/or urine samples may act as a deterrent to participation, making it difficult to achieve a representative sample, and the cost of analysis may make them prohibitively expensive for use in large surveys.

Other methods

Many alternative or slightly adjusted methods to assess dietary intake exist, and we have no intention to be complete here. A few seem worth mentioning. Screening methods are brief questionnaires to collect information on specific aspects of diet or qualitative information of dietary intake. For example, screeners for fat intake, dietary fibre intake or for adherence to a dietary index. Nowadays, the screeners are usually in an online format.

Direct observation of dietary intake has been used in small-scale studies and for validation of less intensive methods of dietary assessment. Researchers observe and record the details of the foods consumed and may weigh or estimate the amount of food consumed. Observation is very labour intensive but is feasible in school or institutional settings, particularly when only specific meals are of interest (e.g. school lunch).

Image-capture-based methods

Researchers at the University of Pittsburgh have developed an e-button that is worn on the chest and records digital images of food intake along with where food and drink are bought and time spent in various activities (Sun *et al.*, 2010). The e-button has two cameras that allow portion size to be estimated automatically. Such

technology makes observation of an individual's total dietary intake more practicable.

On-body sensors have been used to detect eating events based on arm movement, chewing and swallowing (e.g. Amft and Troster, 2009). Chewing Jockey combines a photo-reflector, which detects movement of the lower jaw, along with a sound filter to recognise food texture (Koizumi *et al.*, 2011). Amft and Troster (2009) were able to recognise 19 foods with 80% classification accuracy using chewing strokes detected by an ear-pad microphone and could differentiate between low and high bolus volume using a swallowing sensor around the neck. Bite weight recognition using acoustic chewing recordings has also been shown to be feasible for solid foods (Amft *et al.*, 2009).

Combined methods

Combination of two dietary assessment methods might balance the shortcomings and strengths of different methods. Self-reporting of dietary intake is always subject to error, and biomarkers do not provide insight into the dietary sources of nutrient intake. Combining self-reporting methods with biomarkers, therefore, has important advantages. Food records and 24-h recalls do not provide insight into usual intake of an individual, whereas FFQs cannot estimate the level of intake well. Combining FFQs with recalls and records might balance these shortcomings.

3.3 Selective issues in dietary assessment

Mode of administration

Various modes of administration of dietary assessment methods exist. Traditionally, dietary assessment tended to be interviewer administered. In the 1980s, large-scale epidemiological studies replaced this with paper-administered questionnaires; and later there were computer-assisted or computer-administered questionnaires. In the 21st century, innovative computer, internet, telecommunication and imaging technologies have resulted in further innovation of dietary assessment.

Using new and novel technology to enhance traditional dietary assessment methods reduces the cost and participant burden, potentially increasing participation rates, and improving accuracy and precision. CAPI has benefits, in that the interview and coding process are standardised and the need for manual coding and data entry is reduced, thus limiting the scope for human error. In addition to this, online dietary self-assessment methods, such as ASA24 (Kirkpatrick *et al.*, 2014), have the potential to engage the user and make the task less onerous. They offer increased flexibility, in that the participant can complete the assessment at a time that suits them; and they reduce the amount of researcher time required, and therefore the cost of dietary assessment. Many traditional methods of dietary assessment require an in-depth interview with a nutritionist or dietitian, which may act as a deterrent to participation for many. Replacing the interviewer with a computer may increase participation rates and also accuracy, as the feeling that dietary intake is being judged may be reduced. There is, however, a loss of flexibility, in that an interviewer can tailor their questions to the cognitive skills and level of food knowledge of their respondent. For example, a skilled interviewer may be able to ascertain cooking methods by asking questions such as, 'Was the food made in a pan on top of the cooker or did it go inside the oven?' A computer system does not have the flexibility to respond in this way. Additionally, such methods require subjects to be computer literate and to have access to the internet.

Objective methods such as Sensecam or direct observation (by a researcher) remove the need for the participant to report their dietary intake. They can be used to collect an accurate account of what the subject consumes during the recording period, particularly if observation is paired with weighing of the foods by the observer. There may be changes to usual intake due to the knowledge that food intake is being monitored, and it may not be possible to tell the difference between certain types of foods which are visually similar but nutritionally different (e.g. skimmed milk and whole milk) by observation alone.

Food description and classification

In dietary assessment, the specificity in the description of the foods needs to fit with the purposes of the study. Moreover, in the case of self-reporting, the terminology and food knowledge of the participant are important to consider. Preparation method (e.g. raw, boiled, fried), fat content (e.g. full-fat, skimmed) and sugar content (sugar-sweetened, artificially sweetened, unsweetened) are often important aspects in food description to assess macronutrient intake. Depending on voluntary fortification practices, it might be important to know if a consumed food was fortified or not to assess intake of some micronutrients. However, many participants cannot report this characteristic. When collecting information on specific food and brand names, inspection or pictures of packages might help to obtain this type of information. The EPIC-Soft system of food description is a very systematic way to describe foods according to 18 characteristics (called facets), with a varying number of options (descriptors)

for each facet (Slimani et al., 1999). The system is based on the Langual food description system. A systematic way for food description is helpful in standardisation in data collection across studies and countries. Many food classification systems exist, which are often fit for a specific purpose. Food classifications that are useful for data collection (treating foods within the food group the same during data collection and processing) might differ from classifications to report results or classifications used to study relationships between food (groups) consumption and, for example, health, diseases and determinants of dietary intake.

Dietary supplements

Dietary supplements can be important sources of micronutrient intake for an individual. In affluent populations, for several micronutrients, the contribution at the population level can be substantial. Dietary supplements differ in content and strength; and consumption patterns might be regular or irregular, and in different dosages. For large-scale studies in which diet is related to, for example, diseases, the frequency of use for different categories of dietary supplements may be the most important information to collect. Examples of categories are multivitamins, multivitamins/multiminerals, vitamin C supplements, calcium supplements and so on. When the aim is to assess the level of vitamin and mineral intake on a specific day, information on the exact subtype of dietary supplement, brand and strength is necessary. Since many participants cannot recall this very specific information, inspection of the packages, reading of barcodes and collection of images can be helpful for this purpose.

Amount quantification

In order to convert food intakes into nutrient intakes an estimate or measure of portion size is required. Participants can be supplied with calibrated scales and asked to weigh every item they eat and drink, including any amount leftover. However, this places a large burden on the participant and may result in changes to diet to facilitate recording and low participation rates. Portion size estimation aids have been developed to help participants provide an estimate of the amount of food consumed. These include food photographs (Nelson et al., 1997), food models (Foster et al., 2008), digital images of food (Subar et al., 2010) and two-dimensional drawings (Steyn et al., 2006). See Figure 3.1 for some examples. Estimation of portion size is associated with a range of both over– and underestimation. Portion size assessment aids should contain foods and portion sizes appropriate to the population and should be tested and validated for the

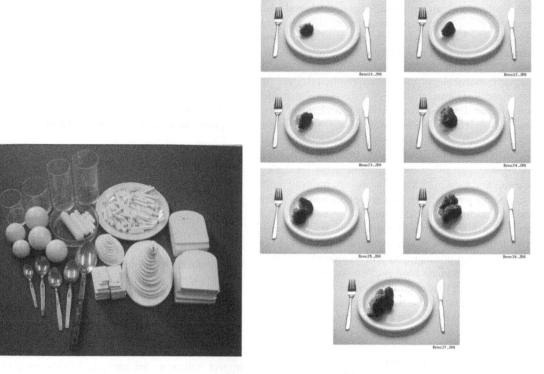

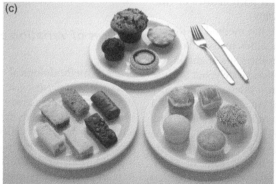

Figure 3.1 Examples of sources for portion size: (a) food models; (b) food photographs; (c) guide photographs.

population in which they are to be used. Household measures can also be used to give an estimate of the amount of food in terms of slices, pieces, spoons and cups. Research has shown that whilst people may be confident in their ability to accurately report portion size using household measures their use may be associated with significant misreporting (Chambers *et al.*, 2000). If no measure or estimate of the amount of food consumed is collected then average portion sizes may be used. There are UK average portion sizes available for adults (Wrieden and Barton, 2006) and children (Wrieden *et al.*, 2008).

Specific population groups

Young children up till the age of 7 years have insufficient abilities to cooperate in dietary assessment procedures. Therefore, often parents or caregivers have acted as surrogate respondents. Studies comparing direct observations with recalls by parents suggest that the latter are reliable reporters of food intake at home, but not for out-of-home consumption.

From the age of 8 years onwards there is a rapid increase in the ability to self-report food consumption.

Issues to take into account are limited memory, concept of time, attention span and knowledge of foods and food preparation. Food preference and the rapidly changing food habits affect the reliability of the recall of food consumption. Of key importance in designing questionnaires is to understand how food-related information is organised in memory and subsequently retrieved in dietary recall. Domel *et al.* (1994) developed a model showing that the most usual retrieval mechanism categories employed by children were visual imagery (the colour of foods and shape), usual practice (familiarity with eating the food previously), behaviour chaining (linking foods to other food items or activities during the meal) and food preference. In order to improve recall accuracy, the time between consumption and reporting must be minimised. For example, for a 24-h recall interview it is preferable that no meals are consumed between the last meal to be reported and the start of the interview. Using photographs and technology, children were found to estimate food portion size with an accuracy approaching that of adults (Domel *et al.*, 1994). By adolescence, cognitive abilities should be fully developed; limiting problems in that age are issues of motivation and body image, and knowledge of food preparation. Techniques including attractive technologies may improve reports by increasing motivation, cooperation and recognition of types of foods and portion sizes of children and adolescents (Baxter, 2009).

Up to the age of around 70, the method of dietary assessment does not need to be different from younger adults. Also, some individuals in their 80s might be able to report their food consumption accurately, but because memory fades with age, dietary assessment in older adults requires particular care. Adaptations of record methods and diet histories have resulted in valid reports for older adults. Similarly, a picture-sort technique including a cognitive processing approach helps elderly people to remember what they usually eat. For FFQs, interviewer-administration or reviewing of completed questionnaires with older participants is important, especially to check omitting answers on questions. For 24-h dietary recalls it might be useful to combine these with a food record as a memory aid (De Vries *et al.*, 2009).

Dietary assessment in minority groups with a strong ethnic and cultural identity needs to be adjusted to the foods consumed, eating habits, and social and cultural background of the group. Structured questionnaires or records need to be adapted to the foods and culinary habits. Such adaptations can best be made after initial data collection using an open method such as dietary recalls or food records and focus group discussions with individuals from the minority groups. If relevant, questionnaires in the language or interviewers with the same background are of great help. Food composition databases should be checked for completeness regarding ethnic foods and recipes. Photo books often are necessary in identifying foods. Dietary assessment in remote areas or developing countries with limited facilities is outside the scope of this chapter.

It is a well-known problem that people who are overweight and obese tend to underreport their diet. Particularly for this group, objective ways of dietary assessment are preferred over self-reporting methods.

Nutrient intake and other impacts of diet

Total nutrient intake per person can be calculated by multiplying the nutrient content of the foods reported with the quantity consumed, and them summing intake over all foods. In case dietary supplements are taken, intake from dietary supplements should also be considered to obtain total nutrient intake. Chapter 6 describes various aspects of importance when working with nutrient databases. Similarly, exposure to food chemicals (relevant for food safety assessment) and the environmental impact of diets can be assessed by merging collected food consumption data with databases of chemical concentrations in foods and environmental impact indicators for consumed foods respectively.

Sources of variation and measurement error

From a methodological point of view, four types of measurement error exist: random within-person error, systematic within-person error, random between-person error and systematic between-person error. Systematic error is also called bias. The types and size of error vary with the particular dietary assessment method, study design and with the population in which it is applied. Many participants have some kind of dietary pattern, with daily and seasonal variation on top of that. These aspects should be taken into account in the study design for a specific objective. For example, covering different days of the week and seasons, including sufficient repeated measurements and study participants. See Chapter 4 for more information on study design.

A validation study provides insight into the type and size of measurement error. Conducting a validation study requires the availability of a gold-standard or reference method. Few such gold standards are available, and at the moment it is impossible to evaluate the validity of dietary assessment of all dietary components in large-scale real-life settings. The assessment of energy intake can be validated using doubly labelled water, and assessment of nitrogen, potassium and sodium intake with 24-h dietary urinary excretions of these components. For other dietary components, relative or congruent validity against another dietary assessment method of accepted quality can be studied. In this case, it is important that the error structures of the test and reference method are as different as possible; for example, to compare an FFQ that asks for long-term dietary intake with repeated 24-h recalls of food records that assess short-term dietary intake. An example of a well-conducted validation study, with gold standards, is the OPEN-study (Kipnis *et al.*, 2003).

In the evaluation of dietary intake of populations, researchers are often interested in the usual intake (i.e. the long-term average intake). One relevant objective, where usual rather than short-term dietary intake is important, is in the assessment of nutrient adequacy of populations. Approaches for such evaluation can be found in Chapter 7. In food consumption surveys, dietary intake is often collected with short-term measurements; for example, 24-h recalls or food records. The random within-person variation in intake is random within-person error from the perspective of usual intake assessment. Short-term measurements repeated on non-consecutive days can be used to estimate the distribution of usual intake for a population by analytically estimating and removing the effects of within-person variation in the observed intake (Dodd *et al.*, 2006). Similarly, for many epidemiological studies usual intake of participants is of relevance. Based on validation study results, it is recommended to estimate usual intake based on a food propensity questionnaire and repeated non-consecutive short-term dietary assessment for each participant. However, it should be noted that the assumption in usual intake estimation is that the applied short-term method is unbiased. This assumption is often not true for self-reported dietary assessment.

Each type of dietary assessment method has its strengths and weaknesses and method-specific measurement error. Moreover, even one type of method can be developed and applied in a variety of ways; so, using the same type of method does not mean that the results can be pooled or compared. In standardised methods, each detail and step of dietary assessment and subsequent data handling are the same. However, in harmonised methods, the general approach, procedures and outcomes are similar but not necessarily all details. When dietary assessment in different countries or groups with different culinary habits needs to be conducted, harmonisation is often a better option than standardisation, since differences in consumed foods and eating habits are usually incompatible with fully standardised methods, such as the same food items in FFQs, or the same pictures for portion size assessment.

3.4 Conclusions

It is important that, for each study, a dietary assessment method is chosen which is appropriate for the study objectives, study population and study setting. In many cases an existing method needs to be adapted or a dietary assessment method needs to be specifically developed. For each new study, thorough preparation of the dietary assessment part is essential. In the case of a new dietary assessment, sufficient time allotted for development and pilot testing is essential. When the work is done by interviewers, an extensive training period is required. Meanwhile, if (new) technologies are applied, testing these in different field circumstances, appropriate study populations and settings that might occur in the study is strongly recommended. Dietary assessment with new technologies potentially offers advantages, such as increased participation rates, and improving accuracy and precision. In addition, technology offers the opportunity to collect rich contextual information, such as location of eating events, how many other potential outlets a person passed before settling on their eating destination, duration of eating events, whether the TV was on and whether they were eating in company or alone – all without any additional burden to the participant. Feasibility and validity studies are needed to obtain insight into the type and size of measurement error of dietary assessment with new technologies. This will establish whether the potential advantages (such as reduced cost, increased participation and reduced underreporting) are achieved and check the impact on the quality of the dietary data.

References

Amft, O. and Troster, G. (2009) On-body sensing solutions for automatic dietary monitoring. *IEEE Pervasive Computing*, **8**, 62–70.

Amft, O., Kusserow, M. and Troster, G. (2009) Bite weight prediction from acoustic recognition of chewing. *IEEE Transactions on Biomedical Engineering*, **56**, 1663–1672.

Baxter, S.D. (2009) Cognitive processes in children's dietary recalls: insight from methodological studies. *European Journal of Clinical Nutrition*, **63** (Suppl 1), S19–S32.

Chambers E. IV, Godwin, S.L. and Vecchio, F.A. (2000) Cognitive strategies for reporting portion sizes using dietary recall procedures. *Journal of the American Dietetic Association*, **100**, 891–897.

Conway, J.M., Ingwersen, L.A. and Moshfegh, A.J. (2004) Accuracy of dietary recall using the USDA five-step multiple-pass method in men: an observational validation study. *Journal of the American Dietetic Association*, **104**, 595–603.

De Vries, J.H., de Groot, L.C. and van Staveren, W.A. (2009) Dietary assessment in elderly people: experiences gained from studies in the Netherlands. *European Journal of Clinical Nutrition*, **63** (Suppl 1), S69–S74.

Dodd, K.W., Guenther, P.M., Freedman, L.S. *et al.* (2006) Statistical methods for estimating usual intake of nutrients and foods: a review of the theory. *Journal of the American Dietetic Association*, **106**, 1640–1650.

Domel, S.B., Thompson, W.O., Baranowski, T. and Smith, A.F. (1994) How children remember what they have eaten. *Journal of the American Dietetic Association*, **94**, 1267–1272.

EFSA (2009) General principles for the collection of national food consumption data in the view of a pan-European dietary survey. *EFSA Journal*, **7**, 1435.

Foster, E., Matthews, J.N.S., Lloyd, J. *et al.* (2008) Children's estimates of food portion size: the development and evaluation of three portion size assessment tools for use with children. *British Journal of Nutrition*, **99**, 175–184.

Hercberg, S., Castetbon, K., Czernichow, S. *et al.* (2010) The Nutrinet-Santé Study: a web-based prospective study on the relationship between nutrition and health and determinants of dietary patterns and nutritional status. *BMC Public Health*, **10**, 242.

Jenab, M., Slimani, N., Bictash, M. *et al.* (2009) Biomarkers in nutritional epidemiology: applications, needs and new horizons. *Human Genetics*, **125**, 507–525.

Kipnis, V., Subar, A.F., Midthune, D. *et al.* (2003) Structure of dietary measurement error: results of the OPEN biomarker study. *American Journal of Epidemiology*, **158**, 14–21; discussion 22–26.

Kirkpatrick, S. I., Subar, A. F., Douglass, D. *et al.* (2014) Performance of the automated self-administered 24-hour recall relative to a measure of true intakes and to an interviewer-administered 24-h recall. *The American Journal of Clinical Nutrition*, **100**, 233–240.

Koizumi, N., Tanaka, H., Uema, Y. and Inami, M. (2011) Chewing jockey: augmented food texture by using sound based on the cross-modal effect. In T. Romão, N. Correia, M. Inami *et al.* (eds), *ACE '11 Proceedings of the 8th International Conference on Advances in Computer Entertainment Technology*. ACM, New York; article no. 21.

Lloyd, A. J., Fave, G., Beckmann, M. *et al.* (2011) Use of mass spectrometry fingerprinting to identify urinary metabolites after consumption of specific foods. *The American Journal of Clinical Nutrition*, **94**, 981–991.

Mensink, G., Haftenberger, M. and Thamm, M. (2001) Validity of DISHES 98, a computerised dietary history interview: energy and macronutrient intake. *European Journal of Clinical Nutrition*, **55**, 409–417.

Nelson, M., Atkinson, M. and Meyer, J.A. (1997) *A Photographic Atlas of Food Portion Sizes*. MAFF Publications, London.

O'Loughlin, G., Cullen, S. J., McGoldrick, A. *et al.* (2013) Using a wearable camera to increase the accuracy of dietary analysis. *American Journal of Preventive Medicine*, **44**, 297–301.

Slattery, M.L., Murtaugh, M.A., Schumacher, M.C. *et al.* (2008) Development, implementation, and evaluation of a computerized self-administered diet history questionnaire for use in studies of American Indian and Alaskan native people. *Journal of the American Dietetic Association*, **108**, 101–109.

Slimani, N., Deharveng, G., Charrondière, R.U. *et al.* (1999) Structure of the standardized computerized 24-h diet recall interview used as reference method in the 22 centers participating in the EPIC project. *Computer Methods and Programs in Biomedicine*, **58**, 251–266.

Slimani, N., Casagrande, C., Nicolas, G. *et al.* (2011) The standardized computerized 24-h dietary recall method EPIC-Soft adapted for pan-European dietary monitoring. *European Journal of Clinical Nutrition*, **65** (Suppl 1), S5–S15.

Steyn, N.P., Senekal, M., Norris, S.A. *et al.* (2006) How well do adolescents determine portion sizes of foods and beverages? *Asia Pacific Journal of Clinical Nutrition*, **15**, 35–42.

Subar, A.F., Crafts, J., Zimmerman, T.P. *et al.* (2010) Assessment of the accuracy of portion size reports using computer-based food photographs aids in the development of an automated self-administered 24-hour recall. *Journal of the American Dietetic Association*, **110**, 55–64.

Sun, M., Fernstrom, J. D., Jia, W. *et al.* (2010) A wearable electronic system for objective dietary assessment. *Journal of the American Dietetic Association*, **110**, 45–47.

Wrieden, W.L. and Barton, K.L. (2006) Calculation and collation of typical food portion sizes for adults aged 19–64 and older people aged 65 and over. Final Technical Report to the Food Standards Agency.

Wrieden, W.L., Longbottom, P.J., Adamson, A.J. *et al.* (2008) Estimation of typical food portion sizes for children of different ages in Great Britain. *British Journal of Nutrition*, **99**, 1344–1353.

4

Assessment of Nutritional Status in Public Health Nutrition Settings

H David McCarthy

Key messages

- A number of anthropometric measurements are used to assess nutritional status of individuals and groups. In contemporary public health nutrition practice, measures of overweight and obesity and how they relate to metabolic risk are particularly important. Body mass index (BMI), waist circumference (WC) and percentage body fat measurement are all used in this context.
- Despite a number of advantages, BMI has several drawbacks, the most important being that it is not a measure of adiposity and is unable to differentiate between fat and lean tissues. This can lead to misclassification of individuals.
- WC measurement is a proxy for visceral adipose tissue accumulation which is linked to risk for metabolic disease.
- Assessment outcomes in children and adolescents are influenced by growth and therefore measures including height, BMI and WC

are evaluated using percentile charts based on population reference data.
- Self-reporting of heights and weights are prone to bias which can lead to underestimation of BMI and in public health settings, an underestimation of true prevalence of overweight and obesity.
- More recent measures including body fatness and skeletal muscle mass offer opportunities to move beyond BMI in order to better rate individuals based on the fat and lean components of the body.
- Further validation studies are needed to establish whether these newer measures offer greater advantage over the simpler methods to identify individuals and groups at greater risk of metabolic and degenerative diseases.

4.1 Introduction

Anthropometry and related measures are key to the assessment of the nutritional status of individuals and populations, whether in a public health, clinical or research setting. The range of anthropometric measurements includes height, weight and circumferences, and individual measures serve similar or specific purposes across the life cycle, depending on the particular need at that time. Obesity and metabolic disease are now major public health issues, while undernutrition remains an important issue in selected population groups. Additionally, sarcopenia – an age-related loss of skeletal muscle mass and function – is an emerging clinical and public health issue. Anthropometric measures are critical for the surveillance of these conditions and in evaluating the efficacy of interventions. In this chapter, the range of anthropometric measures is described, including more

recent developments in this area, their role in a public health setting and addressing their strengths, weaknesses and measurement error. The knowledge gained from reading this chapter should help practitioners and researchers select the measurement(s) most appropriate for the purpose of their work and target population group.

4.2 Anthropometric measures

Standing height

Measurement of height represents cumulative linear growth and body size and comprises the lengths of the lower limbs, trunk, and neck and head. It is thus the maximum distance between the floor and the vertex of the head. Across childhood and adolescence, height measurements are a sensitive marker of growth, which in

Public Health Nutrition, Second Edition. Edited by Judith L Buttriss, Ailsa A Welch, John M Kearney and Susan A Lanham-New.
© 2018 by The Nutrition Society. Published 2018 by John Wiley & Sons, Ltd.
Companion website: www.wiley.com/go/buttriss/publichealth

extremis reflects nutritional stunting and at the other end of the spectrum excessive linear growth. In adults, final achieved height is linked to morbidity, including metabolic risk and cancer risk. Standardised measurement protocols aim to ensure an accurate value is obtained when using a calibrated stadiometer, and height should be taken in stockinged feet and measured to 0.1 cm. A minimum of two readings should be taken, and where the difference between the two is greater than 0.4 cm a third measurement should be included. A critical element of height measurement is the correct positioning of the head, which should be placed in the Frankfurt plane – an imaginary straight line passing between the inferior margin of the orbit and the upper margin of the ear canal. While height measurements are usually used in conjunction with weight to obtain a body mass index (BMI; see Section 4.5), the components of total height or stature can be assessed to obtain a measure of body proportionality.

Sitting height

Sitting height is obtained using a specialised table which measures the length of the trunk, neck and head. Subtracting this value from standing height gives an estimation of leg length, which can be incorporated into a ratio of leg length to height. Although not a routine measure in public health nutrition practice, in research settings a measure of proportionality indicates the relative growth of the upper and lower body which has been linked to risk of metabolic disease.

Body weight

Body weight is a simple measure to perform, and its accuracy will depend on a range of factors, including the calibration of the scales, the subject's clothing and hydration status. In a weight management context, weight loss is a simple marker of fat loss, although this will be accompanied by some loss of fat-free tissue.

Weight/height ratio: body mass index

Height and weight measures are usually combined to provide a measure for classifying an individual's weight relative to their height in order to give an indication of fatness. The BMI, a term coined in 1972, is also known as Quetelet's index. It is derived as weight (kilograms)/ height squared (square metres). Taking the square of height is intended to remove the height–weight relationship, thus making BMI independent of height. It is more correctly a measure of overweight and obesity, and the accuracy and precision of BMI measurements are dependent on the accuracy and precision of height and weight measurements. BMI correlates reasonably well with body

Table 4.1 BMI categories.

BMI range	Category
<18.5	Underweight
18.5–24.9	Normal (healthy) weight
25.0–29.9	Overweight
30–34.9	Obese
35–39.9	Severe obese
≥40	Morbidly obese

fat (kilograms) and to a lesser degree with body fat (per cent). Table 4.1 show the BMI ranges which relate to categories of underweight, normal weight, overweight and obese, as well as further divisions of obesity.

BMI is used for the clinical assessment of individuals and in population surveys. BMI exhibits a 'J'-shaped curve with mortality, with a high BMI being strongly associated with significantly increasing mortality. Likewise, a high BMI is linked with increased morbidity, including type 2 diabetes, hypertension and coronary heart disease. The World Health Organization (WHO) and national bodies such as the Centers for Disease Control (CDC, USA) and the National Institute for Health and Care Excellence (UK) recommend the use of BMI as a measure of overweight and obesity but also recognise that caution must be exercised when interpreting BMI as it is not a direct measure of adiposity.

Practitioners and researchers in public health nutrition therefore need to be aware of the strengths and limitations of BMI, which are summarised in Table 4.2. Critically, BMI represents only a crude proxy for body

Table 4.2 Strengths and limitations of BMI.

Strengths	Limitations
Non-invasive	A measure of weight, not fatness
Quick to perform	Does not differentiate between fat mass and fat-free mass (FFM)
Inexpensive	Gives no indication of body fat distribution
Simple to undertake	No indication of skeletal muscle mass (sarcopenia/sarcopenic obesity)
Equally useful clinically/ epidemiologically	Risk of misclassification of individuals
Easy to interpret (?)	Does not treat all ethnicities equally
Accounts for expected differences in weights in individuals of different height	Not a simple calculation for the general public to perform
Values are independent of age and sex in adults	

fatness and can lead to significant misclassification of individuals. While it can incorrectly classify a small number of individuals with a high FFM (particularly skeletal muscle mass) as overweight, a far greater problem is the misclassification of individuals with a high fat mass into the normal or healthy BMI range. For the same reasons, it is important to recognise that, as a measure of overweight and obesity or as a measure of disease risk, BMI does not treat individuals of different ethnicities equally. This is largely due to ethnicity-related variations in body proportions and composition. For example, certain Asian populations typically can be characterised by a shorter height, with relatively shorter legs for their height compared with European populations. Additionally, the South Asian phenotype is characterised by a lower skeletal muscle mass, greater fat mass and a more centralised distribution of body fat for a given BMI compared with individuals from a European background. Consequently, lower BMI cut-offs have now been adopted to define overweight (BMI = 23) and obesity (BMI = 25) in certain South Asian populations, including India. Some South-East Asian countries, such as Singapore, have also adopted similar lower cut-offs. In national surveys such as the Health Survey for England, where BMI is used, obesity prevalence figures between ethnic groups (with associated morbidity risk) must be interpreted with caution when a single set of BMI cut-offs is used to define different weight categories.

In summary:

- BMI is a widely used measure of overweight and obesity.
- Its use is recommended by several authorities on health and nutrition.
- It has a number of advantages and drawbacks.
- Public health nutrition practitioners need to be aware of its limitations and interpret individual results with caution.
- BMI should be used in combination with other simple measures (e.g. WC).

In a research setting, and depending on the purpose of the study, BMI is sometimes partitioned into two components: the fat mass index and FFM index. However, to obtain these values, knowledge of the fat mass and FFM is required, which is usually obtained from technologies such as bioelectrical impedance (BIA), air-displacement plethysmography or dual energy X-ray absorptiometry. Such divisions of BMI may be useful when evaluating growth across childhood and adolescence and the partitioning of dietary energy and nitrogen into fat and lean tissues.

Waist circumference

Jean Vague (1947) first described sex differences in body fat distribution and demonstrated that an excess abdominal body fat accumulation was related to increased risk for type 2 diabetes and atherosclerosis. Metabolic syndrome (MS), a clustering of risk factors for coronary heart disease, is now considered of major global importance. The International Diabetes Federation consensus worldwide definition of MS (IDF, 2006) places central or abdominal obesity, measured by waist circumference (WC – with ethnicity-specific values), as the core defining component of MS – WC being more indicative of the MS profile than BMI. Any two of the following four factors together with central obesity would constitute a person being defined as having MS:

- raised triglycerides;
- reduced high-density lipoprotein cholesterol;
- raised blood pressure;
- raised fasting plasma glucose.

While measures of abdominal obesity correlate reasonably well with BMI, the degree of association is variable, which suggests that BMI and waist indices may provide different information regarding metabolic risk. However, the WHO argues there is convincing evidence that measures of abdominal fatness which incorporate WC are useful for predicting risk for non-communicable diseases, including hypertension, insulin resistance, type 2 diabetes, dyslipidaemia, non-alcoholic fatty liver and coronary heart disease. Specifically, in adults, WC is an indicator of visceral adipose tissue accumulation, although subcutaneous fat is also captured by a waist measurement. Visceral fat differs from subcutaneous fat in that it is drained by the portal blood system and free fatty acids released from visceral fat are delivered directly to the liver. It is thought that it is this excess free fatty acids delivery to the liver which underpins the insulin resistance which drives MS.

Waist measurement

WC is measured using a flexible, non-elastic tape. However, a key issue is that there is no universally agreed definition of the measurement site. The sites range from the level of the umbilicus, midway between the 10th rib and iliac crest, to a point at around 4 cm above the umbilicus. In a public health context this can make comparisons between populations difficult when different measurement sites are employed at different centres. Additional problems include sensitivity issues due to the perceived invasiveness of the measurement. While it is preferable to take the measurement directly over the surface of the skin, this can be addressed, in part, by establishing protocols where the measurement is taken over a single layer of indoor clothing, such as a vest or t-shirt, and then subtracting the contribution of the clothing to the circumference reading. Additionally, with very

Table 4.3 International Diabetes Federation criteria for ethnic or country-specific values for WC.

Country/ethnic group	Sex	WC (cm)
Europid	Male	>94
	Female	>80
South Asian	Male	>90
	Female	>80
Chinese	Male	>90
	Female	>80
Japanese	Male	>90
	Female	>80

obese individuals, it can be difficult to locate the true waist site, leading to greater measurement errors and poor precision. Indeed, the measurement error, particularly between-observer errors, could invalidate the waist measurement as an effective public health assessment tool. This potential error emphasises the importance of training the practitioner and researcher in the waist measurement technique. In skilled hands, a low technical error of measurement can be achieved with a within-observer error as low as 1%, and a true measurement to within ±1 cm for most individuals.

Gender-specific cut-offs have been established for WC to define individuals at different degrees of metabolic risk. As for BMI, these cut-offs have been revised downwards for individuals from Asian backgrounds (Table 4.3). In clinical and public health practice, WC and BMI are usually collected together, and between the two indices a level of risk can be established (Table 4.4).

Table 4.4 Combined recommendations of BMI and WC cut-off points made for overweight or obesity, and association with disease risk.

	BMI	Obesity class	Disease risk (relative to normal weight and WC)	
			Men <102 cm Women <88 cm	Men >102 cm Women >88 cm
Underweight	<18.5			
Normal	18.5–24.9			
Overweight	25.0–24.9		Increased	High
Obesity	30.0–34.9	I	High	Very high
	35.0–39.9	II	Very high	Very high
Extreme obesity	≥40.0	III	Extremely high	Extremely high

Source: adapted from NHLBI Obesity Education Initiative Expert Panel (2000).

Hip circumference and waist/hip ratio

The use of the ratio of WC to hip circumference (WHR) dates back to the middle of the 1980s with the concept pioneered by Per Björntorp, the rationale being that this ratio distinguishes between fat accumulation in the lower (subcutaneous, hip and buttocks) body and upper (abdominal/visceral) areas. WHR varies with age, gender and degree of overweight and is strongly associated with an increased risk for type 2 diabetes, coronary heart disease and stroke. Mean WHR can vary between 0.87 and 0.99 (for men) and 0.76 and 0.84 (for women), and WHR cut-offs for increased risk of cardiovascular disease risk have been accepted for international use, although ethnic-specific cut-offs may be required. WHR has gained more significance since the recent recognition that subcutaneous fat on the hips, buttocks and thighs acts as a reservoir for triglycerides. Indeed, hip circumference appears to acts as an independent marker of glucose tolerance, with a higher hip circumference being protective against cardiometabolic disease risk and associated with better health outcomes. Hip should be measured at the site of greatest circumference, and although it is reported that intra-observer measurement produces acceptable levels of error, there can be strong between-observer differences. This limitation could reduce the potential of the WHR as an alternative to waist alone.

Waist/height ratio

A more recent development in the use of WC as a measure of metabolic risk is its incorporation with height into the waist/height ratio (WHtR; Browning et al., 2010). One immediate advantage of this index over BMI is the lack of requirement to measure body weight, thus eliminating the need for scales and removing any sensitivity issues around collecting body weight data. The rationale underpinning the WHtR is that, for a given height, there is an acceptable degree of fat stored on the upper body and so WHtR acts a measure of abdominal fatness corrected for height. Ashwell and Gibson (2014) have proposed a boundary value of 0.500 to indicate whether the amount of abdominal fat accumulation is excessive and poses an increased risk for hypertension and coronary heart disease. The WHtR offers a number of additional advantages in that the boundary value appears to function independent of age, gender and ethnicity and can be incorporated into the simple public health message to 'keep your waist to less than half your height'.

Skinfold thickness

Skinfold thickness measurements using callipers have been a mainstay for predicting body fat levels in both clinical (individual) and public health (populations) practice. More recent technology, particularly BIA, has superseded skinfold measurements given its improved precision and predictive ability. Indeed, certain BIA instruments have practically eliminated both within- and between-observer error. As a result, skinfold measurement tends to be less routinely employed in contemporary public health nutrition practice. However, given the relative low cost of callipers, their portability and perceived ease of technique, they can still be favoured in some assessment contexts, such as in health clubs and for weight management programmes. However, practitioners need to be fully aware of the limitations of the technique and its poor validity. Also, training the measurer in the technique is essential.

Bioelectrical impedance analysis

BIA technology is finding a greater role in public health nutrition practice, such as in community weight management programmes. Unlike BMI, BIA provides an indication of body fat levels. BIA passes a small electrical current through the body and relies on the differential conductance/impedance properties of the fat and fat-free tissues. Algorithms based on age, gender, height, weight and impedance are employed to predict total body water, and hence FFM. Body fat can be obtained by subtracting FFM from body weight.

In the same way as for skinfold thickness measurement, BIA is a predictive technique, but current BIA technology has superior precision, coupled with an acceptable degree of accuracy. Additionally, it meets many of the requirements of a suitable assessment tool, in that it is relatively inexpensive and quick to perform (compared with laboratory techniques), is portable, non-invasive and safe.

Body fat ranges have been established with cut-offs to define underfat, normal, overfat and obese. Thus, BIA should allow better population monitoring compared with BMI as misclassification of individuals is substantially reduced. Furthermore, most BIA systems now provide an indication of skeletal muscle mass, which in the near future may offer potential for surveillance of sarcopenia (a loss or deficit of skeletal muscle mass, strength and function) in the ageing population.

Self-assessment of height, weight and waist

In certain large-scale surveys, the complexity of the study as well as constraints on resources may require participants to self-report body measurements. While instructions and tools such as a waist tape can be made available, considerable bias and error can be introduced, thus making the anthropometric measures invalid. Error can be

random, but also result from overestimation of height and underestimation of weight, resulting in a BMI outcome closer to healthy range from overweight individuals.

4.3 Assessment in children and adolescents: references, norms and percentile charts

The measurement tools and their techniques described herein are as equally applicable to assessing nutritional status in children and adolescents as they are in the adult population. Height measurement is probably more important in this age group as it is an essential marker of growth. Equally, it is important that weight status is assessed in younger people due to the recent rapid increase in the prevalence of overweight and obesity in this age group. However, a critical difference exists for children and adolescents when using and interpreting these assessment tools since unlike in adults, fixed cut-offs cannot be used. This is because all anthropometric measures are highly age dependent due to the process of growth across infancy, childhood and adolescence. Measures are also usually gender dependent. Thus, most often, measurements are interpreted through the use of percentile charts – a series of curves that graphically represent the distribution of the variable of interest in a reference population against age and which are specific for each sex (Cole, 2012). Percentile curves are usually derived from a normally distributed variable; however, modern statistical tools used to construct these charts are able to handle variables that are not normally distributed. Percentile charts are used with most anthropometric variables of interest, including height, weight, BMI, WC and body fat. An individual percentile indicates a child's position relative to a reference population (for age and gender), with the percentile representing the percentage of children below this value for age and sex. The 50th percentile represents the median value, whereas the 98th percentile, for example, represents the top 2% of the population distribution, and the second percentile representing the bottom 2%. Cut-offs to define, for example, underweight, healthy weight, overweight and obese are statistical in nature rather than being linked directly to morbidity. Practitioners should note that percentile charts are population references rather than standards – the latter term suggesting some ideal or desirable distribution. Percentile charts are mostly used in a clinical environment with individual children, whereas for population-based surveys a standard deviation score (SDS) is more often calculated. An SDS represents by how many standard deviations an observation or data point lies either above (positive SDS) or below (negative SDS) the median. Thus, an SDS of +1.0 or −1.0 respectively equals one

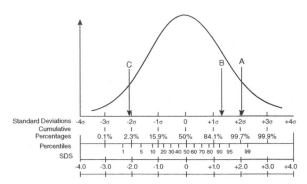

Cut-offs are used to define borders between categories. Using BMI as an example, the arrow at point A identifies a SDS = +2.05, which equates to the 98th percentile – the clinical cut-off to define obesity. The arrow point at B identifies a SDS = +1.34, the 91st centile and the clinical cut-off to define overweight. At point C lies the cut-off to define underweight set at the 2nd percentile or a SDS = -2.05

Figure 4.1 Relationship between percentiles and standard deviation scores (SDS) in a normally distributed variable.

standard deviation above or below the median, and each SDS is equivalent to a percentile on a chart. An SDS equal to zero represents the median value. The relationship between percentiles and SDSs for a normally distributed variable is represented in Figure 4.1.

Specific cut-offs on percentile charts to designate a certain anthropometric condition vary between sources of the charts and their purpose. Using BMI as an example, US CDC charts employ the 85th and 95th percentiles to represent overweight and obese respectively. Equivalent BMI cut-offs on UK charts use the 85th and 95th percentiles for epidemiological purposes and the 91st and 98th percentiles for clinical referral. In recognition that these statistically based cut-offs do not relate either to morbidity or adult BMI cut-offs, an additional set of curves has been generated known as the International Obesity Task Force cut-offs (Cole et al., 2000). These curves have been derived from selected multi-ethnic international populations and relate to the percentiles which at age 18 years pass through the adult BMI cut-offs of 25 (overweight) and 30 (obesity). Despite the clear advantage these percentile curves offer, there is an assumption that adult weight and final height are achieved by age 18 years. Although in boys the mean age of adult height attainment is around 18 years, this can vary by up to 3 years in either direction. In addition, adult height is on average achieved in girls some 2 years earlier than in boys.

Despite having a high specificity (i.e. identifying only a few non-overweight children as being overweight), the use of BMI suffers from poor sensitivity – that is, it fails to correctly identify relatively large numbers of children with excess body fat. This sensitivity–specificity trade-off is largely a function of the choice of cut-offs, and so in public health situations BMI can underestimate the prevalence of overweight and obesity through the creation of false negatives. Given the high prevalence of overweight and obesity in the paediatric population worldwide, these limitations of BMI have led to calls for improved assessment tools for both epidemiological and surveillance purposes. WC percentile charts have been developed for several paediatric populations around the world, and these go some way to addressing these calls despite their use not yet being fully endorsed by national health governing bodies. WC is related to several components of the MS in children and adolescents, including an adverse atherogenic lipoprotein profile, adverse insulin concentration, higher blood pressure and non-alcoholic fatty liver (IDF, 2007). WC levels in children and adolescents have increased at a greater rate than BMI over the past 20 years, indicating that abdominal adiposity has increased greater than general adiposity has. Given the strong link between WC and morbidity, greater attention needs to be paid to this measure.

Newer percentile charts: body fat and muscle mass

As for adults, BIA technology has provided the opportunity to characterise and quantify specific body components linked to morbidity in children and adolescents, and reference norms for body fat and skeletal muscle mass are now available (McCarthy, 2014). The body fat percentile charts reveal gender differences in fat patterning that are obscured by BMI. Cut-offs to define underfat, healthy, overfat and obesity have been selected and these references allow practitioners to track body fatness in individuals and groups. They could identify for example, those children who have high fat mass and low skeletal muscle mass but a BMI within the healthy range and potentially signal the early origins of sarcopenic obesity. Additionally, a low skeletal muscle mass is linked to poor glucose disposal and reduced insulin sensitivity. A clear advantage of these charts over BMI equivalents is the reduction in misclassification of children.

4.4 Conclusions

Measures of growth, weight status and risk for metabolic disease are important components of public health nutrition surveys and interventions. For each particular study, practitioners must select appropriate assessment methods that meet their objectives as well as considering the study population, including age group and ethnicity. The validity of the assessment method must be considered, and adequate training of the data collection team in measurement techniques is essential. Sufficient consideration of the limitations of self-measurement and reporting of height and weight must be taken if the study necessitates this approach to data collection.

Practitioners need to be aware of the limitations associated with using BMI as the method to assess overweight and obesity, especially when used with children and adolescents and in populations with different ethnic groups. An understanding of population references and percentile curves is required when conducting studies in children and adolescents. If newer technologies such as BIA are to be employed, then the cost, strengths and limitations in comparison with the more established methods must be considered. Newer technologies in assessment can offer the opportunity to distinguish between fat and fat-free components of body weight and BMI that can be collected with little additional burden to the participant.

References

Ashwell, M. and Gibson, S. (2014) A proposal for a primary screening tool: 'keep your waist circumference to less than half your height'. *BMC Medicine*, **12**, 207.

Browning, L.M., Hsieh, S.D. and Ashwell, M. (2010) A systematic review of waist-to-height ratio as a screening tool for the prediction of cardiovascular disease and diabetes: 0.5 could be a suitable global boundary value. *Nutrition Research Reviews*, **23**, 247–269.

Cole, T.J. (2012) The development of growth references and growth charts. *Annals of Human Biology*, **39**, 382–394.

Cole, T.J., Bellizzi, M.C., Flegal, K.M. and Dietz, W.H. (2000) Establishing a standard definition for child overweight and obesity worldwide: international survey. *BMJ*, **320**, 1240–1245.

IDF (2006) *The IDF Consensus Worldwide Definition of the Metabolic Syndrome*. International Diabetes Federation, Brussels. https://www.idf.org/webdata/docs/IDF_Meta_def_final.pdf (accessed 25 November 2016).

IDF (2007) *The IDF Consensus Definition of the Metabolic Syndrome in Children and Adolescents*. International Diabetes Federation, Brussels. http://www.idf.org/webdata/docs/Mets_definition_children.pdf (accessed 25 November 2016).

McCarthy HD. (2014) Measuring growth and obesity across childhood and adolescence. *The Proceedings of the Nutrition Society*, **73**, 210–217.

NHLBI Obesity Education Initiative Expert Panel (2000) *The Practical Guide: Identification, Evaluation, and Treatment of Overweight and Obesity in Adults*. NIH Publication Number 00–4084.

National Heart, Lung, and Blood Institute, Bethesda, MD. https://www.nhlbi.nih.gov/files/docs/guidelines/prctgd_c.pdf (accessed 4 January 2017).

Vague, J. (1947) La diffférenciacion sexuelle, facteur déterminant des formes de l'obésité. *La Presse Médicale*, **30**, 339–340.

5
Food Composition

Mark Roe, Jenny Plumb, U Ruth Charrondierre and Paul Finglas

Key messages

- Food composition data are essential for food-based nutrition and nutrition-sensitive agriculture. Studies into the relationship between intake of food components and diet and health, food safety and food security depend on the availability of high-quality food composition data.
- Food composition data are an important tool for researchers, nutritionists, dietitians, the food industry, health practitioners, policy makers and consumers.
- Food composition databases are intended to provide data for prioritised foods that are commonly consumed or are nutritionally important.

- Nutrient composition databases are produced in most countries and many are freely available online. Specialist datasets are available for bioactive compounds, contaminants and dietary supplements.
- There are many factors that lead to variation in the composition of foods, and composition of individual foods may differ from published values.
- There are limitations in the use of food composition data and these should be considered by users, particularly when using data to calculate nutrient intake.

5.1 Introduction

A knowledge of the chemical composition of foods is the first essential in the dietary treatment of disease or in any quantitative study of human nutrition (McCance and Widdowson, 1940).

This statement was originally published in 1940 as part of the first sentence in the introduction to a book that evolved into the McCance and Widdowson series of UK Food Composition publications. The statement is just as true today, and although it is often not obvious, food composition data underpin almost all research into the links between diet and health. Food composition data are therefore used by researchers, policy makers, the agri-food industry, dietitians, health practitioners and consumers.

Published food composition data can be traced back over 200 years to when Hofmann published data on the composition of mineral waters. Data on vegetable substances was published in book form by Johann John in 1814. Food composition tables (FCTs) in the format used today were not published until the latter part of the 19th century. The first European composition table was published in Germany by König in 1878, and the first North American tables (Atwater and Woods) followed in 1896. UK interest in food composition can be traced back to the First World War when the British War Office analysed common foods, with the results being published in 1921. In 1925, R.A. McCance was awarded a Medical Research Council grant to analyse carbohydrates in raw and cooked vegetables. Further analytical studies followed, and the results were combined into the first edition of what became *The Composition of Foods*. Since then, UK data have been published in a series of analytical reports, books and electronic data files, the most recent publication being the *McCance and Widdowson's The Composition of Foods, Seventh Summary Edition* (Finglas *et al.*, 2015a), and the *Composition of Foods Integrated Dataset* (Finglas *et al.*, 2015b).

Many countries produce their own national food composition datasets, and most of them are available online, searchable and free of charge. Most European datasets are updated regularly and available directly from the organisations that produce them and also through

Public Health Nutrition, Second Edition. Edited by Judith L Buttriss, Ailsa A Welch, John M Kearney and Susan A Lanham-New.
© 2018 by The Nutrition Society. Published 2018 by John Wiley & Sons, Ltd.
Companion website: www.wiley.com/go/buttriss/publichealth

the European Food Information Resource (EuroFIR). In developing countries, the picture is very different as many countries do not have a national FCT/food composition database (FCDB) or only an outdated one of inadequate quality according to international standards. Therefore, they very often use FCDBs from other countries, especially the United States Department of Agriculture (USDA) database as it is comprehensive and easily accessible. The International Network of Food Data Systems (INFOODS) was established in 1984 with the objective to improve the quality and availability of relevant food composition data worldwide. INFOODS also maintains an inventory of international food composition resources.

5.2 Uses of food composition data

Food composition data are used by a wide selection of individuals and organisations working at both national and international levels. The diversity of users means that there are differing requirements, depending on use, and it is challenging for data producers to provide information in a form that satisfies all users. Many users have to adapt published datasets and modify the data to suit their own requirements as the national or regional FCT/FCDB does not include all foods, recipes or components of interest, or has missing values and/or documentation. The publication of data in electronic form makes their use easier but has resulted in further challenges related to data quality, data exchange formats and documentation. All users require high-quality data on foods and recipes that are commonly consumed or are nutritionally important to specific populations. Information on an increasingly wide range of food components is also required, including nutrients, bioactive compounds, contaminants, toxicants and allergens. There is also an increasing need for data on food supplements that are consumed and can contribute dramatically to nutrient intake. Dietary supplements are traditionally not included in FCT/FCDB, but several countries have included supplements in separate databases that are used for national consumption surveys.

Dietary monitoring, food safety and food security assessment

Many national food composition datasets are produced and maintained to provide data for national dietary monitoring programmes. For example, the *UK Composition of Foods* data underpins Public Health England's

Nutrient Databank, which is linked to consumption survey data to produce results for the National Diet and Nutrition Survey. The Department for Environment Food and Rural Affairs Family Food Survey in the UK also uses food composition data to derive nutrient intakes from household food purchases. Similar food composition and consumption survey programmes are in place in other countries and are likely to be implemented in countries that do not yet have a national FCT/FCDB.

Variability in FCTs/FCDBs can lead to errors in estimation of nutrient intake that affect the assessment of intakes of proportions of the population experiencing nutrient inadequacy or who have intakes above toxic thresholds. Individuals may also be misclassified, leading to errors in correlations between nutrient intakes and diseases or nutritional interventions. Sources of variability between foods included in an FCT/FCDB and the foods actually consumed by individuals include natural variations (e.g. differences in plant varieties, growing conditions, post-harvest storage, animal species) and extrinsic variations due to differences in production and processing. Systematic errors may also occur; for example, where fortification or supplementation is not taken into account. FCTs/FCDBs contain values for the total amounts of nutrients in food and do not consider bioavailability, so calculations of intake based on composition data represent the maximum amount of a nutrient that is available to the body (Gibson, 2005).

Nutrition epidemiology and research

Epidemiological and other research studies are also dependent on food composition data that provide representative data for foods consumed by the populations being studied. Data are needed for all nutrients of interest but are unlikely to be available for all nutrients for all foods. The use of more standardised datasets and linking between data available in different datasets helps to improve the quantity of information available and aid development of modified datasets for specific users. In recent years datasets from European countries have been combined for use in pan-European studies (European Prospective Investigation into Cancer, European Food Safety Authority Food Composition Dataset). However, it is to be noted that data from other countries are very likely to be different from the composition of local foods, and use of such data can lead to random errors that result in misclassifications, leading to the underestimation of true correlations between nutrient intakes and diseases or nutritional interventions.

Industry

The agri-food industry uses food composition data and supporting information to develop new and modified products that will conform to nutrition policy; for example, reduction of salt, sugar, saturated and trans fatty acids in processed foods. The European Food Information Regulation (EU 1169/2011) made nutrient labelling mandatory from December 2016 and applies to all foods intended for the final consumer, including foods delivered by mass caterers, and foods intended for supply to mass caterers.

In the international arena, Codex Alimentarius recommends that nutrient labelling should be mandatory for protein, total fat, saturated fat, available carbohydrate, sugars, sodium and energy for all pre-packed foods. Codex Alimentarius also recommends that nutrient values should be provided for any other nutrient for which a nutrition or health claim is made and any other nutrient considered to be relevant for maintaining a good nutritional status, as required by national legislation or national dietary guidelines (e.g. trans fatty acids). In Europe, in addition to protein, total fat, saturated fat, available carbohydrate, sugars, salt and energy, nutrient values can also be declared for, monounsaturates, polyunsaturates, polyols, starch, dietary fibre and a defined range of minerals and vitamins. It is also compulsory to declare nutrient values for any substance on which a nutrition or health claim is made. Those values can derive from chemical analysis or from 'recognised' national food composition datasets. Nutritional information on food labels enables consumers to make informed choices based on nutrient composition of food products. In addition, retailers and manufacturers often make nutrient labelling information available on their web sites. Food composition is a very important marketing tool, and producers and manufacturers are very aware of changes in composition that may imply that a food product is more or less healthy. There is a trend in making more food composition data available on branded foods with complete nutrient profiles in FCTs/FCDBs. Branded foods represent an increasing proportion of food worldwide, so this would be a very important step forward in allowing improved nutrient estimations, providing that the quality of data can be maintained and datasets can be kept up to date. Data for branded foods are usually only available for those nutrients for which nutrition labelling is mandatory, and to provide information for other nutrients it is necessary to link branded foods to composition data for generic products. The large quantity of branded products available and the frequency of changes in products available to consumers makes the task of maintaining good quality data, for minerals and vitamins in particular, very challenging for national food composition data compilers. Composition data are currently usually available either as generic datasets of nationally representative foods with comprehensive nutrient coverage or as distinct datasets of branded foods with limited nutrient coverage.

Agricultural practice can also be influenced by nutrition policy, and it is important that food composition data adequately reflect biodiversity of plant-based foods and reflect trends in production of crops that have been bred to have higher amounts of micronutrients; for example, cereal crops with enhanced content of iron, zinc or vitamin A.

Health practitioners and policy makers

Results from national monitoring surveys and research studies inform nutrition policy at national and international levels. Food industry and health practitioners (dietitians, nutritionists, doctors) will respond to policy changes. National FCTs/FCDBs should include not only commonly consumed foods but also those of high micronutrient content, and those consumed by specific population groups to be able to tailor advice to their tradition, culture, preference and health conditions. Food composition data must reflect changes by industry to enable health practitioners to base decisions and advice on good quality and up-to-date information.

Consumers

Consumers may use food composition data directly but are more likely to use information that is presented in modified forms. Consumer interest in food composition and nutrition will require composition data to be made available in more easily accessible forms. Many software applications already include food composition data and can be delivered using web-based mobile applications. Increasing consumer interest in diet and health has encouraged the development of many such software applications that rely on food composition data to help consumers monitor their nutrient intake against either recommended or personal target intakes. Some software is aimed at particular consumer groups (e.g. school children) where education in food composition and healthy diets is an important feature. Developers of these applications should inform users on the underlying sources of food composition data so that users can select the application that most likely reflects their foods consumed.

5.3 Food and component coverage and description

Most users would like FCTs/FCDBs to be 'comprehensive'; however, the range of foods and components, and the continual changes in products that may be consumed, means that the development and maintenance of a truly comprehensive database is not possible. The costs of food analysis are high, and human resources are needed to compile, manage and maintain FCTs/FCDBs. The investment in food composition programmes is proportional to the coverage of foods and nutrients and their quality and relevance. The high demands on comprehensive and high-quality food composition data are not met by almost all existing FCTs/FCDBs as national and international investments in these fundamental data are usually insufficient. This means that often only values for commonly consumed foods are included for a limited selection of nutrients.

Foods are usually prioritised based on national consumption statistics, consumption in specific population subgroups (e.g. infants, elderly, ethnic) and on changes in food production and processing. The concept of key foods (Haytowitz et al., 1996) has been developed in the USA (i.e. those foods that together contribute approximately 80% of the population intake of a nutrient); these can be used as a basis to identify the foods that are most important in population diets. Some key foods may only be key contributors to one or two nutrients, but a significant number may be key contributors to intake of 10 or more nutrients. An alternative approach is to base the choice of foods on consumption data and make subjective assessments of a food's importance. Ideally, a wide range of users, including researchers, government departments and industry, should be consulted to ensure that priorities meet the demands of users.

More data from samples collected to reflect population consumption and analysed using standard analytical methods in accredited laboratories need to be generated, compiled and disseminated in comprehensive databases, especially in developing countries, to allow all stakeholders to make well-informed decisions.

In addition to national FCTs of generic foods, data for branded food products are also widely available. European Union labelling regulations require that nutrient content of energy, fat, saturated fat, carbohydrate, sugars, protein and salt must be provided on labels of pre-packaged foods with the option of providing data for some additional nutrients (e.g. fibre, minerals, vitamins – see 'Industry' in Section 5.2). This information is also usually available from manufacturer and retailer web sites as well as a range of web-based applications targeted at consumers.

Food composition databases should be continually revised to provide data for new foods and for foods where composition has changed. In practice, most FCTs/FCDBs are revised based on foods that are identified as priorities. Priorities may be based on food type (e.g. surveys of eggs, meat, fish, fruit or vegetables), or in some cases based on nutrients that are expected to have changed – for example, as was the case with the 2012 UK survey of processed foods that may have contained trans fatty acids from partially hydrogenated fats.

The differing needs of users, requires that compositional data should be provided for raw foods, processed foods and for foods as prepared for consumption. The different states of foods included means that careful consideration should be given to the description of each food, particularly where differences impact on nutrient composition: for example, vegetables, raw or cooked; vegetables boiled with or without added salt; fruit canned in juice or syrup; fish canned in brine or oil. Publication of data in book or table form allows for additional descriptive text to be added to distinguish between foods where necessary, but the move to electronic datasets and database searching means that this additional information may not always be available alongside the food name.

Faceted systems have been developed to describe foods and to distinguish between different foods that may not be fully described by the food name alone: for example, to describe the plant or animal source of a food in more detail; specify parts analysed and/or inedible waste; describe food processing such as cooking method, preservation method or addition of ingredients. These systems also aid the comparison of data between different datasets, particularly those from different countries or those that were intended for a different purpose. The LanguaL™ (Langua alimentaria) system was developed by the US Food and Drug Administration in the 1970s and has been modified and adopted for use in European countries as part of the EuroFIR initiative to better standardise approaches for food description used for foods in national FCDBs in European countries. The European Food Safety Authority (EFSA) has also developed a similar system of facet descriptors for use with the FoodEx2 food list that is used as the basis for dietary intake, exposure and risk assessments. See Table 5.1.

Wherever possible, food composition data sources should describe foods as unambiguously as possible, and faceted description systems are useful tools for that purpose. It is not essential that the same systems have been used, but the system used should be mapped to other systems to allow data to be exchanged between users.

Table 5.1 Characteristics used for identification of foods.

Characteristic	LanguaL facet	FoodEx facet
Common name	Original food name/English food name	Food hierarchy
Food classification	Product type	Food hierarchy
Scientific name: genus, species, variety	Food source	Source
		Raw source of derivative
Kind/type (e.g. animal or plant source)	Food source	Source
Part (e.g. seed, stem, leg, wing)	Part of plant or animal	Part nature (e.g. part of plant or animal)
	Adjunct characteristics of food e.g. (cut of meat, colour of flesh, plant maturity)	Part consumed/analysed
Portion analysed (e.g. with/without peel/skin, fat/lean)	Part of plant or animal	Part consumed/analysed
	Adjunct characteristics of food (e.g. extent of fat trim, drained or not drained, presence of rind or crust)	
Origin (country, region)	Geographic places and regions	None
Processing technique	Extent of heat treatment	Dough mass
	Treatment applied	Process technology
		Treatment modifying structure (e.g. milling, fermentation, curing, drying, dilution)
Preparation technique	Cooking method	Cooking method
		Final preparation
		Extent of cooking
Special descriptors (e.g. low fat, salt, sugar)	Consumer group/dietary use/label claim	Fat content
		Sweetening agent
		Qualitative information
Physical state, shape, size, form, temperature	Physical state, shape or form	Physical state
Ingredient added	Treatment applied	Ingredients
		Sweetening agent
		Fortification agent
Packaging medium (e.g. brine, oil, juice, syrup)	Packing medium	Surrounding medium (e.g. brine, oil, juice, syrup)
	Adjunct characteristics of food (e.g. drained, not drained)	
Preservation method	Preservation method	Preservation technique
Packaging	Container or wrapping	Packaging format

Source: adapted from Greenfield and Southgate (2003).

5.4 Components

Food composition databases should aim to include values for all nutrients and non-nutrient food components that are known or believed to be important for human health. As with food coverage, it is rarely possible to achieve ideal nutrient coverage within a single dataset. Analysis of some food components, particularly vitamins and bioactive components, is specialised and consequently expensive. Since resources are usually limited, many datasets concentrate on components that have been selected as priorities and are more selective in providing data for additional components; for example, information on water, protein, fats, carbohydrates and energy are core to all nutrient datasets and some minerals and vitamins are likely to be included based on nutritional requirements for health (e.g. iron and vitamin A).

Priorities are often set at a national or regional level and depend primarily on known diet-related health problems and on current concerns in nutritional and toxicological sciences. The availability of alternative sources of data could be taken into account, where the data can reasonably be applied to the population of interest, particularly in databases that are developing with limited resources. The existence of legislation related to food information also has an impact on data available for specific nutrients because food will be routinely analysed where data provision is required by law. Researchers are often the users most interested in components where nutritional and health interest is more recent and data are more limited and may need to produce modified datasets with data obtained from additional sources (e.g. scientific literature).

Correct identification of components (e.g. dietary fibre or vitamins that are composed of different vitamers) is essential but not always straightforward. Both INFOODS and EuroFIR have systems for component identification but take different approaches. Analytical method can be critical to correct component identification, and the method used is included within component identifiers used by INFOODS. The EuroFIR system does not take into account different analytical methods in the component identifier but captures method information separately so that data for components analysed using different methods may be combined more easily. Some food components are calculated from contributing components, either with or without the use of conversion factors. Examples are protein, which is not analysed directly but is calculated from total nitrogen, using conversion factors, and energy, which is calculated from food components that contribute to energy, including protein, fat, carbohydrate, fibre, alcohol, polyols, organic acids and short- and long-chain acyl triglyceride molecules (salatrims – additives used as a fat substitute in reduced-calorie foods).

Nutrients

The extent of the coverage of nutrient components in FCTs/FCDBs varies between countries. The number of components included in European databases varies from about 30 to around 300, although the coverage for components (i.e. the percentage of all food items for which a value is given) varies considerably between databases. It should however be noted that low coverage does not necessarily mean a large number of missing values, because some components do not naturally occur in all food groups. EuroFIR defined a range of 42 prioritised nutrients based on coverage in EC directives and nutrition recommendations, and those components would be expected to form the basis of most FCTs/ FCDBs. Table 5.2 lists the nutrients included in the *UK Composition of Foods* dataset.

The *UK Composition of Foods* series of publications and analytical laboratory reports associated with the series have also published data, for a limited range of foods, for other nutrients, including: 'Southgate' dietary fibre, cellulose, lignin, resistant starch, phytic acid, sulphur, choline, vitamin K_2 (menaquinone) and amino acids.

FCDBs from other countries generally contain data for a similar range of components, although, as in the UK, data for some inorganic components, some vitamins, phytosterols and organic acids may be limited to key foods only.

Bioactive compounds

Bioactive compounds are essential and non-essential compounds that occur in nature and have an impact on health. Some essential bioactive compounds are commonly included in FCTs (e.g. vitamins, oligosaccharides,

phytosterols), but most are not included and data are available either in specialist datasets or from scientific literature. There is a growing interest in bioactive compounds and an increasing body of scientific literature investigating their impact on human health. Since bioactive compounds are found in plant-based foods, the association between intake of fruit and vegetables and prevalence or risk of chronic disease is a common focus of research. Table 5.3 shows examples of classes of bioactive compounds and their plant sources.

There are several online databases of bioactives available, including the USDA Database for the Flavonoid Content of Foods Release 3.2, eBASIS and Phenol-Explorer. Each of these databases contains different examples of bioactive classes, and all use quality systems to extract data from peer-reviewed scientific publications.

The EuroFIR eBASIS database (Bioactive Substances in Food Information System) is a collation of data relating to bioactive compounds in plant-based foods. The database is divided into two principal sections: composition data and bioeffects data. eBASIS consists of a user-friendly interface for searching, extracting and exporting the data, including the references. The entire database includes data from over 1100 peer-reviewed publications, forming 39 000 data points, covering 750 compounds in over 250 food plants, with the data linked to authoritative plant and plant-part lists. eBASIS also includes the LanguaL food description system to aid clear description of the plant foods included. The data are extracted from critically evaluated scientific publications, and the database contains only data that meet quality requirements for factors including identification of plant, sample treatment and analytical method.

The Phenol-Explorer database is a comprehensive phenols database and contains more than 35 000 content values for 500 different polyphenols in over 400 foods. These data are derived from the systematic collection of more than 60 000 original content values found in more than 1300 scientific publications. Each of these publications has been critically evaluated before inclusion in the database. The Phenol-Explorer database also contains information on polyphenol metabolism and on the effects of processing and cooking. Values are given as weighted mean content values and standard deviations which take into account the different number of samples used to generate original data collected from the publications.

Contaminants

The main focus of food composition has traditionally been on components that are beneficial to health, but foods can also contain contaminant substances that are not intended to be present. Sources of contamination include environmental (e.g. soil, water, atmosphere),

Table 5.2 Nutrients included in the *UK Composition of Foods* dataset.

Proximates

Water
Total nitrogen
Protein (calculated from total nitrogen)
Alcohol
Energy (calculated[a])

Fats

Fat, total
Saturated fatty acids, total
Monounsaturated fatty acids, total
Polyunsaturated fatty acids, total
Trans fatty acids, total
Individual fatty acid isomers[b]
Cholesterol

Carbohydrates

Carbohydrate, available (glycaemic), total[c]
Starch
Sugars, total
Sugars: glucose, galactose, fructose, maltose, lactose
Oligosaccharides
Dietary fibre: non-starch polysaccharides, AOAC

Inorganics

Sodium, potassium, calcium, magnesium, phosphorus, iron, zinc, copper, chloride, manganese, selenium, iodine

Vitamins, fat soluble

Retinol (*all-trans*-retinol, 13-*cis*-retinol, retinaldehyde)
Carotene, beta carotene equivalents (α-carotene, β-carotene, cryptoxanthins)
Lutein[b]
Lycopene[b]
Vitamin D (cholecalciferol, 25-hydroxyvitamin D_3)
Vitamin E, α-tocopherol equivalents (tocopherols and tocotrienols)
Vitamin K_1

Vitamins, water soluble

Thiamin
Riboflavin
Niacin
Tryptophan
Vitamin B_6
Vitamin B_{12}
Folate, total
Pantothenate
Biotin
Vitamin C

Phytosterols[b]

Phytosterols, total
Phytosterol
β-Sitosterol
Brassicasterol
Campesterol
δ-5-Avenasterol
δ-7-Avenasterol
δ-7-Stigmasterol
Stigmasterol

Organic acids[b]

Citric acid
Malic acid

[a] Calculated from protein, fat, carbohydrates and alcohol.
[b] For a limited selection of foods only.
[c] Sum of total sugars, oligosaccharides and complex carbohydrates (dextrins, starch and glycogen).

Table 5.3 Examples of bioactive compound classes, common compounds and their plant sources.

Compound class and examples of compounds	Common plant sources
Glucosinolates: glucoraphanin, progoitrin, sinigrin, glucotropaeolin, gluconasturtiin	Broccoli, cabbages (white cabbage, Chinese cabbage), Brussels sprouts, watercress, horseradish, capers and radishes
Capsaicinoids: capsaicin, dihydrocapsaicin, nordihydrocapsaicin, nonivamide	Peppers, chilli peppers
Lignans: secoisolariciresinol, lariciresinol, pinoresinol, medioresinol, syringaresinol, matairesinol	Lignans are widely distributed in the plant kingdom. Grains: wheat, barley and oats; legumes: beans, lentils and soybeans; and vegetables: garlic, asparagus, broccoli and carrots
Phytosterols: sitosterol, stigmasterol, campesterol	Cereal grains, cereal-based products, nuts and seeds
Flavonoids	
Anthocyanidins: cyanidin, delphinidin, malvidin, pelargonidin, peonidin, petunidin	Blueberries, red wine, strawberries
Flavonols: isorhamnetin, kaempferol, myricetin, quercetin	Blueberries, garlic and onions, kale, broccoli, spinach, tea, red wine, cherry tomatoes
Flavones: apigenin, luteolin	Celery, garlic, green peppers, peppermint, parsley family
Isoflavones: daidzein, genistein, glycitein, formononetin, biochanin A	Soy products, peanuts, beans, legumes
Flavanones: eriodictyol, hesperetin, naringenin	Citrus fruits and juices, peppermint
Flavan-3-ols: epicatechin, epicatechin 3-gallate, epigallocatechin, epigallocatechin gallate, catechin, gallocatechin	Apples, apricots, peaches, pears, strawberries, black and green teas, blueberries, cranberries, chocolate, grapes and red wine
Proanthocyanidins: monomers, dimers, trimers, 4–6 mers, 7–10 mers, polymers	Apples, apricots, peaches, pears, strawberries, black tea, blueberries, cranberries, chocolate, peanuts, grapes, red wine, pecans and walnuts

production processes and packaging or storage. Contamination is associated with potential health risks depending on exposure levels, and many countries therefore monitor the food chain for substances of concern and apply policies to limit exposure. The EU has established maximum intake levels for contaminants, including mycotoxins, metals (cadmium, lead, mercury, inorganic tin), dioxins, polychlorinated biphenyls and polycyclic aromatic hydrocarbons.

EFSA is mandated to collect all available data from member states on the occurrence of chemical contaminants in food and feed. Data are submitted from national authorities, research institutions, academic organisations and other stakeholders and used in EFSA scientific opinions and reports that are publicly available. This data, along with data from other countries, can be submitted to the World Health Organisation's Global Environment Monitoring System – Food Contamination and Assessment Programme (GEMS Food). The GEMS Food database was established in 1976 and is available online as a searchable database that includes more than 400 000 analytical results on the occurrence of about 300 chemicals in food, as well as individual food consumption data from more than 40 countries and regions.

Food/dietary supplements

Food supplements are significant sources of some nutrients and bioactive components for a growing proportion of the population in developed countries, and it is therefore important to consider their impact in any dietary survey. Many national organisations that monitor diet collect information on supplements and their ingredients but these data are not often publicly available. The USDA Nutrient Data Laboratory publishes the Dietary Supplement Ingredient Database, which contains data from analysis of representative samples of multivitamin/mineral and omega-3 fatty acid supplements. The samples analysed are prioritised, based on intake prevalence data identified from the National Health and Nutrition Examination Survey in the USA. The US National Institutes of Health's Dietary Supplement Label Database is also available online and contains information from a wide range of dietary supplement products marketed in the USA. Food Standards Australia New Zealand also publishes a database for supplements, containing nutrient values from product information for over 2000 supplements recorded during 2011–2013 Australian Health Surveys. Data for European supplements are collected by some European countries, but published data are limited. Supplement data from eight countries was provided to EFSA for use in the EFSA food composition database for nutrient intake used for European dietary monitoring (Roe *et al.*, 2013). The ePlantLIBRA database (Plumb *et al.*, 2016) also contains information about plant and plant food supplements, specifically bioactive compounds, in botanicals and herbal extracts with putative health benefits and adverse effects.

5.5 Sources of data and data quality

Food composition data can be derived from a variety of sources, and most food composition datasets contain values produced in a range of different ways. Data quality is associated with a variety of factors (including food description, component identification, sample collection, sample handling, analytical method and laboratory performance) related to derivation of values, but national food composition datasets are compiled by experts and all published values are judged to be reasonable estimations of the nutrient composition of foods. There have been many collaborative projects and networks of food composition data compilers that have aimed to improve consistency and harmonisation of composition databases, so that values from different datasets are of comparable quality. In Europe, a quality framework for use with food composition data has been developed by the EU-funded network EuroFIR and tested with food database compiler organisations in Europe (Castanheira et al., 2009), and this system generally gives a reasonable estimate of data quality that is compatible with other systems; for example, the system used by the USDA (Holden et al., 2002). In addition, EuroFIR has produced a range of tools to help data compilers, including procedures for documenting data values, and has supported the development and publication of a European standard for food data (EN 16104:2012, Food data – structure and interchange format) and also provides a range of training opportunities (http://www.eurofir.org). INFOODS also produces guidelines for data compilation, online resources and coordinates training activities (http://www.fao.org/infoods/infoods/en/).

Sources of food composition data are:

- **Analytical values derived by direct analysis** Direct analysis of food samples is the preferred data source, but the process of sample collection and analysis is expensive and few data compilers have the resources to analyse all foods for all nutrients. Ideally, a range of representative samples are collected and analysed individually so that descriptive statistics (e.g. mean, range, standard deviation) can be produced, but the cost is often prohibitive and therefore samples may be pooled into a composite sample with only a single value being published. The composite sample approach (where a single sample for analysis is produced from a number of subsamples that represent typical consumer intake of a food) means that analytical data can be provided for a larger range of foods and nutrients, and this is considered by many data compilers to be preferable to publishing more values for the same type of food. In some situations, analysis may be carried out specifically for the purpose of compiling a database, but carefully evaluated analytical data from other types of survey and from other sources (e.g. scientific literature, manufacturer's data) can also be used.
- **Imputed values** Original analytical data may be used as the basis for calculation of values for a similar food or a different form of the same food (e.g. values for foods that are cooked may be calculated from raw values based on known dry matter content). Some nutrients may be calculated from other nutrients that have been analysed (e.g. chloride calculated from sodium) or calculated from a combination of nutrients (e.g. moisture calculated by difference).
- **Calculated values** Values for many foods are calculated from recipes, based on the nutrient content of ingredients and on weight loss or gain during cooking. Values for heat-labile vitamins are usually corrected for losses that are likely to occur during cooking. The recipes used for calculation are usually representative of recipes that would be commonly used in the home or are based on traditional recipes. In practice, the amounts and types of ingredients used and the preparation procedures employed are likely to be very variable, so these calculated values may not always compare well with the composition of foods prepared by individual consumers.
- **Borrowed values** Food composition database compilers are not able to produce data for all foods consumed, so values for some foods or nutrients may be taken from another country's food composition tables. In this case the values should be referenced back to their original source wherever possible. In some cases, the original values may be modified to match the known water or fat content of the food they are intended to represent.

To enable users to evaluate the data they are using and to allow further investigation of the data sources, it is important that published values should be traceable to their original source wherever possible. Datasets should at least provide a reference to value sources so that more information can be retrieved by users (e.g. on sampling or analytical method) if needed. Most European databases provide additional documentation of their values, much of which can be found in national datasets published online or through EuroFIR. The 2015 updates of UK composition data include main data sources and the year of sampling and/or analysis for each food. Many of the analytical reports referred to can be accessed online from either government archives or from the Institute of Food Research Food Databanks National Capability (http://fooddatabanks.ifr.ac.uk/). Approximately 70% of the data in the 2015 UK food composition dataset is derived from direct analysis (including imputed values), with approximately 21% calculated from recipes and the remainder from literature (mainly other food composition databases) or other sources.

5.6 Biodiversity

In recent decades there has been a worldwide trend in dietary simplification, with possible negative impacts on food security, nutrition and health. The range of plant varieties cultivated has reduced significantly. For example, in most Asian countries, the number of rice varieties being grown has dropped from thousands to just a few dozen, and diets rely on a limited number of energy-rich foods. Biodiversity in nutrition is increasingly important to encourage promotion of a diverse and sustainable diet that includes different foods and different species of plants and animals. In some cases the variation in nutrient content within species can be as high as the variation between species, and those differences can potentially make the difference between nutritional adequacy and inadequacy; for example, the protein content of rice varieties range between 5–14 g/100 g and the carotenoid content of sweet potatoes can differ by a factor of 200 or more. Crops that are currently underutilised may be important nutritional alternatives to mainstream crops, and there is growing evidence that food-based approaches to nutrition can be useful alternatives to fortification or supplementation.

Nutrient composition can differ enormously between different varieties/cultivars/breeds of the same species, and the availability of food composition data reflecting those differences is needed to underpin the link between biodiversity and nutrition. Food composition databases, particularly in developed countries, often do not include data that reflect the biodiversity of foods because they are usually based on foods that are commonly consumed and are the most widely available commercial varieties. Data for less commonly consumed varieties and species are available in the scientific literature and also in specialist databases such as the Food Composition Database for Biodiversity compiled by FAO/INFOODS (http://www.fao.org/infoods/infoods/en/).

5.7 Limitations of food composition data and their use

There are two schools of thought about food tables. One tends to regard the figures in them as having the accuracy of atomic weight 'determinations'; the other dismisses them as valueless on the ground that a foodstuff may be so modified by the soil, the season or its rate of growth that no figure can be a reliable guide to its composition. The truth, of course, lies somewhere between these two points of view (Widdowson and McCance, 1943).

The variability of nutrients in foods means that the reported composition of a food is unlikely to be precisely the same as any particular food item. The reported values should therefore be considered as estimates. Unprocessed foods such as cereals, dairy products, eggs, meat, fish, fruits and vegetables are subject to natural variations, including plant variety, country of origin, growing conditions, season, plant/animal feed, plant/animal maturity and storage. In general, nutrients that are closely related to structure and metabolic function show less variation than nutrients that accumulate in particular parts of plants or animals; for example, nitrogen and phosphorus tend to be less variable than iron, vitamin A or vitamin C. Water content can also be important in plant foods where water is the main component. Processed foods are subject to further differences in composition that can result from processing changes introduced by manufacturers (processing techniques, use of different types or amounts of ingredients), caterers or in-home preparation.

Food composition data should be updated on a regular basis to ensure that published values are a reasonable estimation of the foods they are intended to represent. Public health initiatives in many countries have led to reductions in the amounts of total fat, saturated fat, trans fatty acids, sugar and salt in food. These changes have necessitated the update of many processed food items and the 2015 *UK Composition of Foods* dataset produced new values or reviewed and validated existing data for all processed foods. Maintenance of food composition databases is a constant challenge, and it is inevitable that a proportion of published values will not be up to date.

There are some potential issues and challenges that users of food composition datasets should be aware of:

- Missing values should not be treated as zero. Major nutrients are usually reported for most foods, but values are not always included for some nutrients, particularly inorganics (e.g. chloride, manganese, iodine), vitamins (e.g. biotin, pantothenate, vitamin D, vitamin E), individual sugars and individual fatty acids. Treating missing values as zero can lead to underestimation of nutrient intake.
- Food names and descriptions should be carefully checked to ensure that data for the correct types of foods are used; for example, raw/cooked, full fat/reduced fat, with or without skin, peel, pips.
- Values for generic foods may be different to values for specific branded products.
- Bioavailability of nutrients is not usually considered in food composition data, so composition values generally represent the maximum amount of a nutrient that is available to the body. There are many factors that can influence nutrient bioavailability, both dietary and physiological, and factors that estimate the proportion

of a nutrient that is likely to be absorbed should be used if bioavailability is to be taken into account.

- Comparison between values for similar foods from different datasets or between values published at different times should carefully consider the following points:
  ○ samples analysed will be different;
  ○ foods analysed may not be the same, even if food names are identical or very similar;
  ○ analytical methods may be different;
  ○ units or conversion factors used in calculations may be different.
- Estimations of nutrient intake rely on the combination of food composition data and on estimates of food intake. The accuracy of intake estimations is affected by limitations in the dietary assessment methods used, including measurement of quantities of foods consumed (see Chapter 4).

References

Castanheira, I., Roe, M., Westenbrink, S. *et al.* (2009) Establishing quality management systems for European food composition databases. *Food Chemistry*, 113(3): 776–780.

Finglas, P.M., Roe, M.A., Pinchen, H.M. *et al.* (2015a) *McCance and Widdowson's The Composition of Foods, Seventh Summary Edition*. Royal Society of Chemistry, Cambridge.

Finglas, P.M., Roe, M.A., Pinchen, H.M. *et al.* (2015b) *McCance and Widdowson's The Composition of Foods Integrated Dataset.* https://www.gov.uk/government/publications/composition-of-foods-integrated-dataset-cofid (accessed 25 November 2016).

Gibson, R.S. (2005) *Principles of Nutritional Assessment*, 2nd edn. Oxford University Press, New York.

Greenfield, H. and Southgate, D.A.T. (2003) *Food Composition Data: Production, Management and Use*, 2nd edn. Elsevier, London.

Haytowitz, D.B., Pehrsson, P.R., Smith, J. *et al.* (1996) Key foods: setting priorities for nutrient analysis. *Journal of Food Composition and Analysis*, 9(4), 331–364.

Holden, J.M., Bhagwat, S.A., Patterson, K.Y. (2002) Development of a multi-nutrient data quality evaluation system. *Journal of Food Composition and Analysis*, 15, 339–348.

McCance, R.A. and Widdowson, E.M. (1940) *The Chemical Composition of Foods*. His Majesty's Stationery Office, London.

Plumb, J., Lyons, J., Nørby, K. *et al.* (2016) ePlantLIBRA: a composition and biological activity database for bioactive compounds in plant food supplements. *Food Chemistry*, 193, 121–127.

Roe, M.A., Bell, S., Oseredczuk, M. *et al.* (2013) Updated food composition database for nutrient intake. *EFSA Supporting Publication* 2013 10(6), EN-355.

Widdowson, E.M. and McCance, R.M. (1943) Food tables. Their scope and limitations. *Lancet*, 241, 230–232.

6
Dietary Reference Values

Peter J Aggett

Key messages

- Dietary reference values (DRVs) are a set of values providing an upper, a median or average, and a lower value for nutrient intakes against which population food supplies and intake may be gauged.
- DRVs are public health tools. They relate to nutrients and not to diets, but they can be used to plan diets and food programmes.
- DRVs, individually and as a set, are risk markers. They are not diagnostic thresholds of deficiency or excess either for individuals or populations.
- DRVs are not recommendations.
- DRVs are precautionary and overestimate requirements.
- DRVs are derived from an incomplete database that is especially weak at intake levels relevant to using markers of incipient deficiency and toxicity to establish their values.

- DRVs should only be used for individual or therapeutic purposes if this done in the overall context of the intended application.
- DRVs inform the construction and monitoring of dietary standards and guidelines by national and international agencies.
- DRVs and their use will probably need to be adapted to meet the needs of developments in risk assessment of nutrient deficiency and excess in communities, in food programmes and in the agri-food industry and global market.
- A system to support public health nutrition may evolve in which the roles of DRVs and recommendations are more clearly defined and more complementary.

6.1 Introduction

Dietary reference values (DRVs) are a set of reference standards, based on the best contemporary nutritional science, intended to inform, assess, and implement and monitor public health policy relevant to nutrition and overall strategic planning and risk assessment and management (Harper, 1987; Committee on Medical Aspects of Food Policy, 1991; King and Gaza, 2007; EFSA Panel on Dietetic Products, Nutrition, and Allergies (NDA), 2010). In short, they have evolved to help policy makers and planners at all levels of government to ensure that people, from individuals through to communities and nations, have an adequate logistic supply and consumption of nutrients. This chapter will relate to DRVs as they are currently being updated in the EU (EFSA Panel on Dietetic Products, Nutrition, and Allergies (NDA), 2010) and to those produced in the UK in 1991 (Committee on Medical Aspects of Food Policy, 1991).

Specific terminology for DRVs in public health nutrition is outlined in the following. This list is taken from the preparatory opinion of the Nutrition, Dietetics and Allergy Panel (NDA) of the European Food Safety Agency, which is producing a series of thorough opinions on DRVs for macro- and micronutrients (EFSA Panel on Dietetic Products, Nutrition, and Allergies (NDA), 2010):

- *Population reference intake* (PRI) – the level of nutrient intake that is enough for virtually all healthy people in a group.
- *Average requirement* (AR) – the level of nutrient intake that is enough for half of the people in a healthy group, given a normal distribution of requirement.
- Lower threshold intake – the level of intake below which, on the basis of current knowledge, almost all individuals will be unlikely to maintain 'metabolic integrity', according to the criterion chosen for each nutrient.
- *Adequate intake* (AI) – the value estimated when a PRI cannot be set because an AR cannot be determined.
- *Reference intake range for macronutrients* – the reference intake range for macronutrients expressed as a percentage of energy intake, defined by a lower and upper bound.

Public Health Nutrition, Second Edition. Edited by Judith L Buttriss, Ailsa A Welch, John M Kearney and Susan A Lanham-New.
© 2018 by The Nutrition Society. Published 2018 by John Wiley & Sons, Ltd.
Companion website: www.wiley.com/go/buttriss/publichealth

• *Tolerable upper intake level* – the maximum level of total chronic daily intake of a nutrient (from all sources) judged to be unlikely to pose a risk of adverse health effects to humans (Expert Group on Vitamins and Minerals, 2003; Scientific Committee on Food Scientific Panel on Dietetic Products, Nutrition and Allergies, 2006). These will not be considered further, but are particularly relevant to assessments of the safety of supplements.

This terminology has a commonality with that of the COMA report of 1991 (Committee on Medical Aspects of Food Policy, 1991). These and other terms that are either in use or proposed as a basis for facilitating future international developments (King and Gaza, 2007) in DRVs are listed in Table 6.1.

The derivation of DRVs traditionally assumes a normal distribution of requirements and sets a range of references by first determining an EAR. This is usually based on a specific criterion of adequacy. Then an RNI and an LRNI are calculated respectively two standard deviations (SDs) above and below the EAR. The RNI provides a value at which the needs of 97.5% or nearly all the healthy population would be met. Conversely, intake values consistently at the lower end of the distribution curve (i.e. the LTI) are presumed to indicate an inadequate intake and risk of deficiency for the population (Figure 6.1). An exception to this profile is energy, for which an EAR is set.

In some instances there is inadequate information to allow the derivation of DRVs. Where this is the case, an SI value (or the similar adequate intake (AI) value) is set at which it is judged there is very little risk of deficiency or of toxicity in the population. Separate DRVs are set for subpopulations based on age, gender and physiological development. There are no DRVs for the first 6 months of life, at which time babies are predominately breast or

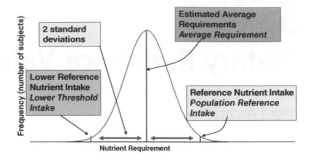

Figure 6.1 Dietary Reference Values (*UK and EU*).

formula fed and it is assumed that the nutrient content of breast milk in the first half of infancy would be adequate for most babies, and the composition of infant formulas is regulated to match the nutritional profile and outcomes of breast-fed infants.

DRVs enable assessments of food supply, dietary surveys, dietary composition and planning, the impact of novel foods, changes in food composition and formulation, assessing and planning meal provision and food labelling. They can be used for dietary guidelines, nutritional information and education – the European Food Safety Authority (EFSA) opinions on individual nutrients and substrates are invaluable educational resources and can be accessed through http://www.efsa.europa.eu/en/publications/efsajournal. DRVs may also underpin the development of dietetic strategies for the management of disease and of foods for special medical purposes (i.e. foods that are designed for the therapeutic support of patients who are unable to consume conventional diets and foodstuffs), and standards for food and renutrition programmes. They therefore provide guidance for health

Table 6.1 DRVs and intake terminologies.

Reference term	UK	EU	USA and Canada	United Nations University (UNU) harmonised
Overarching collective term	DRVs	Dietary reference intake	Nutrient intake values	
Average requirement (AR) meets the average physiological requirement	Estimated average requirement (EAR)	AR	EAR	Average nutrient requirement
Value that would be expected to meet the needs of most healthy people	Reference nutrient intake (RNI)	PRI	Recommended dietary allowance (RDA)	Individual nutrient level (INL$_x$); set to meet the x centile of the population of interest
Lower reference intake	Lower reference nutrient intake (LRNI)	Lower threshold intake (LTI)		Lower reference nutrient level
Safe intake (SI) or AI when DRVs cannot be set	SI	AI	AI	

Sources: Committee on Medical Aspects of Food Policy (1991), King and Gaza (2007), EFSA Panel on Dietetic Products, Nutrition, and Allergies (NDA) (2010).

professionals, food planners, the agri-food industry and any government authorities and agencies that are responsible for public health nutrition.

DRVs relate to nutrients and not to diets, and to healthy people rather than those with disease or metabolic abnormalities. DRVs apply to populations and subpopulations and not to individuals. They are risk indicators, and, as such, values in DRVs are not diagnostic thresholds of deficiency or excess either in the population or in individuals. Currently, they do not accommodate adjustments to account for lifestyle, smoking or alcohol consumption.

Unfortunately, many 'users' of these values seem not to appreciate their derivation or intended use, although these points are elaborated in dietary reference reports. Such users seem only to base their interpretation and use of these values on the summary tables alone, rather than reading the narrative text. It is therefore very important to read the accompanying text, which will explain how the DRVs were derived and include an account of the assumptions and uncertainties involved.

Although one cautions against injudicious use of DRVs for assessing an individual's intakes, requirements and risks of deficiency, DRVs can be used to do this when this assessment is informed by the nutrient-specific account in a DRV report, and by more knowledge about the individual's state. Similar caveats apply to using DRVs to assess the risks of excess or deficiency in therapeutic nutrition. Nevertheless, using a DRV alone without any insight on its derivation and quality is inappropriate.

Inappropriate uses and misapprehensions of reference values probably stemmed from early reports in which the term 'recommendations' was used. 'Reference' was not used until 1991 (Committee on Medical Aspects of Food Policy, 1991). Ironically, 'reference' had been rejected in the past because, it was thought, it inferred too much of an element of finality and absolutism. 'Reference' intakes are now considered to reflect better their intended use than do recommended intakes.

However, many national and international sets of reference values still include 'recommendation' in their terminology, including both the Institute of Medicine in North America, and Food Standards Australia and New Zealand. Nonetheless, both agencies support the concept of reference values and warn against the potential misinterpretation of 'recommendation'.

6.2 Evolution of dietary standards, recommendations and reference values

The character, usage and terminology of guidance on nutrient intakes has developed in the wake of advances in nutritional sciences and changing perspectives of regulators for strategies for risk management and communication in public health nutrition. The early history of this progress has been reviewed, as follows, by Harper (1987).

An early regulatory dietary standard was the British Merchant Seamen's Act of 1835, which required the compulsory provision of lime or lemon juice for sailors. This qualitative measure was intended to reduce the morbidity and mortality of sailors from scurvy. A quantitative guideline appeared in 1862, when the British Privy Council produced quantitative advice on the diet of the working population. This guidance was intended to manage starvation and related diseases among workers and was based on observed carbon and nitrogen intakes of apparently healthy factory workers at that time. Overall, the guidance approximated 3000 kcal of energy and 80 g of protein per day.

Many similar standards in the latter half of the 19th century devised similar values for the management of famine. However, in France and Prussia, for example, there was an increasing appreciation that food supply and diet were important influences on the health and work performance of the citizenry and military alike; and that a population's physical welfare and economic performance relied on the prevention of endemic chronic malnutrition.

Dietary and nutrient guidance focused on the macronutrients because, apart from antiscorbutic factor, iron and iodine (the antigoitrogenic effect of which had been demonstrated in 1850), little was known about any other nutrient. However, the burgeoning knowledge of the chemistry and biochemistry of protein and amino acids (including inborn errors of metabolism, calorimetry and energy metabolism) and enzymology carried nutritional science forward and led to the discovery of micronutrients, which underpinned substrate and energy metabolism, survival, growth and optimal function of animals, including humans (Todhunter, 1976). Only the major nutrients were considered (with scaling for women and children) by the Royal Society when it assessed food aid needed from North America to compensate the loss of agricultural production in western Europe at the end of the First World War. However, in the 1930s, newly recognised nutrients began to be incorporated in dietary standards (Todhunter, 1976).

Vitamin B_1, riboflavin, calcium, phosphate, iron, vitamins A and C and energy needs based on activity levels were included in a guide for the nutrient composition of US Department of Agriculture food programmes by Stiebling (1933). These standards were extended by the League of Nations between 1936 and 1938 to improve the diets of infants, children and mothers. The figures provided were regarded as being 'average needs', but Stiebling and Phipard (1939) proposed that, when applied to a population, ARs should be increased by 50% to allow for individual variability; this also compensated the uncertainties involved in the estimation of the requirements. Then, when it was appreciated that most biological variables have a normal (Gaussian or bell-shaped) distribution with an SD of 10–15%, the use of a 50% increment was dropped and 'average needs' were adjusted by two SDs by multiplying them by either 1.2 or 1.3 to provide a top of the range value that would match the needs of nearly all the population. Subsequently, some committees have used 1.2 and others have used 1.3 as a multiple (see later). As yet there is no common agreement on which value to use.

Thus, by 1940, nutritional knowledge had evolved from being derived from observed intakes to being based on the best contemporary scientific knowledge; and, as a consequence, had become quantitative guidance to support general public health nutrition rather than just food programmes for the management of malnutrition. In 1941 the Food and Nutrition Board of the US National Research Council produced the first set of RDAs. These RDAs were regarded as 'levels of intake of essential nutrients that, on the basis of scientific knowledge, are judged . . . to be adequate to meet the known nutrient needs of practically all healthy persons' (Food and Nutrition Board, National Research Council, 1943), and they were described as 'yardsticks'.

Many national agencies used very much the same core nutritional knowledge to derive their own independent sets of nutrient standards coupled with their own terminology. The many 'recommendations', definitions and terms became to be seen as potentially confusing and confounding in the context of the need for effective governance of the increasingly globalised agri-food industry and trade (Aggett *et al.*, 1997; King and Gaza, 2007).

The 1989 American Food and Nutrition Board Report on RDAs included a complete range of vitamins and trace elements, as did the 1991 COMA report on DRVs (Committee on Medical Aspects of Food Policy, 1991). Each micronutrient was included irrespective of whether or not a deficiency of it was thought to be likely. The inclusion of a wider range of nutrients accommodated a need for a reference base to enable nutritional and labelling claims.

The 1991 COMA report produced the DRV terminology, the principle of which was adopted by the Scientific Committee on Food (SCF) of the European Commission in 1993. The SCF improved on the UK nomenclature by replacing the RNI with the PRI, thereby re-emphasising that the reference values applied to populations and groups of people and not to individuals (EFSA Panel on Dietetic Products, Nutrition, and Allergies (NDA), 2010).

6.3 Principles of deriving reference values

The process of developing reference values involves:

1. Reviewing the literature thoroughly and identifying the most appropriate data to use for setting DRVs.

2. Determining a physiological requirement, which is the amount needed to be absorbed and retained systemically for a defined marker of adequacy.
3. Translating that physiological requirement to a dietary intake (the EAR) that would meet the physiological requirement.
4. Deriving the reference values using, if possible, distribution data to set a PRI.

Literature review

The first stage of deriving a reference value is a full and critical appraisal of the relevant literature. This would enable creating a strategy informed by up-to-date knowledge on the absorption, internal exposure and distribution, metabolism and excretion of each nutrient and substrate in order to characterise systemic changes to various intakes of nutrients and substrates. This review would aim to identify appropriate validated markers of nutrient intake, and to detect, in response to various intakes, markers of adaptations in absorption, altered urinary and faecal losses, altered systemic depots, changes in circulating distribution mechanisms (e.g. carrier proteins), nutrient and substrate turnover and metabolism, and of functional and architectural tissue damage. The objective of this exercise is to identify a dose (i.e. dietary intake)–response 'curve' for outcomes on the spectrum of deficiency to adequacy to toxicity (Figure 6.2), ideally finding markers of incipient deficiency and excess.

The background to the range of markers in Figure 6.2 is shown as a set of U-shaped curves. This is a set of hypothetical dose–response curves representing degrees of deficiency and excess. In reality these curves are not as balanced as they are shown. The curves on the left of the figure represent degrees of deficiency and show how a progression from early depletion to marked deficiency can theoretically be traced from a failure in homeostasis following reduction of stores, reduced excretion or systemic degradation and an inadequate absorption of the nutrient. For micronutrients, such as vitamins and trace elements, reduced systemic depots (stores) can be detected by measuring circulating markers of systemic depots (e.g. ferritin) or key metabolites (25-hydroxycholecalciferol). Early dysfunction can be detected as loss of saturation of a key functional protein (selenoprotein P) or of an enzyme activity (e.g. caeruloplasmin for copper; or a zinc-dependent enzyme).

Dysfunctional or disease outcomes have become used as markers to enable the estimation of levels intakes that are not associated with a particular disease. This approach depends on the meta-analyses of multiple observational studies of disease associations with long-term intakes of nutrients. An example is the exploration of the association of potassium and sodium or of lipids with raised blood

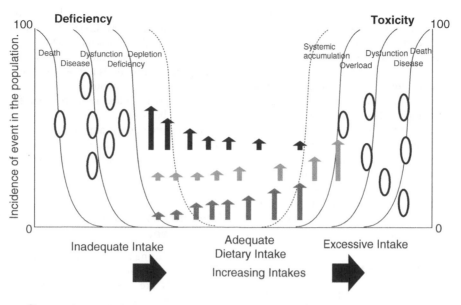

Figure 6.2 The spectrum of nutrient deficiency and excess and the range of potential markers that could be used to set DRVs for ideal nutrient intakes, and markers that could be used to set safe upper levels and to gauge the risk of toxicity associated with high intakes of nutrients.

pressure and cardiovascular disease. The latter approach skips the identification of a physiological requirement but is arguably more representative for the assessment of population intakes than are the traditional setting of DRVs. These points are revisited later.

The right-hand side of Figure 6.2 shows the progression of events related to nutrient safety at excessive intakes and to assessing upper levels or safe upper levels in EFSA or UK terminology respectively. Approaches analogous to those used to identify markers of inadequate intakes are used to identify markers of excess exposure. However, the data available are poorer than those on deficiency, and the estimation of upper levels usually needs to use toxicological approaches involving large margins of safety to set levels for SIs. These values are called health guidance values, and they are more precautionary than DRVs. Collective experience with setting DRVs and upper levels suggests that setting these values in the future will benefit from the use of proteomics to identify and validate markers of homeostatic adaptation to inadequate and excessive intakes.

Many of the markers used in developing reference values are outside the range of intakes at which homeostasis is effective. This is because, although homeostatic

mechanisms are known for nearly all nutrients, there are few dose–response data which are characterised sufficiently to enable the derivation of DRVs based on adaptive phenomena.

This paucity of information applies to studies in animal models as much as to those on humans, but many of the mechanisms and markers in the spectrum shown in Figure 6.2 have been derived from studies in animal models. The knowledge on which DRV requirements are based comprises a miscellany of data derived from studies in vitro and in vivo, studies in animal models as well as in humans, inborn errors of metabolism, clinical nutrition including malnutrition, parenteral and enteral nutrition and disease states, and epidemiological information from observation as well as prospective controlled intervention trials. This literature is also of a variable quality; and its exploitation requires expert judgement, and a significant degree of metabolic insight, to integrate, explore and critique the available data in a competent fashion. Such an approach is exemplified in the Functional Food Science in Europe report (Diplock et al., 1999), which shows how a large array of information could be explored, integrated and used effectively and intelligently in an evidence-based mechanistic approach without uncritically imposing a hierarchy of data. Such an analysis of the data would also help explain the uncertainties in the determinations of the DRVs, and to identify and prioritise the knowledge needs.

Additionally, this information needs to be explored according to the particular needs of specific age and gender groups for which DRVs are being prepared; thus, the influences of life stage, such as early and late infancy, early childhood, preadolescence, adolescence, maturity, pregnancy and lactation, and older age groups, need to be included in the background search. Usually, DRVs are derived on a body weight basis, but for some nutrients, whose functions relate to energy metabolism, opportunities are sought to see if any values could be based on a denominator such as body surface area.

Physiological requirement

The idealised concept of a physiological requirement is the amount and chemical form of a nutrient which is needed systemically to maintain normal health and development without extreme adaptation and without disturbance of the metabolism of any other nutrient or substrate; the supply of other nutrients is considered to be adequate. This, of course, implies that an AR/EAR is similarly independent.

Physiological requirements and reference values are based factorially on a summation of estimations of compositional data and size of body compartments and on metabolic balance studies. Balance studies provide data on basal losses, such as those from hair, skin, and urinary, gastrointestinal and respiratory tracts. Information from balance study data can be improved by the use of radioisotopic and stable isotopic tracers, which improve information about the turnover of endogenous pools, intestinal uptake and transfer, obligatory losses of nutrients and determine true and apparent absorption and whole-body retention of nutrients, particularly of inorganic nutrients such as trace elements and calcium.

Tracers have been used:

- to monitor zinc, iron and calcium utilisation and turnover;
- to complement nitrogen balances in estimating needs for protein;
- to follow the metabolic transitions of lipids, nitrogen sources and carbohydrates; and
- to measure energy production.

DRVs for energy are ARs only and are based on assessed total energy expenditure, which is derived factorially from estimates of resting energy expenditure plus the energy needed for various levels of physical activity.

Body composition data have been enhanced by non-invasive techniques and imaging technology, but are of an uncertain value in assessing DRVs.

DRVs for fats are difficult to set because of the heterogeneity of lipids as a group and the limited quantitative information about deficiencies of certain fatty acids. A reference intake range for total fat of 20–35% of energy has been set.

Unfortunately, most approaches to assessing physiological requirements do not have sufficient sensitivity or specificity to make extensive use of measurements of either homoeostasis or systemic depots of nutrients.

Estimated average requirement/average requirement

Rather than using an estimated bioavailability to extrapolate from a physiological requirement to an EAR/AR, most DRVs are based on outcomes associated with observed dietary intakes.

Approaches used to derive the precursors of reference values have relied on analogies with the observed dietary intakes of populations who were presumed to be healthy. This method now involves matching such observed intakes with the same type of endpoints described in Section 6.2, and the correlation between intake data and outcomes from epidemiological studies are being explored statistically using models of distributions and interactions that do not assume first-order linear relationships. With sufficient good-quality data it is possible to detect the existence of inflexions that could be indicative of homeostatic adaptation. The distributions of data are not necessarily normal, and median as well as average data points can serve to identify an AR. Furthermore, these analyses aid assessments as to whether the data can provide a secure EAR/AR or that setting an AI would be the better choice.

Population reference intake/reference nutrient intake

Classically, as has been said, a multiple based on an assumed Gaussian distribution has been used to derive from an 'average value' a value which would be expected to cover the needs of nearly all the population. This is used to create a PRI/RNI from the AR/EAR. The Institute of Medicine, using an SD of 10%, would use a factor of 1.2, whereas the UK, FAO, and France using a 15% SD would multiply the AR/EAR by 1.3. However, this is not a default approach. More information about the distributions of intake data enables tighter SDs to be assessed, and sometimes such data show that at lower intakes of micronutrients the distributions of outcome data below the median or average intakes are tighter or smaller, consistent with concepts of homeostasis, and thus the SD with which to set an LRNI/LTI could be smaller. The adjustment from EAR/AR to PRI/RNI probably does cover the elements of human population variability. These include homeostatic adaptation, functional polymorphisms, epigenetic effects, and the qualitative and quantitative uncertainties and defects of the data on which the EAR is based.

6.4 Uncertainties in setting dietary reference values

A principal source of difficulty in setting DRVs is confidence in the methodologies being used to acquire the information and data being used.

DRVs need to undergo reality checks to ascertain whether or not they correspond to observed intakes, and, in the context of customary dietary patterns, if they are both achievable and reconcilable with the DRVs for other nutrients. These assessments and validations should be done using data that were not used to determine the DRVs in the first place.

EAR/AR and PRI/RNI for the various life stages are derived from extrapolations from adult data or interpolations between adult data and data applicable in late infancy and early childhood. Adjustments to set PRI/RNIs for life stages are often precautionary and are thus arguably generous. This compensates for concern about not setting appropriate DRVs to cover such vulnerable groups. This attitude applies particularly to setting DRVs for pregnancy and lactation, during which there is considerable adaptation in systemic metabolism. This adaptation involves, amongst other things, an increase in plasma volume, which, for example, results in an apparent anaemia, although there is, in fact, an increased red cell mass. This dilutional phenomenon distorts other markers which are used to assess functional and compositional status. Unfortunately, these are commonly misinterpreted as evidence of impending deficiency and of an insufficient intake. The COMA DRV report (Committee on Medical Aspects of Food Policy, 1991) advocated that DRVs should be set to address the needs of women between pregnancies, and therefore set nearly all its values to meet the needs of all women in their reproductive years, and did not set additional DRVs for pregnancy and lactation.

The major uncertainty in setting DRVs, however, is the data used in the process. The Diplock *et al.* (1999) report emphasised the key criteria for the validation of markers in nutritional science. Unfortunately, against the criteria for a good marker, many of the markers used in deriving DRVs are not appropriately validated. The most

fundamental of these is the measurement of intake (i.e. dietary exposure).

Most exposure data are based on weighed, reported or recalled intakes. Even if these were free of the well-appreciated deficiencies of such data (see Chapter 4), there are uncertainties arising from the period over which the information is captured. Since people have different consumption patterns, their actual intakes of some nutrients might vary widely, and at the time of sampling they may have a seemingly low intake whereas on another day their intake of that nutrient could be relatively high. Three-day studies try to include a weekend day to capture some of this variability. The time needed to acquire reasonably accurate estimates of 'true average intakes' varies by nutrient. There are few details on this because the necessary studies are very demanding on resources. For example, gaining a true average intake of iron probably needs 18–130 days (median 68 days) of intake data, whereas 23–72 days are needed for protein and 27–140 days may be needed to assess sodium intake. Thus, short-term studies may provide good estimates of mean or median nutrient intakes (true average intakes) but they give a poor indication of the pattern and distribution of such intakes (Basiotis *et al.*, 1987).

6.5 Critique

Setting DRVs is a challenging process; expert and experienced judgement is needed to evaluate critically and use existing nutritional knowledge. The exercise demonstrates the variable quality of the nutritional database. There is a lot of information about the effects of markedly deficient and excessive intakes, but there are few validated dose-related outcomes relevant to understanding intestinal and systemic adaptations to intakes of nutrients, and the functional sequelae of marginal deficient and excessive intakes (Aggett *et al.*, 1997; King and Gaza, 2007).

It is often claimed that DRVs are too low or too high; however, those involved with preparing them appreciate that they are highly conservative and it is more likely that PRIs, for example, may be high. The DRVs are based on more cautious criteria than the simple avoidance of clinical deficiency, and derived values are usually approximations and precautionary, in that they are often devised for safety rather than for precision. If this is the case, then this should be made clear in the explanation of the assessment. In some instances (e.g. iron) a reality check demonstrates that there is a discrepancy between customary dietary intakes and the PRI value set for adolescents. However, there is so much uncertainty about the variability of requirements during adolescence that a seemingly high yardstick for assessing a population's adequacy of iron intakes was set.

Almost certainly, most teenagers do not need such a high intake. This illustrates an important distinction between a DRV and a recommendation. The DRV narrative for iron, and that for other nutrients, should explain this. Similarly, reports should highlight crucial knowledge gaps which are prioritised for resolution. Thus, DRVs, although uncertain or insecure for vulnerable groups such as children and adolescents, are almost certainly generous or conservative and are not marginal. Another fallacy arising from a lack of appreciation of the precautionary nature of DRVs is the notion that failure to achieve a DRV, usually the PRI or RNI but sometimes the LRNI or LTI, is evidence of deficiency.

Arguments that DRVs are low are usually based on misinterpretation of markers of status or of a risk of deficiency, commonly as a result of not understanding how such markers are confounded by physiological effects and intercurrent infections. The haemodilutional effect on haemoglobin, iron and zinc values during pregnancy is an example of the former, and the alteration of values as a result of the acute phase reaction is an example of the latter.

Often, setting DRVs involves inductive extrapolation from limited observations in small numbers of individuals who might not be representative of the target population; for example, many data are acquired from studies on a few male participants. The increasing use of observed intake data offsets these problems. Furthermore, prospective long-term monitoring of the effects of energy and nutrient intakes will validate, or otherwise, current DRVs by facilitating reality checks. An example is that of determining whether the DRVs for energy or protein are compatible with the DRVs for micronutrients; during the deliberations of some panels it has been realised that matching DRVs for iron and zinc would entail intakes of protein that exceed both observed intakes and PRIs.

Many interested bodies, including government agencies, policy makers and risk managers, and communicators and advisory bodies, need to understand better the nature of DRVs and their limitations and use; and there is increasingly a need to harmonise internationally their development, and to monitor their use to enable their validation and implementation in public health nutrition at all levels of public health activity. Doing this would need to be sensitive to the cost–benefit analysis of DRVs. This means that future exercises on DRVs should have very clear purposes and, because of implications for trade and claims, a wide applicability. This could not be done without international collaboration and pooling of data combined with a standardisation or harmonisation of approaches.

The UNU 'Nutrient Based Dietary Standards' initiative developed from concerns, such as those discussed

Population distribution of requirements for a nutrient

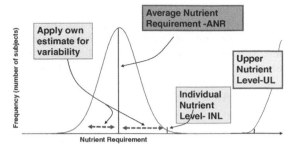

Figure 6.3 International Harmonisation of Approaches for Developing Nutrient-Based Dietary Standards. King, Gaza (2007).

here, raised by members who served on one or more of the several national and international reference value panels that worked in the 1980s and 1990s (Aggett *et al.*, 1997). These concerns are captured in the UNU report (King and Gaza, 2007), which took up the point made by Professor A.E. Harper (1987) in his classic review, that there should be a set of dietary standards named 'adequate intakes of essential nutrients' and that these should not be seen as 'recommendations'. The UNU initiative's essential premise was that the terminology should relate to nutrients, and it proposed that the reference values could simply be called nutrient intake values (Figure 6.3) and that the pivotal element of these would be an average nutrient requirement. Research and data should focus on establishing this as a core, universally agreed value. It should then be possible for other panels and agencies to determine and apply their own estimates of possible variability and variance within their populations. Such an initiative may seem aspirational, but DRVs will need to become more transparent and adaptable to different emerging evidence bases and needs. For example, whereas single key values may be needed for regulatory or labelling purposes, a simple range of sufficient intakes previously termed in some way as an 'adequate range' might suffice to inform competent authorities about the risk of deficient or excess nutrient intakes in their communities, and about the design of food programmes.

Additionally, in the context of the evolution of the derivation and use of DRVs, it is increasingly necessary to resolve the confusion between DRVs and 'recommendations'. Close consideration of the explanations of the derivations of DRVs demonstrates that, in many cases, the values being derived are de facto recommendations. This represents a transition of DRVs from being monitoring tools to becoming a component of a more targeted and specific system for public health nutrition. Future developments will need to accept this realisation and produce a research strategy and a public and population health approach within which DRVs and recommendations have separate but complementary roles within public health nutrition.

Thus, in the future, there may be an altered dependence on DRVs; even so, they and applications derived from them will persist, and the same may be said about DRVs, as Ruth Leverton (cited by Harper (1987)) said about RDAs: 'DRVs are not for amateurs'.

References

Aggett, P.J., Bresson, J., Haschke, F. *et al.* (1997) Recommended dietary allowances (RDAs), recommended dietary intakes (RDIs), Recommended nutrient intakes (RNIs) and population reference intakes (PRIs) are not recommended intakes. *Journal of Paediatric Gastroenterology and Nutrition*, **25**, 236–241.

Basiotis, P.P., Welsh, S.O., Cronin, F.J. *et al.* (1987) Number of days of food intake records required to estimate individual and group nutrient intakes with defined confidence. *Journal of Nutrition*, **117**, 1638–1641.

Committee on Medical Aspects of Food Policy (1991) *Dietary Reference Values of Food Energy and Nutrients for The United Kingdom. Report On Health and Social Subjects.* HMSO, London.

Diplock, A., Aggett, P.J., Ashwell, M. *et al.* (1999) Scientific concepts of Functional Foods in Europe (FUFOSE) consensus statement. *British Journal of Nutrition*, **81**, S1–S27.

EFSA Panel on Dietetic Products, Nutrition, and Allergies (NDA) (2010) Scientific Opinion on principles for deriving and applying dietary reference values. *EFSA Journal*, **8**(3), 1458–1487.

Expert Group on Vitamins and Minerals (2003) *Safe Upper Levels for Vitamins and Minerals.* Food Standards Agency. https://cot.food.gov.uk/sites/default/files/vitmin2003.pdf (accessed 28 November 2016).

Food and Nutrition Board, National Research Council (1943) *Recommended Dietary Allowances.* Report of the Food and Nutrition Board, Reprint and Circular Series No. 115. National Research Council, Washington, DC.

Harper, A.E. (1987) Evolution of recommended dietary allowances – new directions? *Annual Reviews of Nutrition*, **7**, 509–537.

King, J.C. and Gaza, C. (eds) (2007) International Harmonisation of Approaches for Developing Nutrient-Based Dietary Standards. *Food and Nutrition Bulletin*, **28**(1 Suppl 1), S1–S154.

Scientific Committee on Food Scientific Panel on Dietetic Products, Nutrition and Allergies (2006) *Tolerable Upper Intake Levels for Vitamins and Minerals.* European Food Safety Authority. http://www.efsa.europa.eu/sites/default/files/efsa_rep/blobserver_assets/ndatolerableuil.pdf (accessed 28 November 2016).

Stiebling, H.K. (1933) *Food Budgets for Nutrition and Production Programs.* USDA Miscellaneous Publication no. 183. USDA, Washington, DC.

Stiebling, H.K. and Phipard, E.F. (1939) *Diets of Families of Employed Wage Earners and Clerical Workers in Cities.* USDA Circular no. 507. USDA, Washington, DC.

Todhunter, E.N. (1976) Chronology events in the development and application of the science of nutrition. *Nutrition Reviews*, **34**, 353–365.

7
Assessment of Physical Activity

Bjørge H Hansen and Ulf Ekelund

Key messages

- Physical activity is a complex human behaviour comprising type of activity, intensity, frequency, duration and the context of where activity takes place (domain).
- The validity of any given measurement indicates the degree to which a method actually measures what it purports to measure.
- Reliability is an integral part of validity and represents the extent to which a method gives the same result on different occasions.
- To understand the relationship between physical activity, sedentary behaviour and health, accurate measures are needed for assessing the total amount and the patterns of physical activity.
- Currently, no single physical activity assessment method can assess simultaneously all dimensions, types and domains of physical activity.

- Objective methods provide a reasonably accurate assessment of time spent in ambulatory activities, total physical activity, time spent in different activity intensities, and time spent being sedentary.
- Currently, available objective methods cannot assess domains and types of physical activity
- Subjective methods can effectively rank categorise individuals into levels of physical activity, but have limited ability to quantify physical activity.
- Careful considerations must be given to the aims of the study, study population, and the pros and cons of available assessment methods before selecting a method to assess physical activity.

7.1 Nutrition, physical activity and public health

For the majority of adults, the most significant manageable risk factors for non-communicable diseases are what they eat and how physically active they are. Traditionally, nutrition and physical activity have been considered as two different specialties. However, as the links between diet and physical activity and their combined impact on health are being elucidated, researchers and public health workers are increasingly adopting a more holistic view in preventative research and when implementing public health programmes. Physical inactivity (defined later) has been identified as the fourth leading risk factor for non-communicable diseases, accountable for more than 3 million preventable deaths annually worldwide (World Health Organization, 2009); and others have recently suggested that physical inactivity accounts for about 9%, or more than 5.3 million, premature deaths globally (Lee et al., 2012). Despite different estimates of the consequences of physical inactivity on premature mortality it

is obvious that physical activity is a key determinant of health and longevity.

Although much is known of the health benefits of regular physical activity, the specific dose–response relationship between activity and different health outcomes remains unclear, and the magnitude of the relationships between physical activity, sedentary behaviour and health vary considerably. This is at least partly due to challenges surrounding accurate measurement of the exposure in observational research. An imprecise measure of physical activity and/or sedentary behaviour will attenuate the true effect, thus underestimating or masking the true association between the exposure and outcome. Therefore, accurate measurement of physical activity and sedentary behaviour is crucial for understanding basic characteristics of human movement and its relationship with various health outcomes (Chen and Bassett, 2005). Furthermore, sensitive, valid and reliable assessment methods are required when assessing population levels of physical activity behaviours and how they vary by time, and when evaluating the effects of interventions (Wareham and Rennie, 1998).

Public Health Nutrition, Second Edition. Edited by Judith L Buttriss, Ailsa A Welch, John M Kearney and Susan A Lanham-New.
© 2018 by The Nutrition Society. Published 2018 by John Wiley & Sons, Ltd.
Companion website: www.wiley.com/go/buttriss/publichealth

The assessment of physical activity and sedentary behaviour should involve the recording of daily physical activity patterns individually. Physical activity is a behaviour that varies substantially between individuals and is inherently difficult to measure due to its complex nature, making the measurement of physical activity (and sedentary behaviour) a truly challenging task. This chapter describes the fundamental aspects of physical activity and sedentary behaviour, defines the modern terminology used and focuses on available methodology for the assessment of physical activity and sedentary behaviour in individuals and populations.

7.2 Physical activity definitions

Physical activity is a complex construct that includes many terms associated with movement of the body. The construct includes work, leisure activities, exercise, physical fitness, sedentary behaviour and energy expenditure. These terms are often used interchangeably and are defined as follows in this chapter.

Physical activity is defined as any bodily movement produced by skeletal muscles that require energy expenditure (Caspersen *et al.*, 1985). It is a complex multidimensional form of human behaviour that includes all bodily movement from fidgeting to participating in very vigorous exercise. It is an integral and complex part of human behaviour that occurs in a variety of modes and domains, with modes referring to the different specific activities (e.g. walking, running, carrying loads or cycling) and domains referring to the context or reason for the physical activity (e.g. transportation, occupational physical activity, leisure-time physical activity, household activities or exercise) (Welk, 2002). It varies along three dimensions: *frequency* (number of bouts of activity), *duration* (time spent in a single bout of activity) and *intensity* (how strenuous the activity is).

Total energy expenditure (TEE) refers to the sum of basal metabolic rate (BMR), thermic effect of food and activity thermogenesis (or activity energy expenditure (AEE), the energy expenditure of physical activity). BMR is defined as the energy expended when an individual is lying at complete rest, and is usually measured by indirect calorimetry in a post-absorptive state in the morning. BMR is under most circumstances accountable for the largest proportion of TEE. The thermic effect of food is the increase in energy expenditure associated with digestion, absorption and storage of food, and accounts for approximately 10% of TEE. AEE displays the largest inter-individual differences and varies from 5% in a sedentary individual to 45–50% of TEE in highly active individuals (Westerterp, 2003). A *metabolic equivalent of task* (MET) is commonly used to classify the intensity of

physical activity and is expressed as multiples of resting energy expenditure (REE) in relation to body weight (Montoye *et al.*, 1996). One MET is by definition the equivalent of REE, and commonly considered equal to an oxygen uptake of 3.5 mL per kilogram body weight per minute in adults (American College of Sport Sciences, 1998). Although extensively used, one should keep in mind that this is an estimated value, and newer studies suggest that this value may be overestimated (Byrne *et al.*, 2005). Additionally, REE expressed per body weight is higher in young children and decreases by age and maturity and also is influenced by the body composition of an individual; that is, the relative proportion of fat mass and fat-free mass. Finally, METs is an absolute definition of intensity, and being active at a 5 METs intensity may be considered light by a young, fit person whereas the same MET level may be maximal for an older person. Thus, categorising intensity of physical activity according to *METs* should take the aforementioned into consideration. Nevertheless, physical activity recommendations are based on MET intensity levels, and moderate intensity physical activity and vigorous intensity physical activity are commonly defined as 3 METs and 6 METs respectively.

Exercise is defined as a subset of physical activity that is planned, structured and repetitive and has as a final or an intermediate objective that is the improvement or maintenance of physical fitness. Thus, exercise is a minor part of the total volume of physical activity and is performed with a specific purpose. *Physical fitness* refers to a set of attributes, either health or skill related, and this is not synonymous with physical activity. *Cardiorespiratory fitness* refers to the ability of the circulatory and respiratory systems to supply and utilise oxygen during sustained physical activity, and is a set of attributes rather than a behaviour (Caspersen *et al.*, 1985). Cardiorespiratory fitness, defined as maximal oxygen uptake (VO_2max), is generally considered to be the best marker for functional capacity of the cardiorespiratory system. Because larger persons normally have higher absolute VO_2 by virtue of larger muscle mass, the term is often expressed relative to body weight (millilitres per kilogram per minute). Cardiorespiratory fitness is determined by physical activity and exercise and non-modifiable factors, such as sex, age and genotype (Shvartz and Reibold, 1990; Blair *et al.*, 2001; Nokes, 2009; Nelson *et al.*, 2010; Aspenes *et al.*, 2011).

Sedentary behaviour is typically defined as a range of human endeavours that result in an energy expenditure of no more than 1.5 METs in a sitting or reclining posture (Owen *et al.*, 2000; Healy *et al.*, 2008; Matthews *et al.*, 2008). Common sedentary behaviours include TV viewing, video game playing, computer use (often referred to as 'screen time'), passive transportation (driving automobiles, public transportation) and reading. In this context, an individual may be described as sedentary if they engage in large amounts of sedentary behaviour. On the other hand, it is common for researchers to describe an individual as *physically inactive* when not meeting physical activity recommendations (Tremblay *et al.*, 2010).

7.3 Validity and reliability

Validity and reliability are crucial concepts in all types of research. They represent different concepts, but are sometimes erroneously used interchangeably. The *validity* of any given measurement indicates the degree to which a method actually measures what it purports to measure. *Logical validity* (or *face validity*) refers to the degree of which a method obviously involves the outcome of interest – whether a test appears (at face value) to measure what it claims to be measuring. Logical validity is sometimes used in research studies, but a more objective indication of validity is preferred. *Criterion validity* is the degree of association between the method tested and some recognised standard and more accurate method, sometimes referred to as 'gold standard'. The main types of criterion validity are concurrent validity and predictive validity. *Concurrent validity* refers to the degree to which an outcome of a method correlates with the criterion that is administered at the same time. Concurrent validity is typically used to assess whether a shorter, more easily administered method (e.g. self-reported physical activity) can replace a criterion (e.g. physical activity assessed by direct observation) that is more difficult to measure. On the other hand, when the criterion is some later behaviour, the *predictive validity* of a method is the major concern. *Absolute validity* refers to the agreement between the absolute outcome of a measure (i.e. physical activity energy expenditure or time spent sitting) and the criterion measure which provides the same outcome measure.

Correlation coefficients (Pearson product-moment correlation coefficient or Spearman's rank correlation coefficient) are often used as the outcome variable in validity studies, but might not be the most appropriate statistical methods to use for reporting validity. Intraclass correlation coefficients are considered a more appropriate measure for continuous measures on the same scale, whereas weighted kappa is a better choice of method for categorical measures (Terwee *et al.*, 2007). Another common way of reporting validation results is by means of Bland–Altman plots with limits of agreement that can be used to determine systematic error (Figure 7.1a) and estimate heteroscedasticity (see Figure 7.1b).

Reliability is an integral part of validity and may be defined as the consistency of measurements or the absence of measurement error (Rennie and Wareham, 1998) – the extent to which a method gives the same result on different occasions (Bland and Altman, 1986). A test cannot be considered valid if it is not reliable. There are several types of reliability. *Test–retest reliability* refers to the comparison of repeated administrations of the same method to the same population, at different time points. It is normally used for self-report methods such as questionnaires and commonly presented as intraclass correlation coefficients, which refers to estimates of systematic and error variance. *Inter-investigator reliability* is the degree to which different investigators agree on measurement, which is highly relevant to studies using investigator-determined subjective information (i.e. direct observation) including several investigators. Degree of reliability can be presented in various ways, including intra- and interclass correlation coefficients, absolute differences in actual units of measurement, as a proportion of the measured values and as Bland–Altman plots.

7.4 Methods to assess physical activity and sedentary behaviour

Accurate, valid and reliable assessments of habitual physical activity are important for several reasons:

- To document the frequency and distribution of physical activity in population groups; to monitor time trends in physical activity.
- To gain insight into the interactions between habitual physical activity and health; to identify correlates and determinants of physical activity that might be targets for interventions or health programs aimed at increasing physical activity.
- To evaluate the efficacy and effectiveness of interventions or health programs aimed at increasing physical activity (Wareham and Rennie, 1998; Westerterp, 2009).

A wide range of methods for assessment of physical activity are available and the method of choice is a function of several parameters. Factors such as the extent of participant interference and participant effort of a particular method should be evaluated, whether that method provides information on activity context and activity structure, the objectivity of the data, as well as the time and cost involved for the researcher. The available methods are commonly divided into subjective and objective methods, based on whether the method is relying on an individual's ability to recall physical activity (subjective) or if the method objectively records physical activity performed by the individual by the use of instruments or monitors (objective). In the following section, the most commonly used techniques for assessing physical activity will be presented.

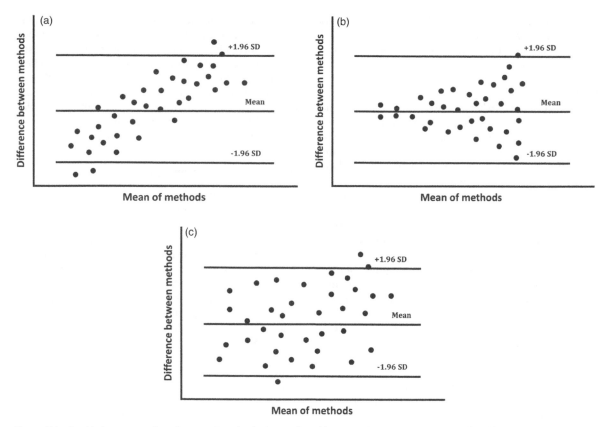

Figure 7.1 Graphical representation of error using Bland–Altman plots: (a) systematic errors are errors introduced by measurement bias or human factors; (b) heteroscedasticity occurs when the variance of the error terms differs across observations; and (c) random error indicates the size of the measurement errors and is randomly distributed.

Criterion methods

Any method proposed for assessing physical activity and sedentary behaviour should preferably be tested against a 'gold standard' (criterion validity) in the population of interest before implementation in a research study or a surveillance system. Commonly used criterion methods include direct behavioural observation, direct or indirect calorimetry, and the doubly labelled water (DLW) method. Direct observation can theoretically validate all the dimensions and domains of physical activity by following and observing free-living individuals. DLW and calorimetry both derive their estimate of physiological energy expenditure from oxygen consumption and/or carbon dioxide production, but they are estimated from different sources. The DLW method relies on estimated carbon dioxide production for calculation of TEE during free-living, while calorimetry relies on measurement of oxygen consumption and carbon dioxide production when calculating energy expenditure.

Direct observation

Direct behavioural observation was one of the first methods used to assess physical activity, involving an observer that records observations while watching an individual. Although considered the gold standard for physical activity assessment, the method has not been validated due to lack of criterion methods. However, face validity appears to be good (Montoye *et al.*, 1996), and direct observation is often used as the criterion method in validation studies of other assessment methods (Welk, 2002). The strength of the method comprises providing quantitative and qualitative information on physical activity behaviour, including contextually rich data that helps researchers to understand how physical activity is influenced by surrounding physical and social factors. The method is limited by its time-consuming nature, large participant intrusiveness and risk of reactivity, as observing someones behaviour might be behaviour-altering (Welk, 2002). Further, direct observation is usually limited to a specific location (e.g. school or work place) and time (e.g. school-day) and may be prone to the Hawthorne effect, suggesting that individuals may modify their behaviour as a consequence of being observed.

Calorimetry

Room calorimetry, whether direct or indirect, is not suitable for assessing habitual physical activity in free-living settings as it requires confinement to a metabolic chamber. The direct method uses the heat transfer from the body to the environment and the indirect method uses the measurement of expired gases to calculate energy expenditure. Both methods are able to very accurately estimate energy expenditure, but unfortunately in unnatural environments and at a high cost. A similar but more feasible method to assess energy expenditure is indirect calorimetry, a method that collects expired air via a face mask, mouthpiece or hood covering the head, and uses standardised equations to predict energy expenditure from oxygen consumption and carbon dioxide production. Indirect calorimetry is frequently used to validate other assessment instruments (e.g. activity monitors) under controlled and free-living conditions and to determine the energy cost of specific activities.

The doubly labelled water method

The DLW method was developed in the early 1940s and 1950s (Lifson et al., 1955). Researchers observed that the oxygen in respired carbon dioxide was in rapid isotopic equilibrium with the oxygen in body water and concluded that isotopically labelled oxygen (^{18}O) in body water would exit the body as water and as carbon dioxide, whereas isotopically labelled hydrogen (^{2}H) in body water would exit the body as water. Consequently, the turnover rates of isotopic hydrogen-and oxygen-labelled water would differ, and the difference would be proportional to carbon dioxide production. Thus, energy expenditure (and other components of energy metabolism) can be calculated by the use of standard indirect calorimetric equations and an estimation of the respiratory quotient (Schoeller and van Santen, 1982). The DLW method had not been used to assess human energy metabolism until relatively recently and is currently considered the gold standard for assessing TEE in free-living settings. In practice, a known quantity of enriched ^{2}H and ^{18}O atoms are ingested as water by the participant and the difference in the rates of disappearance of the two isotopes usually measured from collected urine samples are used to estimate carbon dioxide production. The DLW method measures energy expenditure over longer periods (1–3 weeks), thereby providing a good estimate of daily energy expenditure, with an accuracy of 4–7% (Schoeller and van Santen, 1982). The method is non-invasive, is applicable across all age groups, and

individuals can maintain their daily activities without restriction. However, the high cost of the stable isotopes and the sophisticated analysis technique limits the usefulness of the DLW method in epidemiological studies. The method does not provide the researcher with any information of the day-to-day variation of physical activity, nor the patterns of activity throughout the day, and the precision of the method is increased by individual registration of energy intake.

Objective assessment methods

Heart rate monitoring

Heart rate (HR) monitoring does not measure physical activity directly, but is a marker of the physiological stress on the cardiopulmonary system during physical activity. The method originates from the observations made by Berggren and Christensen (1950) that HR responds to increasing levels of physical activity in a linear fashion and proportional to the intensity of the activity. Consequently, HR is often used to predict TEE and AEE; to determine time spent being physically active, with HR above a certain threshold as an indicator of activity and to determine time spent at various intensities of physical activity (e.g. moderate-intensity physical activity).

The method is socially acceptable and can be applied for periods long enough to provide representative estimates of energy expenditure. However, owing to individual variations in resting HR and physical fitness, assessing physical activity using HR monitoring requires some sort of individual calibration for estimating physical activity energy expenditure and time spent at different intensity levels. The individual relationship between HR and energy expenditure (oxygen uptake) is usually established in the laboratory during lying, sitting, standing and then during various intensities of walking and running. HR is affected by several factors other than physical activity (such as age, physical fitness, emotional state and food intake), and the relationship between HR and energy expenditure is less robust while at rest or performing activities at lower intensities (Livingstone et al., 1990). Although HR monitoring has been validated in both controlled and free-living settings and shows good agreement with energy expenditure measured by DLW at group level (Livingstone et al., 1992; Eston et al., 1998), research using HR to assess physical activity has not been anywhere as prolific as the use of motion sensors. This is due to the complex process of calibrating each individual for the HR and energy expenditure relationship.

Movement sensing

When a person moves, the limbs and body are accelerated. Theoretically, the acceleration of body segments is proportional to the muscular forces responsible for the accelerations, and thus to energy expenditure (John and Freedson, 2012). Since almost all forms of physical activity involve movement of the trunk or limbs, the direct measurement of movement using sensors attached to one or more locations of the human body is attractive. The most common motion sensors are pedometers and activity monitors that contain accelerometers. Such devices provide objective measures of motion that can be used in their raw form or transformed into estimates of overall levels of physical activity, intensity or energy expenditure.

Pedometers

The pedometer is a relatively simple device for counting steps or estimating distance travelled. Pedometers use three basic mechanisms for counting steps. The most basic model is a spring-suspended horizontal lever arm that moves up and down in response to vertical displacement of the waist (e.g. the Yamax DigiWalker SW-701). Newer models have incorporated a glass-enclosed magnetic reed proximity switch (e.g. the Omron), while a third type has an accelerometer consisting of a horizontal beam and a piezoelectric crystal that counts steps by registering number of zero crossings of the instantaneous acceleration versus time curve (Crouter et al., 2003).

Numerous studies have established the validity and reliability of pedometers under controlled laboratory conditions and free-living settings (Bassett et al., 2000; Tudor-Locke et al., 2002a,b; Crouter et al., 2003, 2005; John et al., 2010). In general, pedometers provide a low-cost estimate of the number of steps taken. They are less accurate for assessing walking or running distance and for estimating energy expenditure associated with physical activity. The method is further limited by its inability to quantify intensity and duration of physical activity, and several studies have suggested that pedometers might underestimate physical activity at slower speeds due to the actual vertical acceleration being below the devices' sensitivity thresholds (Crouter et al., 2003; Schneider et al., 2004). Nonetheless, pedometers can be used as a motivational tool aimed to increase physical activity in the experimental group in a physical activity intervention study (Craig et al., 2007; Merom et al., 2007).

Accelerometers

Accelerometry refers to the measurement of the amplitude and frequency of accelerations and decelerations of human movement by accelerometers. The accelerations recorded while moving are proportional to the net internal muscular forces used, and therefore directly reflect the energy cost of movement (Freedson and Miller, 2000; Mathie et al., 2004). There are many commercially available brands of activity monitors that contain accelerometers, and at least 18 different

brands of activity monitors containing accelerometers that have been validated against the DLW method (Plasqui et al., 2013). Accelerometers measure the acceleration in one or more directions. Uniaxial accelerometers measures the acceleration in one plane, usually in the vertical plane, biaxial in two planes, most often the vertical and anterioposterior plane, and triaxial in the vertical, anterioposterior and mediolateral planes. The underlying scientific principles and technical specifications have been comprehensively described by Chen and Bassett (2005).

Most commonly, accelerometers are enclosed in solid casings and attached to the body at the hip, lower back, ankle, wrist or thigh. The choice of placement depends on the type of monitor and feasibility. They can be affixed to the participant using elastic belts, waistband clips or adhesive pads placed on the skin. They can be worn under or over clothing, but should be fitted snugly against the body. Recently, there has been a shift from waist-worn accelerometers to wearing the devices on the wrist. While the wrist placement has obvious advantages – being less obtrusive that the hip placement – the waist and wrist outputs are not comparable (Routen et al., 2012). Acceleration data are usually either sampled over a 24-h period or during waking. The latter approach is perhaps more common, and some consensus has emerged around the use of a minimum 10 h per day measurement period to determine adequate wear. Furthermore, a 7-day monitoring period has been recommended and routinely used in in physical activity studies because this provides activity data for both week and weekend days. This is important, as activity patterns differ between week and weekend days (Kolle et al., 2010; Hansen et al., 2011). Furthermore, a 7-day protocol has been shown to provide data that could be regarded as reflective of an individual's normal activity pattern as the between-day intraclass correlations usually exceed 80% in most populations.

The primary outcome from accelerometry is body acceleration, often expressed as a count value. A count is a brand-specific, arbitrary value that is influenced by the amplitude and frequency of acceleration. Secondary outcomes are estimates of bouts of frequency, duration and intensity of activity (see Table 7.1). The most common method for validation and calibration studies has been to compare activity counts and measured oxygen consumption during specific activities selected to mimic key elements of daily living, typically walking and running. Freedson et al. (1998) developed some of the first regression equations to estimate energy expenditure from activity counts, deriving specified activity count cut-points corresponding to different intensity levels (i.e. light, moderate, hard and very hard). More recently, studies have included both dynamic and static

Table 7.1 Common output variables obtained from accelerometers.

Outcome variables	Types of summary variables	
	Absolute	Relative
Acceleration	g-force units or m/s^2	
Activity counts	Total counts (counts/day)	Average counts (counts/min per day)
Expenditure-based measures		
TEE	kcal/day	kcal per hour monitored
Physical AEE	MET-min/day or MET-h/day	MET-min/day per hour monitored
Intensity-based measures		
Sedentary (<1.5–2.0 METs)	h/day or min/day	% wear/monitored time
Light (1.5/2.0–2.9 METs)	h/day or min/day	% wear/monitored time
Moderate (3.0–5.9 METs)	h/day or min/day	% wear/monitored time
Vigorous (≥6.0 METs)	h/day or min/day	% wear/monitored time

activities that are more generalisable to the full range of activities encountered in daily life (Ainsworth *et al.*, 2000a; Bassett *et al.*, 2000; Hendelman *et al.*, 2000; Swartz *et al.*, 2000). This use of such a wide range of activities and intensities has produced variation in the published equations and intensity thresholds. In effect, data obtained using a relatively robust technology have been splintered by the calibration process into a wide range of summary measures that are much less comparable than preferable, and this inconsistency hampers the ability to interpret results from studies across the lifespan, populations and different brands of accelerometers (Matthews, 2005). For example, available intensity thresholds for sedentary vary from <100 cpm to <800 cpm, and from >200 cpm to >3000 cpm for moderate intensity. Both Crouter *et al.* (2006) and Rothney *et al.* (2008) have compared published regression equations, and they both conclude that one equation is unable to estimate energy expenditure for all activities accurately and that equations developed to measure energy expenditure during walking are not accurate for most other activities.

In general, accelerometers have been shown to provide a reasonably accurate assessment of time spent in ambulatory activities, time spent in different activity intensities and time spent being sedentary. The method is less accurate in predicting energy expenditure, especially in free-living environments, generally showing large variability when compared with the DLW method (Plasqui and Westerterp, 2007; Plasqui *et al.*, 2013). Limitations include an underestimation of the energy cost of several activities due to their limited ability to detect arm movement (e.g. upper body strength training), external work (carrying heavy loads) or activity with little or no movement of the body segment where the monitor is placed (e.g. the hip during cycling) (Westerterp, 2009).

Advances in technology and memory capacity now make it possible to collect the raw acceleration signal at high frequency (e.g. 80 Hz) for up to 20 days. Therefore, the newest generations of accelerometers provide their output in raw accelerations expressed as units of gravity *g* in three planes. The raw data allow increased control over data processing and in theory enables comparisons between acceleration data regardless of monitor brands. By increasing the number of acceleration samples per minute, more analytically sophisticated approaches relying on automated pattern recognition and machine learning have been applied to several aspects of physical activity monitoring. Examples include the identification of different types of physical activity (Pober *et al.*, 2006) and the use of neural networks to estimate energy expenditure (Rothney *et al.*, 2007). Promising results of this emerging field yield high probabilities of correct identification of types of activity (Pober *et al.*, 2006) and reduced estimation errors from minute-by-minute energy expenditure (Rothney *et al.*, 2007). However, computational complexity and the need for a large number of annotated examples of activities limit the current feasibility of the method. Providing access to the raw acceleration signal by a given monitor, and the specifics of the calibration studies used to translate raw acceleration signals into relevant behavioural outcomes, is needed and would serve to enhance comparability across studies. A repository of standardised and publicly available calibration data collected from representative samples is needed to facilitate the development of algorithms that can be applied in population-based studies.

Combined sensing

The accuracy of currently available equations for estimating energy expenditure vary greatly, which is at least partly due to the fact that identical accelerations may not result in the same metabolic costs for different individuals, although the activity count values may be the same (Rothney *et al.*, 2007). Recent developments in technology are rapidly pushing the field of physical activity assessment forward. Such developments include improved accuracy and precision in energy expenditure prediction by the combined analysis of accelerometer data and a physiological measure like HR (Corder *et al.*, 2008). This method minimises the limitations associated with each method. At lower levels of intensity, HR is less accurate in determining energy expenditure whereas accelerometers perform better and vice versa. The combination of accelerometry and HR also makes the identification of non-wear time less prone to misclassification, and the method has been validated in adults and children (Corder *et al.*, 2005; Crouter *et al.*, 2008). Brage *et al.* (2004) used branched equation modelling of simultaneously recorded physiological (HR) and biomechanical (acceleration) data and individual calibration of the HR–physical AEE relationship to reduce the error of predicted physical AEE. In general, the combined accelerometer and HR monitor method has better accuracy and precision than either method alone. Relatively simple calibration techniques achieve acceptable levels of accuracy for this combined device to be feasible for use in large-scale studies (Warren *et al.*, 2010). Limitations with the method include the high cost and that some individuals are allergic to the electrodes used to attach the monitor to the torso.

Subjective assessment methods

Subjective assessment methods rely on information obtained from individuals using some sort of self-report. Self-report methods are the most commonly used tools for the assessment of physical activity, and include diaries, logs and self- or interviewer-administered questionnaires (Warren *et al.*, 2010). They provide a practical and low-cost method for assessing physical activity in large-scale studies and surveillance systems. However, the method is associated with numerous limitations, including difficulties in capturing the frequency, duration and intensity of physical activity, ascertaining all domains of physical activity, the complex cognitive process underlying the recall of physical activity, and social desirability bias (Sallis and Saelens, 2000; Warren *et al.*, 2010). Furthermore, available self-report methods generally show limited reliability, validity and sensitivity (Shephard, 2003; Chinapaw *et al.*, 2010; Warren *et al.*, 2010; Helmerhorst *et al.*, 2012). Nevertheless, self-report offers an assessment of physical activity by domains, which is currently not possible by objective assessment of physical activity (Warren *et al.*, 2010).

Activity diaries

To try to diminish the bias of recall error in physical activity questionnaires (PAQs), researchers have used physical activity diaries as a more direct measure of physical activity. In contrast to retrospective questionnaires, an activity diary requires the participant to code the predominant activity or intensity of activity periodically in specified time segments (e.g. every 15 min). By accumulating the information from each time segments across the whole day, detailed patterns of habitual physical activity, time spent in different intensities (including sedentary time) as well as estimated energy expenditure can be obtained. The Bouchard diary (Bouchard *et al.*, 1983) is an example of an activity diary that has been used in observational research (Eisenmann *et al.*, 2003; Garcia *et al.*, 2004). The method estimates daily energy expenditure by a factorial approach in which the entire day is divided into periods of 15 min each. Energy expenditure for each period is qualified on a scale from 1 to 9 corresponding to the energy cost of the dominant activity for that period, and completed for 3 days.

Activity diaries are inexpensive, feasible for use in large populations, do not require an observer, and lists of activities and their respective energy cost are available. The diary method provides reasonable estimates of physical activity when compared with objectively measured physical activity (Wickel *et al.*, 2006), and has frequently been used as a validation criterion for other types of PAQs (Ainsworth *et al.*, 2000b). However, there is a relatively high participant burden associated with completion of an activity diary that could possibly affect habitual behaviour (Hawthorne effect). The amount of detail provided might vary between individuals, and the recall error might still be considerable as a paper diary does not allow for any monitoring of how frequently the participants actually record their activities (Sternfeld *et al.*, 2012). Furthermore, activity diaries do not consider time segments other that what is predetermined, and recall periods shorter than 15 min have been found to be too intensive. Thus, activities of shorter durations will be missed entirely or misclassified. In order to try to reduce the sources of error associated with activity diaries, cell-phone-based physical activity diary are increasingly being used (Sternfeld *et al.*, 2012). The benefits of a cell-phone-based diary compared with a paper diary include increased compliance. This is important, as the advantage of real-time diary data collection is lost if the diary is completed retrospectively.

Physical activity questionnaires

PAQs are the most widely used self-report method to assess physical activity and have been used extensively. The method has low costs, is relatively easy to administer, poses a small burden on the participant and is feasible for use in very large populations. PAQs include self- or interviewed-administered global, recall and quantitative questionnaires, and they also provide researchers with a practical method for physical activity assessment in relation to categorisation of physical activity levels and risk stratification, in surveillance systems when monitoring physical activity in populations and for examining the aetiology of disease (Helmerhorst *et al.*, 2012).

Global physical activity questionnaires

PAQs typically capture details on the frequency, intensity and duration of physical activity. They are therefore relatively long, and thus time consuming and potentially burdensome for the respondents. In order to collect data in large populations, in different settings (e.g. worksites and community settings) and across a range of interventions (e.g. initiatives to increase walking or active travel initiatives), shorter measurement tools have been developed. These global PAQs generally consist of one to four items and aim to stratify population into main categories of activity. A review by Milton *et al.* (2011) identified 14 validated global PAQs. These PAQs assess physical activity and sedentary behaviour in different ways, including asking whether respondents participated in regular physical activity using a binary (yes/no) scale, assessing current physical activity levels by asking respondents to consider whether they are more or less active than their peers, and assessing the frequency of activity that makes them sweat. The global PAQs tend to inquire about activity over a long time frame (e.g. 1 year), which reduces systematic bias due to season and day of the week. An example of a global PAQ is the EPIC-PAQ, used in the European Prospective Investigation into Cancer and Nutrition (EPIC). The EPIC-PAQ includes four items that refers to the past year's activity, allowing for the derivation of physical activity indices to categorise individuals as inactive, moderately inactive, moderately active and active. Global PAQs appear to effectively rank individuals into levels of physical activity (Peters *et al.*, 2012). Their main use is for surveillance or broad classification of exposure in epidemiological studies. In most cases it is not possible to calculate total physical activity, nor are domains or context of activity assessed (Wanner *et al.*, 2013).

Surveillance physical activity questionnaires

Comparisons of physical activity levels and sedentary behaviours across countries and regions were unachievable until a decade ago, mainly due to the absence of standardised PAQs suitable for international use. During the 1990s, the International Physical Activity Questionnaire (IPAQ) was developed to assess activity worldwide. After showing acceptable reliability (correlation coefficients generally around 0.8) and criterion validity (correlation coefficients generally around 0.3) in a large multinational validation study (Craig *et al.*, 2003), the IPAQ has been used in numerous national and regional prevalence studies. An extended version of IPAQ is the Global Physical Activity Questionnaire, which also includes questions about occupational physical activity. Data from 122 of the194 member states of the World Health Organization were recently compiled and suggested that more than 30% on the world's adult population did not achieve the recommended levels of physical activity according to current guidelines for public health (Hallal *et al.*, 2012). The IPAQ is available in a short form recommended for surveillance systems and in a longer form in which more detailed physical activity information is collected, including different domains of activity (e.g. occupation, leisure, transport).

Aetiological physical activity questionnaires

This category of PAQs comprises comprehensive questionnaires designed to assess all dimensions and domains of physical activity in order to investigate the relationships between lifestyle factors and major chronic diseases, including cancer, cardiovascular disease, type 2 diabetes and osteoporosis. The EPIC-Norfolk Physical Activity Questionnaire 2 is a comprehensive questionnaire to assess physical activity in different domains of life aimed at assessing physical activity energy expenditure, using the last year as the time frame of reference. The questionnaire consists of three sections: activity at home, work and recreation. In order to facilitate large-scale use, the questions are closed rather than open-ended. The criterion validity and test–retest reliability were tested against objective measures of energy throughout the time frame of reference and showed results comparable to other PAQs used in large epidemiological studies (Wareham *et al.*, 2002). A further development of this questionnaire is the Recent Physical Activity Questionnaire with a shorter time frame (4 weeks), which likely improves the accuracy of reporting (Besson *et al.*, 2010). More detailed information on the validity and reliability of PAQs is available in a number of comprehensive reviews (Pereira *et al.*, 1997; Chinapaw *et al.*, 2010; Forsen *et al.*, 2010; van Poppel *et al.*, 2010; Helmerhorst, *et al.*, 2012).

Limitations of subjective methods

Before any self-report method is employed in a study, the reliability and validity should be tested in the population under investigation. This is because questionnaires that have been developed for a specific group (e.g. adults) are inappropriate to use in other age groups (e.g. elderly). Further, unlike objective methods, self-report questionnaires are culturally specific, and a questionnaire developed in one cultural setting may not perform well in another setting or geographical region. The advantages and problems of subjective methods for assessing physical activity (emphasis on questionnaires) have been extensively reviewed (Jacobs *et al.*, 1993; Paffenbarger *et al.*, 1993; Warnecke *et al.*, 1997; Sallis and Saelens, 2000; Helmerhorst *et al.*, 2012). The method relies entirely on the participants' abilities to provide the researcher with accurate information on their level of physical activity, thereby introducing several potential sources of errors. Individuals who knowingly do not participate in recommended amounts of regular physical activity are prone to overreport their level of physical activity (social desirability bias). Further, to recall physical activity is a highly complex cognitive task, which may limit the validity of information provided by some individuals (recall bias). Lastly, one should be aware that leisure activities with high intensity (e.g. soccer, jogging or aerobics) are associated with a well-known terminology, whereas the terminology associated with activities of light or moderate intensity vary more (domestic activities and office work), which consequently may lead to imprecise estimates of such activities (Jacobs et al., 1993; Paffenbarger et al., 1993; Warnecke et al., 1997; Sallis and Saelen, 2000; Helmerhorst et al., 2012). The validity correlation coefficients from the majority of available questionnaires are considered poor to moderate and in most cases only acceptable when results were given as Pearson or Spearman correlation coefficients, suggesting that most questionnaires may be valid for ranking an individual's behaviour but their absolute validity is limited to quantifying physical activity

(Chinapaw et al., 2010; Forsen et al., 2010; van Poppel et al., 2010; Helmerhorst et al., 2012). Owing to the limitations of self-report, a certain degree of exposure misclassification will always be present. One should keep in mind, however, that non-differential misclassification attenuates rather than exaggerates any observed relationship in observational research (Bellavia et al., 2013).

Selecting the most appropriate assessment method

Because of the diversity in available methods for the assessment of physical activity and sedentary behaviours, choosing the most suitable method for any given task is a complicated process (Chinapaw et al., 2010). Selecting an appropriate assessment method depends not only on the specific purpose of the study, but also on the characteristics of the population under study, the outcome of interest and what the theoretical link between the exposure and outcome is. Furthermore, a thorough understanding of the pros and cons of each method is vital, and these should be evaluated. Table 7.2 lists several

Table 7.2 Considerations for researchers when assessing physical activity.

Method	Considerations
Pedometer	The primary outcome of the study should be carefully considered to ascertain whether a pedometer would be an adequate measure of activity.
	What type of activities is the population to be studied likely to engage in?
	How many days will be measured?
	Higher quality and therefore more expensive models have been shown to be superior to cheaper models of pedometers.
Accelerometer	Will activity be assessed in one, two, or three axes?
	Decide the primary outcome of the study; total activity, time spent at different intensities, or estimates of physical activity energy expenditure.
	What is the minimal wear time that will constitute a valid day?
	What epoch period will be selected?
	How many days will be measured?
	How will the accelerometers be distributed: face-to-face or by mail?
	Has sufficient instruction on placement and wearing been supplied?
	Will participants keep concurrent activity logs or detail wearing/non-wearing times?
Combined sensing	What level of calibration is needed?
	Is the participant confident and competent at placing the device, and have sufficient explanation and written instructions been given?
PAQs	What is the PAQ designed to assess?
	What is the time frame for the PAQ?
	Has the PAQ been tested for validity and reliability?
	Was the validation undertaken in a similar population?
	What is the primary outcome of the PAQ and does this fit with the research question?
	How will the PAQ be distributed (face to face, by telephone, internet, through post)?
	Clear completion and return instructions must be provided.
	How will data be cleaned and analysed?
	For which population has the PAQ been designed?
	What is the responsiveness of the PAQ?

Source: adapted from Warren et al. (2010).

considerations that must be taken into account when selecting the most appropriate assessment method (Warren *et al.*, 2010).

For further information on selecting a method for a specific research question, the reader is referred to the Medical Research Council Diet and Physical Activity Toolkit: http://www.dapa-toolkit.mrc.ac.uk/choosing-a-method/physical-activity/index.php.

References

Ainsworth, B.E., Bassett, D.R., Jr, Strath, S.J. *et al.* (2000a) Comparison of three methods for measuring the time spent in physical activity. *Medicine and Science in Sports and Exercise*, 32(9 Suppl), S457–S464.

Ainsworth, B.E., Sternfeld, B., Richardson, M.T. and Jackson, K. (2000b) Evaluation of the Kaiser physical activity survey in women. *Medicine and Science in Sports and Exercise*, 32(7), 1327–1338.

American College of Sport Sciences (1998) *ACSM's Resource Manual for Guidelines for Exercise Testing and Prescription*. Williams and Wilkins.

Aspenes, S.T., Nilsen, T.I., Skaug, E.A. *et al.* (2011) Peak oxygen uptake and cardiovascular risk factors in 4631 healthy women and men. *Medicine and Science in Sports and Exercise*, 43(8), 1465–1473.

Bassett, D.R., Jr, Ainsworth, B.E., Swartz, A.M. *et al.* (2000) Validity of four motion sensors in measuring moderate intensity physical activity. *Medicine and Science in Sports and Exercise*, 32(9 Suppl), S471–S480.

Bellavia, A., Bottai, M., Wolk, A. and Orsini, N. (2013) Physical activity and mortality in a prospective cohort of middle-aged and elderly men – a time perspective. *The International Journal of Behavioral Nutrition and Physical Activity*, 10, 94.

Berggren, G. and Christensen, E.H. (1950) Heart rate as a means of measuring metabolic rate in man. *Arbeitsphysiologie*, 14, 255–260.

Besson, H., Brage, S., Jakes, R.W. *et al.* (2010) Estimating physical activity energy expenditure, sedentary time, and physical activity intensity by self-report in adults. *The American Journal of Clinical Nutrition*, 91(1), 106–114.

Blair, S.N., Cheng, Y. and Holder, J.S. (2001) Is physical activity or physical fitness more important in defining health benefits? *Medicine and Science in Sports and Exercise*, 33(6 Suppl), S379–S399.

Bland, J.M. and Altman, D.G. (1986) Statistical methods for assessing agreement between two methods of clinical measurement. *The Lancet*, 1(8476), 307–310.

Bouchard, C., Tremblay, A., Leblanc, C. *et al.* (1983) A method to assess energy expenditure in children and adults. *The American Journal of Clinical Nutrition*, 37(3), 461–467.

Brage, S., Brage, N., Franks, P.W. *et al.* (2004) Branched equation modeling of simultaneous accelerometry and heart rate monitoring improves estimate of directly measured physical activity energy expenditure. *Journal of Applied Physiology*, 96(1), 343–351.

Byrne, N.M., Hills, A.P., Hunter, G.R. *et al.* (2005) Metabolic equivalent: one size does not fit all. *Journal of Applied Physiology*, 99(3), 1112–1119.

Caspersen, C.J., Powell, K.E. and Christenson, G.M. (1985) Physical activity, exercise, and physical fitness: definitions and distinctions for health-related research. *Public Health Reports*, 100(2), 126–131.

Chen, K.Y. and Bassett, D.R., Jr (2005) The technology of accelerometry-based activity monitors: current and future. *Medicine and Science in Sports and Exercise*, 37(11 Suppl), S490–S500.

Chinapaw, M.J., Mokkink, L.B., van Poppel, M.N. *et al.* (2010) Physical activity questionnaires for youth: a systematic review of measurement properties. *Sports Medicine*, 40(7), 539–563.

Corder, K., Brage, S., Wareham, N.J. and Ekelund, U. (2005) Comparison of PAEE from combined and separate heart rate and movement models in children. *Medicine and Science in Sports and Exercise*, 37(10), 1761–1767.

Corder, K., Ekelund, U., Steele, R.M. *et al.* (2008) Assessment of physical activity in youth. *Journal of Applied Physiology*, 105(3), 977–987.

Craig, C.L., Marshall, A.L., Sjöström, M. *et al.* (2003) International physical activity questionnaire: 12-country reliability and validity. *Medicine and Science in Sports and Exercise*, 35(8), 1381–1395.

Craig, C.L., Tudor-Locke, C. and Bauman, A. (2007) Twelve-month effects of Canada on the Move: a population-wide campaign to promote pedometer use and walking. *Health Education Research*, 22(3), 406–413.

Crouter, S.E., Schneider, P.L., Karabulut, M. and Bassett, D.R., Jr (2003) Validity of 10 electronic pedometers for measuring steps, distance, and energy cost. *Medicine and Science in Sports and Exercise*, 35(8), 1455–1460.

Crouter, S.E., Schneider, P.L. and Bassett, D.R., Jr (2005) Spring-levered versus piezo-electric pedometer accuracy in overweight and obese adults. *Medicine and Science in Sports and Exercise*, 37(10), 1673–1679.

Crouter, S.E., Churilla, J.R., and Bassett, D.R., Jr (2006) Estimating energy expenditure using accelerometers. *European Journal of Applied Physiology*, 98(6), 601–612.

Crouter, S.E., Churilla, J.R. and Bassett, D.R., Jr (2008) Accuracy of the Actiheart for the assessment of energy expenditure in adults. *European Journal of Clinical Nutrition*, 62(6), 704–711.

Eisenmann, J.C., Katzmarzyk, P.T., Perusse, L. *et al.* (2003) Estimated daily energy expenditure and blood lipids in adolescents: the Quebec Family Study. *The Journal of Adolescent Health*, 33(3), 147–153.

Eston, R.G., Rowlands, A.V. and Ingledew, D.K. (1998) Validity of heart rate, pedometry, and accelerometry for predicting the energy cost of children's activities. *Journal of Applied Physiology*, 84(1), 362–371.

Forsen, L., Loland, N.W., Vuillemin, A. *et al.* (2010) Self-administered physical activity questionnaires for the elderly: a systematic review of measurement properties. *Sports Medicine*, 40(7), 601–623.

Freedson, P.S. and Miller, K. (2000) Objective monitoring of physical activity using motion sensors and heart rate. *Research Quarterly for Exercise and Sport*, 71(2 Suppl), S21–S29.

Freedson, P.S., Melanson, E. and Sirard, J. (1998) Calibration of the Computer Science and Applications, Inc. accelerometer. *Medicine and Science in Sports and Exercise*, 30(5), 777–781.

Garcia, K., Eisenmann, J.C. and Bartee, R.T. (2004) Does a family history of coronary heart disease modify the relationship between physical activity and blood pressure in young adults? *European Journal of Cardiovascular Prevention and Rehabilitation*, 11(3), 201–206.

Hallal, P.C., Andersen, L.B., Bull, F.C. *et al.* (2012) Global physical activity levels: surveillance progress, pitfalls, and prospects. *The Lancet*, 380(9838), 247–257.

Hansen, B.H., Kolle, E., Dyrstad, S.M. *et al.* (2011) Accelerometer-determined physical activity in adults and older people. *Medicine and Science in Sports and Exercise*, 44(2), 266–272.

Healy, G.N., Wijndaele, K., Dunstan, D.W. *et al.* (2008) Objectively measured sedentary time, physical activity, and metabolic risk:

the Australian Diabetes, *Obesity and Lifestyle Study (AusDiab)*. *Diabetes Care*, **31**(2), 369–371.

Helmerhorst, H.J., Brage, S., Warren, J. *et al.* (2012) A systematic review of reliability and objective criterion-related validity of physical activity questionnaires. *The International Journal of Behavioral Nutrition and Physical Activity*, **9**, 103.

Hendelman, D., Miller, K., Baggett, C. *et al.* (2000) Validity of accelerometry for the assessment of moderate intensity physical activity in the field. *Medicine and Science in Sports and Exercise*, **32**(9 Suppl), S442–S449.

Jacobs, D.R., Jr, Ainsworth, B.E., Hartman, T.J. and Leon, A.S. (1993) A simultaneous evaluation of 10 commonly used physical activity questionnaires. *Medicine and Science in Sports and Exercise*, **25**(1), 81–91.

John, D. and Freedson, P. (2012) ActiGraph and Actical physical activity monitors: a peek under the hood. *Medicine and Science in Sports and Exercise*, **44**(1 Suppl 1), S86–S89.

John, D., Tyo, B. and Bassett, D.R. (2010) Comparison of four Actigraph accelerometers during walking and running. *Medicine and Science in Sports and Exercise*, **42**(2), 368–374.

Kolle, E., Steene-Johannessen, J., Andersen, L.B. and Anderssen, S.A. (2010) Objectively assessed physical activity and aerobic fitness in a population-based sample of Norwegian 9- and 15-year-olds. *Scandinavian Journal of Medicine & Science in Sports*, **20**(1), e41–e47.

Lee, I.M., Shiroma, E.J., Lobelo, F. *et al.* (2012) Effect of physical inactivity on major non-communicable diseases worldwide: an analysis of burden of disease and life expectancy. *The Lancet*, **380**(9838), 219–229.

Lifson, N., Gordon, G.B. and McClintock, R. (1955) Measurement of total carbon dioxide production by means of D_2O^{18}. *Journal of Applied Physiology*, **7**(6), 704–710.

Livingstone, M.B., Prentice, A.M., Coward, W.A. *et al.* (1990) Simultaneous measurement of free-living energy expenditure by the doubly labeled water method and heart-rate monitoring. *The American Journal of Clinical Nutrition*, **52**(1), 59–65.

Livingstone, M.B., Coward, W.A., Prentice, A.M. *et al.* (1992) Daily energy expenditure in free-living children: comparison of heart-rate monitoring with the doubly labeled water ($^2H_2^{18}O$) method. *The American Journal of Clinical Nutrition*, **56**(2), 343–352.

Mathie, M.J., Coster, A.C., Lovell, N.H. and Celler, B.G. (2004) Accelerometry: providing an integrated, practical method for long-term, ambulatory monitoring of human movement. *Physiological Measurement*, **25**(2), R1–R20.

Matthews, C.E. (2005) Calibration of accelerometer output for adults. *Medicine and Science in Sports and Exercise*, **37**(11 Suppl), S512–S522.

Matthews, C.E., Chen, K.Y., Freedson, P.S. *et al.* (2008) Amount of time spent in sedentary behaviors in the United States, 2003–2004. *American Journal of Epidemiology*, **167**(7), 875–881.

Merom, D., Rissel, C., Phongsavan, P. *et al.* (2007) Promoting walking with pedometers in the community: the step-by-step trial. *American Journal of Preventive Medicine*, **32**(4), 290–297.

Milton, K., Bull, F.C. and Bauman, A. (2011) Reliability and validity testing of a single-item physical activity measure. *British Journal of Sports Medicine*, **45**(3), 203–208.

Montoye, H.J., Kemper, H.C.G., Saris, W.H.M. and Washburn, R.A. (1996) *Measuring Physical Activity and Energy Expenditure*. Human Kinetics, Champaign, IL.

Nelson, M.D., Petersen, S.R. and Dlin, R.A. (2010) Effects of age and counseling on the cardiorespiratory response to graded exercise. *Medicine and Science in Sports and Exercise*, **42**(2), 255–264.

Nokes, N. (2009) Relationship between physical activity and aerobic fitness. *The Journal of Sports Medicine and Physical Fitness*, **49**(2), 136–141.

Owen, N., Leslie, E., Salmon, J. and Fotheringham, M.J. (2000) Environmental determinants of physical activity and sedentary behavior. *Exercise and Sport Sciences Reviews*, **28**(4), 153–158.

Paffenbarger, R.S., Jr, Blair, S.N., Lee, I.M. and Hyde, R.T. (1993) Measurement of physical activity to assess health effects in free-living populations. *Medicine and Science in Sports and Exercise*, **25**(1), 60–70.

Pereira, M.A., FitzerGerald, S.J., Gregg, E.W. *et al.* (1997) A collection of physical activity questionnaires for health-related research. *Medicine and Science in Sports and Exercise*, **29**(6 Suppl), S1–S205.

Peters, T., Brage, S., Westgate, K. *et al.* (2012) Validity of a short questionnaire to assess physical activity in 10 European countries. *European Journal of Epidemiology*, **27**(1), 15–25.

Plasqui, G. and Westerterp, K.R. (2007) Physical activity assessment with accelerometers: an evaluation against doubly labeled water. *Obesity.(Silver Spring)*, **15**(10), 2371–2379.

Plasqui, G., Bonomi, A.G. and Westerterp, K.R. (2013) Daily physical activity assessment with accelerometers: new insights and validation studies. *Obesity Reviews*, **14**(6), 451–462.

Pober, D.M., Staudenmayer, J., Raphael, C. and Freedson, P.S. (2006) Development of novel techniques to classify physical activity mode using accelerometers. *Medicine and Science in Sports and Exercise*, **38**(9), 1626–1634.

Rennie, K.L. and Wareham, N.J. (1998) The validation of physical activity instruments for measuring energy expenditure: problems and pitfalls. *Public Health Nutrition*, **1**(4), 265–271.

Rothney, M.P., Neumann, M., Beziat, A. and Chen, K.Y. (2007) An artificial neural network model of energy expenditure using nonintegrated acceleration signals. *Journal of Applied Physiology*, **103**(4), 1419–1427.

Rothney, M.P., Schaefer, E.V., Neumann, M.M. *et al.* (2008) Validity of physical activity intensity predictions by ActiGraph, Actical, and RT3 accelerometers. *Obesity (Silver Spring)*, **16**(8), 1946–1952.

Routen, A.C., Upton, D., Edwards, M.G. and Peters, D.M. (2012) Discrepancies in accelerometer-measured physical activity in children due to cut-point non-equivalence and placement site. *Journal of Sports Sciences*, **30**(12), 1303–1310.

Sallis, J.F. and Saelens, B.E. (2000) Assessment of physical activity by self-report: status, limitations, and future directions. *Research Quarterly for Exercise and Sport*, **71**(2 Suppl), S1–S14.

Schneider, P.L., Crouter, S.E. and Bassett, D.R. (2004) Pedometer measures of free-living physical activity: comparison of 13 models. *Medicine and Science in Sports and Exercise*, **36**(2), 331–335.

Schoeller, D.A. and van Santen, E. (1982) Measurement of energy expenditure in humans by doubly labeled water method. *Journal of Applied Physiology*, **53**(4), 955–959.

Shephard, R.J. (2003) Limits to the measurement of habitual physical activity by questionnaires. *British Journal of Sports Medicine*, **37**(3), 197–206.

Shvartz, E. and Reibold, R.C. (1990) Aerobic fitness norms for males and females aged 6 to 75 years: a review. *Aviation, Space, and Environmental Medicine*, **61**(1), 3–11.

Sternfeld, B., Jiang, S.F., Picchi, T. *et al.* (2012) Evaluation of a cell phone-based physical activity diary. *Medicine and Science in Sports and Exercise*, **44**(3), 487–495.

Swartz, A.M., Strath, S.J., Bassett, D.R., Jr. *et al.* (2000) Estimation of energy expenditure using CSA accelerometers at hip and wrist sites. *Medicine and Science in Sports and Exercise*, **32**(9 Suppl), S450–S456.

Terwee, C.B., Bot, S.D., de Boer, M.R. *et al.* (2007) Quality criteria were proposed for measurement properties of health status questionnaires. *Journal of Clinical Epidemiology*, **60**(1), 34–42.

Tremblay, M.S., Colley, R.C., Saunders, T.J. *et al.* (2010) Physiological and health implications of a sedentary lifestyle. *Applied Physiology, Nutrition, and Metabolism,* **35**(6), 725–740.

Tudor-Locke, C., Ainsworth, B.E., Thompson, R.W. and Matthews, C.E. (2002a) Comparison of pedometer and accelerometer measures of free-living physical activity. *Medicine and Science in Sports and Exercise,* **34**(12), 2045–2051.

Tudor-Locke, C., Williams, J.E., Reis, J.P. and Pluto, D. (2002b) Utility of pedometers for assessing physical activity: convergent validity. *Sports Medicine,* **32**(12), 795–808.

Van Poppel, M.N., Chinapaw, M.J., Mokkink, L.B. *et al.* (2010) Physical activity questionnaires for adults: a systematic review of measurement properties. *Sports Medicine,* **40**(7), 565–600.

Wanner, M., Probst-Hensch, N., Kriemler, S. *et al.* (2013) What physical activity surveillance needs: validity of a single-item questionnaire. *British Journal of Sports Medicine,* **48**(21), 1570–1576.

Wareham, N.J. and Rennie, K.L. (1998) The assessment of physical activity in individuals and populations: why try to be more precise about how physical activity is assessed? *International Journal of Obesity and Related Metabolic Disorders,* **22**(Suppl 2), S30–S38.

Wareham, N.J., Jakes, R.W., Rennie, K.L. *et al.* (2002) Validity and repeatability of the EPIC-Norfolk Physical Activity Questionnaire. *International Journal of Epidemiology,* **31**(1), 168–174.

Warnecke, R.B., Johnson, T.P., Chavez, N. *et al.* (1997) Improving question wording in surveys of culturally diverse populations. *Annals of Epidemiology,* **7**(5), 334–342.

Warren, J.M., Ekelund, U., Besson, H. *et al.* (2010) Assessment of physical activity – a review of methodologies with reference to epidemiological research: a report of the exercise physiology section of the European Association of Cardiovascular Prevention and Rehabilitation. *European Journal of Cardiovascular Prevention and Rehabilitation,* **17**(2), 127–139.

Welk, G.J. (2002) *Physical Activity Assessments for Health-related Research.* Human Kinetics, Champaign, IL.

Westerterp, K.R. (2003) Impacts of vigorous and non-vigorous activity on daily energy expenditure. *Proceedings of the Nutrition Society,* **62**(3), 645–650.

Westerterp, K.R. (2009) Assessment of physical activity: a critical appraisal. *European Journal of Applied Physiology,* **105**(6), 823–828.

Wickel, E.E., Welk, G.J. and Eisenmann, J.C. (2006) Concurrent validation of the Bouchard diary with an accelerometry-based monitor. *Medicine and Science in Sports and Exercise,* **38**(2), 373–379.

World Health Organization (2009) *Global Health Risks. Mortality and Burden of Disease to Selected Major Risks.* World Health Organization, Geneva.

Part Two

Current State of Evidence

8
Poor Dietary Patterns

Judith L Buttriss and Anne P Nugent

Key messages

- Most countries have some form of assessment of intake of key foods and nutrients that provides information about current dietary patterns of intake and underpins public health policy. But, owing to considerable differences in methodology, it is difficult to make inter-country comparisons.
- Up-to-date food composition data are critical in the translation of information about food intake into nutrient intakes, which can be compared with dietary reference values.
- The increasing use of information about intake of nutrients allows us to overcome a dependence on information about foods, which can differ between countries. Nutrient-based analysis has the potential to inform policy across countries, particularly with increasing harmonisation of methodologies.
- The most recent analysis in the UK shows improvements over the past decade in intakes of sugars (especially among young children), salt, saturated fat and trans fatty acids; but except for trans fatty acids, intakes remain above recommended levels. Fibre intakes remain below recommendations.
- Indeed, in the UK, Ireland and elsewhere in Europe the prevailing dietary patterns are characterised by excessive intakes of saturates, free sugars, salt, low intakes of fibre and, particularly in teenagers and young adults, there is evidence of low intakes of some minerals and vitamins, notably iron, calcium, folate and vitamin A. There is also widespread evidence of low vitamin D status, and evidence of low folate status, which is of special concern in women of childbearing age.

- Many of the concerns reflect the global situation, where intakes of salt, saturates and free sugars are already too high (or rising) and iron, iodine, vitamin A and vitamin D are recognised as nutrients of concern.
- Among babies under 1 year old in the UK, there is limited adherence to the advice to breastfeed exclusively for the first 6 months, but nutrient intakes are generally adequate (with the exception of vitamin D and iron). Energy intakes are higher than recommended, and protein intakes are relatively high.
- Although children under the age of 11 typically have adequate micronutrient intakes, average intakes of free sugars, saturates and salt exceed recommendations, and fibre intakes are low.
- Teenage girls and women of childbearing age seem to be particularly vulnerable from a dietary perspective, particularly in terms of the micronutrient density of their diets. The importance of this is particularly noteworthy as evidence emerges about the importance of nutrition during early life on the health prospects of the unborn child.
- Older adults often have better diets than younger adults; it is as yet unclear whether the dietary patterns reported in younger adults will continue (track) as they age or improve over time.
- Food-based dietary guidelines and related tools have been developed in most western countries and can be used to help people move towards a more healthy diet.

8.1 Introduction

Most countries have some form of assessment of intake of key foods and nutrients, which vary in extent and sophistication and are a key tool in understanding current patterns of intake, and addressing and monitoring issues relating to the safety of food and nutrient intake. They also underpin public health policy, and in some countries they inform food reformulation initiatives to offer healthier choices. Government-funded surveys, such as the UK's National Diet and Nutrition Surveys (NDNS) that measure the food and drinks consumed by individuals and the UK's Family Food survey that measures household purchases, can be used to explore the food and nutrient intakes and dietary patterns of population groups of different age or sex, socio-economic circumstance or ethnicity (see Chapter 4). The predecessor of the annual Family

Public Health Nutrition, Second Edition. Edited by Judith L Buttriss, Ailsa A Welch, John M Kearney and Susan A Lanham-New.
© 2018 by The Nutrition Society. Published 2018 by John Wiley & Sons, Ltd.
Companion website: www.wiley.com/go/buttriss/publichealth

Food survey, the National Food Survey, began more than 60 years ago and allows the tracking of trends in household food supply during this period.

The NDNS is a nationally representative programme of surveys designed to assess the diet, nutrient intake and nutritional status of the general population aged 1.5 years and over living in private households in the UK. It began in 1992 and comprised a series of cross sectional surveys of different age groups, but since 2008 it has been a rolling programme (data are collected in a continuous manner). Recently, a national survey of UK children aged 4–18 months, the Diet and Nutrition Survey of Infants and Young Children (DNSIYC), has been published, and UK Infant Feeding surveys are conducted every 10 years. More information about such surveys, including their limitations, such as underreporting, is given in Chapter 4.

Using food composition data (see Chapter 7), the dietary information collected can be transformed into information about the nutrient composition of the diets of different groups. By comparing this information with food-based dietary guidelines and the dietary reference values (DRVs) established by national governments and other competent bodies, such as the World Health Organization (WHO) and the European Food Safety Authority (EFSA) (see Chapter 8), an idea of the appropriateness of nutrient intakes and their associated dietary patterns can be established for various population groups. This chapter focuses primarily on inadequate/ 'poor' dietary patterns in the UK, with some comparison with Ireland.

Thus, using this sort of survey data it is relatively easy to identify average intakes of individual nutrients or specific foods or components in the general population or subpopulations, and potential inadequacies can be identified. However, until recently, less work has been done to capture information about dietary patterns: the combinations of foods consumed by individuals. Using either complex statistical techniques (e.g. principal component (factor) or cluster analysis) or by creating theoretically driven measures of dietary quality, dietary patterns can be identified. These patterns allow investigation of the types of foods consumed by those who do/ do not achieve food-based dietary guidelines and can be used to improve the efficacy of public health recommendations (Hu, 2002). Use of such techniques is discussed briefly later in the chapter.

Before considering the evidence from dietary surveys, it is worth noting that the comparisons in this chapter are made using current dietary and nutrient population-orientated recommendations that have often been established using surrogate markers of disease (e.g. the association with raised blood cholesterol levels in the case of saturated fatty acids) rather than a direct association with a disease outcome. It is recognised that the presence of markers of disease risk does not necessarily translate into disease, especially when dietary components can affect risk factors in different directions, as in cardiovascular disease (Sanders, 2014). Also, DRVs can differ nationally, globally and also change from time to time within the one country. For example, the Scientific Advisory Committee on Nutrition that advises the government in the UK proposed in June 2014 that the DRV for fibre should be increased (to 30 g AOAC fibre per day in adults) and that, on average across the population, intakes of free sugars (all added sugars plus those in fruit juice, honey and syrups) should not exceed 5% of total dietary energy. These recommendations, among others concerning carbohydrate, were subject to public consultation during 2014, have since been confirmed (SACN, 2015a) and adopted by ministers, and will in due course be adopted in the reporting of dietary surveys in the UK.

8.2 Overview of current diets in the UK

Children aged 0–18 months

The data on breastfeeding incidence, duration and frequency of feeding from the DNSIYC (Lennox et al., 2013) is similar to the findings of the 2010 Infant Feeding Survey (McAndrew et al., 2012), in which 78% and 76% respectively were breastfed at least once. In the DNSIYC, of those who were breastfed, the majority (57%) were not breastfed beyond 3 months of age and a further 22% had their last breast milk between 4 and 6 months. Despite the recommendation to breastfeed exclusively for the first 6 months, very few babies (1%) were exclusively breastfed to the age of 6 months in the 2010 Infant Feeding Survey (Figure 8.1). Associated with advice about breastfeeding, the advice on the introduction of complementary foods is that it should start at about 6 months. Yet as shown in Table 8.1, the majority of babies receive foods other than milk well before this age, although the situation has improved since 2005 – see British Nutrition Foundation (2013). In the 2010 Infant Feeding Survey and DNSIYC, 75% of children had received complementary foods by 5 months of age

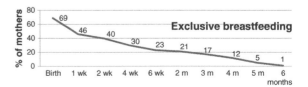

Figure 8.1 Prevalence of exclusive breastfeeding up to 6 months in the UK in 2010 (Infant Feeding Survey 2010). *Source:* McAndrew *et al.* (2012). Reproduced under OGL.

Table 8.1 Proportion of mothers introducing solids during different age periods: 2005 versus 2010.

Age of solids introduction	Mothers introducing solids (%)	
	2005	2010
6 weeks	1	2
8 weeks	2	2
3 months	10	5
4 months	51	30
5 months	82	75
6 months	98	94
9 months	100	99

Data extracted from Infant Feeding surveys: see British Nutrition Foundation (2013) for a more detailed summary for different parts of the UK.

and 94% by 6 months in the Infant Feeding Survey (97% in DNSIYC).

In the DNSIYC, the majority of children (75% of boys and 76% of girls) exceeded the estimated average requirements (EARs) for energy established in 2011, which are lower than the 1991 EARs. Protein intakes were higher than the reference nutrient intake (RNI) for 1- to 3-year-olds (14.5 g/day) in both the DNSIYC and NDNS of young children: 38 g and 42 g respectively in children aged 12–18 months and 18–36 months (Table 8.2).

With the exception of vitamin D and iron, children generally met the dietary recommendations for micronutrients. Vitamin D intakes (including supplements) averaged only 55% of the RNI in children aged 12–18 months and 33% of the RNI for those aged 18–35 months, raising concern about suboptimal vitamin D status during the winter months for the majority of

children in this age group, especially when skin exposure during the summer is limited. At the time of the surveys, UK health departments recommended that all infants and young children aged 6 months to 3 years take a daily vitamin D supplement (8.5 µg for 0–6 months and 7 µg for 6 months to 3 years) as it is difficult to achieve the recommended amount of 5 µg/day from diet alone. Yet, during the 4-day recording period, only around 1 in 10 children aged 12–36 months received any vitamin D from supplements. In children aged 10–12 months, 88% received a vitamin-D-fortified milk (infant formula or follow-on formula), but this fell to 39% in children aged 12–18 months (Lennox *et al.*, 2013). Vitamin D recommendations have since been increased to 10 µg per day for those over 4 years of age (8.8-10 µg/day for children under 4 years (SACN 2016).

Over the 4-day food diary period of the survey, the proportion of children given a micronutrient supplement ranged from 5% for those aged 4–6 months to 10% for those aged 12–18 months. This was most often a multivitamin supplement and was more likely in children of South Asian and 'other' ethnicities (versus white children). Usage was low despite the long-standing recommendation regarding use of supplements providing vitamins A, C and D.

Figure 8.2 shows the vitamin D intakes in children aged 4–18 months compared with the RNI in place at the time. For children who are breastfed, intakes are generally low, while in non-breastfed children the vitamin D intakes fall as the child moves from a predominantly milk-based diet to a mixed diet. By comparison, in countries where cows' milk is routinely fortified with vitamin D, such as the USA, children aged 12–35 months have mean vitamin D intakes of 8–9 µg/day (Butte *et al.*, 2010; Dwyer *et al.*, 2010). The implications of these findings have recently been considered by the UK

Table 8.2 Macronutrient intakes in children aged 4–36 months.

	Age group (months)				
	4–6	7–9	10–11	12–18	18–36*
Protein (g)	18.1	24.7	29.5	37.7	42.0
Total fat (% energy)	40.5	36.2	35.4	35.4	34.1
Saturated fatty acids (% energy)	17.9	15.7	15.2	16.3	15.1
Total carbohydrate (% energy)	49.7	51.6	51.1	49.0	59.6
Total sugars (% energy)	38.4	32.7	29.4	25.8	N/A
NMES (% energy)	4.3	6.2	6.2	7.7	11.5
NSP (g)	4.6	6.3	7.2	7.3	8.1

Sources: DNSIYC (Lennox *et al.*, 2013); *NDNS Rolling Programme (Bates *et al.*, 2014).

NMES: non-milk extrinsic sugars; NSP: non-starch polysaccharides.

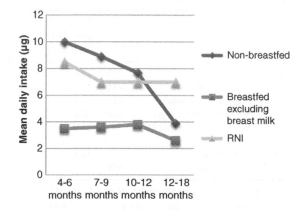

Figure 8.2 Vitamin D intake of breastfed versus non-breastfed babies. *Source:* Lennox *et al.* (2013: table 6.20). Reproduced under OGL.

Government's Scientific Advisory Committee on Nutrition (SACN); a draft report recommending revised recommendations was published in 2015 (SACN, 2015b) (see Chapter 20 on bone health); the final report was published in 2016 (SACN, 2016).

Iron deficiency is the most commonly reported nutritional disorder during early childhood across most of Europe as well as globally. Intakes of iron were below the EAR in more than 30% of children aged 18–35 months living in the UK and 7% had intakes below the LRNI (the lower reference nutrient intake – LRNI – for a vitamin or mineral is set at a level of intake considered likely to be sufficient to meet the needs of only 2.5% of the population). The DNSIYC food consumption data showed that iron intakes fall after age 12 months in line with a reduction in (fortified) formula milk consumption; in children aged 12–18 months, cereal foods provide 41% of the daily intake of 6.4 mg.

So, overall, a picture is painted of limited adherence to the advice to breastfeed exclusively for the first 6 months coupled with adequate nutrient intakes in the main (with the exception of vitamin D and iron) but higher energy intakes than recommended and relatively high protein intakes. Nutrition for this age group is discussed in more detail in Chapter 12.

The survey does not specifically provide information on the dietary patterns associated with poor or adequate nutrient intakes. Of interest, it is evident that fruit and vegetable intakes are relatively high compared with older children, as discussed in more detail later. There is currently no recommendation for the number of portions of fruit and vegetables consumed per day or recommended portion sizes for young children, but data from DNSIYC show that children aged 4–18

months are on average consuming about one to two adult portions (100–170 g) a day.

Older children and adults

Macronutrients and dietary fibre

Results from the NDNS rolling programme show that diet and nutrient intakes of the UK population are largely similar to findings from previous assessments but, where trends exist, they are largely in the direction of UK dietary recommendations. For example, expressed in food energy terms, trans fatty acid, saturated fatty acid, total fat and NMES intakes have continued to fall over the past decade. For example, in the 1986–1987 survey, saturates provided 16.5% energy in men and 17% in women, and total fat 40.4% and 40.3% energy respectively. Table 8.3 illustrates changes among adults over the past decade, in terms of the DRVs existing at the time.

Since these data were published, new recommendations for dietary fibre and a new recommendation of <5% dietary energy from free sugars (SACN, 2015a) have been adopted by the UK Government. Free sugars are those added by the manufacturer, cook or consumer plus those present in fruit juices, honey and syrups (i.e. those not present in intact fruit/vegetables or in milk). A detailed definition of free sugars is expected to be published in 2017, but for the purposes of this chapter it can be assumed that NMES and free sugars values are similar. Mean energy intakes were: 2111 kcal/day and 1613 kcal/day in men and women respectively aged 19–64; 1935 kcal/day and 1510 kcal/day in men and women respectively aged 65 and over; 1126 kcal/day in children aged 1.5–3 years; 1532 kcal/day in children aged

Table 8.3 Macronutrient intakes in adults, 2000–2001 compared with 2008–2012.

	DRV	Men and women (combined) aged 19–64 2008–2012	Men, 19–64 years		Women, 19–64 years	
			2000–2001	2008–2012	2000–2001	2008–2012
Total fat (% food energy)	<35	34.6	35.8	34.8	34.9	34.5
Saturated fat (% food energy)	<11	12.6	13.4	12.6	13.2	12.6
Trans fatty acids (% food energy)	<2	0.7	1.2	0.7	1.2	0.7
Total carbohydrate (% food energy)	>50	48.0	47.7	47.8	48.5	48.2
Starch and sugars in milk and fruit (% food energy)	>39	35.8	34.9	35.1	37.0	36.6
NMES[a] (% food energy)	<11	12.1	13.6	12.7	11.9	11.6
Dietary fibre, NSP[b] (g/day)	>18	13.7	15.2	14.7	12.6	12.8

Source: data extracted from Henderson *et al.* (2002) and Bates *et al.* (2014).

[a] In 2015, a new reference value for free sugars (<5% of total dietary energy) was adopted (SACN, 2015a).

[b] In 2015, new reference values for fibre for people of different ages were adopted (SACN, 2015a). For adults the new recommendation is 30 g AOAC fibre per day; the old value of 18 g/day (expressed as NSP fibre) equates to 23–24 g/day AOAC fibre and current intakes are about 18 g AOAC fibre per day in adults.

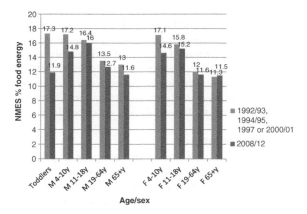

Figure 8.3 NMES intakes as a percentage of food energy in NDNS 2008–2012, compared with previous surveys. *Source:* Bates *et al.* (2014). Reproduced under OGL.

4–10 years; and 1776 kcal/day in 11- to 18-year-olds (Bates *et al.*, 2014). The NDNS report notes the fact that underreporting is a feature of all dietary surveys (see Chapter 4 for a more detailed discussion). Intake of total fat met the recommendation (no more than 35% food energy) in all age/sex groups except men aged 65 and over (36.0%). Mean daily intakes of saturated fatty acids exceeded the 11% food energy recommendation: 12.6% of energy in adults, 12.5% for those aged 11–18 years and 13.2% for those aged 4–10 years. Milk and milk products were the main contributors for younger children (46% for children aged 4–10 years versus 22% for older children and adults); the major contributor within this group was cheese. In older children and adults, the major contributor was meat and meat products, providing about a quarter of intake. Cereals and cereal products also made a substantial contribution, ranging from 18% for the youngest children to 20% in adults and 25% in

children aged 4–18 years. Mean daily trans fatty acid intakes are now well below the recommended upper limit of 2% of energy at 0.6–0.7% of energy for all age groups.

Mean daily NMES intakes exceeded the 11% food energy (excluding alcohol) recommendation in all age groups, most notably children aged 11–18 years (15.6% food energy). Contributions of NMES to energy intake were reduced compared with past surveys in all groups except women (see Figure 8.3) but have remained fairly static over the period 2008–2012 (Bates *et al.*, 2014). For toddlers (1.5–3 years), there was a marked fall in energy from NMES from 17.3% of food energy in a previous survey to 11.9%, reflecting a marked fall in soft drink consumption in this age group. Table 8.4 shows the main dietary sources of NMES for different age groups.

In general, the major sources of NMES were non-alcoholic beverages, cereals and cereal products, confectionery and fruit juice. Soft drinks contributed 16% of NMES intake for adults, 17% for children aged 4–10 years, 12% for toddlers (a fall from 32%) and 30% for those aged 11–18 years. Except for toddlers, these contributions were similar to previous surveys. Cereals and cereal products together contributed 21% of NMES intake for adults, 29% in children aged 4–10 years and 22% in 11- to 18-year-olds. Sugars, preserves and confectionary together provided about 26% for adults and slightly less for children, compared with over 30% in previous surveys.

Energy-dense diets, such as those high in sugars, can contribute to excess energy intake, which if sustained can lead to excess weight gain. Obesity prevalence has become a major public health concern (see Chapter 16), with a marked relationship with deprivation in the UK, especially among children (Public Health England, 2014a). Sugars intake is also of concern in relation to dental health; almost a third of 5-year-olds in England

Table 8.4 Major contributors to total NMES intake in the UK.

Source	Contribution to total NMES intake by age (%)				
	1.5–3 years	4–10 years	11–18 years	19–64 years	≥65 years
Soft drinks[a]	12	17	30	16	8
Fruit juice	14	13	10	8	8
Biscuits	8	8	7	6	7
Buns, cakes, pastries and fruit pies	6	9	6	7	13
Breakfast cereals	6	8	6	6	5
Puddings	3	3	2	2	4
Table sugars and preserves	7	7	8	17	21
Confectionery	12	14	13	9	5
Alcoholic drinks	—	—	2	10	6

Source: Bates *et al.* (2014). Reproduced under OGL.

[a] Soft drinks includes carbonated drinks, squashes, cordials.

have tooth decay (Public Health England, 2013). As a result, Public Health England is placing particular emphasis on 'free' sugars reduction; namely, those sugars not present in intact fruit or in milk. They announced a work package in June 2014 (Public Health England, 2014b) and published a package of recommendations to achieve sugar reduction in October 2015 (Public Health England, 2015a). For a discussion of these recommendations, see Chapter 24.

Dietary fibre intakes published in 2014 remained below the recommendation of at least 18 g/day NSP (equivalent to 23–24 g fibre measured by the AOAC method required in EU legislation), at 13.8 g/day in adults (equivalent to about 18 g AOAC fibre), 11.8 g/day in children and 8.2 g/day in toddlers (1.5–3 years). This means that intakes in children have risen slightly and adult intakes have remained the same. Cereal and cereal products provided 39% of intake in adults and 42% in children aged 4–10 and 11–18 years. Vegetables and potatoes were the second major contributor, with contribution increasing with age from 24% to 32%.

Recommendations from SACN, recently adopted by the UK Government, indicate that evidence for the relationship between dietary fibre intake and health (especially digestive health and cardiovascular health) has strengthened and that the population DRV should be increased from approximately 23–24 g/day to 30 g/day of AOAC fibre for adults (with proportionately lower daily values for children of 15 g, 20 g and 25 g for those aged 2–5 years, 5–11 years and 11–16 years respectively) (SACN, 2015a). Achieving the new DRVs will mean that men would on average need to increase their fibre intake by 50% (current mean intakes are 10–11 g below the proposed reference value) and women by around 75% (current mean intakes are 13 g below the proposed reference value). For children, the shortfalls are estimated to be 4–6 g/day for those aged 2–10 years and 9 g/day for those aged 11–16 years (SACN, 2015a). SACN advises that the 30 g could be achieved by consuming all of the following on a daily basis: five portions of fruit and vegetables, two slices of wholemeal bread, a portion of high-fibre breakfast cereal, a baked potato and a portion of whole-wheat pasta. To put this advice in context, the NDNS shows that only 30% of adults (and less than 10% of 11- to 18-year-olds) are currently achieving the five a day recommendation. The top 20 foods contributing to current fibre intakes in a range of age groups in the UK are shown in Table 8.5. Examples of diets providing 30 g of fibre and <5% dietary energy as free sugars can be found at https://www.nutrition.org.uk/attachments/article/881/SACN%20guidelines%20meal%20planner.pdf.

For both sugars and dietary fibre, there is evidence in the NDNS and other surveys of a socio-economic gradient, with higher intakes of NMES as a percentage of energy for adults and lower intakes of dietary fibre for both adults and children in the lower income groups. Achieving these proposed targets will require substantial changes in the dietary patterns of many, incorporating more high-fibre starchy foods, pulses, fruits and vegetables to bring them closer to the dietary pattern illustrated in the government's Eatwell Guide, described later.

Micronutrient intakes

Micronutrient intakes are mainly adequate in primary school-age children, but low intakes of some micronutrients are evident, especially among girls in the teenage years and young women (see later). Sodium intakes are higher than recommendations (expressed as salt, sodium chloride) in all age groups.

Salt intakes have fallen by an average of 1.5 g in adults over the past decade. NDNS data from 2011 give the average intake in adults as 8.1 g/day against a target of <6 g/day; a more recent estimate of intake in older adults aged 65 years and older is 7.2 g/day (SACN, 2015a). Intakes in children are 3.7 g/day (children aged 4–6; target <3 g/day); 5.0 g/day (children aged 7–10 years; target <5 g/day); 6.6 g/day (children aged 11–18 years; target <6 g/day).

Mean daily intakes of vitamins (except vitamin D) from food sources were close to or above the RNI for all groups. Intakes of vitamin D were well below the RNI (which existed at the time for children under 4 years and for adults over 65) even when contribution from dietary supplements was taken into account: 32% of the RNI for children aged 1.5–3 years and 51% of the RNI for adults aged 65 years and over. The group of foods comprising meat and meat products was the major contributor for all age groups except children aged 1.5–3 years, providing 23–35% of intake. Milk/milk products were the major source for those aged 1.5–3 years, providing 24%. Fat spreads, most of which contain added vitamin D, contributed 19–21% across the age groups, cereals/cereal products provided 13–20% and fish/fish dishes provided 17–23% in adults and 8–9% in children. In 2015, SACN proposed a new population-wide reference value for vitamin D of 10 µg/day for those aged 4 years and over, and a safe intake of 8.5–10 µg/day for those under the age of 4 years (SACN, 2015b). For further information, see Chapter 20.

As shown in Table 8.6, among children aged 11–18 years, 11% of boys and 14% of girls had vitamin A intakes below the LRNI; the contribution of dietary supplements did not reduce the proportions below the LRNI. For riboflavin, 9% of boys and 21% of girls aged 11–18 years had riboflavin intakes below the LRNI.

Mean daily intakes of minerals from the diet were below the RNI for some age groups, in particular children

Table 8.5 Top 20 contributors to NSP fibre intake in different age groups.

	Contribution to daily NSP fibre intake (g [%])				
	1.5–3 years	4–10 years	11–18 years	19–64 years	≥65 years
Vegetables and vegetable-based dishes	1.5 [18.5]	2.1 [18.4]	2.1 [18]	3.3 [24.2]	3.3 [25.0]
Fruit	1.3 [16.3]	1.5 [13.1]	0.9 [7.2]	1.4 [10.2]	1.8 [13.5]
White bread	0.5 [6.1]	0.9 [8.1]	1.2 [10.1]	1.0 [7.6]	0.9 [6.6]
Wholemeal bread	0.4 [4.8]	0.4 [4.0]	0.4 [3.4]	0.9 [6.6]	0.9 [6.6]
Wholegrain and high-fibre breakfast cereals	0.8 [10.1]	0.9 [7.7]	0.5 [4.6]	0.8 [6.1]	1.1 [8.5]
Chips, fried potatoes and potato products	0.4 [5.2]	0.8 [7.3]	1.2 [10.3]	0.9 [6.3]	0.6 [4.9]
Boiled, mashed, baked potatoes	0.3 [3.9]	0.4 [3.9]	0.5 [4.6]	0.7 [5.3]	0.9 [6.8]
Brown, granary and wheatgerm bread	0.4 [5.2]	0.6 [5.3]	0.5 [4.1]	0.6 [4.0]	0.6 [4.2]
Pasta and pasta-based dishes	0.4 [5.1]	0.5 [4.4]	0.6 [4.9]	0.5 [3.3]	0.2 [1.5]
Biscuits	0.3 [3.2]	0.3 [3.1]	0.4 [3.2]	0.4 [2.7]	0.4 [2.7]
Savoury sauces, pickles and condiments	0.1[1.2]	0.2 [1.5]	0.3 [2.3]	0.3 [2.3]	0.2 [1.3]
Crisps and savoury snacks	0.1 [1.8]	0.4 [3.3]	0.5 [4.2]	0.3 [2.0]	0.1 [0.7]
Pizza	0.1 [1.2]	0.3 [2.5]	0.5 [3.9]	0.3 [1.9]	Not top 20
Other cereals (e.g. couscous, oats, semolina)	0.1 [1.1]	0.1 [1.2]	0.2[1.3]	0.2 [1.8]	0.2 [1.7]
Buns, cakes, pastries	0.1 [1.4]	0.3 [2.6]	0.2 [2.1]	0.2 [1.8]	0.4 [2.9]
Sausages and sausage-based dishes	0.2 [2.3]	0.3 [2.3]	0.2 [2.1]	0.2 [1.5]	0.1 [1.0]
Nuts and seeds	Not top 20	Not top 20	Not top 20	0.2 [1.2]	0.1 [0.9]
Rice	Not top 20	Not top 20	Not top 20	0.1 [0.9]	Not top 20
Other breakfast cereals (not high fibre)	0.1 [1.2]	0.2 [1.7]	0.2 [1.8]	0.1 [0.9]	0.1 [0.7]
Chocolate confectionery	Not top 20	Not top 20	0.1 [1.2]	0.1 [1.0]	Not top 20
Meat pies and pastries	0.1 [0.9]	0.1 [0.7]	0.1 [1.0]	Not top 20	Not top 20
Milk and cream	0.1 [1.8]	Not top 20	Not top 20	Not top 20	Not top 20
Commercial toddler foods	0.1 [0.9]	Not top 20	Not top 20	Not top 20	Not top 20
White fish, coated or fried	Not top 20	0.1 [0.7]	Not top 20	Not top 20	Not top 20
Fruit juice	Not top 20	0.1 [0.7]	Not top 20	Not top 20	Not top 20
Burgers and kebabs	Not top 20	Not top 20	0.1 [1.1]	Not top 20	Not top 20
Soup	Not top 20	Not top 20	Not top 20	Not top 20	0.2 [1.4]
Cereal-based puddings (including sponge and rice)	Not top 20	Not top 20	Not top 20	Not top 20	[1.1]
Other bread (e.g. rye, gluten free, oatmeal)	Not top 20	Not top 20	Not top 20	Not top 20	0.1 [0.8]

Source: SACN (2015a).

NDNS 2008–2009 and 2009–2010 combined.

Table 8.6 Micronutrient intakes in different age and sex groups, showing the percentage with intakes below the LRNI.[a]

	Male (% below LRNI)				Female (% below LRNI)			
	4–10 years	11–18 years	19–64 years	≥65 years	4–10 years	11–18 years	19–64 years	≥65 years
Vitamin A	5	11	11	4	7	14	5	1
Riboflavin	0	9	5	5	1	21	12	3
Folate	0	4	2	1	0	8	4	1
Iron	1	7	1	2	1	46	23	2
Calcium	1	8	5	3	3	19	8	4
Magnesium	0	28	16	19	3	53	11	8
Potassium	0	16	11	13	0	33	23	14
Zinc	7	12	9	10	11	22	4	1
Selenium	0	22	12	30	2	46	51	52
Iodine	2	9	6	1	4	22	10	3

Source: Bates *et al.* (2014). Reproduced under OGL.

[a] The LRNI for a vitamin or mineral is set at a level of intake considered likely to be sufficient to meet the needs of only 2.5% of the population. Bates *et al.* (2014) note that DRVs for some nutrients – such as magnesium, potassium, selenium and zinc – are based on very limited data and so caution should be used when assessing adequacy of intake using the LRNI.

Table 8.7 Prevalence of intakes of iron, calcium and folate below the LRNI, by age group.

	Those with intakes below the LRNI (%)			
	11–15 years	16–24 years	25–49 years	50–64 years
Females				
Iron	44	40	29	5
Calcium	18	16	8	7
Folate	7	9	4	2
Males				
Iron	6	4	1	2
Calcium	7	9	6	2
Folate	4	3	2	1

Source: Bates *et al.* (2014). Reproduced under OGL.

Table 8.8 Prevalence of low vitamin D status (plasma 25-hydroxyvitamin D <25 nmol/L).

	Males (%)	Females (%)
1.5–3 years	7.5 (males and females combined)	
4–10 years	12.3	15.6
11–18 years	19.7	24.4
19–64 years	24.0	21.7
≥65 years	16.9	24.1

Source: Bates *et al.* (2014). Reproduced under OGL.

aged 11–18 years. Furthermore, a substantial proportion of this age group, particularly girls, has intakes below the LRNI (Table 8.6). Mean daily intakes of iron were below the RNI in girls aged 11–18 years and women aged 19–64 years, and 46% of girls and 23% of women (19–64 years) have intakes below the LRNI (Table 8.6). Use of supplements had little effect on the proportions below the LRNI. The low intakes of iron reported in teenage girls continued into early adulthood (Table 8.6). The proportion of teenage girls with intakes below the LRNI for iodine is also of concern, not least because of the importance of iodine during pregnancy. Mean daily intakes of all minerals were above the RNIs in children under 11 years, and few children in this age group had intakes below the LRNI.

In girls aged 11–15 years, the median intake of iron was 55% of the RNI, rising slightly to 58% in 16- to 24-year-old women. Calcium intakes (expressed as per cent RNI) in these age groups were 81% and 84% respectively. By comparison, median intakes of iron for males aged 11–15 years and 16–24 years were 93% and 111% of the RNI respectively. For calcium in males, values were 83% and 111% respectively. Table 8.7 provides information for three nutrients of particular concern – calcium, iron and folate – illustrating that the low intakes of iron and calcium evident in teenage girls persist into early adulthood (and beyond for iron).

Micronutrient status

There is evidence of low vitamin D status (a plasma 25-hydroxyvitamin D below 25 nmol/L; see Table 8.8), and during the months January to March, 40% of children aged 11–18 years had low vitamin D status (Bates *et al.*, 2014).

Some ethnic groups living in the UK are particularly prone to vitamin D deficiency due to the dark pigmentation of their skin coupled with the lower level of sun

irradiation at UK latitudes, as well as cultural clothing norms that limit skin exposure. This was confirmed in the reanalysis of 1997 NDNS data, with 85% of non-white children having inadequate vitamin D levels (as judged by plasma levels below 50 nmol/L) compared with 30% of white children (Absoud *et al.*, 2011). In recent years a number of additional functions of vitamin D have been identified, over and above its role in bone health, and debate continues as to the best threshold to use as an indicator of inadequate status. This matter was considered by SACN, the UK Government's advisory committee. See Chapter 20 for more information.

The time spent exercising and playing outdoors has also been associated with vitamin D status. Children who exercise and play outdoors for at least 60 min a day had significantly higher vitamin D levels compared with those who spend less than 30 min per day outdoors. In contrast, spending more time watching TV was associated with lower vitamin D levels (Absoud *et al.*, 2011).

There also seem to be socio-economic differences, with children from families receiving income support having significantly lower vitamin D levels compared with those in families who do not receive income support (Absoud *et al.*, 2011). Dietary supply may be a factor (dietary sources include margarines/spreads, oily fish, vitamin-D-fortified breakfast cereals, eggs and meat), but the main contributor to vitamin D levels is considered to be sunlight exposure during the summer months – see Spiro and Buttriss (2014).

In the UK, people with dark skin and those who cover up have for some time been advised to take vitamin D supplements (10 μg/day). A daily 5 μg supplement has also been recommended for many years for all under-5s and 10 μg/day for pregnant and breastfeeding women; new population-wide recommendations were published by SACN in 2016.

The latest findings of the NDNS rolling programme indicate that 35.1% of children aged 1.5–3 years, 20.5% girls aged 4–10 years and 27.5% of 11- to 18-year-old girls have low plasma ferritin levels, suggestive of low iron stores; fewer boys of these ages are affected (11.7%

and 8% respectively). Among adults aged 19–64 years, 2.2% of men and 15.5% of women have low ferritin levels; among those aged 65 years and over the respective prevalences are 6.4% and 5.8% respectively. Low haemoglobin levels, indicating iron-deficiency anaemia, were found in 12.9% of children aged 1.5–3 years, 5.7% of girls aged 4–10 years and 7.4% of girls aged 11–18 years (the figures in boys were 3.1% and 1.8% aged 4–10 years and 11–18 years respectively) (Bates *et al.*, 2014). Prevalence was 1.5% in men aged 19–64 years and 15.2% in older men. In women, the prevalence was 9.9% and 12.3% respectively in those aged 19–64 years and 65 years and over. Iron deficiency (using an index that combines ferritin and haemoglobin measurements) was estimated to be present in 5.2% of children aged 1.3–3 years, 4.9% of girls aged 11–18 years, 4.7% of women aged 19–64 years and 3.1% of women over 65 years (prevalence was lower in other age/sex groups).

Another nutrient of concern is folate. One in five teenage girls and young women aged 16–24 years in the UK are deficient in the B vitamin folate, according to figures from NDNS, published in March 2015 (Public Health England, 2015b). Median blood levels are about half those in the USA, where flour is now fortified with folic acid, and similar to concentrations in the USA in the mid-1990s prior to the introduction of fortification. Folate deficiency results in a form of anaemia, and blood levels in early pregnancy predict risk of fetal neural tube defects (Chapter 11). The NDNS reveals that 85.5% of UK women aged 16–49 years fail to meet the blood folate level that minimises risk of a neural tube defect affected pregnancy.

Adherence to dietary recommendations

There is some evidence of an increase in consumption of fruit and to a lesser extent vegetables in children since previous NDNS surveys, but little change in adults. Intakes of fruit and vegetables combined (including that from composite dishes but not including juice) were higher in 4- to 10-year-olds (205 g/day) than in 11- to 18-year-olds (172 g/day). This was mainly due to a higher intake of fruit in the younger compared with the older age group (108 versus 60 g/day), although vegetable intake was lower in 4- to 10-year-olds compared with the older age group (97 versus 112 g/day). Only 9% of 11- to 18-year-olds achieved the recommended five portions a day – this information is not provided in the NDNS report for younger children because there is no set definition of what constitutes a portion of fruit or vegetables for young children. However, data from the DNSIYC show that children's mean consumption of fruit and vegetables (excluding juice) ranged from 100 g/day for children aged 4–6 months to 170 g/day for those aged 12–18 months; the equivalent of about one to two adult portions.

In the NDNS rolling programme (see Section 8.1 for a description and Chapter 4), adults on average consumed 4.1 portions of fruits and vegetables per day (including those provided by composite dishes and including up to one portion each of fruit juice and baked beans/pulses per day), with a range of 0.8 portions a day (lower 2.5 percentile) to 9.7 portions/day (upper 2.5 percentile) for men and 0.7–8.8 for women. For those aged 11–18 years, mean consumption was 3.0 portions a day for boys and 2.7 for girls. The proportion who met the five-a-day guideline was 7% of girls, and 10% of boys aged 11–18 years, 30% of women and 30% of men. In past surveys, the contribution of vegetables and fruit from composite dishes had not been taken into account; this underestimated vegetable intake by 25–35 g/day for children and 40–50 g/day for adults (and fruit intake by 2–6 g/day).

Two servings of fish each week are recommended, one of which should be an oily type (and hence a rich source of omega 3 fatty acids). Mean consumption of oily fish was well below the recommendation of one (140 g) serving a week; average intake was 54 g/week in adults and 14 g/week among children.

A disaggregation approach was also used for meat from all sources to separate meat and non-meat (e.g. pastry, vegetables) components of meat-based dishes. This resulted in estimates of meat intake falling considerably (as previous estimates had included all components of the meat dish, not just the meat itself). Total meat intake (including poultry) in 2008–2012 using the new method was 42 g/day for toddlers (under 4 years), 72 g/day for girls, 95 g/day for boys, 89 g/day for women and 130 g/day for men (compared with 64 g/day, 132 g/day, 159 g/day, 161 g/day and 217 g/day respectively), representing an approximate 40% reduction in reported consumption across all age/sex groups. The proportion of the meat that was 'red' meat ranged from 63% of the total for women to 71% for toddlers, and was 66% for men and 62% for children aged 11–18 years. The government recommendation for red and processed meat consumption is 70 g/day.

Income comparisons in the National Diet and Nutrition Surveys rolling programme

Energy and macronutrients

The 2014 NDNS report provides an analysis by equivalised household income (that takes account of household size and composition) divided into quintiles, with quintile 1 being the lowest equivalised income group and quintile 5 the highest. Some differences were observed in food consumption and intakes of energy and nutrients intakes, particularly for fruit and vegetable intake. Differences were clearest between the lowest and highest quintiles but were not seen in all age/sex groups. They were most evident in women aged 19–64 years, with total energy and protein significantly lower in quintiles 1, 2 and 3 than in quintile 5. Men and women aged 19–64 years had a lower percentage of energy from saturated fatty acids but a higher percentage energy from NMES in the lowest quintile compared with the highest, although intakes exceeded recommended levels (at that time, <11% food energy) in almost all quintiles. For example, in women aged 19–64 years, intakes of NMES in quintiles 1 (13.1%) and 2 (12.1%) were significantly higher than in quintile 5 (10.6%). In men aged 19–64 years, NMES intake was significantly higher in quintile 1 (15.5% food energy and 79.5 g/day) than in quintile 5 (12.4% food energy and 66 g/day). Conversely, in boys aged 4–10 years the mean percentage of food energy from NMES and intake in absolute terms were significantly lower in quintile 1 (14.0% and 59.1 g) than in quintile 5 (16.1% and 69 g). NSP intakes were significantly lower in the lowest quintile groups than in the highest in all age/sex groups, but intakes for adults were below the recommended 18 g NSP in all quintiles (the recommendation has since been increased; see earlier). For example, in women aged 19–64 years, mean intake was significantly lower in quintiles 1 (11.8 g), 2 (11.9 g) and 3 (12.6 g) than in quintile 5 (13.7 g).

Mean iron intake for girls aged 11–18 years and women aged 19–64 years was below 90% of the RNI in all income quintiles. In women, but not girls, the lowest income quintile had a significantly lower mean intake (8.7 mg) than the highest quintile (10.4 mg), and a significantly higher proportion had intakes below the LRNI: 39% in quintile 1, 29% in quintile 2, 20% in quintile 3 and 12% in quintile 5. No clear pattern was seen for girls aged 11–18 years.

For both men and women aged 19–64 years, mean intake of calcium increased from the lowest to highest quintile. In men, the mean intake was significantly lower in quintile 1 (768 mg) than in quintile 5 (940 mg). A similar pattern was observed in women, with mean intakes in quintiles 1 (686 mg), 2 (711 mg) and 3 (709 mg) being significantly lower than quintile 5 (748 mg). This pattern was also seen in girls aged 4–18 years, for whom intake in quintile 1 (686 mg) was significantly lower than in quintile 5 (748 mg). A substantial proportion of girls aged 11–18 years (15–21%) in all income quintiles had calcium intakes below the LRNI. There were clear differences in intakes of both vitamin C and folate by income quintile, with lower intakes in the lowest quintile. For vitamin C, mean intake was above the RNI in all quintiles, but girls aged 11–18 years had a mean folate intake below the RNI in the lowest income quintile.

Comparing income quintiles 1 and 5, mean fruit and vegetable consumption expressed in grams was significantly lower in children and in adults aged 19–64 years and was also significantly lower in children aged 11–18 years and adults aged 19–64 years when expressed as 'five-a-day' portions. The percentage achieving five portions of fruit and vegetables per day was significantly lower in boys aged 11–18 years in quintiles 1 (3%) and 2 (5%) than those in quintile 5 (18%). Similarly, the percentage of men aged 19–64 years achieving five portions was significantly lower in quintiles 2 (26%) and 3 (26%) than in quintile 5 (39%) and in women aged 19–64 years in quintiles 1 (23%) and 2 (23%) than in quintile 5 (36%). These findings are consistent with those of the Low Income Diet and Nutrition Survey that looked specifically at dietary intakes of families with low income (Nelson et al., 2007).

No clear pattern in total meat or red meat consumption was observed, with the exception of children aged 1.5–3 years, where mean consumption of total meat was significantly higher in income quintiles 1 and 2 than in quintile 5. Oily fish consumption increased from the lowest to highest quintile for men and women aged 19–64 years.

8.3 Micronutrient intakes in Europe

National nutrition surveys and the EU-funded EURRECA project (http://www.eurreca.org) have suggested there may be micronutrient insufficiencies in the European region, but lack of harmonisation of the survey approaches has hampered interpretation of the available data. Nutrition survey data from a range of European countries (Belgium, Denmark, France, Germany, Netherlands, Poland, Spain and the UK) have been used to investigate intakes of a number of micronutrients (calcium, copper, iodine, iron, magnesium, potassium, selenium, zinc; vitamins A, B1, B2, B6, B12, C, D, E and folate). Using a harmonised approach, the mean and fifth percentile intakes were defined for various age and sex groups, and compared with reference intakes derived from UK and Nordic Nutrition Recommendations (Mensink et al., 2013). For vitamins, with the exception of vitamin D, there was a low risk of low intakes. However, for minerals, there was evidence of an increased risk of low intakes in some groups. As in the UK, there is far less of a problem among 4- to 10-year-olds, but more than 5% of 11- to 17-year-olds had intakes below the LRNI for calcium, iron, magnesium, potassium, selenium and vitamin A (Mensink et al., 2013), and in some countries (for some nutrients) this rose to above 10%, showing that poor micronutrient intakes in sections of the population is not exclusively a UK problem.

So, even in the midst of an abundant dietary supply, concerns remain about the prevalence of suboptimal micronutrient intakes across the region.

Nutrient intakes in Ireland

For comparison with the predominantly UK data presented, the findings of recent dietary surveys in Ireland are now discussed. Over the past decade there have been a series of nationally representative food surveys in the Republic of Ireland in adults, children, teenagers and most recently young children aged 1–4 years, the top line results of which are summarised in Table 8.9 – for full details see Walton *et al.* (2014, 2017) and www.iuna.net. Direct comparisons with the UK surveys cannot easily be made as the methodologies are different and the recommendations used to benchmark intakes can differ between the two countries (e.g. comparison with macronutrient intake is typically as a percentage of total energy rather than of food energy (i.e. excluding alcohol) as used in the UK. However, some general observations can be made.

Macronutrients and dietary fibre

In Ireland, although intakes of macronutrients are typically adequate, imbalances were observed for total fat, saturated fat, fibre and sugars (Table 8.9). Mean daily intakes of total fat and saturates for Irish adults were higher (34% and 13%) than the UK dietary guidelines of ≤33% and ≤10% total energy and intakes observed currently in the UK. A similar pattern is identified across

all age groups, with the highest intakes of total fat and saturates observed in preschool children. Intakes of saturates in adults typically arise from meat and meat products (16%), biscuit, cakes pastries and buns (8%), cheese (8%) and whole milk (7%). Broadly similar patterns emerge for other population groups, but with whole milk providing the greatest contribution in preschool children (22%), children (21%) and teenagers (15%). Intakes of trans fatty acids were 0.5–0.7% total energy – that is, well within recommended levels (WHO/FAO, 2003) – and with the major contributing sources for adults being cheese (17%) and fresh meat (14%). In contrast, intakes from biscuits, cakes, pastries and buns contributed 6% of total energy from trans fatty acids. This indicates that intakes of trans fats were predominately from natural sources, rather than the synthetic (artificial) forms which were historically produced during the hardening of vegetable oils (this practice is no longer used in the production of spreading and cooking fats in Europe (Li *et al.*, 2016)).

As in the UK, imbalances in carbohydrate intake are also observed, whereby fibre intakes are typically lower than recommended and sugar intakes higher. In Ireland, dietary fibre intakes were compared with the EFSA recommendation of 25 g/day or 2 g/MJ for children (EFSA Panel on Dietetic Products, Nutrition, and Allergies (NDA), 2010a)), based on the AOAC measurement method (this roughly equates to the 18 g/day NSP recommended at the time in the UK). Except for preschool children, where intakes are 11–13 g/day (2.4–2.5 g fibre

Table 8.9 Overview of dietary intakes for Irish population groups[a].

	NPNS				NCFS	NTFS	NANS	
	1y	2y	3y	4y	5–12y	13–17y	18–64y	>65y
Energy (MJ)	4.2	4.7	4.8	5.3	7.0	8.3	8.6	7.4
Protein (% TE)[b]	15.6	15.3	14.9	15	13.6	14.8	16.9	17.9
Carbohydrate (% TE)	50.4	52.4	53.7	54.0	52.0	49.0	43.0	44.0
Total Sugars (%TE)	26.2	24.8	24.9	24.7	23.9	20.4	16.6	17.9
Sugars[c] (% TE)	9.0	11.0	13.4	14.4	14.6	12.4	n/a	n/a
Fibre (g/d)	10.5	11.6	12.0	12.8	12.5	15.5	19.2	18.9
Total Fat (% TE)	34	32.9	32.1	31.9	33.9	35.7	34.1	34.9
Saturates (% TE)	15.8	14.9	14.7	14.2	14.7	14.4	13.3	14.3
Monounsaturates (% TE)	12.1	11.1	10.7	10.8	11.6	12.7	12.5	12.2
Polyunsaturates (% TE)	3.7	4.3	4.4	4.5	4.9	5.8	6.1	5.9
Trans fatty acids (% TE)	0.7	0.6	0.6	0.6	n/a	n/a	0.5	0.6
Salt (g/d)[d]	2.3	3	3.1	3.6	5.3	6.3	7.4	6.3
Fruit & vegetables (g/d)[e]	195	216	244	259	204	203	235	271

n/a: not assessed; NANS: National Adult's Nutrition Survey; NCVS: National Children's Food Survey; NPNS: National Preschool Nutrition Survey. TE: total energy. Values are % unless otherwise stated
[a] details of all surveys available at www.iuna.net
[b]

[c] relates to 'free' sugars for NPNS and 'added sugars' for NCFS and NTFS.
[d] refers to salt from food sources only.
[e] includes fruit juice; value for preschool children includes intakes from composite dishes. n/a not assessed. TE, total energy.

per megajoule), current intakes are generally inadequate for all population groups, with 81% of adults aged 18–64 years and 80% of those aged 65 years and over failing to achieve this level of intake. The main sources in adults aged 18–64 years were bread (26%), vegetables (17%), potatoes (13%), fruit juice (10%) and breakfast cereals (9%).

Sugars intake has been estimated using a variety of approaches, which include assessments of total, free and added sugars. In general, irrespective of the approach taken, intakes across all population groups, except 1 year olds, at approximately 11–15% of energy, are higher than the UK recommendation for NMES of 10% total energy, with the highest intakes recorded for children aged 4–12 years (up to 15% of total energy). Although the major contributing sources to total sugars in preschoolers were fruit, fruit juices and beverages, with increasing age there were increasing contributions observed for biscuits, cakes, pastries and buns (5–8%), confectionary (2–8%) and beverages (3–7%). Micronutrient dilution has been reported for Irish children aged 5–12 years with the highest intakes of sugar (Joyce and Gibney, 2008).

Micronutrients

Based on comparison with the estimated average requirements (i.e. the amounts sufficient for 50% of the population) published by EFSA (EFSA Panel on Dietetic Products, Nutrition, and Allergies (NDA, 2010b)) (rather than the RNIs and LRNIs used in the NDNS), intakes of most vitamins in Ireland were judged to be adequate. The most notable exceptions were iron and folate in women, and vitamin D in both sexes, which broadly reflects the situation in the UK. Around two-thirds of adult men and women had mean daily intakes of vitamin D below 5 μg/day, with 7% of adults having vitamin D status deemed to be deficient using the US Institute of Medicine threshold of <30 nmol/L (25 nmol/L is used in the UK). Furthermore, 40% of adults had 25-hydroxyvitamin D status below the level deemed to cover the vitamin D requirements of nearly all (97.5%) of a general healthy population (Institute of Medicine (US) Food and Nutrition Board, 2011) (i.e. <50 nmol/L) (Cashman *et al.*, 2010). Major dietary sources were meat (30%), fish (12%) and fat spreads (10%). Inadequate dietary vitamin D intakes were observed across all population groups: 70–84% of 1- to 4-year-olds had intakes of less than 5 μg/day and 17–35% had intakes of less than 1 μg/day (IUNA, 2011). Respective values for children and teenagers are 34% below 5 μg/day and 22% with intakes less than 1 μg/day.

As in the UK, almost half of women (48%) aged 18–64 years had inadequate intakes of iron; among women of childbearing age the percentage rose to 61%. Again, it should be noted that the Irish data compare intakes with the estimated average requirement (sufficient for the

needs of 50% of the population), rather than the LRNI value used in data presented for the UK (i.e. the amount appropriate for only the 2.5% with the lowest needs). The prevalence of inadequate intakes among the 10% of females who took an iron supplement was much lower at 20%, compared with 80% in those who did not. Reflecting this, approximately 12% of women aged 36–50 years had haemoglobin concentrations deemed to be 'low' (<12 g/dL) and 20% had low serum ferritin concentrations (<15 μg/L). This phenomenon of inadequate dietary iron intake in females was observed at all ages, whereby 23% of 1-year-olds had dietary intakes below the EAR rising to 34% for girls aged 5–12 years and 74% for teenage girls. Among women aged 65 years and over, 17% had inadequate intakes. For folic acid, poor adherence was observed to the recommendation that all women of childbearing age consume a 400 μg supplement daily – only 2% of 18- to 35-year-olds and 1% of 36- to 50-year-olds took such a supplement. Other nutrients where dietary intake was identified to be less than the average requirement were calcium in women only and vitamin A in both sexes. Supplement use was typically approximately 20-30% across all surveys, with 28% of adults reporting taking a supplement during the recording period.

In contrast, intakes of sodium (assessed as dietary sodium chloride (salt)) were higher than recommended across all age groups. For adults, mean daily intakes of salt (7.4 g/day) were higher than the recommended value of 6 g/day and this excess intake was reflected in urinary analysis. Chief contributing sources were meat and meat products (27% of sodium intakes) and breads and rolls (22%).

Fruit and vegetable intakes were relatively constant across all age groups, typically <300 g/day, and well below the WHO recommendation of 400 g/day. Of note, contributions of juices to this value increased with age, and approximately half of fruit and vegetable intakes in older children and teenagers arose from fruit juice.

In summary, patterns of intakes of many nutrients in Ireland are broadly in line with those of the UK. Some of the greatest imbalances in dietary intake are evident among women, who often have inadequate micronutrient intakes yet some of the highest intakes of fat and saturated fatty acids.

8.4 Food-based dietary guidelines and tools for delivering healthy eating advice

Surveys such as the NDNS in the UK and the Irish surveys characterise diets consumed in terms of nutrients and food sources, thus enabling comparison with dietary guidelines. Food-based dietary guidelines can be used to help people move towards a healthier and more sustainable diet.

Food-based dietary guidelines illustrate food choices that will meet nutritional needs within appropriate energy allowances and include a variety of foods to accommodate personal preferences. They rely on consumption of foods rich in nutrients rather than energy-dense micronutrient-poor options, with only limited allowance for additional energy from foods rich in added sugars and saturated fatty acids, particularly in populations that are sedentary. A best practice stepwise guide to setting food based dietary guidelines was published by EFSA in 2010.

When setting dietary recommendations, Maki *et al.* (2014) stress the importance of applying a hierarchical approach to the evaluation of evidence (see Chapter 7), with emphasis on randomised controlled trials that use clinical events as endpoints where such data exist but noting that in some cases the best available evidence will be from intervention trials with disease surrogates or risk markers as endpoints. Prospective cohort (observational) data are considered the next best option, the methodological limitations of which (chance, bias, confounding) are summarised by Maki *et al.*, along with a discussion of measurement errors and substitution/displacement effects and collinearity (foods that are high in dietary fibre, for example, are often also good sources of B vitamins and magnesium, making it more difficult to identify possible mechanisms of effect).

In the UK, the *eatwell plate* (originally developed in the 1990s and known as the *Balance of Good Health*) has for about 20 years provided the basis for delivering healthy eating advice to the general UK population. It has been a guide to the overall balance of the diet that should be achieved over a day or even a week, and was replaced by the new Eatwell Guide in 2016. Many countries have a guide of this type and associated food-based dietary guidelines (http://www.eufic.org/article/en/expid/food-based-dietary-guidelines-in-europe/), but the extent of supporting information varies considerably. For example, the USA's *My Plate* tool defined by the Dietary Guidelines for Americans 2015–2020 (http://health.gov/dietaryguidelines/2015/) has a web site and detailed information on portion sizes (http://www.choosemyplate.gov/). Health Canada's guide (http://www.hc-sc.gc.ca/fn-an/food-guide-aliment/index-eng.php) and the Irish approach (https://www.fsai.ie/newrecommendationsforfoodbaseddietaryguidelinesforhealthyeatinginireland.html; https://www.healthpromotion.ie/hp-files/docs/HPM00796.pdf) are also very comprehensive. The UK's Eatwell Guide does not provide detailed information for all food groups on portion size and frequency of consumption. However, examples of meals and snacks that, over the course of a day, are in line with the Eatwell Guide and with Government guidance

on energy intake at different meal occasions can be found at https://www.nutrition.org.uk/nutritionscience/nutrients-food-and-ingredients/carbohydratesandhealth.html. The Eatwell Guide is not designed for those under the age of 5 years. The British Nutrition Foundation has published a guide for younger children, following similar principles to the Eatwell approach (https://www.nutrition.org.uk/healthyliving/toddlers/5532.html).

Analyses in the UK (Harland *et al.*, 2012; Defra, 2015; Scarborough *et al.*, 2016) and also in the USA (Britten *et al.*, 2012) reveal that there is currently a gap between current consumption patterns and the respective food-based dietary guidelines.

Data from the Family Food survey have been used to estimate the extent to which current dietary patterns in the UK are in accord with dietary recommendations depicted in the *eatwell plate* (Defra, 2015). Data on household food and drink purchases during the survey period were grouped approximately into the five *eatwell plate* groupings. Neither low-income households nor the average for all households is close to the recommendations of the *eatwell plate*. For example, the *eatwell plate* depicts 33% of the diet being provided by fruit and vegetables, but in fact this grouping provides only 25% of the average diet and 21% of the diets of low-income groups, reflecting the findings of the NDNS referred to earlier. Purchases of starchy foods also fall short of recommendations, reflecting the findings of the NDNS for fibre intake. The group of foods high in fat and/or sugar is intended to comprise just 7% of the diet but contributes 21% on average and 24% in low-income households. Sources of NMES in the British diet are shown in Table 8.4. NDNS data has also been used to assess compliance with the Eatwell Guide (Scarborough *et al.*, 2016).

Breakfast consumption has been considered in a number of studies, and the importance of an appropriate breakfast for school-aged children has recently been emphasised, with a focus on provision of school breakfast clubs in the UK. A healthy breakfast can contribute to essential nutrient intake, and there is some evidence to suggest it can also improve attention and cognitive performance during lessons (see Chapter 13); breakfast skipping and breakfasts of poor nutritional quality have been reported to be more common in children in lower income households. By 2012, breakfast clubs were available in almost half of schools in England, with delivery concentrated in areas of deprivation (Hoyland *et al.*, 2012). In Wales, a Government-supported free breakfast scheme for primary schools was initiated in 2005 and was taken up by an estimated 75% of schools.

According to Moore *et al.* (2013), there is tentative evidence that actions based on education, information provision and promotion of voluntary change are more likely to increase health inequalities as they will be adopted by those in least need, whereas altering higher level factors that change the environment to make healthy behaviours easier may be more likely to reduce inequalities (see references in Moore *et al.* (2013)). Breakfast provision represents an attempt to improve behaviour by altering the environment to make the behaviour easier, and the study by Moore *et al.* (2013) looked at the differential effectiveness by socio-economic status of universal breakfast provision and reported support for the notion that universal interventions may be more likely to reduce inequalities (i.e. disproportionately benefit children from poorer backgrounds) than to make them worse.

8.5 Dietary patterns and pattern analysis

Converging evidence from prospective observational studies and clinical trials indicates that, in the prevention and management of widespread conditions such as type 2 diabetes, the quality of dietary fat (in particular, replacement of saturated fatty acids by *n*-6 polyunsaturated fatty acids) and carbohydrate (especially types rich in fibre, especially cereal fibre) is more important than the quantity consumed of these macronutrients. Diets rich in fruit and vegetables, whole grains, legumes and nuts, moderate in alcohol consumption and lower in refined grains, red/processed meats and sugar-sweetened beverages have been reported to decrease the overall risk of type 2 diabetes and improve glycaemic control and blood lipids in patients with diabetes. Dietary patterns based on traditional Mediterranean-style eating, and low glycaemic index, moderate carbohydrate (though not 'low' carbohydrate) and vegetarian diets can be tailored to personal/cultural food preferences and appropriate energy intake for weight control and prevention and management of type 2 diabetes (Ley *et al.*, 2014). The so-called DASH dietary pattern, characterised by fruit and vegetables, low-fat dairy products, whole grains, poultry, fish and nuts and low in saturates and salt, has also been shown to reduce risk of type 2 diabetes and also cardiovascular disease, and is used as an exemplar within the *Dietary Guidelines for Americans 2015–2020* (USDA, 2015).

Various techniques have been developed to study established dietary patterns; for example, data-driven methods such as factor and cluster analysis, investigator-driven methods such as indices and scores, and methods combining the two, such as reduced rank regression (Michels and Schulze, 2005). There is growing interest in dietary pattern analysis for two reasons. First, because people eat meals consisting of a variety of foods and many combinations of nutrients, the traditional approach (focusing on single foods or nutrients) may be inadequate for taking account of interactive effects on the bioavailability, circulating levels and metabolism of nutrients. Second, dietary pattern analysis is useful in situations where several dietary exposures are simultaneously associated with disease risk (e.g. cardiovascular disease), potentially exerting their effects in opposing directions (Mozaffarian *et al.*, 2011). Culturally acquired food habits in countries across Europe appear to have stronger effects on dietary patterns than factors such as socio-economic status or lifestyle (e.g. smoking). Overall food patterns (Slimani *et al.*, 2002) are much more diverse than the overall nutrient pattern; this is not surprising, as a number of foods are sources of each nutrient and several nutrients are ubiquitous in many foods. So, another option is to study nutrient patterns, and this may have several advantages, particularly in international contexts. Nutrients are functionally not exchangeable, unlike foods, and the same nutrients are consumed across populations with only low rates of non-consumers, which should facilitate the use and generalisation of nutrient pattern approaches across populations.

Until recently, the study of differences in nutrient patterns between countries was hampered by a lack of standardisation of dietary methods and nutrient databases. Using standardised procedures (the same standardised computerised dietary software, EPIC-Soft, was used to collect a single 24-h dietary record that was analysed for energy and nutrients using a standardised food composition database), the EPIC cross-sectional study, comprising over 36 000 randomly selected people aged 35–74 years, was used to compare dietary patterns between and within 10 European countries (a total of 27 regions) (Freisling *et al.*, 2010).

Freisling *et al.* (2010) identified three main region-specific patterns with a geographical gradient within and between specific European countries. In Mediterranean regions (including Greece, Italy and southern Spain, the nutrient patterns were dominated by relatively high intakes of vitamin E and MUFA, whereas intakes of retinol and vitamin D were relatively low. In contrast, Nordic countries including Norway, Sweden and Denmark reported intake of these same nutrients that resulted in an almost opposite pattern. Germany, the Netherlands and the UK shared a dietary fatty acid pattern relatively high in PUFA and saturates and relatively low in monounsaturated fatty acids, in combination with a relatively high intake of sugars. Within countries, the intakes of nutrients were very similar between men and women with the exception of alcohol.

Recently, Moskal *et al.* (2014) applied principle component analysis to nutrient intake data collected by food frequency questionnaires as part of the EPIC study. Four nutrient patterns explaining 67% of the total variance and distinguished by high or low intakes of plant or animal foods and/or specific nutrients (e.g. calcium, proteins, phosphorus or riboflavin) were identified. These patterns could typically be explained by energy intake and location of research centre and were validated using a 24-h recall. Such analysis adds further evidence to support the notion that meaningful nutrient-based dietary patterns can be identified, these patterns having the potential to further nutrition research as well as to inform public health policy. Other novel approaches involve pattern analysis based on markers of nutritional status (Gao et al., 2003; Knoops et al., 2009) or metabolomics (O'Sullivan et al., 2011; Cheung et al., 2017), with the focus of subsequent analysis being to identify the dietary intakes driving these patterns. Nevertheless, this area of science is still in its infancy, with further research required before it is directly transferrable to public health policy or direct strategies to improve dietary intakes.

Following identification of dietary patterns, approaches such as linear programming can be used to model how food patterns can be improved (Buttriss et al., 2014). For example, a study in France using data from the French national food survey demonstrated that nutrient-based recommendations could be achieved by isocalorically increasing average intakes of plant-based products (fruit and vegetables, starchy foods/grains, and low-fat dairy products) and reducing contributions from the meat/fish/eggs/poultry group, added fats and sweets/savoury products by 15%. Linear programming, especially the recently developed 'individual' diet modelling approach, enables optimisation of diets by changing existing dietary patterns as little as possible (Maillot et al., 2011). The modelling is done within a set of constraints; for example, setting ranges for specific nutrients (e.g. fat or free sugars) and limits on food quantities or portion sizes or cost. In a similar manner, probabilistic modelling can simulate the impact on population dietary intakes of altering the composition of individual foods or groups of foods while accounting for relevant influencing factors. Examples can include fortification, product reformulation or alterations (increases/decreases) in the intakes of a particular nutrient, food or groups of foods. Use of probabilistic modelling can avoid the assumption that all individuals and foods are affected equally and allow for refinements such as inter-person variability, reach, market share, portion size control, seasonality and replacement scenarios.

Finally, there is increasing recognition of the environmental impact of food and drink, and food policy and dietary advice need to go beyond their traditional focus on nutrition to include consideration of environmental impacts. Balancing environmental, economic and social aspects with nutritional ones adds complexity to the task of determining dietary guidelines, as discussed by Garnett (2014). Mathematical modelling techniques can also be used to establish the changes required to make diets more sustainable as well as healthier, and work to date suggests that a move towards current European national food-based dietary guidelines would be a step in the right direction from an environmental perspective (Macdiarmid et al., 2012). Characteristics of dietary patterns with lower environmental impact were increased quantities of legumes as a source of protein, less meat and more cereals and starchy foods, such as potatoes, bread and pasta.

8.6 Conclusions

Most countries use an assessment of dietary intakes to provide information that can be converted to estimates of nutrient intakes. Using relevant, comprehensive and up-to-date food composition data, these estimates can then be compared with DRVs and dietary guidelines to establish the adequacy of dietary patterns and to inform public health policy. This chapter has presented data for the UK and Ireland, but the issues identified are typical of western Europe, and indeed many countries globally. The role of food-based dietary guidelines as tools to deliver healthy eating advice is described. In future, increasing emphasis may be placed on a more holistic approach involving pattern analysis of foods, nutrients and potentially other (bio)markers of health.

Acknowledgements

All data sourced and used under Open Government Licence v3.0. The Irish Food Surveys (NANS, NCFS, NPNS, NTFS) were funded by the Irish Department of Agriculture, Food and the Marine under the Food Institution Research Measure.

References

Absoud, M., Cummins, C., Lim, M.J. et al. (2011) Prevalence and predictors of vitamin D insufficiency in children: a Great Britain population based study. PLoS ONE, 6, e22179.

Bates, B., Lennox, A., Prentice, A. et al. (eds) (2014) National Diet and Nutrition Survey. Results from Years 1, 2, 3 and 4 (combined) of the Rolling Programme (2008/2009–2011/2012). Public Health England, London. https://www.gov.uk/government/uploads/system/uploads/attachment_data/file/310995/NDNS_Y1_to_4_UK_report.pdf (accessed 30 November 2016).

British Nutrition Foundation (2013) Nutrition and Development: Short- and Long-term Consequences for Health. Wiley Blackwell.

Britten, P., Cleveland, L.E., Koegel, K.L. et al. (2012) Updated US Department of Agriculture Food Patterns meet goals of the 2010 dietary guidelines. Journal of the Academy of Nutrition and Dietetics, 112, 1648–1655.

Butte, N.F., Fox, M.K., Briefel, R.R. *et al.* (2010) Nutrient intakes of US infants, toddlers, and pre-schoolers meet or exceed dietary reference intakes. *Journal of the American Dietetic Association*, **110**, S27–S37.

Buttriss, J.L., Briend, A., Darmon, N. *et al.* (2014) Diet modelling: how it can inform the development of dietary recommendations and public health policy. *Nutrition Bulletin*, **39**, 115–125.

Cashman, K.D., Muldowney, S., McNulty, B. *et al.* (2013) Vitamin D status of Irish adults: findings from the National Adult Nutrition Survey. *British Journal of Nutrition*, **109**(7), 1248–1256.

Cheung, W., Keski-Rahkonen, P., Assi, N. *et al.* (2017) A metabolomic study of biomarkers of meat and fish intake. *American Journal of Clinical Nutrition*, epub ahead of print. doi: 10.3945/ajcn.116.146639

Defra (2015) *Family Food 2014*. Department for Environment, Food and Rural Affairs, London. https://www.gov.uk/government/uploads/system/uploads/attachment_data/file/485982/familyfood-2014report-17dec15.pdf (accessed 30 November 2016).

Dwyer, J.T., Butte, N.F., Deming, D.M. *et al.* (2010) Feeding Infants and Toddlers Study 2008: progress, continuing concerns, and implications. *Journal of the American Dietetic Association*, **110**, S60–S67.

EFSA Panel on Dietetic Products, Nutrition, and Allergies (NDA) (2010a) Scientific Opinion on dietary reference values for carbohydrates and dietary fibre. *EFSA Journal*, **8**(3), 1462.

EFSA Panel on Dietetic Products, Nutrition, and Allergies (NDA) (2010b) Scientific Opinion on principles for deriving and applying dietary reference values. *EFSA Journal*, **8**(3), 1458.

Freisling, H., Fahey, M.T., Moskal, A. *et al.* (2010) Region-specific nutrient intake patterns exhibit a geographical gradient within and between European countries. *The Journal of Nutrition*, **140**, 1280–1286.

Gao, X., Yao, M., McCrory, M.A. *et al.* (2003) Dietary pattern is associated with homocysteine and B vitamin status in an urban Chinese population. *Journal of Nutrition*, **133**, 3636–3642.

Garnett T. (2014) What is a sustainable healthy diet? *Food Climate Research Network*, 29 April. http://www.fcrn.org.uk/fcrn/publications/fcrn-discussion-paper-what-sustainable-healthy-diet (accessed 30 November 2016).

Harland, J.I., Buttriss, J. and Gibson, S. (2012) Achieving *eatwell plate* recommendations: is this a route to improving both sustainability and healthy eating? *Nutrition Bulletin*, **37**, 324–343.

Henderson, L., Gregory, J., Irving, K. and Swan, G. (2002) *The National Diet and Nutrition Survey: Adults Aged 19 to 64 Years. Volume 2: Energy, Protein, Carbohydrate, Fat and Alcohol Intake*. TSO, London.

Hoyland, A., McWilliams, K.A., Duff, R.J. and Walton, J.L. (2012) Breakfast consumption in UK schoolchildren and provision of school breakfast clubs. *Nutrition Bulletin*, **37**, 232–240.

Hu, F. (2002) Dietary pattern analysis: a new direction in nutritional epidemiology. *Current Opinion in Lipidology*, **13**, 3–9.

Institute of Medicine (US) Food and Nutrition Board (2011) *Dietary Reference Intakes for Calcium and Vitamin D*. National Academy Press, Washington, DC.

IUNA (2011) *National Adult Nutrition Survey. Summary Report on Food and Nutrient Intakes, Physical Measurements and Barriers to Healthy Eating*. Irish Universities Nutrition Alliance. http://www.iuna.net/wp-content/uploads/2010/12/National-Adult-Nutrition-Survey-Summary-Report-March-2011.pdf (accessed 12 January 2017).

Joyce, T. and Gibney, M.J. (2008) The impact of added sugar consumption on overall dietary quality in Irish children and teenagers. *Journal of Human Nutrition and Dietetics*, **21**(5), 438–450.

Knoops, K.T., Spiro, A., III de Groot, L.C. *et al.* (2009) Do dietary patterns in older men influence change in homocysteine through folate fortification? The Normative Aging Study. *Public Health Nutrition*, **12**, 1760–1766.

Lennox, A., Sommerville, J., Ong, K. *et al.* (eds) (2013) *Diet and Nutrition Survey of Infants and Young Children, 2011*. https://www.gov.uk/government/uploads/system/uploads/attachment_data/file/139572/DNSIYC_UK_report_ALL_chapters_DH_V10.0.pdf (accessed 29 November 2016).

Ley, S.H., Hamdy, O., Mohan, V. and Hu, F.B. (2014) Prevention and management of type 2 diabetes: dietary components and nutritional strategies. *The Lancet* **383**, 1999–2007.

Li, K., McNulty, B.A., Tierney, A.M. *et al.* (2016) Dietary fat intakes in Irish adults in 2011: how much has changed in 10 years? *British Journal of Nutrition*, **115**, 1798–1809.

Maillot, M., Issa, C., Vieux, F. *et al.* (2011) The shortest way to reach nutritional goals is to adopt Mediterranean food choices: evidence from computer-generated personalized diets. *The American Journal of Clinical Nutrition*, **94**, 1127–1137.

Maki, K.C., Slavin, J.L., Rains, T.M. and Kris-Etherton, P.M. (2014) Limitations of observational evidence: implications for evidence-based dietary recommendations. *Advances in Nutrition*, **5**, 7–15.

Macdiarmid, J.I., Kyle, J., Horgan, G.W. *et al.* (2012) Sustainable diets for the future: can we contribute to reducing greenhouse gas emissions by eating a healthy diet? *The American Journal of Clinical Nutrition*, **96**, 632–639.

McAndrew, F., Thompson, J., Fellows, L. *et al.* (2012) *Infant Feeding Survey 2010*. NHS The Information Centre. http://www.hscic.gov.uk/catalogue/PUB08694/Infant-Feeding-Survey-2010-Consolidated-Report.pdf (accessed 29 November 2016).

Mensink, G.B., Fletcher, R., Gurinovic, M. *et al.* (2013) Mapping low intake of micronutrients across Europe. *British Journal of Nutrition*, **110**, 755–773.

Michels, K.B. and Schulze, M.B. (2005) Can dietary patterns help us detect diet–disease associations? *Nutrition Research Reviews*, **18**, 241–248.

Moore, G.F., Murphy, S., Chaplin, K. *et al.* (2013) Impacts of the primary school free breakfast initiative on socio-economic inequalities in breakfast consumption among 9–11-year-old schoolchildren in Wales. *Public Health Nutrition*, **17**(6), 1280–1289.

Moskal, A., Pisa, P.T., Ferrari, P. *et al.* (2014) Nutrient patterns and their food sources in an international study setting: report from the EPIC study. *PLoS ONE*, **9**(6): e98647. doi: 10.1371/journal.pone.0098647.

Mozaffarian, D., Appel, L.J. and Van Horn, L. (2011) Components of a cardioprotective diet: new insights. *Circulation*, **123**, 2870–2891.

Nelson, M., Erens, B., Bates, B. *et al.* (2007) *Low Income Diet and Nutrition Survey. Volume 2: Food Consumption and Nutrient Intake*. TSO, London.

O'Sullivan, A., Gibney, M.J. and Brennan, L. (2011) Dietary intake patterns are reflected in metabolomics profiles: potential role in dietary assessment studies. *The American Journal of Clinical Nutrition*, **93**, 314–321.

Public Health England (2013) *National Dental Epidemiology Programme for England: Oral Health Survey of Five-Year-Old Children 2012*. A Report on the Prevalence and Severity of Dental Decay. http://www.nwph.net/dentalhealth/Oral%20Health%205yr%20old%20children%202012%20final%20report%20gateway%20approved.pdf (accessed 30 November 2016).

Public Health England (2014a) Obesity slide sets. http://www.noo.org.uk/slide_sets (accessed 30 November 2016).

Public Health England (2014b) *Sugar Reduction: Responding to the Challenge*. https://www.gov.uk/government/uploads/system/

uploads/attachment_data/file/324043/Sugar_Reduction_Responding_to_the_Challenge_26_June.pdf (accessed 30 November 2016).

Public Health England (2015a) Sugar reduction: from evidence into action. https://www.gov.uk/government/publications/sugar-reduction-from-evidence-into-action (accessed 30 November 2016).

Public Health England (2015b) NDNS: blood folate supplementary report. https://www.gov.uk/government/statistics/national-diet-and-nutrition-survey-supplementary-report-blood-folate (accessed 30 November 2016).

Sanders, T.A. (2014) Protective effects of dietary PUFA against chronic disease: evidence from epidemiological studies and intervention trials. *The Proceedings of the Nutrition Society*, **73**, 73–79.

SACN (2015a) *Carbohydrates and Health*. TSO, London. https://www.gov.uk/government/uploads/system/uploads/attachment_data/file/445503/SACN_Carbohydrates_and_Health.pdf (accessed 29 November 2016).

SACN (2015b) *Draft Vitamin D and Health Report*. https://www.gov.uk/government/uploads/system/uploads/attachment_data/file/447402/Draft_SACN_Vitamin_D_and_Health_Report.pdf (accessed 29 November 2016).

SACN (2016) *Vitamin D and Health*. https://www.gov.uk/government/uploads/system/uploads/attachment_data/file/537616/SACN_Vitamin_D_and_Health_report.pdf (accessed 29 November 2016).

Scarborough, P. *et al.* (2016) http://bmjopen.bmj.com/content/bmjopen/6/12/e013182.full.pdf.

Slimani, N., Kaaks, R., Ferrari, P. *et al.* (2002) European Prospective Investigation into Cancer and Nutrition (EPIC) calibration study: rationale, design and population characteristics. *Public Health Nutrition*, **5**, 1125–1145.

Spiro, A. and Buttriss, J.L. (2014) Vitamin D: an overview of vitamin D status and intake in Europe. *Nutrition Bulletin*, **39**(4), 322–350.

USDA (2015) *Dietary Guidelines for Americans 2015–2020*, 8th edition. US Department of Agriculture, Washington, DC. http://health.gov/dietaryguidelines/2015/guidelines/ (accessed 11 December 2016).

Walton, J., Kehoe, L., McNulty, B.A. *et al.* (2017) Nutrient intakes and compliance with nutrient recommendations in children aged 1–4 years in Ireland. *Hum Nutr Diet*, doi:10.1111/jhn.12452

Walton, J., McNulty, B., Nugent, A.P. *et al.* (2014) Diet, lifestyle and body weight in Irish children: findings from Irish Universities Nutrition Alliance national surveys. *The Proceedings of the Nutrition Society*, **73**(2), 190–200.

WHO/FAO (2003) *Diet, Nutrition and the Prevention of Chronic Diseases. Report of a Joint WHO/FAO Expert Consultation*. WHO Technical Report Series 916. World Health Organization, Geneva.

9
Minerals and Vitamins of Current Concern

Iron
Peter J Aggett

Iodine
Margaret P Rayman and Sarah C Bath

Vitamin A
Elizabeth J Johnson and Emily Mohn

Iron

Key messages

- Iron is essential for energy and substrate metabolism, mixed function oxidase enzymes that metabolise nutrients and xenobiotics, and for the synthesis of connective tissue, neurotransmitters and hormones.
- Some 80% of the body's iron is in haemoglobin and myoglobin, which respectively distribute to and store oxygen in tissues.
- The features of iron deficiency are protean and difficult to distinguish from other deficiencies and include impaired muscle function, cerebration, lethargy.
- In infants and children, iron-deficient anaemia has been associated with persisting impaired neurodevelopment. This has significant implications for socio-economic development.
- Intestinal absorption of iron is the only way by which systemic iron burdens can be controlled. Usually this is downregulated by hepcidin.
- Hepcidin production is reduced in iron deficiency. It is increased by adequate systemic iron status and by infection and inflammatory

stress, which if constant causes a functional iron deficiency called Anaemia of Chronic Disease.
- Iron deficiency is usually accompanied by other nutritional deficiencies. A major cause of iron deficiency is blood loss from intestinal parasitism.
- The best indicator of iron deficiency is a serum ferritin value $<15\,\mu\text{m/L}$.
- The prevention and management of iron deficiency in populations requires broad interdisciplinary strategies to improve public health and sanitation generally, and to improve agricultural and culinary practices.
- Iron intakes can be increased using fortification and supplementation. The implementation of interventions to improve iron supply needs to be subject to a risk benefit analysis, in which the effects of iron on the utilisation of other micronutrients, and on intestinal bacteria and systemic infections need to be assessed.

9.1 Introduction

Iron is pivotal in the body's use of oxygen for the metabolism of dietary substrates and other food components, to generate energy and for the synthesis of tissues, hormones and neurotransmitters. The switch between ferrous (Fe^{2+}) and ferric states (Fe^{3+}) and their reactivity with nitrogen and sulphur, as well as oxygen, are integral to these functions, examples of which are shown in Table 9.1.

Public Health Nutrition, Second Edition. Edited by Judith L Buttriss, Ailsa A Welch, John M Kearney and Susan A Lanham-New.
© 2018 by The Nutrition Society. Published 2018 by John Wiley & Sons, Ltd.
Companion website: www.wiley.com/go/buttriss/publichealth

Table 9.1 Examples of iron-dependent protein activities.

Type	Function and comment
Iron–sulphur proteins	
Dehydrogenases: isocitrate, NADPH, succinate	Citric acid cycle in mitochondria, serial oxidation producing NADPH, ATP and GTP, and substrates for synthesis of amino acids, lipogenesis and glycogenesis
Aconitase and iron–sulphur-sensing cluster	Aconitase is also involved with regulation of iron kinetics, cell signalling, haem synthesis
Haem proteins	Several variants of haem involved
Cytochromes a, b, c	Electron transfer chain in mitochondria oxidising NADPH from citric acid cycle to drive synthesis
Cytochrome c oxidase	of ATP (i.e. oxidative phosphorylation). The citric acid cycle and respiratory chain involves six different haem proteins and six iron–sulphur clusters
Cytochrome P450 mono-oxygenases	Microsomal. Over 11 000 activities, including synthesis of steroid hormones, metabolism of organic acids, fatty acids, prostaglandins, xenobiotics and sterols, including cholesterol and vitamins A, D and K
Fatty acid desaturases	Long-chain fatty acid synthesis: myelination by oligodendrocytes
Peroxidases	Numerous substrates (e.g. iodide to iodate)
Myeloperoxidase	Neutrophil bactericide
Catalase	$2H_2O_2$ to $2H_2O + O_2$
Tryptophan-2,3-dioxygenase	Neurotransmitters, serotonin 5 HIAA, niacin and nicotinamide metabolism
Reductases	Sulphite, nitrite metabolism
Dcytb ferric reductase	Fe^{3+} to Fe^{2+} on enterocytes
Haem and globin	Haem is embedded in a globin, which enables it to bind dioxygen reversibly
Haemoglobin, myoglobin, neuroglobin	Transport O_2, CO_2, NO. For transport (haemoglobin) and dioxygen storage in muscle and CNS
Iron as a cofactor	
Phenylalanine hydroxylase	Phenylalanine to tyrosine
Tyrosine hydroxylase	Tyrosine to dopaminergic acid
Prolyl and lysyl hydroxylase	Procollagen and collagen synthesis
Ribonucleotide reductase	Ribo- to deoxyribonucleotide; DNA metabolism
Cysteine oxygenase	Cysteine metabolism

5HIAA: 5-hydroxyindoleacetic acid; ATP: adenosine triphosphate; CNS: central nervous system; Dcytb: duodenal cytochrome b; GTP: guanosine triphosphate; NADPH: nicotinamide adenine dinucleotide phosphate (SACN, 2010).

The reactivity of free iron, particularly with lipid membranes, nucleic acids and proteins, can cause oxidative functional and architectural damage to tissues and organs. Therefore, to protect tissues, iron is tightly bound in enzymes, tissue depots such as ferritin, cytoplasmic and mitochondrial carrier proteins or in an extracellular protein, transferrin, which distributes the element systemically. Both Fe^{2+} and Fe^{3+} are poorly soluble at physiological PH and an important benefit of these proteins is that they maintain iron at a high intracellular concentration (10^{-4} M compared with 10^{-18} M in water at physiological pH), whilst keeping free iron low at 10^{-24} M.

9.2 Iron absorption: intestinal mucosal uptake and transfer of iron

Dietary iron is released from food by gastric proteolysis and acidity. The acidity of the proximal small intestine and the coincidently released amino acids and peptides keep both cations of iron in solution and available for adsorption to the intestinal mucosa. Uptake into enterocytes is specific for Fe^{2+}, and any Fe^{3+} is reduced to Fe^{2+} by the mucosal enzyme cytochrome b reductase. Fe^{2+} is transferred by a divalent metal transporter (DMT) into the enterocyte. Some haem iron is taken up in the proximal bowel, but because haem is more soluble in an alkaline environment, it is possible that most haem is absorbed further down the intestine. The mechanism for haem uptake is uncharacterised.

In the enterocyte, haem is degraded by haem oxygenase and the released iron forms a common pool with non-haem iron. Of this, small amounts may be retained in the enterocyte in ferritin or used for the synthesis of haem, but most is transported to a basal membrane transporter (ferroportin 1) which exports iron as Fe^{3+} to apotransferrin in the portal plasma, forming transferrin for distribution to the liver and systemic circulation. Transferrin is the main carrier of iron in the extracellular fluid; it binds one or two Fe^{3+} molecules and delivers them to peripheral organs and tissues, all of which are equipped with cell membrane transferrin receptors (TfR1) that enable the endocytosis of transferrin and the intracellular release of iron. Within cells, iron is either distributed to cytoplasmic functional sites, to ferritin depots, to the mitochondria for incorporation in iron–sulphur clusters and haem, or it is stowed in mitochondrial ferritin. The residual apotransferrin is released into the extracellular fluid; thus, apotransferrin levels can be an indicator of systemic uptake of, and need for, iron.

Eighty per cent of absorbed iron is used for erythropoiesis, and the erythron is highly dependent on TfR1 for iron uptake. Not all other tissues share this dependency, and some (e.g. oligodendrocytes) can acquire iron from ferritin in the extracellular fluid or from iron bound to low molecular weight iron-ligands in the circulation.

Whole-body iron approximates 4.4 g in men and 2.8 g in women (4 g of iron represents 4.3×10^{23} atoms of iron) distributed as haemoglobin 2.5–3.5 g, myoglobin 0.3–0.4 g, haem and non-haem enzymes 100 mg, and the transit pools of extracellular transferrin and intracellular carriers containing around 3 mg and 7 mg of iron. The main systemic depot for iron is a mobile repository of it in hepatic ferritin. There is an additional but immobile pool of iron in hepatic haemosiderin, which is a degraded ferritin. Ferritin and haemosiderin together comprise 1.0 g of iron.

Some 25 mg of iron is recycled daily; this comes from the turnover of tissues, and most comes from the daily breakdown of 10^{11} senescent erythrocytes. The iron is salvaged by the haem-oxygenases of the monocyte–macrophage system which phagocytose effete erythrocytes. The released iron is either exported by the macrophages' ferroportin as Fe^{3+} to apotransferrin, or retained in the cell's ferritin pool. The salvage of endogenous iron is 90% efficient. The other 10% is lost through blood loss and integumental and urinary losses; other than this adventitious route, the body has no way to lose iron. Thus, the body needs sensitive regulation of the intestinal absorption of iron to maintain balance and to prevent overload and the daily requirement for absorption is around 3 mg to compensate these losses, plus any needed for new tissue synthesis (e.g. growth, pregnancy).

The handling of iron within cells and mitochondria is controlled by an iron-sensing system that responds to their iron needs and also to hypoxaemia, and inflammation. Collectively, the iron-sensing systems regulate iron-responsive proteins that in turn control the expression of proteins which regulate the expression of TfR, the endocytosis, deposition in ferritin and export of iron, and the synthesis of haem. This predominantly local cellular response integrates with a systemic response that regulates the intestinal and systemic handling of iron.

Intestinal absorption of iron is usually downregulated; however; absorption increases at serum ferritin concentrations below 60 µg/L. This adaptation is effected by two mechanisms. One involves a hepatic hormone, hepcidin, which is usually produced continuously and which reduces enterocytic uptake of iron by reducing DMT1 activity, and the export of iron to the portal circulation by inducing the degradation of ferroportin. This traps any iron taken up from the gut lumen in the epithelium and the iron is lost in the faeces when the epithelial cells are shed into the lumen. The production of hepcidin is regulated via a system which responds to the sensing by a specific hepatic transferrin receptor (TfR2) of transferrin saturation as a proxy for the systemic need for iron. Thus, hepcidin production is decreased when plasma transferrin concentrations are low, indicating that there is a systemic need for iron for activities such as erythropoiesis. Hepcidin production increases when tissue iron, particularly hepatic iron depots, and circulating transferrin concentrations are high. The response to increased hepcidin takes about 8 h. The second adaptation takes 1–2 days to be effective: in this, an interaction between transferrin and TfR1 on the basolateral surface of enteroblasts programmes the mature enterocytes, the expression of DMT and ferroportin enteroblasts programmes the expression of DMT and ferroportin in the mature enterocytes.

9.3 Iron and women in their reproductive years

Menstrual blood loss is quite constant for individual women but varies a lot between women. The 50th centile of iron losses for women in their reproductive years approximates 1.34 mg/day. The distribution of losses is highly skewed, with a 97th centile, of 3.13 mg/day, reflecting the effect of large menstrual losses of some women.

An estimated 840 mg of iron is required to support a singleton pregnancy, of which 270 mg is for the neonate (i.e. 75 mg/kg body weight), 90 mg for the placenta and umbilical cord, and 175 mg for blood loss at delivery. This requirement is met from endogenous depots, and by an adaptive increased efficiency of non-haem iron absorption. Other adaptations include expansion of the plasma and blood volumes, and of red blood cell mass starting at 6–8 weeks and peaking at 28–34 weeks of gestation, and transferrin changes favouring distribution of iron to the placenta.

There is a difficult challenge when dealing with pregnant adolescents. In this group there is a need for iron to support systemic growth as well as the conceptus, and it is unclear if the adaptations for pregnancy compromise the supply of iron to support growth. Ideally, the pregnancy would be managed specifically as a clinical rather than a public health nutritional issue; unfortunately, many communities do not have the resources to provide such a service. Thus, although there are no specific guidelines, it is prudent for pregnant girls to be provided, as a precautionary measure, a small iron supplement.

9.4 Infants and children

After birth, a newborn's red cells break down and its haemoglobin concentration (15–18 g/L) falls, releasing iron which is stored as ferritin. This reserve of iron can be increased by 30–35 mg by delaying clamping of the umbilical cord until 2 min or later after birth. Overall, these stores suffice to support growth and development until 6 months of age in fully breast-fed infants. In early lactation, the iron concentration in breast milk is 0.5–1.0 mg/L, but it quickly decreases to 0.3 mg/L in mature milk. These amounts do not correlate with maternal dietary or supplementary iron intake.

The iron requirements of children reflect the synthesis of new tissues with growth as well as basal losses. Until puberty, dietary iron requirements increase slowly, but then higher intakes are needed to support the pubertal growth spurt. This may be associated with falls in serum ferritin concentrations in both sexes, and in girls this precedes menarche.

9.5 Dietary sources of iron

Although iron comprises 6% of the Earth's crust it is poorly available. It enters the food chain by virtue of specific chelators (siderophores) released by soil bacteria and fungi, and by plant roots. Organic acids, phenols and flavonoids also enhance iron's availability to plants. Grazing livestock acquire iron from ingested soil as well as from vegetation. In subsistence communities, agricultural practice such as alkalisation of soil by liming can limit the entry of iron into the food chain.

Foods that are relatively good sources of iron include meat, fish, cereals, beans, nuts, egg yolks, dark green vegetables, potatoes and fortified food products; the iron content of dairy products and many fruits and vegetables is lower. In the EU, grains and grain products provide 20–49% of iron intake. Mixed diets provide about 70–90% of the dietary iron as non-haem iron. The proportion of haem in the iron content of meat approximates 69% for beef; 39% for pork, ham, bacon, pork-based luncheon meats and veal; 26% for chicken and fish; and 21% for liver. Cooking may denature haem and cause loss of non-haem iron; on the other hand, iron may be gained from pots and utensils. The daily intakes of iron in European populations are approximately as follows: infants: 2.6–6.0 mg; 1 to <3 years: 5.0–7.0 mg; 3 to <10 years: 7.5–11.5 mg; 10 to <18 years: 9.2–14.7 mg, and in adults >18 years: 9.4–17.9 mg.

Table 9.2 Factors influencing intestinal uptake and transfer of iron.

Enhancers	Inhibitors
Systemic	
Systemic need for iron; iron deficiency, new tissue synthesis (e.g. increased erythropoiesis)	Chronic inflammatory states – part of the Anaemia of Chronic Disease (ACD)
	Iron overload
Fasting	Achlorhydria
Pregnancy	Copper deficiency
Food components	
Amino acids (lysine, cysteine, histidine) peptides	Phosphates; phytate, casein phosphatides, tannins,
Organic acids: citric, ascorbic, lactic, malic, lactic	polyphenols (tea, coffee, cocoa, red wine), vegetables
Fructose, sorbitol, ethanol	(spinach, aubergine), legumes
Additives (e.g. NaFeEDTA)	Soy and legume proteins
	Inorganic elements: Ca, Zn, Cd

Source: EFSA (2016), Hurrell and Egli (2016)

9.6 Bioavailability of iron

Factors influencing the bioavailability of dietary iron are summarised in Table 9.2. The predominant determinant of bioavailability of iron is the systemic need for iron. Algorithms to assess the contribution of this to iron bioavailability have been based on serum ferritin concentrations. This is a valuable tool because dietary factors only become limiting when there is a significant systemic requirement for iron.

Phytate and polyphenols, of which those in tea are most inhibitory, are the major inhibitors of iron uptake, and ascorbic acid is a good enhancer of the uptake of non-haem iron by reducing Fe^{3+} to Fe^{2+} and it can ameliorate most of the inhibitory effects of other food components. It is important to note that much information on bioavailability has been derived from single meal studies performed in individuals who are iron replete. Longer studies show an attenuation, presumably due to intestinal adaptation, of the initial effects of both inhibitors and enhancers over a period of days after their incorporation into diets. It is now realised that bioavailability data need to be interpreted cautiously.

9.7 Iron dietary reference values

The physiological requirement for iron is based on a factorial model of losses, or on a composite of daily losses assessed by monitoring the rate of loss of isotopes used to label the systemic pool. The latter approach informed the dietary reference values (DRVs) in Table 9.3.

Table 9.3 DRVs for iron, European Food Safety Agency, 2016.

Age	Average requirement (mg/day)	Population reference intake (mg/day)
7–11 months	8	11
1–6 years	5	7
7–11 years	8	11
12–17 years (M)	8	11
12–17 years (F)	7	13
≥18 years (M)	6	11
≥18 years (F)		
premenopausal	7	16
postmenopausal	6	11
Pregnancy	As for non-pregnant premenopausal women	
Lactation	As for non-lactating premenopausal women	

Source: EFSA (2016)

9.8 Causes of iron deficiency

It is important to note that a pure iron deficiency is unusual (Table 9.4). It may be encountered in infants and toddlers who are inappropriately fed. More commonly the conditions associated with iron deficiency are invariably associated with other nutrient deficiencies. Blood loss is a significant cause; 1 g of haemoglobin contains 3.39 mg iron. Most enteropathies involve, as well as malabsorption, loss of systemic iron and other trace elements, as well as proteins. Thus, in most instances iron deficiency needs to be regarded as a marker of a multinutritional deficit, particularly in communities where anaemia is endemic. For example, vitamin A can affect several stages of iron metabolism, including erythropoiesis and the release of iron from ferritin stores; riboflavin is involved in the mobilisation of iron from

Table 9.4 Causes of iron deficiency.

Low iron intake relative to systemic needs
Periods of rapid tissue synthesis, such as growth and rehabilitation; pubertal growth, menarche, delayed and inappropriate diversification of diet in later infancy (too much cows' milk displacing other foods in infants and toddlers); inappropriate diets in general; vegetarians: cows' milk, dietary matrix
Maldigestion and malabsorption
Reduced gastroduodenal acidity caused by gastrectomy, gastric bypass, gastric atrophy, proton pump inhibitors, antacids, intestinal resection. Enteropathies (see 'Systemic loss' entry).
Systemic loss
Genitourinary system, menorrhagia, childbirth, trauma, blood loss in the gastrointestinal tract, protein-losing gastroenteropathies, enterocolitis, intestinal parasitism (*Necator americanus, Ancylostoma duodenale, Trichuris trichiura, schistosomiasis, Helicobacter pylori*)

Source: SACN (2010)

ferritin, and folate can often be a limiting factor in the erythropoietic response to iron therapy. Vegetarians have been reported to have lower serum ferritins than omnivores, but their values are usually within the reference range for serum ferritin.

9.9 Features of deficiency

In animal models, iron deficiency, with or without anaemia, is associated with inefficient energy metabolism, altered glucose and lactate utilisation, and reduced muscle myoglobin content, strength and endurance; reduced cytochrome c oxidase activity in muscle and in the intestinal mucosa; impaired collagen synthesis and osteoporosis; altered vitamin A and prostaglandin metabolism. In the brain, dopaminergic and serotonin neurotransmission may be reduced, and neuromyelination, and dendritic and synapse development may be defective and persistent from early life. Associated functional impairments include delayed responses to auditory and visual stimuli, and impaired memory and spatial navigation. There are few data giving a dose–response relationship for these effects, but many accompany relatively more severe iron deficiencies than those usually encountered in human populations. Nonetheless, these manifestations provide plausible but not definitive mechanisms for inferring that iron deficiency, with or without anaemia, may have similar effects in humans.

Some features traditionally attributed to iron deficiency, such as spoon-shaped soft nails, glossitis, dermatitis at the corners of the mouth, mood changes, muscle weakness and impaired immunity, can also be secondary features of other nutritional deficiencies.

Many studies examining relationships between iron deficiency and adverse sequelae in humans use anaemia as a surrogate indicator of iron deficiency and do not characterise the 'deficiency' sufficiently to identify thresholds of anaemia or iron deficiency at which adverse outcomes occur.

Iron-deficient and anaemic infants and children have impaired attention, poor recognition memory, reduced reward-seeking behaviours and impoverished social interactions. Other features are poor motor development, altered auditory responses and a long-lasting poor cognitive and behavioural performance. There is evidence that adolescent girls who were anaemic as toddlers have altered memory and spatial awareness. However, much of this research is confounded by socio-economic and environmental factors and possibly other causes of anaemia. The vulnerable periods for the effects of early-life deficiencies have not been clearly identified. This is problematic, in that many persist and are irredeemable by subsequent iron supplementation, thereby setting affected children on a life course of poor achievement, disadvantage and limited economic productivity, which in many situations affects families, whole communities and subsequent generations.

In adults, low haemoglobin concentrations have been associated with lethargy, impaired concentration and fatigability, reduced voluntary activity, physical work capacity and productivity, and reduced reproductive efficiency. Although many studies have poorly reported outcomes and characterisation of iron deficiency, there is an implication from these data overall that iron-responsive defects occur at haemoglobin concentrations below 80, 95 and 110 g/L. However, these thresholds arise from cut-offs applied during analysis of haemoglobin values, and the outcomes have not been assessed against the degree of anaemia as a continuous variable, so no specific threshold of anaemia (or even the degree of iron deficiency) is really known for these phenomena. A possible exception is that muscle endurance and energetic efficiency decline as haemoglobin concentrations drop below 130 g/L, and the effect becomes greater with every 10 g/L fall in haemoglobin. Additionally iron-responsive impaired muscle endurance has been demonstrated in groups without anaemia but in whom serum ferritin concentrations were <16 µg/L.

9.10 Anaemia of Chronic Disease

Iron turnover and utilisation are disturbed as part of the acute-phase response to infection and inflammation. If such stresses are sustained (e.g. with recurrent infections, persistent infestations, chronic inflammatory disease), a chronic functional iron deficiency including an anaemia (i.e. ACD) develops even though individuals may be iron replete. This condition is attributed to hypoxia, free radicals and, particularly, inflammatory cytokines and interleukins 1 and 6 acting on the cellular iron sensing and regulatory systems to induce a 'shut down' of systemic iron turnover and its absorption. A major part of this phenomenon is the result of increased synthesis of hepcidin, which not only reduces iron uptake and export in enterocytes, but also has the same effect on other cells, including the monocyte–macrophage system responsible for erythropoiesis. Their ferroportin iron export systems are degraded; iron is trapped in the cells and deposited in ferritin. This response overrides any adaptation to an inadequate iron supply. Thus, ACD iron-deficiency anaemia (haemoglobin usually 80–95 g/L) has normal red cell indices and no evidence of new erythrocyte formation, a normal or elevated serum ferritin level and low iron and transferrin and a reduced transferrin saturation. Serum transferrin receptors are usually less affected in ACD. This recompartmentation of iron might be a defence

mechanism to restrict the availability of iron to pathogens. Obesity also induces an ACD via the production of inflammatory mediators and hepcidin.

9.11 Measuring iron inadequacy, adequacy and excess (status)

The development of iron deficiency progresses from depletion of systemic depots coupled with a compensatory increased intestinal absorption of iron, and when this compensation fails, functional iron deficiency ensues. This is usually detected when anaemia is found, by which time other functional effects may be present, particularly in tissues which have shorter turnover times than erythrocytes. There is no single marker of iron status. An assessment of possible iron deficiency depends on an intelligent suspicion and interpretation of the markers of iron adequacy (Table 9.5) in the context of a risk assessment of the diet (i.e. characteristics that might affect the amount and bioavailability of iron), environmental risk, and clinical features in individuals, their families and communities. Once, population surveys measured haemoglobin, serum ferritin, soluble transferrin receptor (sTfR) and/or zinc protoporphyrin, and individuals with two or more abnormal values were considered iron deficient, but now such surveys rely predominantly on measurements of anaemia and iron depots (i.e. haemoglobin and ferritin). Currently, iron deficiency or a significant risk thereof in public health nutrition is regarded as a serum ferritin concentration below 15 µg/L. However, serum ferritin may be elevated as part of an ACD. To distinguish between iron-deficiency anaemia (IDA) and ACD, markers of inflammation (C-reactive protein or α-1-acid glycoprotein) can be measured. A ratio of sTfR to log ferritin >2 is probably indicative of iron deficiency, whereas a ratio <1 suggests an ACD.

There is also limited information on reference values for infants and young children.

9.12 Iron excess

The risk of systemic iron overload from dietary sources is negligible with normal intestinal function. There is no association between high dietary iron intakes and arthritis, diabetes mellitus, neurodegenerative disease and colorectal cancer. However, acute intakes of iron of 20 mg or more elemental iron per kilogram of body weight, particularly without food, damages the intestine, causing diarrhoea and blood loss, which might lead to systemic fluid loss, shock, oxidative tissue and organ damage and failure, and death. Early features of this (gastritis, nausea, abdominal pain and vomiting) have

Table 9.5 Markers of iron adequacy, deficiency and excess.

Marker	Representative reference range (adults)	Diagnostic use Confounding factors
Homeostasis		
Hepcidin		Not yet fully validated. Values correlate with serum ferritin, and are lower in women than in men. Relationship to iron loss (e.g. with menstruation). Potentially very useful but is not yet sufficiently standardised for clinical or public health use.
Tissue iron need		
Serum transferrin receptor	2.8–8.5 mg/L	Inversely related to iron supply to cells and increased with new tissue synthesis (thus increased in growing children) and erythropoiesis. Less perturbed by ACD than serum ferritin but its value for children in regions where malaria and infection are endemic is less certain. Expensive and not well-standardised methodology.
Tissue iron supply and turnover		
Serum transferrin/iron	10–30 μmol/L	Most extracellular iron is bound to transferrin. Subject to diurnal and
Transferrin saturation	15–60%	prandial fluctuations. Reduced with ACD. Raised with iron overload.
Serum total iron binding capacity		Inversely related to transferrin saturation
Iron in tissues		
Serum ferritin		Important marker. In health 1 μg/L represents 8–10 mg Fe in tissues.
females	12–200 μg/L	Elevated in ACD. Raised in iron overload.
males	12–300 μg/L	
Bone marrow:		Stainable iron in aspirate of marrow. Invasive, expensive, and assessment is subjective. Not suitable for population surveys.
Iron-deficient functions		
Haemoglobin		Commonly used. NB: it is a late marker of IDA; poor specificity and selectivity. Good monitor for therapeutic responses.
females	120–160 g/L	
males	130–180 g/L	
Mean corpuscular haemoglobin	27–32 pg	Useful for monitoring therapeutic response. Probably not useful for surveys. Other measures more practical.
Mean cell volume	84–99 fL	
Reticulocyte haemoglobin	<25 pg	Suggestive of iron deficiency
Zinc protoporphyrin	<800 μg/L	Good marker of iron deficiency

Source: SACN (2010), EFSA (2016)

been used to set exposure levels for health guidance. In the UK, a guidance level for supplemental iron intake has been set at 17 mg a day for adults in addition to that in the diet; in North America a guidance value was set at 45 mg.

Iron supplementation might impair physical growth of iron-replete infants and children, but further studies are required to characterise this effect.

Breast milk contains the iron-binding protein lactoferrin, which is thought to protect against pathogenic bacteria by limiting their iron supply and indirectly by favouring a protective intestinal microflora.

An increased incidence of diarrhoeal disease, septicaemia and activation of infections (e.g. malaria) has been observed in communities where iron therapy has been used as a general measure. The World Health Organization (WHO) recommends that children who are anaemic and at risk of iron deficiency should also receive concurrent protection from malaria and other infectious diseases. Furthermore, iron alters the intestinal microflora.

Most bacteria, not just those in the soil, have powerful siderophores. These can strip iron from haem and from iron proteins. If iron is available either in the gut or even systemically, say as a result of the breakdown of red cells by malaria, microbial proliferation and virulence of pathogens may increase and intestinal damage and systemic infections with gut organisms can develop. This is a challenge in devising strategies to prevent and mange iron deficiency/IDA.

9.13 Treatment and prevention of iron deficiency

Routine iron supplementation (30 mg elemental iron a day) as a preventive measure, with a larger dose of 60–120 mg per day to treat anaemia, may be considered enough for routine management of iron deficiency in individuals. The usual iron salts used to provide iron are ferrous sulphate (containing 60 mg of iron/300 mg);

ferrous fumarate (65 mg of iron/200 mg); or ferrous gluconate (35 mg of iron/300 mg). Although this approach might be suitable for an individual with a well-characterised cause for iron deficiency, additional treatments would be needed in circumstances when there may be other nutritional deficiencies or infections to ensure that the iron supplements would be effective. Iron supplements for pregnant women should not be used routinely except for those with haemoglobin values below 110 g/L in the first and second trimester and below 105 g/L from 28 weeks' gestation.

9.14 Addressing iron deficiency as a public health issue

It is estimated that 1.5–2.0 billion people are affected by anaemia; this is often attributed to iron deficiency. These figures are not well verified; nonetheless, the situation is a marker for a global nutritional challenge. Clearly, current understanding of impairments of public health associated with iron deficiency is not as sound as that of understanding those associated with anaemia, and, irrespective of their pathogeneses, anaemias of less than 110 or 130 g/L (see earlier) have adverse effects and thus need to be prevented and managed. This should involve improving iron nutrition along the life trajectory by improving intake and its bioavailability and by preventing recurrent infections and blood loss. At the same time, it is important that associated nutritional deficiencies and other causes of anaemia (thalassaemias, sickle cell disease, haemoglobinopathies, etc.) are not overlooked.

A major strategic approach is to alert and educate the population, appropriate competent authorities and governments to the societal and economic benefits of improved nutrition and public health care. National, regional and local authorities need to appreciate the improved productivity, self-sufficiency and socio-economic benefits arising from reducing the prevalence of IDA/iron deficiency and be given the fundamental economic political and societal will to achieve this. The political will to act on this can be generated by increasing the engagement and empowerment of the citizenry who themselves could undertake some of the basic public health and sanitary measures that would control and eradicate some of the causes of iron deficiency.

To do this, there is a need to characterise the underlying problems and context for deficiencies of iron and other nutrients. These will differ according to social and cultural practices, geography, climate and so on. Vulnerable groups will need to be identified; usually, these would be infants, children and women in their reproductive years, as well as pregnant adolescent girls. Other factors are public sanitation, endemic infectious diseases and intestinal parasitism, agricultural practices and

staple foods, dietary characteristics and culinary practices (Pasricha et al., 2013; Raiten et al., 2016). All will need consideration.

As a general measure, clamping of the cord at birth should be delayed until it has stopped pulsing. Babies should be breast fed, and their weaning diets should be iron rich such as would be achieved with the inclusion of chicken liver or meat-based weaning foods, as are advocated in some WHO regions such as Southeast Asia (WHO, 2006).

Food processing methods such as milling, germination, fermentation and the addition of phytase enzymes can be used to degrade phytate and improve the availability of iron for intestinal uptake from foods. Iron fortification, as part of a wider strategy, is commonly used. The selection of fortificants has to consider oxidative effects of the inorganic iron salts and their effect on the shelf life and organoleptic properties of the foods. Many iron salts, ethylenediaminetetraacetic acid, encapsulated preparations with vegetable oils or stearates, micro-encapsulated 'sprinkles' and a micronutrient powder containing phytase and elemental iron to be added to foods have been tried in studies.

A major intervention should treat the cause of iron deficiency and any coexisting nutritional deficiencies; reduce and eliminate recurrent intestinal infestations; and reduce other underlying infections using measures to combat helminthiasis, schistosomiasis and H. pylori. More often than not, multi-micronutrient supplements, including folate, and the application of approaches as in the rehabilitation from pan-malnutrition and the treatment of infections are best implemented before supplying any iron. These initiatives will, as has been said, differ according to the circumstances in which iron deficiency/IDA are encountered, and measures to monitor the beneficial and adverse effects of any intervention and to inform an improvement cycle are important both in the more immediate context of health and in the broader development and wealth of the communities involved. An emerging challenge is that of applying risk–benefit analyses to these interventions to accommodate the effect that iron fortification and supplementation may have on the intestinal and, possibly, the body's microbiome, as recent animal and clinical studies looking at the relationship between iron supplementation and gut microbiota have reported that supplementation can affect gastrointestinal health (Lee et al., 2016).

9.15 Conclusion

There are many uncertainties concerning human iron nutrition and iron deficiency. Measurement of intakes is compromised by the quality of compositional data, and there are difficulties in measuring and predicting bioavailability of iron from diets and in measuring iron status in people. All of these impair the setting of DRVs. The information needed to address these issues will also enable the characterisation of public health iron deficiency/IDA and its interaction with ACD, along with helping in the risk analysis of, and the interventions to prevent and manage, iron deficiency in public health.

Reference

Hurrell R, Egli I (2010). Iron bioavailability and dietary reference values. *American Journal of Nutrition* **91** 1461–1467.

Lee *et al*, (2016). Oral versus intravenous iron replacement therapy distinctly alters the gut microbiota and metabolome in patients with IBD. *BMJ Gut*; **0**, 1–9.

Lee, T., Clavel, T., Smirnov, K. *et al.* (2016) Oral versus intravenous iron replacement therapy distinctly alters the gut microbiota and metabolome in patients with IBD. *Gut.* doi: 10.1136/gutjnl-2015-309940.

Pasricha S R., Drakesmith H, Black J, Hipgrave D, Biggs B-A (2013) Control of iron deficiency anaemia in low- and middle-income countries. *Blood* **121** 2607–2617.

Raiten DJ, Neufeld LM, De-Regil L-M *et al* (2016) Integration to Implementation and the Micronutrient Forum: A Coordinated Approach for Global Nutrition. Case Study Application: Safety and Effectiveness of Iron Interventions. *Advances in Nutrition* **7** 135–148.

Scientific Advisory Committee on Nutrition (SACN) (2010) Iron and Health. http://www.sacn.gov.uk/pdfs/sacn_iron_and_health_report_web.pdf www.sacn.gov.uk/pdfs/sacn_iron_and_health_report_web.pdf.

Scientific Opinion on Dietary Reference Values for iron. *EFSA Journal 2015*;**13**(10):4254 http://www.efsa.europa.eu/en/efsajournal/pub/4254

World Health Organisation/Food and Agricultural Organisation of the United Nations. 2006 Guidelines on Food Fortification with Micronutrients. WHO Geneva. www.who.int/nutrition/publications/guide_food_fortification_micronutrients.pdf

Iodine

Key messages

- Iodine is essential for the production of thyroid hormones, which are required for growth, development and metabolism. Thyroid hormones, and therefore iodine, are vital for brain and neurological development during gestation and early life.
- The effects of severe iodine deficiency are well known and include goitre, cretinism, reduced IQ and impaired motor skills.
- The WHO-recommended nutrient intake (RNI) for iodine in adulthood is 150 μg/day but rises to 250 μg/day during pregnancy and lactation.
- Excessive iodine intake (>1000 μg/day for adults and 600 μg/day for pregnant women) can lead to thyroid dysfunction and should be avoided.
- Evidence for adverse effects of mild-to-moderate iodine deficiency in pregnancy is sparse, but recent observational data suggest an association between low iodine status in pregnant women and reduced IQ, reading and spelling ability in the child.

- Iodine deficiency has been eradicated in many countries worldwide through salt iodisation programmes.
- National monitoring of iodine status is vital as iodine deficiency has recently re-emerged in some countries that were formerly considered to be iodine sufficient, such as New Zealand, Australia and the UK.
- Iodine is concentrated in the oceans, and therefore seafood (white fish, oily fish and shellfish) and seaweed are rich dietary sources. Some seaweeds are very high in iodine and their consumption can result in excessive iodine intake. Milk and dairy products are major sources of iodine in many countries.
- Iodine deficiency during pregnancy is of considerable public health concern as it affects educational attainment and therefore later employment and earning potential.

9.16 Introduction

Role of iodine

Iodine is a vital component of the thyroid hormones thyroxine (T4) and tri-iodotyrosine (T3). A deficiency of iodine can therefore lead to inadequate thyroid hormone production. T4 is considered to be a pro-hormone that is converted to the biologically active T3 by selenium-dependent iodothyronine deiodinase enzymes. T3 binds to thyroid hormone receptor proteins in target cells (e.g. brain cells) that act as transcription factors, turning on gene transcription and protein synthesis. Thyroid hormones control a range of body functions, including metabolism and thermoregulation, and most importantly fetal neurological development. The WHO considers iodine deficiency to be 'the single most important preventable cause of brain damage' worldwide (WHO *et al.*, 2007).

Global prevalence of iodine deficiency

Iodine deficiency is estimated to affect 241 million school-aged children despite great improvements in global iodine nutrition since the turn of the century (Andersson *et al.*, 2012). This improvement is largely due to successful salt-iodisation programmes (Andersson *et al.*, 2012). Although iodine deficiency is often considered to be a problem of developing countries, it is increasingly recognised that industrialised countries are not immune. The 2012 survey by the WHO found that 32 countries were iodine deficient; no country was classified as severely iodine deficient, but 11 countries had excessive iodine status. Of those countries with iodine deficiency, nine were moderately deficient while 23 were mildly iodine deficient (including the UK) (Andersson *et al.*, 2012). The greatest degree of iodine deficiency in children is in European and African countries, while the Americas and western Pacific have the lowest degree of iodine deficiency.

9.17 Iodine deficiency disorders

Effects of severe deficiency

Goitre

The most recognisable sign of iodine deficiency is goitre (Figure 9.1), an adaptation of the thyroid gland to a very low iodine intake by increasing the iodine-trapping

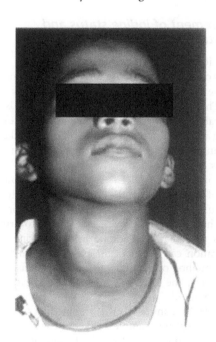

Figure 9.1 Child with goitre.

potential of the thyroid. The thyroid gland initially grows in a diffuse and homogenous manner, but can progress to nodule formation with prolonged iodine deficiency. Nodular goitre is more common in older inhabitants of iodine deficient regions and can pose a risk for iodine-induced hyperthyroidism when excessive iodine is supplied.

Cretinism and mental retardation

Owing to the role of maternal thyroid hormone in fetal brain development, iodine deficiency is associated with varying degrees of brain damage and mental retardation in the child. Severe iodine deficiency is linked to the development of cretinism, which can be categorised as either neurological or hypothyroid (myxedematous), but the two types can present in combination. Neurological cretinism manifests as hearing defects, spasticity of lower limbs and mental retardation; hypothyroid cretinism leads to symptoms of thyroid insufficiency, delayed sexual maturation, dry skin and stunted growth but is associated with less severe mental insufficiency than neurological cretinism (Zimmermann, 2009).

The effect of severe iodine deficiency in a population has been summarised by two meta-analyses of small studies that found a loss of 12–13 IQ points in severely iodine-deficient regions (Zimmermann, 2009).

Effect of mild-to-moderate deficiency

The effects of mild-to-moderate iodine deficiency on cognition are less well known than are those of severe iodine deficiency. Controlled studies of iodine supplementation in pregnancy in regions of mild-to-moderate iodine deficiency (with doses of between 100 and 230 µg/day) found favourable outcomes in terms of parameters of maternal thyroid function, including thyroid volume, but others showed no effect (Zimmermann, 2007). However, none of these studies included measures of infant development, and it was not until 2009 that the effect of iodine supplementation on child cognition was evaluated. Two trials of iodine supplementation in pregnant women from regions of mild-to-moderate iodine deficiency have found benefit on cognition in the offspring up to the age of 18 months (Berbel *et al.*, 2009; Velasco *et al.*, 2009). A later study with three treatment groups that compared the use of iodised salt and two different doses of potassium iodide (200 or 300 µg/day) supplements in pregnancy found no difference between treatments in either maternal thyroid function or neurological function of the child at 18 months (Santiago *et al.*, 2013). However, all these studies had limitations; none was a randomised placebo-controlled trial, so further work is required to establish the benefit, or indeed lack of harm, of iodine supplementation to women in regions of mild-to-moderate iodine deficiency.

Relatively few studies have evaluated the impact on child development of low urinary iodine excretion, rather than suboptimal thyroid function. However, recent studies in Spain (Costeira *et al.*, 2011), the Netherlands (van Mil *et al.*, 2012) and Tasmania (Hynes *et al.*, 2013) have applied such an approach and found an association between low urinary iodine excretion and lower psychomotor and mental scores at 18 months (Costeira *et al.*, 2011), executive functioning at 4 years (van Mil *et al.*, 2012) and spelling ability at 9 years (Hynes *et al.*, 2013).

Mild-to-moderate iodine deficiency in 1000 UK pregnant women was found to be adversely associated with child cognition. After adjustment for 21 confounders, children of women with an iodine-to-creatinine ratio of less than 150 µg/g were significantly more likely to have scores in the lowest quartile for verbal IQ, reading accuracy and reading comprehension than were those of mothers with ratios of 150 µg/g or more (Bath *et al.*, 2013).

Iodine recommendations

Iodine recommendations
The UK DRVs for iodine were set in 1991; 70 µg/day was estimated to be the minimum iodine intake required to prevent goitre in adults, hence the UK RNI was set at twice that value (i.e. at 140 µg/day). Table 9.6 compares UK recommendations for iodine intake with those set by other international bodies. The comparison highlights the fact that the UK does not specify an increment in iodine intake in pregnancy and lactation, in marked contrast to the near-doubling recommended by other authorities. The UK recommendations take no account of the fact that pregnant women require additional iodine for three reasons:

Table 9.6 Iodine recommendations by life stage according to different international bodies.

Life stage	Daily iodine recommendations (µg/day)		
	UK[a] RNI	USA[b] RDA	WHO[c] RNI
15–18 years	140	150	150
19–50 years	140	150	150
Pregnancy	—	220	250
Lactation	—	290	250

Source: Bath and Rayman (2013).
[a] Department of Health (1991).
[b] Institute of Medicine (US) Panel on Micronutrients (2001).
[c] WHO *et al.* (2007).

(i) to facilitate the 50% increase in thyroid hormone production required in pregnancy, (ii) to cover the increase in renal clearance of iodine and (iii) to provide the fetal requirement for iodine after the onset of fetal thyroid function around mid-gestation. Though it may be possible for the higher iodine requirement of pregnancy to be met in part by drawing on thyroidal iodine stores – and possibly placental stores, though it is not known whether these can be utilised by the fetus (Burns *et al.*, 2011) – this is only feasible if these stores are maximised prior to conception, which would not be the case in a region of iodine deficiency.

Excessive intake of iodine
It is worth noting that iodine excess may be as problematic as iodine deficiency, having implications for altered thyroid function, including hypothyroidism and hyperthyroidism. A safe upper limit of 17 µg/day per kilogram body weight, or 1000 µg/day, for adults has been suggested (Department of Health, 1991). The tolerable upper intake level of iodine for pregnant women has been set at 600 µg/day by the European Commission and at 1100 µg/day by the US Institute of Medicine. The upper limit for iodine intake is a somewhat arbitrary cut-off, as some individuals, particularly those with longstanding iodine deficiency, may respond adversely to intakes below the suggested safe level.

Measurement of iodine status and population monitoring

Urinary iodine concentration
Iodine is classified as a micronutrient, the status of which should be assessed by biomarkers rather than by dietary intake. This is because the iodine content of foods varies considerably (e.g. because of farming practice), thus resulting in inaccurate estimates of iodine intake from dietary analysis. It is estimated that over 90% of ingested iodine is excreted via the kidneys; therefore, urinary iodine concentration (UIC) is considered a good biomarker of iodine intake at the population level. However, care should be taken that urine samples used for iodine analysis have not been previously exposed to urine test strips as they may leak iodine into the urine. Iodine concentration can either be measured by the Sandell–Kolthoff method or by inductively coupled plasma mass spectrometry; the latter is considered to be the more accurate method.

The WHO recommends that the median UIC, measured in spot-urine samples, is compared with their published cut-off values to indicate iodine sufficiency in populations (Table 9.7). It is worth highlighting that

Table 9.7 Classification of iodine status of a population according to WHO 2007 criteria.

Life stage	Median UIC (μg/L)	Category of iodine status
School-aged children and non-pregnant adults	<20	Severely deficient
	20–49	Moderately deficient
	50–99	Mildly deficient
	100–199	Adequate
	200–299	More than adequate
	≥300	Excessive
Pregnant women	<150	Insufficient
	150–249	Adequate
	250–499	More than adequate
	≥500	No added health benefit expected

Source: Bath and Rayman (2013).

the cut-off for adults has been assumed to be the same as for school-aged children, but this assumption has been challenged; a median UIC of 60–70 μg/L may be a better reflection of adequate iodine status in adults (Zimmermann and Andersson, 2012).

A spot-urine sample is not suitable for individual iodine assessment due to substantial intra-individual variation in daily urine volume excreted and iodine intake (Zimmermann, 2009). The variation in urine volume can be overcome by measuring urinary creatinine concentration, particularly if adjusted for the age and sex of the individual (Knudsen *et al.*, 2000). Use of the age-and-sex-adjusted iodine-to-creatinine ratio may be preferable to iodine concentration in industrialised countries such as the UK, where subjects are well nourished. However, in malnourished subjects, creatinine excretion is low, and hence the iodine-to-creatinine ratio is not a reliable estimate of iodine excretion.

Thyroid size

Traditionally, the goitre rate in a population was used for assessing iodine nutrition, and iodine sufficiency was assumed if less than 5% of school-aged children had goitre. The use of goitre rate to define the iodine status of a population is problematic as there is a considerable lag-time between an increase in iodine intake and a decline in the goitre rate. Thus, this approach is no longer favoured for population monitoring but can give a long-term estimate of iodine status.

Thyroglobulin

Thyroglobulin (Tg) is a protein that is only produced in the thyroid. Under normal, iodine-sufficient conditions, very little is secreted into the circulation, but in iodine

deficiency the circulating Tg levels increase. Elevated Tg levels have been found in conditions of both iodine deficiency and iodine excess, suggesting its utility as a sensitive marker (more so than thyroid-stimulating hormone or T4) of both low and high iodine intakes (Zimmermann *et al.*, 2013). In addition, Tg levels have been shown to fall in response to iodine supplementation, either with iodised oil or in iodised-salt programmes. Tg can be measured in a dried blood spot, making it a feasible marker for population monitoring. It has been proposed that a median Tg of <13 μg/L or <3% of Tg values >40 μg/L indicates iodine sufficiency in a population (Zimmermann *et al.*, 2013). Antibodies to Tg may confound Tg analysis and interpretation; therefore, these should be measured concurrently, although the prevalence of positive Tg antibodies in school-aged children has been found to be low (<1%).

Correction of iodine deficiency in populations

Iodised salt

The method recommended by the WHO to correct iodine deficiency in a population is universal salt iodisation, which is the iodisation of all salt for human and animal consumption; salt is usually iodised with potassium iodide or iodate. Salt has been the vehicle of choice for iodine fortification programmes as it is relatively inexpensive, easy to monitor and regulate and consumed at constant levels by most people in a population. Many countries have implemented iodised-salt programmes, although it is rare that universal salt iodisation is achieved; many food manufacturers do not use iodised salt, and salt is often not iodised for livestock.

The UK does not currently have a programme for the elimination of iodine deficiency through use of iodised salt. There are obvious potential conflicts between the salt reduction campaigns that have been implemented in many industrialised countries (including the UK) and an iodised-salt programme. However, the WHO suggests that the two public policies can work in harmony, as individual countries can set the concentration of iodine in salt to provide adequate iodine intake from a lower total salt intake.

Alternative vehicles for iodine fortification

As an alternative to salt, other foods can be used as a vehicle for iodine fortification. For example, in Australia and New Zealand there has been a mandatory requirement that all bread should be fortified with iodine (through the use of iodised salt) since 2009, and this has resulted in an improvement in the iodine status of children (Skeaff and Lonsdale-Cooper, 2013; Australian Bureau of Statistics, 2014). Iodine intake can also be improved in a population by indirect or unintentional iodisation; for instance, iodine-enriched milk and dairy produce have improved iodine supply to the UK population as a result of farming practice (Phillips, 1997) and are currently the principal UK dietary sources of iodine intake.

Iodine supplementation in women of childbearing age and pregnant women

The WHO states that in countries where iodised salt programmes cover 90% of the population, pregnant women do not need to take iodine supplements. However, in countries without successful iodisation programmes, pregnant women may be vulnerable to iodine deficiency. Women should ideally ensure adequate iodine intake for several months prior to conception in order to maximise thyroidal stores of iodine. Evidence suggests that optimising iodine stores pre-pregnancy rather than initiating iodine supplementation in pregnancy is preferable for maternal thyroid function (Moleti et al., 2011). Several international bodies (e.g. the American Thyroid Association and the Food Standards Agency of Australia and New Zealand) now recommend that women planning a pregnancy and pregnant or lactating women should take a supplement of 150 μg iodine per day (as potassium iodide/iodate). Kelp supplements should be avoided (see 'Dietary sources of iodine' section). Individual countries need to assess the situation at a local level to ensure that the correct advice is given to women of childbearing age.

Intake

Dietary sources of iodine

The iodine content of foods is dependent on source, whether from sea or land, soil content and farming practice. Fish is a rich source of iodine as fish are able to concentrate iodine from seawater, but there are large variations in iodine content both between species and within species from different sources. However, fish contributes just an estimated 11% of iodine intake in the UK (Henderson et al., 2003) largely because of low fish consumption.

In the UK the most important dietary source of iodine is milk and dairy products, and this food group is also an important source in many European countries, New Zealand and the USA. The iodine concentration of UK organic milk is between 35 and 42% lower than that of conventional milk (Bath et al., 2012; Payling et al., 2015). UK eggs are a reasonably good source of iodine, with a concentration that is similar to that of milk and dairy produce. Although cereals and cereal products, such as

bread, are good sources of iodine in some countries (e.g. the USA and Netherlands), this is not the case in the UK as potassium iodate is not used as a dough conditioner and iodised salt is not used in bread manufacture.

Dietary supplements can make significant contributions to iodine intake, but their suitability depends on the formulation. Kelp supplements have been analysed in both the UK and the USA; the iodine content was found to be highly variable, with most UK kelp supplements providing more than the iodine content declared on the label (Zimmermann and Delange, 2004). As a consequence, kelp and seaweed supplements are an unreliable source of iodine and are not recommended, particularly during pregnancy.

Goitrogens

Goitrogens are dietary or environmental factors that can cause the enlargement of the thyroid. Goitrogens in food exhibit their effects in different ways; thiocyanate and isothiocyanates (produced by ingestion of cassava, cabbage, broccoli and cauliflower) inhibit uptake of iodine into the thyroid (or breast) through competitive inhibition of the sodium-iodide-symporter, while flavanoids (e.g. from soy) impair the oxidation and organification of iodine into thyroid hormones through inhibition of thyroid peroxidise (Gaitan, 1990). Goitrogens only appear to exert an adverse effect if iodine intake is low.

Other nutrients, besides iodine, that are required for adequate thyroid function include selenium and iron. Thyroid peroxidase, the enzyme that catalyses the production of thyroid hormones, is a haem enzyme; hence, iron deficiency is detrimental to the thyroid. Iron deficiency can reduce the effectiveness of iodine supplementation; salt fortified with both iodine and iron benefits thyroid volume and function more than iodine alone in regions with concurrent iron and iodine deficiencies (Hess, 2010). Selenium, as selenoproteins, is required by the thyroid gland; glutathione peroxidase and thioredoxin reductase protect thyrocytes from the hydrogen peroxide generated there, and iodothyronine deiodinases convert T4 to the active form T3 (Kohrle and Gartner, 2009).

Re-emergence of deficiency in developed countries

Iodine deficiency used to be widespread in the UK, as evidenced by endemic goitre in some regions. The UK never introduced a formal iodisation programme but instead experienced iodisation by default as UK milk-iodine concentration increased as a result of changes in the dairy-farming industry that included the use of iodine-fortified cattle feed and iodine disinfectants. Furthermore, the UK Government promoted the consumption of milk for general health. The combined effect of these changes resulted in a threefold increase in iodine intake between the 1950s and the

1980s (Phillips, 1997) that was sufficient to cause a decrease in the incidence of goitre. The population was subsequently assumed to be iodine sufficient. However, this assumption was recently challenged by a number of small-scale, localised studies that found evidence of iodine deficiency in women of childbearing age and pregnant women (Bath and Rayman, 2015). In 2011, the concern for widespread iodine deficiency was heightened when the first national survey for more 60 years revealed mild iodine deficiency in UK schoolgirls (Vanderpump *et al.*, 2011). The median UIC, measured in 737 adolescent schoolgirls (14–15 years) across nine regions in the UK, indicated mild iodine deficiency.

The fact that iodine deficiency has re-emerged in the UK despite the assumption that the problem was confined to history mirrors the experience of other industrialised countries, such as in the USA (where iodine status of women of childbearing age and pregnant women is marginal), Australia and New Zealand (Skeaff *et al.*, 2002; Li *et al.*, 2006). These countries have witnessed a decrease in iodine intake despite being considered iodine replete and having successfully eradicated

iodine deficiency in the past. The declining iodine status in these countries is partly due to the reduced popularity of milk in vulnerable groups such as young girls (e.g. in the UK) and the fact that salt intake from processed foods is largely not iodised (e.g. in Australia and New Zealand). Complacency has been named as the 'greatest enemy in the war against iodine deficiency' (Dunn, 2000) and the experience of these countries highlights the fact that monitoring of population iodine status is critical.

9.18 Conclusions and recommendations

Iodine deficiency, particularly during pregnancy, is of considerable public health concern. Women of childbearing age should endeavour to meet their requirement for iodine prior to conception in order to maximise thyroidal iodine stores and ensure optimal thyroid hormone production in early pregnancy. Population monitoring of iodine status is essential to ensure that both iodine deficiency and iodine excess are avoided.

References

Andersson, M., Karumbunathan, V. and Zimmermann, M.B. (2012) Global Iodine status in 2011 and trends over the past decade. *Journal of Nutrition*, **142**, 744–750.

Australian Bureau of Statistics (2014) Australian Health Survey: Biomedical Results for Nutrients, 2011–12. Feature article: iodine. http://www.abs.gov.au/ausstats/abs@.nsf/Lookup/4364.0.55.006Chapter1202011-12 (accessed 3 December 2016).

Bath, S.C. and Rayman M.P. (2013) Iodine deficiency in the UK: an overlooked cause of impaired neurodevelopment? *Public Health Nutrition*, **72**, 226–235.

Bath, S.C. and Rayman M.P. (2015) A review of the iodine status of UK pregnant women and its implications for the offspring. *Environmental Geochemistry and Health*, **37** (4), 619–629.

Bath, S.C., Button, S. and Rayman M.P. (2012) Iodine concentration of organic and conventional milk: implications for iodine intake. *The British Journal of Nutrition*, **107** (7), 935–940.

Bath, S.C., Steer, C.D., Golding, J. et al. (2013) Effect of inadequate iodine status in UK pregnant women on cognitive outcomes in their children: results from the Avon Longitudinal Study of Parents and Children (ALSPAC). *Lancet*, **382** (9889), 331–337.

Berbel, P., Mestre, J.L., Santamaria, A. et al. (2009) Delayed neurobehavioral development in children born to pregnant women with mild hypothyroxinemia during the first month of gestation: the importance of early iodine supplementation. *Thyroid*, **19** (5), 511–519.

Burns, R., O'Herlihy, C. and Smyth P.P. (2011) The placenta as a compensatory iodine storage organ. *Thyroid*, **21** (5), 541–546.

Costeira, M.J., Oliveira, P., Santos, N.C. et al. (2011) Psychomotor development of children from an iodine-deficient region. *The Journal of Pediatrics*, **159** (3), 447–453.

Department of Health (1991) *Report on Health and Social Subjects: 41. Dietary Reference Values for Food, Energy and Nutrients for the United Kingdom*. The Stationery Office, London.

Dunn, J.T., (2000) Complacency: the most dangerous enemy in the war against iodine deficiency. *Thyroid*, **10** (8), 681–683.

Dietary Reference Intakes for Vitamin A, Vitamin K, Arsenic, Boron, Chromium, Copper, Iodine, Manganese, Molybdenum, Nickel, Silicon, Vanadium and Zinc Gaitan, E. (1990). Goitrogens in food and water. *Annual Review of Nutrition*, **10**, 21–39.

Henderson, L., Irving, K., Gregory, J. et al. (2003) *The National Diet & Nutrition Survey: Adults Aged 19 to 64 Years. Volume 3: Vitamin and Mineral Intake and Urinary Analytes*. HMSO, London.

Hess, S.Y. (2010) The impact of common micronutrient deficiencies on iodine and thyroid metabolism: the evidence from human studies. *Best Practice and Research. Clinical Endocrinology and Metabolism*, **24** (1), 117–132.

Hynes, K.L., Otahal, P., Hay, I. and Burgess J.R. (2013) Mild iodine deficiency during pregnancy is associated with reduced educational outcomes in the offspring: 9-year follow-up of the gestational iodine cohort. *The Journal of Clinical Endocrinology and Metabolism*, **98** (5), 1954–1962.

Institute of Medicine (US) Panel on Micronutrients (2001) *Dietary Reference Intakes for Vitamin A, Vitamin K, Arsenic, Boron, Chromium, Copper, Iodine, Manganese, Molybdenum, Nickel, Silicon, Vanadium and Zinc*. National Academy Press, Washington, DC.

Knudsen, N., Christiansen, E., Brandt-Christensen, M. et al. (2000) Age- and sex-adjusted iodine/creatinine ratio. A new standard in epidemiological surveys? Evaluation of three different estimates of iodine excretion based on casual urine samples and comparison to 24 h values. *European Journal of Clinical Nutrition*, **54** (4), 361–363.

Kohrle, J. and Gartner R. (2009). Selenium and thyroid. *Best Practice and Research. Clinical Endocrinology and Metabolism*, **23** (6), 815–827.

Li, M., Waite, K.V., Ma G. and Eastman C.J. (2006) Declining iodine content of milk and re-emergence of iodine deficiency in Australia. *The Medical Journal of Australia*, **184** (6), 307.

Moleti, M., Di Bella, B., Giorgianni, G. et al. (2011) Maternal thyroid function in different conditions of iodine nutrition in pregnant women exposed to mild-moderate iodine deficiency: an observational study. *Clinical Endocrinology (Oxford)*, **74** (6), 762–768.

Payling, L.M., Juniper, D.T., Drake, C. et al. (2015) Effect of milk type and processing on iodine concentration of organic and conventional winter milk at retail: implications for nutrition. *Food Chemistry*, **178,**: 327–330.

Phillips, D.I. (1997) Iodine, milk, and the elimination of endemic goitre in Britain: the story of an accidental public health triumph. *Journal of Epidemiology and Community Health*, **51** (4), 391–393.

Santiago, P., Velasco, I., Muela, J.A. *et al.* (2013) Infant neuro-cognitive development is independent of the use of iodised salt or iodine supplements given during pregnancy. *The British Journal of Nutrition*, **110** (5), 831–839.

Skeaff, S.A. and Lonsdale-Cooper E. (2013) Mandatory fortification of bread with iodised salt modestly improves iodine status in school-children. *The British Journal of Nutrition*, **109** (6), 1109–1113.

Skeaff, S.A., Thomson C.D. and Gibson R.S. (2002) Mild iodine deficiency in a sample of New Zealand schoolchildren. *European Journal of Clinical Nutrition*, **56** (12), 1169–1175.

Van Mil, N.H., Tiemeier, H. Bongers-Schokking, J.J. *et al.* (2012) Low urinary iodine excretion during early pregnancy is associated with alterations in executive functioning in children. *The Journal of Nutrition*, **142** (12), 2167–2174.

Vanderpump, M.P., Lazarus, J.H., Smyth, P.P. et al. (2011) Iodine status of UK schoolgirls: a cross-sectional survey. *Lancet*, **377** (9782): 2007–2012.

Velasco, I., Carreira, M., Santiago, P. *et al.* (2009). Effect of iodine prophylaxis during pregnancy on neurocognitive development of children during the first two years of life. *The Journal of Clinical Endocrinology and Metabolism*, **94** (9), 3234–3241.

WHO, UNICEF and ICCIDD (2007) *Assessment of Iodine Deficiency Disorders and Monitoring their Elimination.* WHO, Geneva.

Zimmermann, M.B. (2007) The adverse effects of mild-to-moderate iodine deficiency during pregnancy and childhood: a review. *Thyroid*, **17** (9), 829–835.

Zimmermann, M.B. (2009). Iodine deficiency. *Endocrine Reviews*, **30** (4), 376–408.

Zimmermann, M.B. and Andersson, M. (2012) Assessment of iodine nutrition in populations: past, present, and future. *Nutrition Reviews*, **70** (10), 553–570.

Zimmermann, M. and Delange F. (2004) Iodine supplementation of pregnant women in Europe: a review and recommendations. *European Journal of Clinical Nutrition*, **58** (7), 979–984.

Zimmermann, M.B., Aeberli, I., Andersson, M. *et al.* (2013) Thyroglobulin is a sensitive measure of both deficient and excess iodine intakes in children and indicates no adverse effects on thyroid function in the UIC range of 100–299 µg/l: a UNICEF/ICCIDD study group report. *The Journal of Clinical Endocrinology and Metabolism*, **98** (3), 1271–1280.

Vitamin A

Key messages

- Vitamin A is an essential fat-soluble nutrient that is required in vision, gene expression, immunity, and growth and development.
- Two forms of vitamin A are available in the human diet: preformed vitamin A (retinol and its esterified form, retinyl ester) and provitamin A carotenoids. Preformed vitamin A is found in foods from animal sources, including dairy products, fish and meat (especially liver). Provitamin A carotenoids are found in a variety of fruit and vegetables. The provitamin A carotenoid with the highest vitamin A activity is beta-carotene; other provitamin A carotenoids are alpha-carotene and beta-cryptoxanthin.
- Both provitamin A and preformed vitamin A must be metabolised intracellularly to retinal and retinoic acid, the active forms of vitamin A, to support the vitamin's important biological functions.
- Vitamin A deficiency is rare in the USA. However, vitamin A deficiency is common in many developing countries, often because

these populations have limited access to foods containing preformed vitamin A from animal-based food sources and the provitamin A carotenoids food sources have varying conversions to vitamin A. In these areas, infants, young children, and pregnant and lactating women are at particular risk of a vitamin A deficiency.

- Because vitamin A is fat soluble, the body stores excess amounts, primarily in the liver, and these levels can accumulate. Although excess preformed vitamin A can have significant toxicity, large amounts of provitamin A carotenoids from foods are not associated with major adverse effects. However, pharmaceutical doses of beta-carotene supplements in heavy smokers and asbestos workers can increase the risk of lung cancer.

9.19 Introduction

Vitamin A is a generic term for a large number of related compounds. Retinol (an alcohol) and retinal (an aldehyde) are referred to as preformed vitamin A. Retinal can

be converted by the body to retinoic acid, the form of vitamin A known to affect gene transcription. Retinyl esters (retinol bound to fatty acids) are the major forms of vitamin A found in animal food products and in body tissues. Retinol, retinal, retinoic acid and retinyl esters are known as retinoids. Beta-carotene, alpha-carotene and beta-cryptoxanthin can be converted by the body into retinol and are referred to as provitamin A carotenoids (Figure 9.2).

9.20 History

In 1912, Frederick Gowland Hopkins demonstrated that unknown factors found in milk, other than carbohydrates, proteins and fats, were necessary for growth in rats. In 1913, one of these substances was independently discovered by Elmer McCollum at the University of Wisconsin–Madison and by Lafayette Mendel and Thomas Burr Osborne at Yale University, who studied the role of fats in the diet (McCollum and Davis, 1913; Osborne and Mendel, 1913). The factors were termed 'fat

soluble' in 1918 and later 'vitamin A' in 1920. In 1919, Harry Steenbock, from the University of Wisconsin–Madison, noted that yellow corn and 'yellow' vegetables (carrots and sweet potato) eliminated the symptoms of vitamin A deficiency in rats, while white corn, 'white' vegetables (parsnip, potato) and beets did not (Steenbock, 1919; Steenbock and Gross, 1919). The chemical structure of vitamin A was described in 1931 by the Swiss chemist Paul Karrer (Karrer et al., 1931a,b). In 1937, after a 23-year quest, pure vitamin A, 4000 times more potent than cod liver oil, was isolated and crystallised by Holmes and Corbet (1937) of Oberlin College. Vitamin A was first synthesised by the two Dutch chemists Jozef Ferdinand Arens and David Adriaan van Dorp (Van Dorp and Arens, 1947). In this same year the large-scale synthesis by Isler et al. (1947) at Hoffmann-La Roche, made the vitamin available for the prevention and treatment of deficiency. In

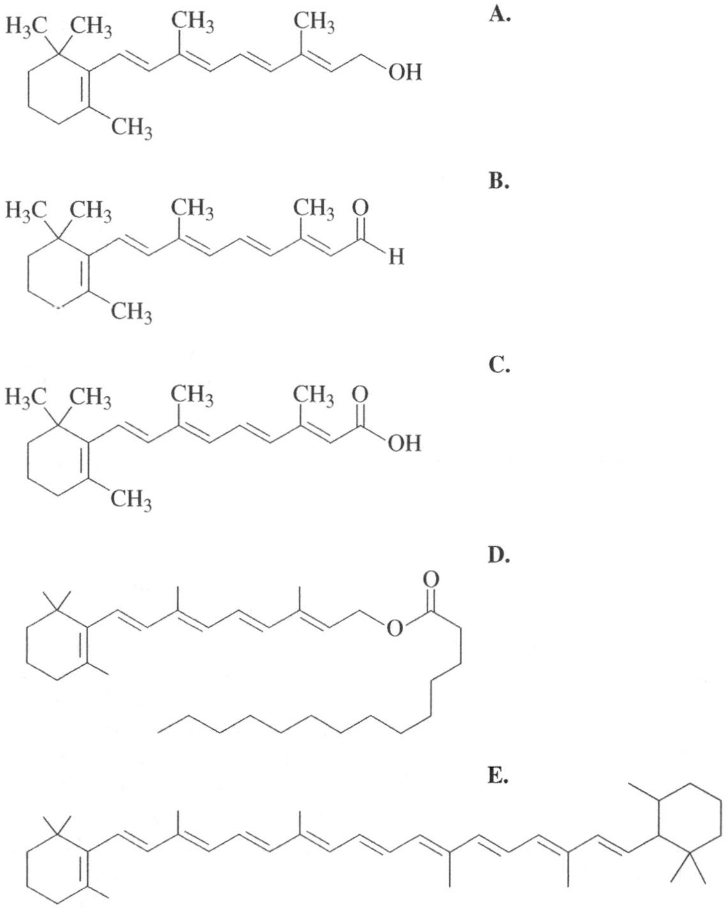

Figure 9.2 Structures of common naturally occuring retinoids and beta-carotene: (a) retinol; (b) retinal (retinaldehyde); (c) retinoic acid; (d) retinyl palmitate; (e) beta-carotene.

the early 1950s, the biochemist George Wald described the role of vitamin A in the visual cycle of the retina (Wald, 1955). This discovery won him a Nobel Prize in Physiology or Medicine in 1967. Vitamin A research continues to this day with evaluations on its specific roles in health and disease.

9.21 Dietary sources

Vitamin A, also known as retinol, is found in a variety of sources as either preformed retinyl esters (retinol esterified with fatty acids, the major form of vitamin in foods and supplements) or provitamin A carotenoids, such as beta-carotene, alpha-carotene and beta-cryptoxanthin (Institute of Medicine (US) Panel on Micronutrients, 2001). These carotenoids may be converted *in vivo* to retinol with varying degrees of efficiency. Dietary beta-carotene is the most efficient, with 12 µg beta-carotene being equal to 1 µg of retinol (or one retinal activity equivalent, RAE). Dietary alpha-carotene and beta-cryptoxanthin are approximately half as efficient, with about 24 µg being equal to 1 RAE (Institute of Medicine (US) Panel on Micronutrients, 2001). A list of food sources of vitamin A is given in Table 9.8. Preformed vitamin A is obtained mostly from animal sources, including meats, cheeses and fortified milk. Provitamin A carotenoids are found in fruits and vegetables, such as cantaloupe, spinach, winter squashes and carrots (USDA, n.d.). Specific sources of alpha-carotene, beta-carotene and beta-cryptoxanthin are listed in Table 9.9. Bioavailability of provitamin A carotenoids varies depending on the food source, processing and preparation (Tanumihardjo, 2002; Yeum and Russell, 2002). For example, staple foods biofortified with provitamin A carotenoids have shown more efficient bioconversion to retinol than generally observed for vegetables (Tanumihardjo *et al.*, 2010). Also, the bioavailability of beta-carotene from vegetables has been shown to be low compared with that of purified beta-carotene added to a simple matrix (e.g. salad dressing) (Van Het Hof *et al.*, 2000). Processing, such as mechanical homogenisation or heat treatment, has the potential to enhance the bioavailability of carotenoids from vegetables (Van Het Hof *et al.*, 2000).

9.22 Absorption and transport

Retinyl esters and provitamin A carotenoids are often bound to other compounds in the food and must be hydrolyzed and freed before uptake into the small intestine (Harrison, 2012). While the process of hydrolysis is thought to begin in the stomach, the majority of it occurs in the small intestine. Both the pancreas and the small intestine are essential for the absorption of vitamin A and carotenoids. The presence of fat, along with vitamin A and carotenoids, in the small intestine stimulates the release of enzymes from the pancreas for conversion of retinyl esters to the vitamin A free form (retinol). Brush border enzymes located on the surface of intestinal cells may also contribute to the release of these nutrients to their free form (Reboul and Borel, 2011; Harrison, 2012). Because of the role of these organs, individuals with diseases of the pancreas (such as cystic fibrosis; Graham-Maar *et al.*, 2026), or intestine (Bousvaros *et al.*, 1998) are highly susceptible to vitamin A deficiencies and have low carotenoid status. A fraction of the provitamin A carotenoids are converted to retinol either in the intestinal lumen prior to absorption, or within intestinal cells (Harrison, 2012). Retinol is then re-esterified and repackaged into chylomicrons along with carotenoids and released into the lymphatic system, where it can be taken up by peripheral tissues until it reaches the liver, which removes the chylomicron remnant from the circulation. The liver is the main storage site of vitamin A, as retinyl esters, and is also responsible for releasing vitamin A to other tissues for use (D'Ambrosio *et al.*, 2011). Upon release from the liver, retinol is bound to retinol-binding protein (RBP) and is transported throughout the bloodstream until it is taken up by the target tissues, which have receptors on the surface that recognise RBP (Institute of Medicine (US) Panel on Micronutrients, 2001). Carotenoids are also stored in the liver, but the major storage site is adipose tissue (Kaplan *et al.*, 1990). In the circulation, carotenoids are found exclusively in lipoproteins (Parker, 1996) (Figure 9.3).

Table 9.8 Food sources of vitamin A.

Food	Common measure	Vitamin A (µg, RAE)	Vitamin A (IU)
Sweet potato, cooked	1 whole	1 403	28 058
Beef liver	3 oz	6 582	22 175
Spinach (cooked, boiled)	1 cup	943.2	18 866
Carrots, raw	1 cup	918.5	18 377
Cantaloupe, raw	1/8 melon	116.6	5 411
Red peppers, raw	1 cup	233.9	4 665
Broccoli, boiled	1 cup	120.1	2 415
Mangos, raw	1 whole	111.8	2 240
Milk, skim, fortified with vitamins A and D	1 cup	149.5	500
Cheddar cheese	1 oz	75.1	284

Source: USDA National Nutrient Database for Standard Reference, Release 25.

IU: international units.

Table 9.9 Food sources of provitamin A carotenoids.

Carotenoid	Food	Amount	
		Common measure	mg
α-Carotene	Pumpkin, canned	1 cup (8 fl oz)	11.7
	Carrot juice, canned	1 cup	10.2
	Carrots, cooked	1 cup	5.9
	Carrots, raw	1 medium	2.1
	Mixed vegetables, frozen, cooked	1 cup	1.8
	Winter squash, baked	1 cup	1.4
	Plantains, raw	1 medium	0.8
	Collards, frozen, cooked	1 cup	0.2
	Tomatoes, raw	1 medium	0.1
	Tangerines, raw	1 medium	0.09
	Peas, edible-podded, frozen, cooked	1 cup	0.09
β-Cryptoxanthin	Pumpkin, cooked	1 cup	3.6
	Papayas, raw	1 medium	2.3
	Sweet red peppers, cooked	1 cup	0.6
	Sweet red peppers, raw	1 medium	0.6
	Orange juice, fresh	1 cup	0.4
	Tangerines, raw	1 medium	0.4
	Carrots, frozen, cooked	1 cup	0.3
	Yellow corn, frozen, cooked	1 cup	0.2
	Watermelon, raw	1 wedge (1/16 melon, 15 in long × 7.5 in in diameter)	0.2
	Paprika, dried	1 tsp	0.2
	Oranges, raw	1 medium	0.2
	Nectarines, raw	1 medium	0.1
β-Carotene	Carrot juice, canned	1 cup	22.0
	Pumpkin, canned	1 cup	17.0
	Spinach, frozen, cooked	1 cup	13.8
	Sweet potato, baked	1 medium	13.1
	Carrots, cooked	1 cup	13.0
	Collards, frozen, cooked	1 cup	11.6
	Kale, frozen, cooked	1 cup	11.5
	Turnip greens, frozen, cooked	1 cup	10.6
	Winter squash, cooked	1 cup	5.7
	Carrots, raw	1 medium	5.1
	Dandelion greens, cooked	1 cup	4.1
	Cantaloupe, raw	1 cup	3.2

Source: USDA National Nutrient Database for Standard Reference, Release 25.

9.23 Functions

Vitamin A is an essential nutrient that has a wide variety of functions in the body. One of its main functions is its role in vision. Vitamin A is stored in the retina, located in the back of the eye, where it is converted to retinal and binds to the protein opsin, forming rhodopsin (Wolf, 2004). When light hits the retina cells, retinal changes conformation and is no longer able to bind opsin. The separation from retinal causes opsin to also change shape. This process generates an electrical impulse in the retina cells, which transfers the signal to nerve cells, and the signal moves to the brain. The brain then interprets the signal as light (Wolf, 2004). This process

is partially regenerative. That is, some retinal can be converted back to its original conformation and can re-bind opsin to form new rhodopsin. However, some retinal is lost during every cycle. Therefore, vitamin A must be replenished through the diet. Because of this role in vision, one of the early signs of a vitamin A deficiency is night blindness (see Section 9.25).

The second major role of vitamin A is its participation in growth and development (Sommer, 2008). In particular, vitamin A is important for eye, limb and heart development. Deficiencies during pregnancy often lead to birth defects and high infant mortality rates (Clagett-Dame and Knutson, 2011). Retinoic acid, a more oxidised form of retinol, plays an important role in gene expression and cell

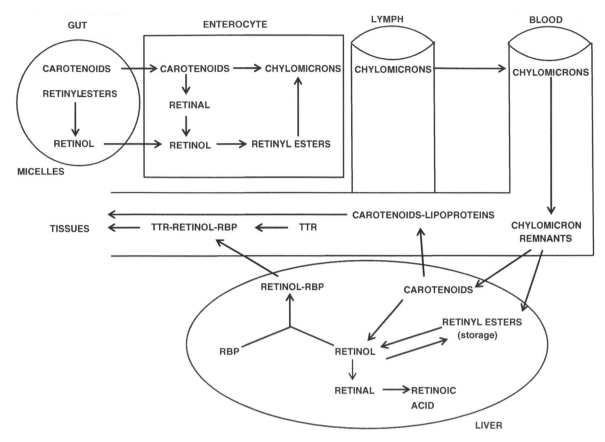

Figure 9.3 Absorption, transport and storage of retinoids and carotenoids. TTR: transthyretin.

differentiation by binding to nuclear receptors that regulate DNA transcription of various genes (Gudas, 2011). This process is vital for differentiating stem cells to epithelial tissues, red blood cells and components of the eye.

Owing to its role in gene expression and cell differentiation, vitamin A also plays an important role in immune function (Cassani *et al.*, 2012; Ross 2012). It does so by maintaining the integrity of the epithelium inside and outside the body, which serves as the body's barrier against foreign pathogens. By promoting the differentiation of epithelial cells, vitamin A helps keep the barrier intact and protects against pathogen invasion.

9.24 Requirements

The dietary requirements for men and women, expressed in both RAE and IU, are listed in Table 9.10 (Institute of Medicine (US) Panel on Micronutrients, 2001). For men, the greatest amount of vitamin A is needed from adolescence and onward throughout adulthood. For women, the

Table 9.10 RDA for vitamin A.

Age	RDA (μg/day) [IU]	
	Male	Female
Infants (0–6 months)[a]	400 [1333]	400 [1333]
Infants (7–12 months)[a]	500 [1667]	500 [1667]
Child (1–3 years)	300 [1000]	300 [1000]
Child (4–8 years)	400 [1333]	400 [1333]
Child (9–13 years)	600 [2000]	600 [2000]
Adolescent (14–18 years)	900 [3000]	700 [2333]
Adult (19–70 years)	900 [3000]	700 [2333]
Adult (≥71 years)	900 [3000]	700 [2333]
Pregnancy (≤18 years)	—	750 [2500]
Breastfeeding (≤18 years)	—	1200 [4000]
Pregnancy (<18 years)	—	770 [2567]
Breastfeeding (≥18 years)	—	1300 [4333]

[a] Adequate intake.

highest need for vitamin A is during pregnancy and breast-feeding. High amounts are necessary during these parts of the life cycle due to its role in growth and development.

9.25 Deficiency

Deficiencies in this fat-soluble vitamin occur primarily in developing nations and account for a large portion of child mortality and morbidity rates in these areas (Ross, 2012). Clinical manifestations of vitamin A deficiency develop once vitamin A stores in the liver are completely or almost completely depleted. One of the earliest and most common consequences of vitamin A deficiency is night blindness (Sommer, 2008). Night blindness occurs when there is insufficient retinal to regenerate rhodopsin in the retina. This leads to an inability to immediately recover vision after flashes of light, as well as loss of vision in dark or dim lighting. Night blindness is reversible with repletion of dietary vitamin A, but not with retinoic acid supplementation, since this form cannot be converted to retinal and used by the retina. In addition to night blindness, vitamin A deficiency also plays a role in complete blindness. This is not due to rhodopsin, but rather it is due to inadequate mucus secretion in the front of the eye. This causes the cells of the cornea to become dry and hard, and keratin (a hard, water-insoluble protein), begins to accumulate through a process called keratinisation, which is a contributor to permanent blindness.

Owing to its role in maintaining epithelium cells to block pathogens, a lack of vitamin A can lead to increased susceptibility to diseases and infection (Russell, 2000). Very severe deficiencies can ultimately lead to death. Currently, one of the priorities in international nutrition policy is supplementation with vitamin A in developing nations, where vitamin A deficiencies are high, in order to decrease infant morbidity and mortality. Just as keratinisation can occur in the eye, prolonged vitamin A deficiency results in keratinisation of external epithelial cells (or skin cells), leading to dry, red, bumpy skin.

In developed countries, the amounts of vitamin A in breast milk are sufficient to meet infants' needs for the first 6 months of life. But in women with vitamin A deficiency, breast milk volume and vitamin A content are suboptimal and not adequate to maintain vitamin A stores in infants who are exclusively breastfed (Oliveira-Menegozzo et al., 2010). In these areas, the prevalence of vitamin A deficiency increases in young children after they stop breastfeeding (Ross, 2005). The most common and readily recognised symptom of vitamin A deficiency in infants and children is xerophthalmia.

Pregnant women need extra vitamin A for fetal growth and tissue maintenance and for supporting their own metabolism (van den Broek et al., 2010). The WHO (2009) estimates that 9.8 million pregnant women around the world have xerophthalmia as a result of vitamin A deficiency. Other effects of vitamin A deficiency in pregnant and lactating women include increased maternal and infant morbidity and mortality, increased anaemia risk and slower infant growth and development.

Other individuals susceptible to vitamin A deficiency include those with pancreatic disease or intestinal disease due to a decreased ability to absorb the fat-soluble vitamin. Research has shown that alcoholics are at an increased risk for vitamin A deficiency as well (Clugston and Blaner, 2012). This is most likely due to the fact that alcohol disrupts retinoid homeostasis by increasing vitamin A mobilisation and depleting liver stores independently of intake and absorption. Retinoid imbalance due to alcohol has been supported by evidence showing higher retinoid levels in the extrahepatic tissues of alcoholics, indicating that alcohol increases the mobilisation of vitamin A out of the liver and into peripheral tissues (Wang, 1999; Clugston and Blaner, 2012).

9.26 Toxicity

Vitamin A toxicity arises only from overconsumption of preformed vitamin A from foods and/or supplements. Conversely, high intakes of provitamin A carotenoids from foods are not toxic (Linus Pauling Institute, Micronutrient Information Center, 2016). However, two randomised clinical trials found pharmaceutical doses of beta-carotene in populations at high risk (smokers, asbestos workers) to increase the risk for lung cancer (The Alpha-Tocopherol, Beta Carotene Cancer Prevention Study Group, 1994; Omenn et al., 1996) (see Section 9.28). Vitamin A toxicity, or hypervitaminosis A, can occur from either extremely high doses over a short period of time or chronic overexposure from a relatively smaller dose. Either situation leads to the saturation of RBP, and free retinol (unbound) begins to damage cells. For this reason, a tolerable upper limit has been set for vitamin A (Table 9.11). Intakes above this limit may

Table 9.11 Tolerable upper level for vitamin A.

Age	Vitamin A (µg/day) [IU]
Infants (0–6 months)	600 [2000]
Infants (6–12 months)	600 [2000]
Children (1–3 years)	600 [2000]
Children (4–8 years)	900 [3000]
Children (9–13 years)	1700 [5667]
Adolescent (14–18 years)	2800 [9333]
Adult (>18 years)	3000 [10 000]

cause liver damage, changes in vision, headache, dry/itchy skin and hair loss (Russell, 2000). For older adults, vitamin A toxicity may occur at doses significantly below the upper limit due to impaired vitamin A metabolism in this population. Studies have also indicated that high doses of preformed vitamin A may also increase the risk of osteoporosis; however, results have been inconsistent in determining the association between vitamin A and skeletal health (Ribaya-Mercado and Blumberg, 2007; Ahmadieh and Arabi, 2011).

9.27 Assessment of status

The majority of vitamin A stores in the body are in the liver in the form of retinyl esters. Therefore, a measure of liver vitamin A is the best index of vitamin A status. Concentrations below 0.07 µmol/g are considered deficient (Sommer and Davidson, 2002). However, vitamin A is not uniformly distributed in the liver (Olson et al., 1979) and liver biopsies are not practical in most cases. Instead, serum vitamin A is more often used. However, serum concentrations do not reflect body stores unless the individual is severely deficient or toxic.

The relative dose response (RDR) test is used to estimate the liver stores of vitamin A. This test is based on the observation that during vitamin A deficiency, when stores are diminished, RBP accumulates in the liver as apo-RBP. Following the administration of a test dose of vitamin A, some of the vitamin A binds to the excess apo-RBP and is then released as holo-RBP in to the circulation (Loerch et al., 1979). Consequently, in vitamin-A-depleted individuals, there is a rapid and sustained increase in serum retinol after a small oral dose of vitamin A, whereas in individuals with normal liver vitamin A stores the rise in serum retinol is very small or does not occur. Typically, a small dose of retinol (450–1000 µg) is given orally in oil and serum is sampled at baseline and again at approximately 5 h later. An increase in plasma retinol of more than 20% compared with baseline concentration is interpreted as an indication that liver vitamin A stores are inadequate for maintaining a normal rate of secretion of holo-RBP.

The modified RDR test requires only one blood sample, which may be an important consideration for field studies on children. For this test, a small dose of vitamin A is administered; usually, 3,4-didehydroretinyl acetate (DRA) is used. This is usually followed by a high-fat, low-vitamin A food to facilitate the absorption of the DRA. DRA combines with RBP in the same way as retinol, but unlike retinol, it is normally found in human plasma or serum. The DRA is hydrolysed in the gastrointestinal tract to 3,4-didehydroretinol (DR), absorbed and re-esterified in the intestinal mucosal cells (Tanumihardjo et al., 1995). The plasma/serum levels of DR and retinol in the single blood sample are measured and the molar ratio of DR to retinol in the sample is a measure of the response. Ratios >0.06 are considered indicative of a subclinical deficiency and those <0.03 are considered to be satisfactory (Tanumihardjo et al., 1996).

9.28 Special considerations

Special attention has been given to the relationship between vitamin A and cancer. It has been well established that vitamin A has a significant effect on cellular growth, differentiation and apoptosis due to its role in the activation of nuclear receptors (RXR and RAR) that control gene expression (Samarut and Rochette-Egly, 2012). It follows, therefore, that vitamin A is instrumental in controlling carcinogenesis. This fact, in addition to the altered vitamin A metabolism that occurs from alcohol, has implicated vitamin A as an important factor in alcohol-induced liver cancer (Wang, 2005). Therefore, vitamin A consumption needs to be carefully monitored in alcoholics.

In addition to research examining the role of preformed vitamin A in cancer prevention, a significant amount of work has been conducted evaluating beta-carotene and cancer. Owing to its antioxidant properties, beta-carotene has been targeted as a possible therapy to combat oxidative stress that can result in carcinogenesis. It became a particular focus for lung cancer in order to remove reactive oxygen species from smoke that damages the lung epithelium. Many human observational studies showed an association between increased dietary and circulating levels of beta-carotene and a decreased cancer risk (Mayne et al., 1994; Comstock et al., 1997). However, human intervention studies showed no effect or a detrimental effect of beta-carotene supplementation on lung cancer (The Alpha-Tocopherol, Beta Carotene Cancer Prevention Study Group, 1994; Omenn et al., 1996). This paradox is due to the fact that the efficacy of beta-carotene depends on its source and the amount given. Beta-carotene works to stop oxidative stress by intercepting free radicals from smoke. Beta-carotene must then be recycled by other antioxidants, such as vitamin E or vitamin C. If it is not, the unstable beta-carotene molecule can act as a pro-oxidant and lead to lipid oxidative damage (Wang and Russell, 1999). Therefore, consuming beta-carotene in fruits and vegetables, which also possess other antioxidants, is much more effective than taking a supplement that only contains beta-carotene. The other reason for the detrimental effect seen in beta-carotene supplementation is due to the fact that subjects were given doses beyond what would normally be consumed from fruits and vegetables. Excess beta-carotene can be harmful because once vitamin A synthesis pathways are saturated, the excess beta-carotene can be cleaved to pro-oxidant metabolites, which activate phase I enzymes that convert procarcinogens, such as smoke, to activate carcinogens that cause DNA damage and mutation (Wang and Russell, 1999; Russell, 2000). Therefore, high doses of beta-carotene supplementation are not recommended for smokers.

9.29 Perspectives on the future

It has been nearly 100 years since the discovery of vitamin A. Since then the role of vitamin A in health has been well investigated. Further work on the role that specific metabolites may have in health or toxicities may provide further insight to the mechanism of vitamin A's action. It is well recognised that a major dietary source of vitamin A is the provitamin A carotenoids. Globally, particularly in areas with a high prevalence of vitamin A deficiency, these carotenoids are the major form of vitamin A. Research has shown that the vitamin A value of individual plant foods rich in provitamin A carotenoids varies significantly among foods and among individuals. Further investigations are warranted to investigate the factors involved in the bioconversion of provitamin A carotenoids to vitamin A.

References

Ahmadieh, H. and Arabi, A. (2011) Vitamins and bone health: beyond calcium and vitamin D. *Nutrition Reviews*, **69**, 584–598.

Bousvaros, A., Zurakowski, D., Duggan, C. *et al.* (1998) Vitamins A and E serum levels in children and young adults with inflammatory bowel disease: effect of disease activity. *The Journal of Pediatric Gastroenterology and Nutrition*, **26**, 129–135.

Cassani, B., Villablanca, E.J., De Calisto, J. *et al.* (2012) Vitamin A and immune regulation: role of retinoic acid in gut-associated dendritic cell education, immune protection and tolerance. *Molecular Aspects of Medicine*, **33**, 63–76.

Clagett-Dame, M. and Knutson, D. (2011) Vitamin A in reproduction and development. *Nutrients*, **3**, 385–428.

Clugston, R.D. and Blaner, W.S. (2012) The adverse effects of alcohol on vitamin A metabolism. *Nutrients*, **4**, 356–371.

Comstock, G.W., Alberg, A.J., Huang, H.Y. *et al.* (1997) The risk of developing lung cancer associated with antioxidants in the blood: ascorbic acid, carotenoids, alpha-tocopherol, selenium, and total peroxyl radical absorbing capacity. *Cancer Epidemiology, Biomarkers & Prevention*, **6**, 907–916.

D'Ambrosio, D.N., Clugston, R.D. and Blaner, W.S. (2011) Vitamin A metabolism: an update. *Nutrients*, **3**, 63–103.

Graham-Maar, R.C., Schall, J.I., Stettler, N. *et al.* (2006) Elevated vitamin A intake and serum retinol in preadolescent children with cystic fibrosis. *The American Journal of Clinical Nutrition*, **84**, 174–182.

Gudas, L.J. (2012) Emerging roles for retinoids in regeneration and differentiation in normal and disease states. *Biochimica et Biophysica Acta*, **1821**, 213–221.

Harrison, E.H. (2012) Mechanisms involved in the intestinal absorption of dietary vitamin A and provitamin A carotenoids. *Biochimica et Biophysica Acta*, **1821**, 70–77.

Holmes, H. and Corbet, R. (1937) The isolation of crystalline vitamin A. *Journal of the American Chemical Society*, **59**, 2042–2047.

Institute of Medicine (US) Panel on Micronutrients (2001) *Dietary Reference Intakes for Vitamin A, Vitamin K, Arsenic, Boron, Chromium, Copper, Iodine, Iron, Manganese, Molybdenum, Nickel, Silicon, Vanadium, and Zinc*. National Academy Press, Washington, DC.

Isler, O., Huber, W., Ronco, A. and Kofler, M. (1947) Syntheses des Vitamin A. *Helvetica Chimica Acta*, **30**, 1911–1921.

Kaplan, L.A., Lau, J.M. and Stein, E.A. (1990) Carotenoid composition, concentrations, and relationships in various human organs. *Clinical Physiology and Biochemistry*, **8**, 1–10.

Karrer, P., Morf, R. and Schöpp, K. (1931a) Zur Kenntnis des Vitamins-A aus Fischtranen. *Helvetica Chimica Acta*, **14**, 1036–1040.

Karrer, P., Morf, R. and Schöpp, K. (1931b) Zur Kenntnis des Vitamins A aus Fischtranen II. *Helvetica Chimica Acta*, **14**, 1431–1436.

Linus Pauling Institute, Micronutrient Information Center (2016) *Vitamin A*. Oregon State University, Corvalis, OR. http://lpi.oregonstate.edu/infocenter/vitamins/vitaminA/ (access 4 December 2016).

Loerch, J.D., Underwood, B.A. and Lewis, K.C. (1979) Response of plasma levels of vitamin A to a dose of vitamin A as an indicator of hepatic vitamin A reserves in rats. *The Journal of Nutrition*, **109**, 778–786.

Mayne, S.T., Janerich, D.T., Greenwald, P. *et al.* (1994) Dietary beta carotene and lung cancer risk in U.S. nonsmokers. *Journal of the National Cancer Institute*, **86**, 33–38.

McCollum, E. and Davis, M. (1913) The necessity of certain lipids in the diet during growth. *Journal of Biological Chemistry*, **15**, 167–175.

Oliveira-Menegozzo, J.M., Bergamaschi, D.P., Middleton, P. and East, C.E. (2010) Vitamin A supplementation for postpartum women. *The Cochrane Database of Systematic Reviews*, (10), CD005944.

Olson, J.A., Gunning, D. and Tilton, R. (1979) The distribution of vitamin A in human liver. *The American Journal of Clinical Nutrition*, **32**, 2500–2507.

Omenn, G.S., Goodman, G.E., Thornquist, M.D. *et al.* (1996) Effects of a combination of beta carotene and vitamin A on lung cancer and cardiovascular disease. *New England Journal of Medicine*, **334**, 1150–1155.

Osborne T, Mendel L. (1913) The relationship of growth to the chemical constituents of the diet. *Journal of Biological Chemistry*, **15**, 311–326.

Parker, R.S. (1996) Absorption, metabolism, and transport of carotenoids. *FASEB Journal*, **10**, 542–551.

Reboul, E. and Borel, P. (2011) Proteins involved in uptake, intracellular transport and basolateral secretion of fat-soluble vitamins and carotenoids by mammalian enterocytes. *Progress in Lipid Research*, **50**, 388–402.

Ribaya-Mercado, J.D. and Blumberg, J.B. (2007) Vitamin A: is it a risk factor for osteoporosis and bone fracture? *Nutrition Reviews*, **65**, 425–438.

Ross, A.C. (2005) Vitamin A and carotenoids. In M. Shils, A.C. Ross, B. Cabellero and R.J. Cousins (eds), *Modern Nutrition in Health and Disease*, 10th edn. Lippincott Williams & Wilkins, Philadelphia, PA; pp. 351–375.

Ross, A.C. (2012) Vitamin A and retinoic acid in T cell-related immunity. *The American Journal of Clinical Nutrition*, **96**, 1166S–1172S.

Russell, R.M. (2000) The vitamin A spectrum: from deficiency to toxicity. *The American Journal of Clinical Nutrition*, **71**, 878–884.

Samarut, E. and Rochette-Egly, C. (2012) Nuclear retinoic acid receptors: conductors of the retinoic acid symphony during development. *Molecular and Cellular Endocrinology*, **348** (2), 348–360.

Sommer, A. (2008) Vitamin a deficiency and clinical disease: an historical overview. *The Journal of Nutrition*, **138**, 1835–1839.

Sommer, A. and Davidson, F.R. (2002) Assessment and control of vitamin A deficiency: the Annecy Accords. *The Journal of Nutrition*, **132**, 2845S–2850S.

Steenbock, H. (1919) White corn vs. yellow corn and a probable relation between the fat-soluble vitamine and yellow plant pigments. *Science*, **59**, 352–353.

Steenbock, H. and Gross, E. (1919) Fat-soluble vitamine. II. The fat-soluble vitamine content of roots, together with some observations on their water-soluble vitamine content. *Journal of Biological Chemistry*, **40**, 501–531.

Tanumihardjo, S.A. (2002) Factors influencing the conversion of carotenoids to retinol: bioavailability to bioconversion to bioefficacy. *International Journal for Vitamin and Nutrition Research*, **72**, 40–45.

Tanumihardjo, S.A., Suharno, D., Permaesih, D. *et al.* (1995) Application of the modified relative dose response test to pregnant Indonesian women for assessing vitamin A status. *European Journal of Clinical Nutrition*, **49**, 897–903.

Tanumihardjo, S.A., Cheng, J.C., Permaesih, D. *et al.* (1996) Refinement of the modified-relative-dose-response test as a method for assessing vitamin A status in a field setting: experience with Indonesian children. *The American Journal of Clinical Nutrition*, **64**, 966–971.

Tanumihardjo, S.A., Palacios, N. and Pixley, K.V. (2010) Provitamin a carotenoid bioavailability:what really matters? *International Journal for Vitamin and Nutrition Research*, **80**, 336–350.

The Alpha-Tocopherol, Beta Carotene Cancer Prevention Study Group (1994) The effect of vitamin E and beta carotene on the incidence of lung cancer and other cancers in male smokers. *New England Journal of Medicine*, **330**, 1029–1035.

USDA (n.d.) *Phytonutrients*. United States Department of Agriculture, National Agricultural Library. https://www.nal.usda.gov/fnic/phytonutrients (accessed 4 December 2016).

Van den Broek, N., Dou, L., Othman, M. *et al.* (2010) Vitamin A supplementation during pregnancy for maternal and newborn outcomes. *The Cochrane Database of Systematic Reviews*, (11), CD008666.

Van Dorp, D.A. and Arens J.F. (1947) Synthesis of vitamin A aldehyde. *Nature*, **160**, 189.

Van Het Ho, K.H., West, C.E., Weststrate, J.A. and Hautvast, J.G. (2000) Dietary factors that affect the bioavailability of carotenoids. *The Journal of Nutrition*, **130**, 503–506.

Wald, G. (1955) The photoreceptor process in vision. *American Journal of Ophthalmology*, **40** (5 Part 2), 18–41.

Wang, X.-D. (1999) Chronic alcohol intake interferes with retinoid metabolism and signaling. *Nutrition Reviews*, **57**, 51–59.

Wang, X.D. (2005) Alcohol, vitamin A, and cancer. *Alcohol (Fayetteville, N.Y.)*, **35**, 251–258.

Wang, X.D. and Russell, R.M. (1999) Procarcinogenic and anticarcinogenic effects of beta-carotene. *Nutrition Reviews*, **57**, 263–272.

WHO (2009) *Global Prevalence of Vitamin A Deficiency in Populations at Risk, 1995–2005: WHO Global Database on Vitamin A Deficiency*. World Health Organization, Geneva.

Wolf, G. (2004) The visual cycle of the cone photoreceptors of the retina. *Nutrition Reviews*, **62**, 283–286.

Yeum, K.-J. and Russell, R.M. (2002) Carotenoid bioavailability and bioconversion. *Annual Review of Nutrition*, **22**, 483–504.

10
Nutrition Pre-conception and during Pregnancy

Sara Stanner

Key messages

- A mother's weight, nutritional status, diet and lifestyle prior to and during pregnancy influence pregnancy outcomes and can have lasting effects on her child's health.
- It is likely that there are periods of fetal development that are particularly sensitive to nutritional imbalance. During these 'critical windows', an offspring's future health can be programmed.
- In many low-to-middle income countries, undernutrition in pregnancy, which is often accompanied by multiple micronutrient deficiencies, is a major determinant of maternal and infant mortality and morbidity.
- Low intakes of some nutrients may also be impacting on health in developed countries. In the UK, for example, despite advice on supplementation, poor folate and vitamin D status amongst many women of childbearing age is of concern. Around 1 in 1000 UK pregnancies are affected by a neural tube defect, and folic acid supplementation prior to and 12 weeks after conception can, in the majority of individuals, prevent these birth defects from occurring. Low vitamin D concentrations have been associated with a wide range of adverse maternal and offspring health outcomes in observational epidemiological studies. Other micronutrients important for fetal growth and development, including iodine, iron and calcium, are also consumed in inadequate amounts in a substantial proportion of women of childbearing age.

- In addition, maternal overweight and obesity are increasing globally and are associated with several adverse pregnancy outcomes, including birth defects, gestational diabetes, pre-eclampsia (a pregnancy complication characterised by high blood pressure) and Caesarean section.
- A mother's consumption of potentially harmful substances, such as alcohol, during pregnancy can have irreversible negative consequences. Pregnant women are also more susceptible to food-borne diseases and their effects and need to take particular care to handle and prepare food safely. Foods that are particularly risky, due to possible contamination with food-poisoning bacteria, should be avoided.
- Only around a third of women of childbearing age in the UK are meeting current physical activity recommendations. Being active helps to maintain an appropriate body weight and has many benefits during pregnancy.
- The antenatal period, with opportunities for regular contact with health professionals, is a good time to intervene as mothers are motivated to make changes that could optimise their health and that of their baby. However, as nutritional status is cumulative over time, improvements in women's nutrition throughout the life course will have the greatest long-term benefits.

10.1 Introduction

Maternal nutritional status and nutrient intake before and during pregnancy can have a profound effect on the health of both mother and child. A woman's nutritional status (and that of her partner) can affect whether or not she conceives, has a major bearing on whether her pregnancy has a healthy course and outcome, and also, to some extent, determines her postpartum nutrient status (e.g. for lactation). In turn, these factors can affect both her short and longer term health. Maternal body composition, nutritional stores, diet and ability to deliver nutrients through the placenta determines nutrient availability for the fetus. The 1000 days spanning from conception to 2 years of life are thought to be a critical period of time when nutritional needs of the fetus must be ensured to avoid adverse impacts on short-term survival, as well as long-term health and development.

Public Health Nutrition, Second Edition. Edited by Judith L Buttriss, Ailsa A Welch, John M Kearney and Susan A Lanham-New.
© 2018 by The Nutrition Society. Published 2018 by John Wiley & Sons, Ltd.
Companion website: www.wiley.com/go/buttriss/publichealth

This chapter summarises the key nutritional issues pre-conception and during pregnancy that influence health outcomes for mother and child. It considers the importance of nutritional status prior to pregnancy and outlines nutritional requirements during pregnancy in relation to energy, macronutrients and micronutrients, linking to critical periods of intake for fetal development. It also considers the current nutritional status of women during pregnancy in the UK and elsewhere, and identifies key issues for certain vulnerable groups. It briefly discusses the main food safety issues for women during pregnancy and summarises current diet and lifestyle messages for women trying to conceive and who are pregnant.

The 'developmental origins of health and disease' hypothesis

A fetus is entirely dependent on its mother for its nutrient supply, which is influenced by her nutritional status prior to conception and in pregnancy. Insufficiency of specific nutrients (e.g. iodine and folate), or excessive intakes (e.g. of vitamin A), have clear developmental effects. Epidemiological studies linking low birth weight (defined as birth weight less than 2500 g) at term (>37 weeks) with adult disease have also suggested that more modest variations in maternal nutrition may increase the risk of offspring developing numerous conditions in later life, including hypertension, obesity, cardiovascular disease (CVD), type 2 diabetes and cancer. Low birth weight serves as a crude proxy for impaired growth during fetal life and indicates a failure of the fetus to achieve its full growth potential (although other measures of fetal growth have later emerged as equally relevant). This led to the development of the 'fetal origins of adult disease' hypothesis or the 'thrifty phenotype hypothesis', a theory put forward by Professor David Barker, Professor Nick Hales and colleagues in the 1990s, which proposed that undernutrition in early development, particularly intrauterine life, could result in lower birth weight and permanent changes in physiology and metabolism, leading to increased disease risk in adulthood.

Barker and colleagues showed that mortality rates for CVD were high in geographical areas that had high infant mortality rates in the past, suggesting that events in fetal life may be important in the origins of CVD. They went on to identify a number of cohorts of adults whose early growth had been recorded. By tracing these men and women they were able to link measures of early growth to disease-specific mortality rates, as well as to risk factors for these conditions. Figure 10.1, for example, shows the risk of dying prematurely from CVD among 15 726 men and women in born in Hertfordshire, UK

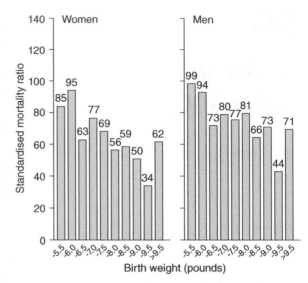

Figure 10.1 Mortality from CVD before 65 years in 15 726 men and women who were born in Hertfordshire. *Source*: Osmond *et al.* (1993). Reproduced with permission of BMJ Publishing Ltd.

(Osmond *et al.*, 1993). This demonstrates a graded inverse association between weight at birth and risk of death from CVD, although risk also increased in those with the highest birth weights, suggesting that excessive fetal growth and early overnutrition may also lead to increased risk of adult disease.

Subsequent cohort studies have replicated these findings, showing associations between low birth weight and increased risk of cardiac events and deaths, as well as with established CVD risk factors such as type 2 diabetes, higher adult blood pressure, reduced adult lean body mass and elevated serum cholesterol. Attempts to quantify the relationship suggest that a 1 kg increase in birth weight is associated with a 10–30% lower risk of type 2 diabetes (Whincup *et al.*, 2008) and a 10–20% lower risk of fatal or non-fatal cardiac events or death (Huxley *et al.*, 2007) (the association was stronger when those weighing >4 kg at birth were excluded). There is an association with growth in infancy and lifestyle habits in later life; for example, risk of CVD is greatest in those born small for gestational age who exhibit fast 'catch-up' growth in early childhood or become overweight or obese in adult life.

More recent evidence has now linked patterns of fetal and infant growth with bone health, gut microbiota, immunity, lung function, mental health and risk of cancer. This area of research is now known as 'developmental origins of health and disease' (DOHaD). It is postulated that the association occurs through the mechanism of 'fetal programming', whereby a stimulus or insult at a critical period in early life development has a permanent effect on the structure, physiology or function

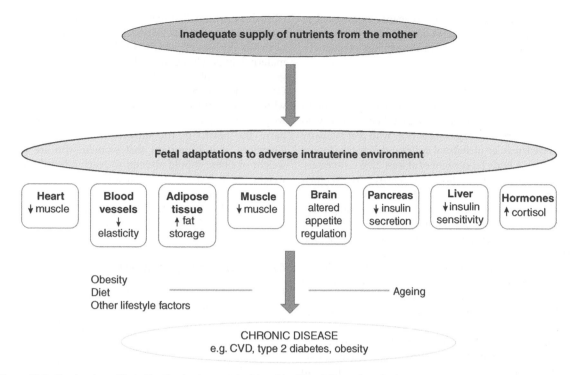

Figure 10.2 Simple schema illustrating the developmental origins of health and disease hypothesis.

of different organs and tissues. The fetus appears to be most susceptible to dietary deficiencies, excesses and toxicity in the first trimester of pregnancy, although programming effects can also occur before and after fetal life. Once the placenta is fully developed it helps to buffer the fetus from extreme fluctuations. However, each organ or tissue has its own phase of rapid growth which, if interrupted, may have long-term consequences if there is no ability to make good any deficit in growth (Figure 10.2). Evidence is emerging to suggest the involvement in epigenetic mechanisms (alterations in gene expression during development), such as altered methylation of specific genes, which can result in programming effects being passed on to future generations.

In animal experiments, a wide range of fetal exposures, including undernutrition (e.g. energy or protein restriction) and overnutrition (e.g. high-fat diets) have been shown to programme long-term metabolism and disease risk. In humans, the DOHaD concept has been tested using 'experiments of history' such as the Dutch Famine, which resulted in poorer health in offspring of mothers exposed to starvation during pregnancy. Cohort studies have also suggested important postnatal effects; notably, that accelerated weight gain (upward crossing of centiles) in childhood or adolescence was associated with an increased risk of adult cardiometabolic disease. However, we are only just beginning to see the hypothesis tested

definitively in humans by following up children born during randomised controlled trials (RCTs) of different exposures *in utero*, infancy or childhood. To date, such trials have provided little evidence of long-term benefits from supplementing undernourished pregnant women with protein, energy or individual micronutrients on offspring cardiometabolic function and disease risk, but limitations to these trials have been noted. Present advice, therefore, is to consume a diet that is adequate and balanced in energy, protein, micronutrients and fatty acids, starting before pregnancy.

10.2 Nutritional status prior to pregnancy

Maternal nutritional status at the time of conception is an important determinant of embryonic and fetal growth. The embryo is most vulnerable to the effects of poor maternal diet during the first few weeks of development, often before pregnancy has been confirmed. Cell differentiation is most rapid at this time, and any abnormalities in cell division cannot be corrected at a later stage. Most organs, though very small, have already been formed 3–7 weeks after the last menstrual period, and any teratogenic effects (including abnormal development) may have occurred by this time.

Good nutrient status prior to pregnancy is essential to ensure adequate fetal supplies during this critical period and to support maternal stores throughout pregnancy.

Pre-pregnancy weight

A vital issue of concern is a mother's weight prior to pregnancy. Women who maintain a low body weight, who have suffered from eating disorders or who diet regularly often have irregular menstrual cycles and may take longer to conceive. A body fat content of at least 22% is necessary for normal ovulatory function and menstruation. Women who are undernourished at the time of conception are unlikely to improve their nutritional status during pregnancy when they have additional demands due to the growing fetus. They may fail to gain sufficient weight during pregnancy and have a higher risk of morbidity, mortality and poor birth outcomes, including stillbirth, preterm delivery (<37 weeks), low birth weight, neonatal mortality (death in the first 28 days of life) and subsequent childhood malnutrition. Maternal short stature has independent adverse effects on pregnancy outcomes.

Maternal undernutrition is a persistent problem in most developing countries, particularly Africa and Asia where the prevalence of low body mass index (BMI) in adult women remains higher than 10% (Black *et al.*, 2013). Although less common in developed countries, a proportion of women are defined as underweight at their first antenatal visit. As well as increasing risk of morbidity and mortality in the newborn infant, low birth weight increases risk of degenerative diseases in later life (see Chapter 11). Inadequate food intake prior to pregnancy also increases risk of inadequate intakes and maternal stores of important nutrients during early pregnancy.

Similarly, men and women who are overweight may encounter problems conceiving, as excessive stores of body fat can impair fertility. In women, obesity contributes to anovulation and menstrual irregularities, reduced conception rate and a reduced response to fertility treatment. Reduction of obesity, particularly abdominal obesity, is associated with improvements in reproductive function. For those with a BMI of 30 or more, losing 5–10% of body weight may increase the chances of conception (NICE, 2010). Obesity in men has also been associated with impaired fertility, by impairing sex hormones, reducing sperm counts, increasing oxidative DNA damage in sperm and changing the epigenetic status of sperm.

Being obese prior to and during pregnancy (BMI $\geq 30\,kg/m^2$ at the first antenatal appointment) is associated with an increased risk of several serious adverse outcomes, including gestational diabetes, pregnancy-induced hypertension, pre-eclampsia, haemorrhage post-delivery, still-birth, miscarriage and birth defects (British Nutrition Foundation, 2013). Maternal obesity leads to increased risk of macrosomia (infants with a birth weight >4 kg), which is believed to be driven by maternal hyperglycaemia. Obesity is also linked to a greater risk of abnormal labour and is a risk factor for Caesarean delivery. Infants born preterm to a mother who is obese are less likely to survive. Dieting to lose weight is not recommended during pregnancy, as it may harm the health of the unborn child (NICE, 2010). Therefore, it is important that women who are overweight or obese should attempt to reach a healthy body weight (i.e. a BMI of 20–25) before trying to conceive. With 40% of adult women overweight or obese globally in 2014 (WHO, 2016a), this is a challenge worldwide and is likely to remain so for the foreseeable future.

Micronutrient requirements

Inadequate intake and status of many micronutrients, including calcium, iodine, iron, folate, zinc and vitamins A and D, is widespread amongst women of reproductive age in low- and middle-income countries. However, in the developed world there is also cause for concern regarding the micronutrient status of mothers-to-be, particularly that of adolescents (see Table 10.1 and Section 10.5: 'Adolescents'). Iron-deficiency anaemia is particularly common; indeed, most women worldwide enter pregnancy with low iron stores. In the UK, the *National Diet and Nutrition Survey* (NDNS) has identified a number of nutrients where intakes amongst teenage girls and women of childbearing age are below the LRNI (the level estimated to be sufficient for only 2.5% of

Table 10.1 Proportion of adolescents and adult women in the UK with intakes of micronutrients below the lower reference nutrient intake (LRNI).

	Proportion (%) below LRNI	
	11–18 years	19–64 years
Vitamin A	14	5
Riboflavin	21	12
Folate	8	4
Iron	46	23
Calcium	19	8
Magnesium	53	11
Potassium	33	23
Zinc	22	4
Selenium	46	51
Iodine	22	10

Data source: Bates *et al.* (2014).

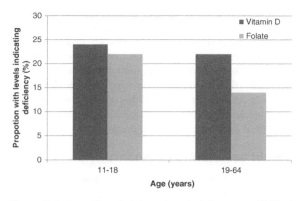

Figure 10.3 Proportion of adolescents and adult women with blood levels of vitamin D and folate indicating deficiency. For vitamin D, the cut-off used is a plasma 25(OH)D concentration below 25 nmol/L (year-round averages). For folate, the cut-off used is a serum total folate concentration below 10 nmol/L, which is the World Health Organization threshold indicating folate deficiency. *Data source:* Bates *et al*, 2014, Bates *et al*, 2015.

the population) (Table 10.1) (Bates *et al.*, 2014). There is also evidence of poor status of some micronutrients, including folate (Figure 10.3) and vitamin D, in these groups (see Section 10.3: 'Vitamins of specific importance during pregnancy' and 'Minerals of specific importance during pregnancy'). National studies indicate similar concerns elsewhere in Europe.

Folate/folic acid

Increased intake of folic acid (the synthetic form of the vitamin folate) is recommended before and during early pregnancy in many countries as this vitamin is of critical importance in protecting against neural tube defects (NTDs) in the developing fetus. NTDs occur when the brain and skull and/or the spinal cord and its protective spinal column do not develop properly within the first 4 weeks after conception (usually between 21 and 28 days following conception). The most common NTDs are

anencephaly, which results in stillbirth or death soon after delivery, and spina bifida, which may lead to a wide range of physical disabilities, including partial or total paralysis.

The initial evidence for the beneficial role of folic acid in NTD prevention came from the Medical Research Council Vitamin Study, an RCT in multiple centres across seven countries which showed that folic acid supplementation (4 mg/day) before conception reduced the risk of an NTD by an estimated 72% (MRC Vitamin Study Research Group, 1991). Subsequently, Wald *et al.* (2001) showed an inverse dose–response relationship between folate status and the risk of NTDs, such that supplementation with 400 μg (0.4 mg) of folic acid per day was estimated to reduce risk by about 36%, 1 mg/day by 57%, and a 5 mg tablet daily by about 85%.

The extra folate required is difficult for women to obtain through diet alone, particularly in countries where folic acid fortification has not been implemented. Mandatory fortification has been introduced in over 70 countries, including the USA, Canada and Australia, but, despite evidence that such fortification is effective (Table 10.2), over 120 countries have not introduced mandatory folic acid fortification, including all countries in the EU. Women of childbearing age therefore need to take folic acid supplements before pregnancy to reduce their risk of an NTD pregnancy. The World Health Organization (WHO) recommends that women who are trying to conceive consume a 400 μg folic acid supplement daily starting 2 months before the planned pregnancy and continue for the first 3 months of pregnancy. It is also recommended that women who have previously had a baby with an NTD or who have diabetes or are taking anti-epileptic medication may need to take a higher dose of folic acid (5 mg daily). This is similar to advice from the UK Department of Health (see Section 10.6: 'Advice regarding nutritional supplements during pregnancy'). Women should also consume foods that are naturally rich in folate (e.g. green vegetables, oranges), as

Table 10.2 Examples of the impact of global folic acid fortification on the prevalence of NTDs.

Country	Introduction of mandatory folic acid fortification	Quantity and delivery method	Decrease in NTDs reported since introduction of folic acid fortification
Canada	1998	150 μg/100 g wheat flour	46% by 2002
Chile	2000	220 μg/100 g wheat flour	40% by 2002
Costa Rica	1999	180 μg/100 g wheat flour	35% by 2000
	2000	180 μg/100 g maize flour	
	2001	40 μg/100 g milk	
South Africa	2003	150 μg/100 g wheat flour	31% by 2005
		221 μg/100 g maize flour	
USA	1998	140 μg/100 g wheat flour	27% by 2000

Data source: British Nutrition Foundation (2013).

well as foods fortified with folic acid, such as some breads and breakfast cereals (see Section 10.3: 'Vitamins of specific importance during pregnancy').

There is some evidence that, even in the absence of NTDs subtle differences in prenatal folate levels may be linked with poorer cognitive function and brain growth in young children. A study of pregnant Dutch women found mild to moderate folate insufficiency in early pregnancy to be associated with a smaller total brain volume and poorer language and visuo-spatial performance in children at 6–8 years (Ars *et al.*, 2016), highlighting the need for women of childbearing age to pay attention to their diet and also take the recommended folic acid supplements prior to pregnancy and during the early weeks.

The Scientific Advisory Committee on Nutrition recommended the introduction of mandatory fortification with folic acid in 2006 and 2009, suggesting controls on voluntary fortification in the UK, and has recently written to the Health Ministers to encourage a decision. However, a formal response from the UK Government is still awaited.

Dietary advice for women planning pregnancy in the UK

The Department of Health (UK) provides dietary advice for women planning a pregnancy. General dietary recommendations are similar to the advice given to non-pregnant women in terms of following a healthy, varied and balanced diet to ensure an adequate intake of energy and nutrients. There is additional emphasis on consuming plenty of iron– and folate-rich foods. Women who may become pregnant are advised to take a folic acid supplement of 400 µg per day until the 12th week of pregnancy (5 mg for women at greater risk). All adults need 10 µg of vitamin D a day and should consider taking a supplement, particularly during the winter months. Those planning for pregnancy should also maintain a healthy weight, avoid alcohol, limit caffeine intake and avoid taking vitamin A supplements, or foods containing high levels of vitamin A (such as liver and liver products) (see Section 10.7).

10.3 Nutritional requirements during pregnancy

A varied, nutrient-dense diet is important for both the mother and baby during pregnancy. The developing fetus obtains all of its nutrients through the placenta, so dietary intake has to meet the needs of the mother, as well as the products of conception (e.g. fetus and placenta), and enable the mother to lay down stores of nutrients required for the development of the fetus and lactation following the birth.

Requirements for a number of nutrients rise in pregnancy, although physiological adaptations during this period mean that recommendations for higher intakes are not always necessary and women should not be encouraged to 'eat for two'. Where requirements cannot be met by diet alone (due to limited food supply or requirements exceeding levels within normal dietary patterns), supplements are advocated (see Section 10.6: 'Advice regarding nutritional supplements during pregnancy').

Weight gain during pregnancy

Weight gain during pregnancy results from products of conception (fetus, placenta and amniotic fluid), increases in various maternal tissues (uterus, breasts, blood and extracellular extravascular fluid) and increases in maternal fat stores.

Weight gain during pregnancy varies considerably amongst women. Excessive weight gain during pregnancy is associated with increased or decreased birth weight and greater postpartum weight retention, but inadequate weight gain also increases risk of low birth weight. High maternal BMI is also associated with increased risk of stillbirth, maternal and infant mortality and birth defects (Tennant *et al.*, 2011; Figure 10.4). Low BMI, indicative of maternal undernutrition, has declined globally in the past two decades but continues to be prevalent in Asia and Africa. In contrast, prevalence of maternal overweight has steadily increased since 1980 (Black *et al.*, 2013) and ranges from 1.8 to 25.3% across different countries (Public Health England, 2016). A national study in 2009 estimated around 5% of the UK maternity population to be severely obese (BMI ≥35); in real terms this equates to around 1 in 20 pregnancies each year (Centre for Maternal and Child Enquiries, 2010).

The amount of weight gain required during pregnancy varies depending on the individual concerned (i.e. initial weight of the mother at the start of pregnancy), with underweight women needing to gain more.

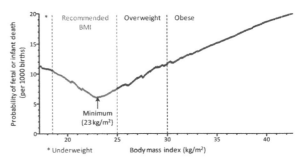

Figure 10.4 Association between maternal BMI and the risk of fetal or infant death. *Source*: Tennant *et al.* (2011). Reproduced with permission of Oxford University Press.

Table 10.3 US Institute of Medicine (IOM) recommendations for total weight gain during pregnancy, based on pre-pregnancy BMI.

Pre-pregnancy weight category	BMI[a]	Recommended range of total weight (kg)	Recommended rates of weight gain[b] in the second and third trimesters (kg) [mean range, kg/week]
Underweight	<18.5	12.5–18	0.51 [0.44–0.58]
Normal weight	18.5–24.9	11.5–16	0.42 [0.35–0.50]
Overweight	25–29.9	7.0–11.5	28 [0.23–0.33]
Obese (includes all classes)	≥30	5.0–9.0	22 [0.17–0.27]

Source: modified from Rasmussen and Yaktine (2009).

[a] BMI calculated as weight in kilograms divided by height in metres squared, or as weight in pounds multiplied by 703 divided by height in inches.
[b] Calculations assume a 1.1–4.4 lb (~0.5–2 kg) weight gain in the first trimester.

There are no evidence-based UK guidelines on recommended weight-gain ranges during pregnancy. However, the US Institute of Medicine (IOM) guidelines, which recommend different levels of weight gain depending on the woman's pre-pregnancy BMI, are typically used (Rasmussen and Yaktine, 2009) (Table 10.3). Evidence suggests that women who gain weight in accordance with these guidelines experience better maternal and infant outcomes compared with those who gain excess weight during pregnancy. Weight gain above the IOM recommendations tends to consist of fat and is therefore undesirable. Women expecting multiple births, such as twins, will gain more weight. Women who are overweight (>100 kg) or underweight (<50 kg) may require more specific advice about how much weight gain is needed.

Weight-loss programmes are not recommended during pregnancy as they may harm the health of the unborn child. However, women should be advised to eat healthily, with the addition of some extra foods to meet the small increase in energy demands (see Section 10.3: 'Energy requirements') alongside the need for some additional macro– and micronutrients (see Section 10.3: 'Macronutrient requirements' and 'Micronutrient requirements'), and to continue to participate in moderate-intensity physical activity (see Section 10.6: 'Physical activity'). Some studies have reported lifestyle interventions (e.g. counselling on healthy eating, physical activity and weight monitoring) during pregnancy to prevent excessive gestational weight gain, although evidence of benefit for longer term effects on postpartum weight, maternal complications or neonatal outcomes is lacking. Appropriate dietary and lifestyle advice should be given at the earliest opportunity; for example, during a pregnant woman's first visit to a health professional (NICE, 2010).

Energy requirements

During pregnancy the maternal diet must provide sufficient energy to ensure the delivery of a full-term, healthy infant of adequate size and appropriate body composition, particularly later in pregnancy. Extra dietary energy is required to make up for the energy deposited in maternal and fetal tissues and the rise in energy expenditure attributable to increased basal metabolism during pregnancy and to changes in the energy cost of physical activity. Internationally, the joint FAO/WHO/UNU Committee (2004) estimated the total energy cost of pregnancy to be around 320 MJ (~77 000 kcal), with highest requirements in the last trimester (Table 10.4). However, average energy requirements during pregnancy must be population specific as the extent to which women are likely to change their habitual activity patterns during pregnancy, for example, will be determined by socio-economic and cultural factors specific to the population. In countries where physical activity is

Table 10.4 Energy cost of pregnancy estimated from increments in total energy expenditure and energy deposition.

	Energy cost (kJ/day)			Total energy cost	
	1st trimester	2nd trimester	3rd trimester	MJ	kcal
Protein deposition	0	30	121	14.1	3 370
Fat deposition	202	732	654	144.8	34 600
Total energy expenditure	85	350	1 300	161.4	38 560
Total energy cost	**287**	**1 112**	**2 075**	**320.2**	**76 530**

Source: FAO/WHO/UNU (2004).

Table 10.5 Recommended intakes of energy, protein, essential fatty acids and micronutrients during pregnancy in the UK.

Nutrient	Daily RNI (EAR for energy) for women aged 19–50 years	Additional requirement during pregnancy	Increase during pregnancy (%)
Energy (per day)	8 MJ; 1940 kcal	+0.8 MJ; +200 kcal[a]	10.3
Protein (g/day)	45	+6	13.3
Essential fatty acids			
Omega-3 (n-3)	one portion of oily fish per week[b]	—	—
Omega-6 (n-6) (g/day)	minimum 2.2		
Vitamin A (μg/day)	600	+100	16.7
Thiamin (mg/day)	0.8	+0.1[a]	12.5
Riboflavin (mg/day)	1.1	+0.3	27.3
Niacin (mg/day) (nicotinic acid equivalents)	13	—	—
Vitamin B$_6$ (mg/day)	1.2	—	—
Vitamin B$_{12}$ (μg/day)	1.5	—	—
Folate (μg/day)	200	+100	50
Vitamin C (mg/day)	40	+10[a]	25
Vitamin D (μg/day)	10 μg	—	—
Calcium (mg/day)	700	—	—
Phosphorus (mg/day)	550	—	—
Magnesium (mg/day)	270	—	—
Sodium (mg/day)	1600	—	—
Potassium (mg/day)	3500	—	—
Chloride (mg/day)	2500	—	—
Iron (mg/day)	14.8[c]	—	—
Zinc (mg/day)	7.0	—	—
Selenium (μg/day)	60	—	—
Iodine (μg/day)	140	—	—

Source: Committee on Medical Aspects of Food Policy (1991); SACN (2016).

EAR: estimated average requirement; RNI: reference nutrient intake – a value which is two notional standard deviations above the EAR, representing an amount that is enough or more than enough for approximately 97.5% of people in a group.

Dashes indicate no increment.

[a] For last trimester only.

[b] Pregnant women and women of childbearing age should eat no more than two portions of oily fish per week (e.g. salmon, fresh tuna, mackerel, trout, sardines).

[c] Insufficient for women with high menstrual losses, where the most practical way of meeting iron requirements is to take iron supplements.

commonly reduced, additional energy requirements will be lower.

In the UK, a small increment of 0.8 MJ/day is required during the third trimester only (Table 10.5) (SACN, 2011). Women who are underweight at the start of their pregnancy and women who do not reduce their activity may require more, whilst women who are overweight at the start of pregnancy may not need such an increment, nor perhaps women who become more sedentary during pregnancy.

Excess energy intake over requirements during pregnancy is associated with excessive gestational weight gain, which is an important contributing factor to the global obesity epidemic in women and associated with multiple maternal and neonatal complications (see Section 10.3: 'Weight gain during pregnancy'). It is therefore important for health professionals to identify women at risk and encourage appropriate changes in diet and lifestyle habits. Undernourished pregnant women are also at increased risk of adverse pregnancy outcomes. In such cases, antenatal nutrition education with the aim of increasing energy alongside protein intakes may be effective in reducing risk of preterm birth and low birth weight (Ota *et al.*, 2015).

Macronutrient requirements

Protein

Protein provides the basic building blocks necessary for the formation of enzymes, muscle, antibodies and collagen. Collagen is used as the framework for skin, bones, blood vessels and other body tissues. Pregnancy increases protein needs due to an increase in hormone production and plasma volume expansion, along with increased tissue formation for the placenta, fetus and breasts. To meet the high demand, a woman's body adapts during pregnancy to conserve protein. Hormones signal a state of anabolism, which causes retention of nitrogen for protein synthesis. The majority of weight gain in the fetus occurs during the latter half of pregnancy. However, many of the maternal adaptations involving protein and nitrogen metabolism occur early in pregnancy, before there is a substantial increase in fetal demand, and recent studies have suggested increased protein needs from early gestation. Inadequate protein intake during pregnancy is associated with intrauterine growth restriction and infant low birth weight, which increases risk of neonatal morbidities and mortality and may impact on risk of chronic disease in later life (see Section 10.1: 'The "developmental origins of health and disease" hypothesis').

The WHO currently recommends that pregnant women consume 1 g, 9 g and 31 g of additional protein daily during the first, second and third trimesters respectively (estimated to support a 13.8 kg gestational weight gain) (FAO/WHO/UNU, 2007). In the UK, the Department of Health recommends an average increment of 6 g/day above the normal daily requirement throughout pregnancy (see Table 10.5).

In developed countries, most diets provide sufficient protein to meet these needs, but concerns remain about the ability of many women in economically deprived regions to meet their protein requirements during pregnancy. In such areas, antenatal nutritional education has been shown to be effective in improving protein intakes during pregnancy and reducing the risk of preterm births and low birth weight (Ota et al., 2015). Balanced protein energy supplementation (i.e. supplements providing less than 25% of total energy from protein) has also been shown to reduce risk of low birth weight, although there is limited evidence of effects on longer term growth. High protein supplements have been shown to reduce birth weight in some groups and are not advised (Ota et al., 2015) (see Section 10.6: 'Advice regarding nutritional supplements during pregnancy').

Carbohydrate

Requirements for starch, sugar and non-starch polysaccharides (dietary fibre) during pregnancy are not increased. However, constipation, which may be party attributed to reduced motility of the gastrointestinal tract, is common at all stages of pregnancy. Women with low intakes of dietary fibre may benefit from increased intakes, along with increased fluid intake and physical activity to encourage regular bowel movement (see Chapter 17).

Fat

There are no additional EU-wide dietary requirements for fat during pregnancy. However, the essential fatty acids linoleic (18:2 n-6) and alpha-linolenic acid (18:3 n-3), and their long-chain derivatives arachidonic acid, eicosapentaenoic acid (EPA) and docosahexaenoic acid (DHA), are important structural components of cell membranes and substrates of eicosanoids which regulate the activities of inflammatory cells and the production of inflammatory cytokines. An adequate supply is essential to the formation of the fetus during pregnancy (Figure 10.5).

Of particular importance in pregnancy is the long-chain n-3 fatty acid, DHA. It can be synthesised from alpha-linolenic acid to a limited and probably variable extent, but the best dietary source is oily fish, in which it is available pre-formed. DHA is essential for the development of the brain and retina of the fetus, particularly during the third trimester of pregnancy.

Research has shown an association between maternal dietary intake of oily fish or supplements (containing n-3 long-chain polyunsaturates) during pregnancy and visual and cognitive function and other functional outcomes in infants. Some studies have also shown that maternal intake of fish, fish oils or n-3 polyunsaturates (e.g. from some vegetable oils) during pregnancy results in a slightly longer gestational period, lower frequency of intrauterine growth retardation and reduced risk of preterm delivery, although the relationship is stronger for fish than for supplements. Prenatal fish consumption has also been associated with lower frequency of maternal depressive and anxiety symptoms (Emmett et al., 2015) (see Section 10.6: 'Advice regarding nutritional supplements during pregnancy'), and there is some evidence that increased maternal intake of long-chain n-3 fatty acids could lower the risk

n-6 family	n-3 family
Linoleic acid	Alpha-linolenic acid
18:2 n-6	18:3 n-3
↓	↓
18:3 n-6	18:4 n-3
↓	↓
20:3 n-6	20:4 n-3
↓	↓
Arachidonic acid (AA)	Eicosapentaenoic acid (EPA)
20:4 n-6	20:5 n-3
↓	↓
22:4 n-6	22:5 n-3
↓	↓
22:5 n-6	Docosahexaenoic acid (DHA)
	22:6 n-3

Figure 10.5 The n-6 and n-3 polyunsaturated fatty acid pathways.

Table 10.6 Recommendations for long-chain *n*-3 polyunsaturated fatty acid intake.

Reference	Year	Recommendation for normal healthy population	Recommendation during pregnancy
EFSA Panel on Dietetic Products, Nutrition and Allergies (NDA) (2010a)	2010	250 mg EPA plus DHA per day (one or two portions of oily fish per week)	+100–200 mg DHA during pregnancy and lactation
WHO/FAO (2010)	2008	250 mg EPA plus DHA per day for adult males and non-pregnant/non-lactating women	300 mg EPA+DHA per day for pregnant and lactating women, 200 mg of which should be DHA
SACN (2004)	2004	Two portions of fish per week, one of which should be oily; these provide approximately 450 mg long-chain *n*-3 polyunsaturated fatty acids per day	

of immunoglobulin-E-related allergic disease in babies and children (Best *et al.*, 2016).

Table 10.6 shows the global recommendations for intake of long-chain *n*-3 polyunsaturated fatty acids, including specific recommendations for women who are pregnant. Such women should aim to achieve an average dietary intake of at least 200 mg DHA per day (EFSA Panel on Dietetic Products, Nutrition and Allergies (NDA), 2010a), which is provided by consuming one or two portions of fish per week, including oily fish. Large predatory species, which may be more likely to be contaminated with methylmercury, and fish oil supplements (e.g. cod liver oil) with a high vitamin A content should be avoided during pregnancy (see Section 10.6: 'Foods to limit or avoid during pregnancy' and ' Advice regarding nutritional supplements during pregnancy').

Micronutrient requirements

Changes in metabolism, leading to more efficient utilisation and absorption of micronutrients, occur during pregnancy, meaning that for many nutrients an increase in dietary intake over usual requirements is not considered necessary. However, recommendations concerning nutrient requirements during pregnancy differ between countries (Table 10.7); in the UK, increments are advised during pregnancy for vitamins A, C and D, thiamin, riboflavin and folate (Committee on Medical Aspects of Food Policy, 1991). Although severe micronutrient deficiency in the UK is rare, mild deficiency of some micronutrients, pre-conceptionally or during pregnancy, may still have adverse effects on maternal and offspring health, many of which are yet to be fully explored.

Table 10.7 Variation in current micronutrient recommendations for pregnant women within Europe.

	Vitamin A (µg/day)	Folate (µg/day)	Vitamin D[a] (µg/day)	Vitamin B$_{12}$ (µg/day)	Iron (mg/day)	Iodine (µg/day)	Zinc (mg/day)
UK	700	300[b]	10	1.5[c]	14.8[c,d]	140[c]	7[c]
Italy	700	400[e]	10[e]	2.2	30[e]	175	7
Nordic countries[f]	800	500	10	2.0	—[g,h]	175	9[i]
Spain[j]	800	600[k]	10	2.2	18	135	20
Germany/Austria/Switzerland	1.1 mg retinol equivalent	600	5	3.5	30	230[l]	10

Source: data taken from Berti *et al.* (2010).

[a] Vitamin D: 10 µg/day equates to 400 IU/day (IU: international units).

[b] 400 µg/day additionally recommended pre-conception and for the first 12 weeks of gestation.

[c] No increment.

[d] Insufficient for women with high menstruation losses, for whom the most practical approach is to take iron supplements.

[e] Dietary supplements or fortified foods may be required.

[f] Denmark, Finland, Iceland, Norway, Sweden.

[g] The composition of the meal influences the utilisation of dietary iron. The availability increases if the diet contains abundant amounts of vitamin C and meat or fish daily, while it is decreased at simultaneous intake of some substances (e.g. polyphenols or phytic acid).

[h] Iron balance during pregnancy requires iron stores of approximately 500 mg at the start of pregnancy. The physiological need of some women for iron cannot be satisfied during the last two-thirds of pregnancy with food alone, and supplemental iron is therefore needed.

[i] Utilisation of zinc is negatively influenced by phytic acid and positively by animal protein.

[j] From the second half of pregnancy.

[k] First and second half of gestation.

[l] Switzerland: 200 µg/day.

Vitamins of specific importance during pregnancy

Vitamin A

Vitamin A deficiency is widespread globally, affecting about 19 million pregnant women worldwide. Vitamin A is essential during pregnancy for cell division, fetal organ and skeletal growth and maturation, maintenance of the immune system and development of vision in the fetus, particularly during the third trimester when fetal growth is most rapid. It is also needed for maintenance of maternal eye health and night vision, as well as normal immune function. In a pregnant woman with moderate vitamin A deficiency, the fetus can still obtain sufficient vitamin A to develop appropriately, but at the expense of the maternal stores. There is, therefore, a small increased dietary requirement during pregnancy (Tables 10.5 and 10.7). Animal foods, such as dairy products and liver, contain preformed vitamin A, whilst vegetables, such as carrots, spinach, sweet potatoes and red peppers, provide provitamin A (e.g. beta-carotene). A varied diet should provide sufficient intake, although the increased requirement during pregnancy can be difficult to achieve in areas where dietary supply is limited. Although the WHO does not advise vitamin A supplementation in pregnancy as part of routine antenatal care for the prevention of maternal and infant morbidity and mortality, in areas where vitamin A deficiency is a severe public health problem it is recommended for the prevention of night blindness amongst women. In excessive amounts, retinol is teratogenic (can cause birth defects). Toxicity generally results from excessive ingestion of vitamin A supplements, but regular intake of large amounts of liver may also result in toxicity due to its potentially high content of vitamin A. Women in countries where vitamin A intakes are likely to be adequate, such as the UK, are therefore advised to avoid supplements containing retinol (unless advised by a practitioner), as well as liver and liver products during pregnancy (see Section 10.6: ' Advice regarding nutritional supplements during pregnancy').

B vitamins

In addition to the recommendation to take a folic acid supplement and consume folate-rich foods in the early stages of pregnancy to reduce risk of NTDs (see Section 10.2: 'Nutritional status prior to pregnancy'), extra dietary folate is needed throughout pregnancy to prevent megaloblastic anaemia. In the UK, an increment of 100 µg/day of folate (i.e. a total intake of 300 µg/day) is recommended for the duration of pregnancy (Committee on Medical Aspects of Food Policy, 1991) (Table 10.5). Higher recommendations have been made in several other European countries (Table 10.7). As an adequate intake (beyond the first 12 weeks of pregnancy)

can be obtained via consumption of a well-balanced diet that includes plenty of folate-rich foods and foods fortified with folic acid, supplements are generally only recommended up to the 12th week of pregnancy. However, in areas where anaemia is a severe public health problem, the WHO recommends daily oral iron and folic acid supplementation throughout pregnancy as part of antenatal care to reduce the risk of low birth weight, maternal anaemia and iron deficiency (WHO, 2016b).

Vitamin B_{12} deficiency can also cause anaemia but is rare in pregnancy, especially where meat consumption is the norm. As with folate, vitamin B_{12} can act as a methyl donor, influencing methylation processes in the body. DNA methylation is an epigenetic modification that plays an important role in regulation of gene expression and is especially important during early fetal development. Although the current UK recommendation for B_{12} is 1.5 µg/L, recommendations in other European countries are slightly higher (2.0 to 3.5 µg/L) (Table 10.7).

Vitamin D

Vitamin D and its active metabolite 25(OH)D have an important role in calcium balance and bone metabolism. Without sufficient 25(OH)D the intestine cannot absorb calcium and phosphate adequately, which leads to an abnormally high concentration of parathyroid hormone in the blood (hyperparathyroidism), resulting in weakening of the bones through loss of calcium. This eventually can result in rickets in children and osteomalacia in adults. Adequate vitamin D status during pregnancy is important for fetal skeletal development, tooth enamel formation and perhaps general fetal growth and development. Although the maternal gut can adapt to vitamin D insufficiency with increased calcium transport, and calcium levels may be normal *in utero* when maternal supply is inadequate, maternal vitamin D deficiency is a cause of neonatal hypocalcaemia (low blood calcium) and other adverse birth outcomes. Insufficiency has been linked with increased risk of gestational diabetes and pre-eclampsia in the mother and low birth weight.

A number of large RCTs have been investigating the possible benefits of vitamin D supplementation during pregnancy on a range of maternal and fetal outcomes. For example, the Maternal Vitamin D Osteoporosis Study (MAVIDOS) was set up to test the hypothesis that vitamin D supplementation of pregnant women in the UK results in improved bone mass at birth and during early childhood, as well as investigating the influence of maternal vitamin D status on other childhood outcomes, such as blood pressure, glucose tolerance and cardiovascular and immune function. Supplementation did not lead to increased offspring whole-body bone mineral content assessed within two weeks at birth (Cooper *et al.*, 2016). However, this study demonstrated the safety of a daily dose of 1000 IU of cholecalciferol and its ability to ensure that most pregnant women were replete in 25 (OH)D. The results of the ongoing childhood follow-up study are awaited. DALI (Vitamin D and lifestyle intervention), a Europe-wide RCT, is testing the effectiveness of a range of interventions, including vitamin D supplementation, on the development of gestational diabetes in overweight and obese women. Such studies will help to clarify the role of supplementation during pregnancy on a range of maternal and fetal outcomes (see Section 10.6: 'Advice regarding nutritional supplements during pregnancy').

The main source of vitamin D is via sunlight exposure (UVB 290–315 nm). However, latitude, sun avoidance, skin pigmentation (i.e. ethnicity) and use of sunscreen all influence ability to achieve adequate status. Vitamin D may also be obtained from the diet, but is found naturally in few foods. Oil-rich fish is the richest source. Eggs, meat and milk contain small amounts, but this varies during the seasons. Fortified foods (e.g. some spreads, breakfast cereals, dairy foods) can make an important contribution to intakes in many countries, including the UK.

Although there is no widespread agreement on the 'optimal' plasma/serum level of vitamin D, in the UK a plasma/serum 25(OH)D concentration of less than 25 nmol/L has been used as an indicator of inadequate vitamin D status, because of the association of these levels with an increased risk of rickets in children and osteomalacia in adults (SACN, 2016). The most recent data from the National Diet and Nutrition Survey (NDNS) showed that just under a quarter (22%) of women aged 19–64 years have plasma levels below this threshold (Figure 10.3) (Bates et al., 2014). In January to March, when the wavelength of sunlight in countries such as the UK does not stimulate vitamin D production, 40% of adolescents aged 11–18 years and 39% of women aged 19–64 years had concentrations below this level (Bates et al., 2014). Studies assessing vitamin D levels in pregnant women across the UK are more limited but suggest that low serum 25(OH)D concentrations are common in this group (SACN, 2016). Studies purport a similar problem across Europe (Spiro and Buttriss 2014). Pregnant non-Western women may be at particularly high risk of deficiency; a study in The Hague, for example, showed serum 25(OH)D levels lower than 25 nmol/L in more than 80% of Turkish and Moroccan immigrants (van der Meer et al., 2006). A UK study reported that serum 25(OH)D levels below 25 nmol/L were highly prevalent in South Asian women of childbearing age in the winter (81%) and autumn (79%) (Darling et al., 2013). Pre-pregnancy obesity has also been associated with lower levels of vitamin D in both pregnant women and their neonates.

Recommendations for vitamin D intakes for the general population and for women during pregnancy vary globally (Table 10.8). In the UK, SACN has recently proposed a reference nutrient intake (RNI) of 10 μg/day for all adults and children aged 4 years and over (SACN, 2016) (see Chapter 24). There has been a national recommendation for pregnant women to take supplements (10 μg/day, or 400 IU/day) for some time (Committee on Medical Aspects of Food Policy, 1991), as well as for other 'at-risk' groups (e.g. those with increased skin pigmentation), but implementation of the recommendation has been limited and the uptake of vitamin D supplements in these population groups is low. Women who receive little sunlight exposure, such as those who cover up their skin when outdoors, are likely to have low vitamin D status, so it is particularly important that they receive supplementary vitamin D during pregnancy.

Whilst vitamin D is toxic at high doses (the safe upper limit is 50 μg/day or 2000 IU/day for adults in Europe and the USA), it is generally accepted that supplementation at recommended levels/treatment of deficiency is safe during pregnancy.

Table 10.8 Dietary reference values for vitamin D for adults and during pregnancy.

Country/region	Dietary reference value (μg/day)	
	Adults	Pregnancy
European:		
Austria[a]	20	20
Belgium	10–15	20
France	5	10
Germany[a]	20	20
Ireland	0–10	10
Spain	15	15
Switzerland	20	20
Turkey	10	
Netherlands	10	10
NNR	10	10
UK	10	10
EC	0–10	10
Other:		
IOM	15	15
WHO/FAO	5	5
NHMRC	5	5

Source: adapted from Spiro and Buttriss (2014). Reproduced with permission of John Wiley & Sons Ltd.

NNR: Nordic Nutrition Recommendations; EC: European Commission; IOM: Institute of Medicine; WHO/FAO: World Health Organization/Food and Agriculture Organization; NHRMC: National Health and Medical Research Council (Australia).

[a] Specified without endogenous synthesis (assumption of lack of sun exposure).

Vitamin C

During pregnancy, the rapidly growing fetus places demand on a mother's tissue stores of vitamin C. Therefore, an increment of 10 mg/day is advised in the UK during the last trimester of pregnancy to ensure that maternal stores are maintained (Committee on Medical Aspects of Food Policy, 1991). Consumption of foods containing vitamin C (e.g. fresh fruits, especially citrus fruits and berries, green vegetables, peppers, tomatoes and potatoes) can also enhance absorption of non-haem iron from plant sources, helping to avoid iron-deficiency anaemia during pregnancy.

Minerals of specific importance during pregnancy

In the UK, requirements for minerals are not considered to increase during pregnancy due to the more efficient absorption and utilisation that occurs during this period (Committee on Medical Aspects of Food Policy, 1991). However, recommendations vary globally, and some minerals deserve particular attention during pregnancy as adequate intakes can have important effects on maternal and fetal outcomes.

Iron

Iron is vital for fetal growth and development because it plays a key role as a cofactor for enzymes involved in oxidation–reduction reactions, which occur in all cells during metabolism. It is also vital to the production of haemoglobin (which is necessary for oxygen transport), and energy production, fetal immunity and development of the central nervous system. Globally, inadequate iron intake is the most common nutrient deficiency, and women of childbearing age are at particularly high risk because of loss of iron during monthly menses. Despite the respite from iron losses from menstruation during pregnancy, iron requirements are high because of the expansion of maternal blood volume and the needs of the fetus to support normal development.

Iron deficiency is the most common cause of anaemia during pregnancy and is thought to occur in around 40% of pregnant women globally (WHO, 2016b). Although it is more common in developing countries, low iron status is also significantly prevalent in industrialised countries. Maternal anaemia is associated with low birth weight and premature delivery (both risk factors for neonatal and infant morbidity and mortality), stillbirth and a host of perinatal complications, especially haemorrhage.

The fetus is relatively protected from the effects of iron deficiency due to fetal haemoglobin having a greater affinity for oxygen than adult haemoglobin in response to low availability of oxygen *in utero* and a higher haemoglobin concentration in the circulation compared with postnatal life. However, evidence suggests that maternal iron depletion increases the risk of iron deficiency in early life. During the last trimester of pregnancy, the fetus accumulates iron for use during early life and stores are meant to last until around 6 months of age when complementary feeding is initiated. If adequate iron is not available during the prenatal period there can be lifelong neurologic effects that cannot be reversed even if iron is supplemented in adequate levels in childhood. Children born to iron-deficient mothers are more likely to suffer from impaired physical and cognitive development, and to have suboptimal immune systems.

The risk of development of iron-deficiency anaemia in pregnancy is dependent on a woman's iron stores at the time of conception and the amount of iron absorbed during gestation. Recommendations for iron intake differ greatly across the globe (Table 10.9), reflecting differences in the likely bioavailability of dietary iron consumed. In most countries (with the notable exception of the USA and Canada), there is no additional increment for iron intake during pregnancy due to the assumption that the extra iron requirement may be met through cessation of menstrual losses, increased intestinal absorption and mobilisation of maternal iron stores. However, it is worth noting that 40% of UK women aged 16–24 years have an average daily intake below the LRNI. Iron status measurements from the NDNS indicate that 8.8% of girls aged 11–18 years and 9.8% of women aged 19–64 years have haemoglobin levels below the desired threshold levels (<120 g/L), whilst plasma ferritin levels are low in 30.2% and 16.6% respectively (below 15 µg/L threshold). Those most at risk of iron deficiency during pregnancy include women from lower socio-economic groups, teenagers who become

Table 10.9 Global dietary reference values for iron for females aged 19–50 years and those who are pregnant.

	Dietary reference value (mg/day)			
	UK[a]	USA and Canada[b]	FAO/WHO[c]	EU[d]
Women aged 19–50 years	14.8	18.0	20.7/31.0	20.7
Pregnancy[e]	—	27.0	—	—

Source: adapted from Geissler and Singh (2011).

Dashes indicate no change in requirement.
[a] DH (1991); recommended nutrient intake (based on 15% absorption).
[b] National Academy of Sciences (2001); recommended dietary allowance (based on 18% absorption).
[c] FAO/WHO (2002); recommended nutrient intake (based on 15% and 10% absorption respectively).
[d] Scientific Committee on Food (1993); population reference intake (based on 15% absorption).
[e] Bioavailability in the first trimester is as estimated for non-pregnant females, in the second and third trimesters it is increased to 25%.

pregnant and women having successive births with short intervals. There is a strong inverse correlation between parity and iron status, suggesting that short intervals between pregnancies (<18 months) may provide insufficient time for maternal stores to be replenished.

Owing to the persistently high burden of disease, international guidelines recommend universal iron (alongside folic acid) supplementation throughout pregnancy in areas where anaemia is highly prevalent. A Cochrane review found pregnant women taking iron supplements to have a 70% lower risk of anaemia and a 57% lower risk of iron deficiency. In addition, they were less likely to have low-birth-weight babies and their offspring had better iron status in infancy (Peña-Rosas et al., 2012). However, iron supplementation and higher iron status may adversely modify risk of infections, including malaria, complicating a universal policy of routine supplementation in malaria-endemic areas. The benefits of such an approach must therefore be carefully weighed against the possibility of adverse consequences in certain settings, and, where necessary, iron supplements should be provided alongside malaria prevention strategies (see Section 10.6: 'Advice regarding nutritional supplements during pregnancy'). Lower quantities of iron (eg via fortified food) may offer a safer alternative in most cases (Prentice et al., 2017).

In the UK, the National Institute for Health and Care Excellence (NICE) guidance is that all women should have their iron status tested at booking and at 28 weeks and that supplementation should be considered in those with haemoglobin concentrations below 110 g/L in the first trimester and below 105 g/L at 28 weeks (NICE, 2008). As iron status is often poor in this age group, in practice, many women are prescribed iron supplements during pregnancy. All women should be given dietary advice to maximise iron intake by eating iron-containing foods (e.g. red meat, pulses, nuts, eggs, dried fruit, poultry fish, wholegrains and dark-green leafy vegetables) and iron absorption (e.g. via consumption of foods containing vitamin C with plant sources of iron).

Iodine

Iodine is required for the production of thyroid hormones and normal functioning of the central nervous system, as well as cognitive function and normal growth of children (see Chapter 9). Severe iodine deficiency, which mostly affects those living in iodine-deficient areas of Africa and Asia, can result in cretinism (severely stunted physical and mental growth) and intellectual impairment in children. It also increases risk of infant mortality, miscarriage and stillbirth. Iodised salt is recommended by the WHO as the first line of defence in combating conditions caused by iodine deficiency, but supplementation may be required before or during early pregnancy to prevent fetal damage in some countries (see

Section 10.6: 'Advice regarding nutritional supplements during pregnancy').

Although overt deficiency is uncommon in developed countries, pregnant women are still at risk of mild-to-moderate deficiency, which is evident in parts of Europe. In the UK, studies assessing iodine status have indicated that a substantial proportion of adolescent girls, women of childbearing age and pregnant women may be mild-to-moderately deficient. Consistent with this, the NDNS has also reported low intakes in a significant proportion of females, especially those aged 11–18 years (Table 10.1). However, it should be noted that UK food composition data for iodine are uncertain, have not been systematically updated and are unlikely to provide a reliable contribution to assessments of iodine intake. Levels in cereals vary depending on the environmental conditions and iodine content of the soil in which they are grown, and levels in meat, chicken, eggs and dairy products reflect the iodine content of the animal feed and farming practices used. Whether mild-to-moderate deficiency in pregnancy produces more subtle changes in cognitive function in offspring remains unclear, but lower iodine status during the first trimester of pregnancy has been associated with lower verbal IQ and reading ability in UK children at age 8–9 years (Bath et al., 2013).

The UK reference intake for iodine for pregnant women is 140 µg/day (the same recommendation as for non-pregnant women) (Committee on Medical Aspects of Food Policy, 1991), although some researchers suggest this is inadequate. Guidance in the USA is similar to the UK, with a recommendation for 150 µg/day, increased to 220 µg/day during pregnancy (Institute of Medicine (US) Panel on Micronutrients (2001), as well as Australia and New Zealand (NHMRC, 2006). The WHO recommends 250 µg/day during pregnancy (WHO et al., 2007).

Calcium

During pregnancy, calcium moves from mother to fetus to help mineralise the baby's skeleton, particularly during the last trimester. Babies born at full term contain approximately 20–30 g of calcium, most of which is laid down during the last trimester. Inadequate consumption of this nutrient by pregnant women can lead to adverse effects in both mother and fetus, including low bone mineral density (osteopenia), tremor, muscle cramping, tetanus, delayed fetal growth, low birth weight and poor fetal bone mineralisation. Tooth formation begins in the womb, and there is some evidence that increased maternal intake of dairy products during pregnancy may reduce the risk of childhood dental caries. Calcium supplements for women with a low calcium intake have been suggested to reduce the risk of hypertensive disorders in pregnancy (such as pre-eclampsia), although evidence is limited.

A dietary intake of 1200 mg/day of calcium for pregnant women is recommended by the WHO (WHO/FAO, 2004). However, recommendations for calcium intake during pregnancy vary across countries – for example, recommendations in the USA, Australia and New Zealand are 1300 mg/day for those aged 14–18 years and 1000 mg/day for older women (NHMRC, 2006; Ross et al., 2011), whereas in Europe an intake of 700 mg/day has long been established (since 1993) (Hermoso et al., 2011), which is also the current UK RNI for women aged over 19 years (Committee on Medical Aspects of Food Policy, 1991). As there appears to be a doubling in the rate or efficiency of intestinal calcium absorption during pregnancy, the UK dietary reference value panel did not consider any increment in calcium intake to be necessary during pregnancy, although higher maternal calcium was considered advisable for adolescent pregnancies. According to the NDNS, intakes of calcium are likely to be inadequate in a significant proportion of females, especially those aged 11–18 years – 19% estimated to be below the LRNI (Table 10.1) (Bates et al., 2014). As calcium is particularly important during childhood and adolescence for the growth and development of normal bones, an inadequate supply during these life stages may increase the risk of osteoporosis in later life.

Zinc

Zinc is essential for normal fetal development and for brain development before birth and in neonatal life. Zinc deficiency may compromise infant development and lead to poor birth outcome. Low maternal plasma zinc concentrations may affect the supply of zinc to the fetus and alter circulating levels of a number of hormones associated with the onset of labour. As zinc is essential for normal immune function, deficiency may contribute to systemic and intrauterine infections, both major causes of preterm birth.

Zinc deficiency is common, affecting one in five of the world's population, especially in regions with low consumption of animal foods and high intakes of foods rich in phytates, which can inhibit zinc absorption. In such areas, zinc supplementation has been shown to reduce the risk of premature birth (but not of low birth weight), and may be particularly beneficial for preterm and low-birth-weight infants in terms of growth and motor development.

In the UK, a substantial proportion of boys and girls aged 11–18 years have been found to have intakes below the LRNI for zinc (Table 10.1) (Bates et al., 2014). Mild deficiency (i.e. not clinically overt) may still increase the risk of infection and poor growth. However, owing to limitations of micronutrient intake assessment and lack of a reliable biomarker of zinc status, both the level and effect of mild deficiency within the population is relatively hard to quantify.

10.4 Fluid requirements in pregnancy

General fluid needs increase during pregnancy in order to support fetal circulation, amniotic fluid and a higher blood volume. An adequate fluid supply is also necessary to ensure reserves to tolerate blood loss during delivery.

Guidelines for total water intake vary greatly among countries (Table 10.10). There is no specific recommendation about fluid intake in pregnancy in the UK, and data on water intakes of pregnant women is lacking in European populations. However, the European Food Safety Authority (EFSA) has advised a small increase to take account of weight gain and the increase in energy intake in the later stages of pregnancy. Assuming an increase in energy intake of 15% (i.e. 300 kcal/day) in the second trimester, EFSA recommends an additional total water intake of 300 mL/day (EFSA Panel on Dietetic Products, Nutrition and Allergies (NDA), 2010b). The total requirement is therefore 2300 mL/day (as foods provide around 20% of fluid requirements, this equates to around 1850 mL from beverages). In the USA and Canada, recommendations for adequate water intakes are based on the median total water intake observed in the Third National Health and Nutrition Examination Survey (NHANES III) for pregnant women, equating to

Table 10.10 Reference values for water intake in pregnant and lactating women.

	Water intake (mL/day)			
	World[a]	Europe[b]	USA and Canada[c]	Australia and New Zealand[d]
Adult women	2200	2000	2700	2800
Pregnant women	4800	2300	3000	3100

Total water intake refers to water from fluid (water and beverages) and the water in food.
[a] Howard and Bartram (2003).
[b] EFSA Panel on Dietetic Products, Nutrition and Allergies (NDA) (2010b).
[c] Institute of Medicine of the National Academies (2004).
[d] NHMRC (2006).

3000 mL/day (Institute of Medicine of the National Academies, 2004). In Australia and New Zealand, adequate intakes are also based on median water intake. Needs increase amongst those who are very physically active or living in hot climates.

Constipation is a common complaint during pregnancy and can be exacerbated by decreased gut motility and iron supplementation. Increased fluid intake can help to alleviate symptoms, alongside increased dietary fibre intake. It is also important to replenish any loss due to morning sickness, as this is a common cause of dehydration during pregnancy.

Water contamination is of particular concern during pregnancy, particularly for women with conditions that further compromise the immune system (e.g. HIV infection).

10.5 Vulnerable groups within the UK population

Adolescents

Pregnant adolescents are at a greater nutritional risk as they themselves are undergoing an intense period of growth and development. It has been suggested this creates competition for nutrients between a pregnant adolescent and her fetus as both are in critical stages of growth during the gestational period. Adolescents are also more likely than adults to consume, micronutrient-poor diets and to experience adverse pregnancy outcomes, particularly fetal growth restriction and preterm delivery. The proportion of women taking folic acid supplements is smaller amongst pregnant teenagers than older women. They may also be disconcerted by body shape changes associated with pregnancy.

Rates of teenage pregnancy in the UK are high compared with other parts of Europe. NDNS data show nutrient shortfalls in the diets of girls aged 11–18 years (Table 10.1), as well as young women in their later teens and twenties (Bates *et al.*, 2014). This may be exacerbated by socio-economic deprivation and smoking (which is known to cause further depletion of micronutrients). The About Teenage Eating (ATE) Study found poor micronutrient intakes and status, as well as higher rates of iron-deficiency anaemia, which was associated with higher risk of low-birth-weight offspring (Baker *et al.*, 2009). Against this background, it is evident that many adolescent females need guidance on how to eat healthily, even in the absence of pregnancy.

Ethnic minority groups

Some ethnic minority groups are at increased risk of poor pregnancy outcome in the UK. The risk of low birth weight is higher in South Asian pregnancies compared with white Europeans (SACN, 2011). Among those of Indian origin, those who are Hindu (and predominantly vegetarian) have been found to have smaller babies than Muslim women of South Asian origins. Young women from minority ethnic groups and lower socio-economic backgrounds are least likely to take folic acid supplements, and those following a vegetarian diet may require dietary advice to ensure sufficient intakes of other important micronutrients during pregnancy (such as iron and zinc), as well as *n*-3 fatty acids for those excluding oil-rich fish from their diets (British Nutrition Foundation, 2013). Vitamin D deficiency is also particularly common in South Asian women due to reduced skin synthesis (see Section 10.3: 'Vitamins of specific importance during pregnancy').

Lower socio-economic groups

Low socio-economic status is associated with many risk factors for poor pregnancy outcome, including short stature, low pre-pregnancy BMI, low weight gain during pregnancy and higher maternal obesity. Babies born to mothers from lower socio-economic backgrounds are more likely to be of low birth weight and preterm (British Nutrition Foundation, 2013). Mothers in deprived areas, on low incomes, younger mothers and those with lower educational attainment are less likely to take the recommended nutritional supplements before and during pregnancy. The Infant Feeding Survey in 2011, for example, reported 71% of UK mothers from managerial and professional occupation groups to take some form of dietary supplements during their pregnancy compared with 59% of mothers from routine and manual occupations, and use of folic acid before and during pregnancy was lower in mothers who had never worked (McAndrew *et al.*, 2012).

Obese women

Obesity in pregnancy is associated with an increased risk of adverse outcomes for both mother and child (see Section 10.3: 'Weight gain during pregnancy' and Chapter 14). Women with raised BMI are at higher risk of NTDs (see Section 10.3: 'Vitamins of specific importance during pregnancy'), are less likely to use nutritional supplements and have lower folate intakes and serum levels. This has led to suggestions that obese women should receive higher doses of folic acid supplementation prior to and in the first 12 weeks of pregnancy to minimise the risk of NTDs (see Section 10.2: 'Micronutrient requirements'). Pre-pregnancy BMI has also been shown to be associated with serum vitamin D concentrations in pregnant women, and obese women are at increased risk of vitamin D deficiency compared with women with a healthy weight. Cord serum vitamin D levels in babies of obese women have been found to be lower than in babies born to non-obese women. It is therefore particularly important to encourage vitamin D supplementation in this population group.

Smokers

Smoking is associated with lower mean birth weight and increased risks of preterm delivery and stillbirth. Despite a decline in recent years, a substantial proportion of pregnant women in the UK smoke. According to the Infant Feeding Survey (McAndrew et al., 2012), a quarter (26%) of mothers in the UK smoked at some point in the year immediately before or during their pregnancy. Of these mothers, just over half (54%) gave up at some point before the birth, while 12% smoked throughout their pregnancy. Rates were higher among those in manual occupations and younger age groups (<24 years).

Smoking negatively impacts on nutritional intake and status of several micronutrients. In particular, studies have shown lower intakes of vitamin C and carotenoids amongst smokers compared with non-smokers and lower folate status in newborns of smoking mothers (British Nutrition Foundation, 2013).

10.6 Diet and lifestyle advice for a healthy pregnancy

Dietary patterns associated with a positive pregnancy outcome

Most studies investigating the role of diet in pregnancy have assessed the effect of single nutrients, but, of course, individuals consume meals composed of a wide variety of foods that interact with each other. This interrelated nature of dietary exposures makes it difficult to separate out the specific effects of nutrients or foods in relation to birth weight, disease risk or other relevant health outcomes. Dietary pattern analysis facilitates the study of the whole diet and has been adopted in studies in different countries, often involving large prospective cohorts, to look at dietary patterns during pregnancy associated with better outcomes for both mother and child. Whilst different dietary patterns have been identified (e.g. traditional versus western, prudent, health conscious or Mediterranean-style diets), these studies have tended to show that consumption of 'healthier' dietary patterns including foods such as fruit, vegetables, whole grains, low-fat dairy, lean meats, fish and legumes throughout pregnancy appears beneficial in reducing risk of having a low-birth-weight baby and possibly risk of preterm

delivery, gestational diabetes, pre-eclampsia and other adverse obstetric outcomes. Such foods provide a range of important nutrients during pregnancy, including protein, fibre, iron, zinc, calcium and folate. Longer term effects on childhood health have also been investigated. For example, dietary patterns consistent with advice for healthy eating in the UK during pregnancy have been linked with higher bone mass in offspring at 9 years of age (Cole et al., 2009). A recent study of pregnant women from an area of low socio-economic status in Australia has also carried out dietary pattern analysis to assess pre-conception diet on a range of perinatal outcomes (Grieger et al., 2014). This study found no association between any of the dietary patterns identified with low birth weight but reported a 50% reduced risk of preterm delivery following a high protein and fruit pattern, and a 50% increased risk following a high fat, sugar and takeaway pattern. Similarly, in a 9-year follow-up of participants in the Australian Longitudinal Study on Women's Health, pre-pregnancy consumption of a Mediterranean-style diet (characterised by vegetables, legumes, nuts, tofu, rice, pasta, rye bread, red wine and fish) was associated with a 42% lower risk of developing hypertensive disorders during pregnancy (Schoenaker et al., 2015). The study of food patterns is helpful in determining the type of dietary advice that should be provided to women before and during pregnancy in order to promote the best health for themselves and their babies.

Foods to limit or avoid during pregnancy

Food-borne antenatal infections can cause death or serious fetal damage. Pregnant women are advised to pay particular attention to food hygiene when preparing, cooking and storing food during pregnancy and to avoid certain foods, in order to reduce the risk of exposure to substances that may be harmful to the developing fetus. Potentially harmful substances include food pathogens (e.g. listeria and salmonella), toxic food components (e.g. dioxins and polychlorinated biphenyls (PCBs)), as well as alcohol, caffeine and high doses of some dietary supplements (e.g. vitamin A). Table 10.11 summarises food safety advice for pregnant women from the Department of Health in the UK.

Advice regarding nutritional supplements during pregnancy

Although the increased requirements for most nutrients during pregnancy can be achieved by consumption of appropriate amounts of foods in a balanced and varied diet, this can be a challenge for many women in low– and middle-income countries. In areas where undernutrition

Table 10.11 Foods to avoid or limit during pregnancy.

Foods to avoid	Reason
Some types of cheese (although these are safe if well-cooked): • mould-ripened cheeses (e.g. Camembert, Brie and goats' cheese) • soft blue cheeses (e.g. Danish blue, Roquefort, Gorgonzola)	To minimise risk of listeriosis
All types of pâté (including vegetable pâté)	
Unwashed fruit and vegetables	To minimise risk of toxoplasmosis
Raw/rare/undercooked meat	
Cured meats (e.g. Parma ham and salami)	
Unpasteurised goats' milk or goats' cheese	
Raw or partially cooked eggs or foods made from them[a]; for example, homemade mayonnaise, soft-whip ice cream, cake mix, mousses and hollandaise sauce	To minimise risk of food poisoning from *Salmonella* and *Campylobacter*
Raw or undercooked meat, poultry, shellfish (e.g. oysters) and fish (e.g. smoked salmon, trout, sushi)	
Undercooked ready meals and ready-to-eat poultry (unless they have been reheated to a very high temperature)	
Unpasteurised milk and milk products	
Untreated water	
Liver and liver products and supplements containing vitamin A or fish liver oils	To avoid excess vitamin A intake
Some types of fish: shark, swordfish, king mackerel, tilefish and marlin	To avoid high intakes of mercury and other contaminants
Limit intake of tuna; no more than two tuna steaks a week (about 140 g cooked or 170 g raw each) or four medium-size cans of tuna a week (about 140 g when drained)	
No more than two portions of oily fish per week; for example, fresh tuna (not canned tuna – see above), salmon, mackerel, sardines and trout	

Source: adapted from British Nutrition Foundation (2013).

[a] The Advisory Committee on the Microbiological Safety of Food has recently recommended changing this advice, as the risk is very low for eggs produced under the lion code or equivalent standards.

and micronutrient deficiencies are common, provision of nutrition education and food or fortified food products to pregnant women is likely to reduce the prevalence of poor fetal growth. Protein/energy supplementation has also been shown to promote gestational weight gain and reduce risk of low birth weight and stillbirth in undernourished women, and a number of micronutrient supplements may offer benefit for maternal and child health (Table 10.12). National advice regarding supplementation varies according to the public health issues and diets of individual countries and must consider any potential harmful effects associated with high/increased intakes (Table 10.12).

In the UK, all pregnant women are advised to take folic acid (200 µg/day) before conception and during the first trimester of pregnancy. Vitamin D supplements (10 µg/day) are also advised (see Section 10.3: 'Vitamins of specific importance during pregnancy'). Healthy Start vitamins, containing vitamins C and D and folic acid, are available free of charge for pregnant women on a low income who qualify for the scheme. Other supplements (e.g. iron) may be prescribed based on evidence of poor status (Table 10.12). Although some women may choose to take a multivitamin/mineral supplement to ensure all requirements are met, these are not considered a suitable substitute for a

healthy diet. Pregnant women are advised not to take vitamin A supplements, cod liver oil supplements or multivitamin supplements containing vitamin A.

Advice regarding food allergies

Although allergen avoidance during pregnancy has been recommended to prevent allergies, there is little evidence that this offers any benefit. Indeed, such a strategy may be counterproductive because it has been suggested that exposure to foreign proteins that cross the placenta is important to establish a normal immune response that enables the infant to develop normal tolerance to the many foreign proteins in the environment. Because restrictive diets may limit the supply of essential nutrients, these should be practised under medical supervision. Inappropriate and unnecessary exclusion of foods could prevent both mother and baby from receiving the nutrients they need, resulting in significantly reduced weight gain and increased risk of lower birth weights.

Owing to the severity of reactions from peanut allergy, some countries have issued specific advice around intake during pregnancy. Unlike many other food allergies that tend not to persist beyond childhood, peanut allergy is typically a lifelong problem that can cause severe anaphylactic reactions to very small amounts of peanut,

Table 10.12 Summary of evidence of benefits of nutrient supplementation during pregnancy to maternal and infant health and associated safety issues.

Nutrient(s)	Risks associated with inadequacy	Summary of evidence for benefit	Current population-based recommendations regarding supplementation for pregnant women	Safety issues/side effects during pregnancy
Energy/protein	Undernutrition during pregnancy is associated with an increased risk of a range of adverse pregnancy outcomes.	Balanced protein and energy supplementation (supplements providing <25% energy from protein) promotes gestational weight gain, improves fetal growth and reduces risk of stillbirth (Ota *et al.*, 2015), although the effect appears more pronounced in underweight women in low– and middle-income countries and there is limited evidence of effects on longer term growth. Isocaloric-protein supplementation alone has not shown benefits on perinatal outcomes. High-protein supplementation during pregnancy does not appear to be beneficial and may be harmful to the fetus (Ota *et al.*, 2015).	The WHO has concluded that further research is needed before specific recommendations can be made.	High protein supplements may reduce birth weight (Ota *et al.*, 2015).
Long-chain omega 3 fatty acids/ fish oil supplements	Omega-3 fatty acids are critical building blocks of fetal brain and retina. They therefore contribute to the development of normal brain function and vision.	Prospective studies in pregnant women consuming fish or receiving supplements of fish oil have generally demonstrated a beneficial effect on neurodevelopmental outcomes of offspring, but at present there are not enough data to recommend supplementation for reducing risk of preterm birth or preventing perinatal depression.	Consumption of oily fish is recommended during pregnancy.	High intakes of some fish raise concerns about mercury toxicity, as well as PCB exposure. Fish oil supplements containing vitamin A are not advised in the UK during pregnancy (see Section 10.6: 'Foods to limit or avoid during pregnancy').
Vitamin A	Vitamin A is important for visual health, immune function and fetal growth and development. Low intake has been associated with complications in pregnancy, such as maternal and neonatal infections, early delivery, low birth weight and birth defects.	There is good evidence that antenatal vitamin A supplementation reduces maternal night blindness and maternal anaemia in areas where vitamin A deficiency is common. There is some evidence of reductions in maternal infection, but studies to date have not been of high quality. Studies investigating effects on maternal or perinatal mortality have had mixed findings and been carried out in populations with different vitamin A status.	The WHO and other international agencies do not advise supplementation as part of routine antenatal care. However, where deficiency is a severe public health problem, it is recommended for the prevention of night blindness amongst women. In countries where intakes are likely to be adequate, such as the UK, women are advised not to take retinol supplements during pregnancy.	In excessive amounts, retinol is teratogenic (can cause birth defects). Symptoms of toxicity include dizziness, nausea, vomiting, headaches, blurred vision and fatigue. In the UK, pregnant women are advised not to take supplements containing vitamin A including fish liver oil.

(continued)

Table 10.12 (*Continued*)

Nutrient(s)	Risks associated with inadequacy	Summary of evidence for benefit	Current population-based recommendations regarding supplementation for pregnant women	Safety issues/side effects during pregnancy
Folic acid	Folate deficiency has adverse consequences for mothers (e.g. anaemia, peripheral neuropathy) and fetuses (e.g. birth defects).	Supplementation around the time of conception reduces the risk of NTDs in the offspring (MRC Vitamin Study Research Group, 1991).	In most countries, women are advised to take a folic acid supplement (400 μg/day) prior to and during the first 12 weeks of pregnancy. Women at high risk of having a child with an NTD (e.g. having a personal or family history of the condition) are advised to take higher doses (5 mg/day). In areas where anaemia is a severe public health problem, the WHO recommends intermittent iron and folic acid supplementation as part of antenatal care.	Folic acid supplementation can mask vitamin B_{12} deficiency.
Iron	Moderate and severe anaemia during pregnancy increases risk of low birth weight. Deficiency is also linked with increased risk of premature delivery, maternal and child mortality, and infectious diseases. Children born to iron-deficient mothers are more likely to have low iron stores and to suffer from impaired physical and cognitive development.	Supplementation lowers risk of maternal anaemia.	The WHO recommends prenatal use (with folic acid) in low– and middle-income countries where anaemia is a severe public health problem. This is also recommended in some high-income countries. Other countries encourage targeted supplementation; for example, NICE guidance in the UK is for all women to be tested at booking and at 28 weeks, with supplements considered for those with haemoglobin concentrations below 110 g/L in the first trimester and below 105 g/L at 28 weeks (NICE, 2008).	Supplementation may increase risk of infections, including malaria (Prentice et al., 2017). Malaria prevention strategies should therefore be considered alongside supplementation policies. Gastrointestinal symptoms (e.g. constipation, nausea, vomiting) are commonly experienced by women consuming large amounts of supplemental iron, particularly on an empty stomach.
Vitamin D	Vitamin D has a key role in fetal growth via its interaction with calcium homeostasis. Studies have shown positive correlations between maternal and child vitamin D levels, and between prenatal and postnatal vitamin D levels and bone mineralisation. Deficiency has been suggested to increase risk of pre-eclampsia, gestational diabetes mellitus, preterm birth, low birth weight and	Supplementation during pregnancy increases circulating 25(OH)D concentrations in both maternal and cord serum compared with non-supplemented controls (SACN, 2016).	Supplementation is recommended in many countries. The recommended dose is 10 μg/day for pregnant women in the UK (Committee on Medical Aspects of Food Policy, 1991). The WHO does not advise routine supplementation in pregnancy for improving maternal and infant health outcomes (due to limited RCTs). In cases of deficiency, supplements are recommended	Most experts agree that supplemental vitamin D is safe in doses up to 4000 IU/day during pregnancy.

	Caesarean section, but RCTs are lacking (a number of trials are ongoing).	(5 µg/day or 200 IU/day or as per national guidelines).	
Vitamin C	Deficiency has been associated with increased risk of preterm delivery and an early rupture of membranes in the womb. Poor intake is also linked with risk of maternal anaemia via the ability of this vitamin to enhance non-haem iron absorption. There is no evidence to support routine vitamin C supplementation alone, or in combination with other supplements, for the prevention of fetal or neonatal death, poor fetal growth, preterm birth or pre-eclampsia. However, further research is required to elucidate the possible role of vitamin C in the prevention of placental abruption and pre-labour rupture of membranes.	Routine supplementation is not advised.	Normal doses are considered safe in pregnancy, but some studies have shown high-dose supplements to increase the risk of preterm birth. Supplements should be used cautiously in those at risk of high blood pressure during pregnancy. Excessive vitamin C can cause gastrointestinal problems.
Iodine	Severe iodine deficiency can cause goitre, miscarriages, increased infant mortality and birth defects. The effect of mild-to-moderate deficiency during pregnancy is less certain, but lower maternal iodine status has been suggested to impair neuro– and psychomotor development in childhood. Iodised salt or iodine supplements have been shown to be effective in improving the iodine status of pregnant women and preventing iodine-deficiency-related problems worldwide. However, RCTs demonstrating effects of supplements in areas of mild-to-moderate deficiency are limited.	WHO/UNICEF recommend supplementation for pregnant women in countries where less than 20% of households have access to iodised salt. Few Western countries have adopted this recommendation, although iodisation of salt and other vehicles (e.g. bread) is practised in some European countries as a mandatory (e.g. Denmark) or voluntary (e.g. UK) measure.	Intakes around the daily recommended amounts are considered safe during pregnancy. High intakes should be avoided.
Calcium	Inadequate calcium consumption during pregnancy may be associated with delayed fetal growth, low birth weight and poor fetal mineralisation. Supplementation has been shown to lower risk of pre-eclampsia, particularly in women at high risk. The results of trials evaluating the effect on maternal bone mineral density, fetal mineralisation and preterm birth are less conclusive.	The WHO recommends supplementation in populations where calcium intake is low, for the prevention of pre-eclampsia, particularly among women at high risk.	Even quite large doses of calcium appear safe in pregnancy.
Zinc	Maternal zinc deficiency may compromise infant development and lead to poor birth outcomes (e.g. increased risk of preterm birth). Limited trials, primarily involving women of low income, have shown some reduction in preterm births in those receiving zinc supplements versus placebo, but most trials have not found any reduced risk of low birth weight with maternal supplementation.	The WHO has made no recommendation as evidence of public health benefit is limited.	Supplement studies have not reported any harmful effects.
Multivitamins/ mineral supplements	Limited food supply can lead to inadequate intakes of a number of micronutrients in low-income countries. Multiple-micronutrient supplements containing folic acid and iron have been shown to reduce risk of low birth weight compared with iron and folic acid supplementation in low income countries.	The WHO is due to make a recommendation in 2017. In developed countries, micronutrient supplements are not considered a suitable substitute for a healthy diet but can be useful if dietary intake may be poor (e.g. during illness, prolonged morning sickness).	High doses of some micronutrients may cause harm. In the UK, pregnant women are advised to avoid all supplements containing vitamin A.

triggering severe, sometimes fatal, allergic reactions in susceptible people. The only means of managing the condition currently is avoidance of peanut, which is difficult to achieve. In the UK, the Committee on Toxicity had previously issued cautionary advice that women may wish to avoid peanuts during pregnancy and breast-feeding. However, in 2010 the UK Government revised its advice based on a systematic review that found no clear evidence that eating or not eating peanuts during pregnancy affects the chances of a child developing an allergy. Current advice in the UK is that mothers who are not allergic to peanuts and would like to eat peanuts or foods containing peanuts during pregnancy can do so as part of a healthy diet, irrespective of whether there is a family history. This advice is in keeping with many other countries, including the USA.

Caffeine

Caffeine is a naturally occurring substance found in some plant-based food and drink ingredients, such as tea, coffee and cocoa beans. It is added to drink products like cola-based and energy drinks and is also found in a number of prescription and over-the-counter medicines. The typical caffeine contents of several foods and drinks are shown in Table 10.13. A dose-dependent, positive association between caffeine intakes during pregnancy and risk of adverse birth-weight-related outcomes (i.e. fetal growth retardation, small-for-gestational age) in the offspring has been demonstrated. However, EFSA has concluded that regular caffeine consumption of up to 200 mg per day is safe for the unborn child (EFSA Panel on Dietetic Products, Nutrition and Allergies (NDA), 2015). This is equivalent to just over two cups of filter coffee or four cups of tea.

Alcohol

Whilst the damaging effects of excessive alcohol intake on birth defects, miscarriage and developmental

Table 10.13 Caffeine contents of commonly consumed beverages and food.

Food	Caffeine content (mg)
One mug of instant coffee	100
One mug of filter coffee	140
One mug of tea	75
One can of 'energy' drink	80
One can of cola	40
One 50 g bar of plain chocolate	50
One 50 g bar of milk chocolate	25
One mug of drinking chocolate	1–8[a]

Source: Food Standards Agency (2008).

[a] Depending on brand.

abnormalities have been recognised for many years, the question of whether moderate alcohol consumption during pregnancy is linked to health risks for the off-spring has been widely debated. Although there is limited evidence of detrimental effects on outcomes at low intake, many professionals err on the side of caution. From a global perspective, the WHO recommends complete abstinence from alcohol during pregnancy, which is similar to guidance in North America (USA and Canada) and Australia. This is also the case in the UK, where pregnant women or women trying to conceive are advised that the safest approach is to avoid drinking alcohol. Currently, most women either do not drink alcohol (19%) or stop drinking during pregnancy (40%). Binge drinking may be particularly harmful because it exposes the fetus to high blood alcohol concentrations over relatively short periods of time and may be associated with repeated withdrawal episodes.

Smoking

The adverse consequences of smoking whilst pregnant are well documented and include low birth weight, increased risk of preterm delivery and stillbirth (British Nutrition Foundation, 2013). Smoking can also impact on maternal micronutrient status (see Section 10.5: 'Smokers').

Physical activity

In developed countries, many women become less active in pregnancy, and this is of concern given the increasing prevalence of maternal obesity. Whilst vigorous physical activity may increase risk of low birth weight, moderate-intensity physical activity during pregnancy (e.g. swimming, walking) appears to be safe and provides many health benefits, including reduced risk of excessive gestational weight gain, gestational diabetes, pre-eclampsia, preterm birth, perinatal depression and common complications during pregnancy (e.g. varicose veins, swelling of the feet and legs). There is also some evidence that physical activity during pregnancy is associated with a reduced length of labour and delivery complications. Women who are active during pregnancy are more likely to continue physical activity after delivery.

The WHO recommends that all adults aged 18–64 years should engage in at least 150 min of moderate intensity aerobic activity throughout the week (in bouts of at least 10 min), or at least 75 min of vigorous intensity aerobic activity, or an equivalent combination of the two (WHO, 2010). The guideline states that pregnant women may need extra caution and should seek medical advice before striving to achieve the recommendations. In the UK, at least 30 min/day of moderate-intensity activity is recommended on at least 5 days a week for all women (Department of Health, Physical Activity, Health Improvement and Protection, 2011). Only around 30% of women of childbearing age are meeting this recommendation (Craig and Mindell, 2012). Pregnant women who do no exercise routinely are advised to begin with no more than 15 min of continuous exercise, three times per week, gradually increasing to daily 30-min sessions four times a week or more (NICE, 2010), and these should be accompanied by warm-up and cool-down phases. Contact sports or those with risk of falling (e.g. horse riding) are not advised, and hormonal changes cause joints to be more mobile, increasing the risk of injury with weight-bearing activities. After 16 weeks of pregnancy, physical activities that involve lying on the back are not recommended as the womb is likely to put pressure on major blood vessels. Remaining well hydrated and avoiding hot, humid conditions when exercising are important.

10.7 A summary of diet and lifestyle recommendations before and during pregnancy in the UK

The current diet and lifestyle recommendations for women before and during pregnancy in the UK are summarised in Tables 10.14 and 10.15.

10.8 Improving the nutrition status of women of childbearing age

Maternal nutritional status before and during pregnancy is a strong predictor of growth and development in early life and may influence susceptibility to non-communicable diseases in adulthood. This suggests that measures to improve the nutritional intake of women of childbearing age can improve the health of future generations, alter the long-term health of a population and reduce the burden of non-communicable disease.

The antenatal period, with opportunities for regular contact with health professionals, is considered an ideal time to intervene as mothers are motivated to make changes that could optimise their outcome and that of the baby. In low-income countries, where undernutrition is common and micronutrient deficiencies are widespread, improving maternal nutrition can prevent both infant and maternal mortality alongside many other adverse birth outcomes. Diets and lifestyles of women of childbearing age in developed countries, such as the UK, suggest that many aspects also require improvement. These include the micronutrient status of women before and during pregnancy, awareness and use of recommended supplements (e.g. folic acid and vitamin D), and the proportion of women that achieve a healthy weight gain and are physically active during pregnancy.

Table 10.14 Pre-pregnancy: diet and lifestyle messages.

Diet and lifestyle aspect	Key messages
Body weight	Maintain or attain a healthy body weight (BMI 18.5–25).
Folate/folic acid	Take a 400 µg folic acid supplement daily and eat folate-containing foods on a daily basis (e.g. green leafy vegetables, brown rice, some breads, berries, beans, peas, oranges, fortified breakfast cereals, nuts). Larger supplements (5 mg daily) are needed by women who have already had an NTD-affected pregnancy, those with type 1 diabetes and possibly by obese women and smokers.
Iron	Build up iron stores prior to conception by eating plenty of iron-containing foods (e.g. red meat, fish, pulses, wholemeal bread, dried fruit, nuts, seeds, fortified foods) and consuming plant foods containing iron with foods or drinks containing vitamin C, such as fruit or vegetables, or a glass of fruit juice to assist iron absorption.
Vitamin D	Include vitamin-D-containing foods in the diet (e.g. oily fish, eggs and fortified foods) and practice safe sun exposure. Asian women and those who conceal most of their skin from sunlight exposure are vulnerable to poor vitamin D status and should consider taking a 10 µg daily supplement.
Zinc	Ensure an adequate dietary supply (e.g. from meat, cheese, shellfish, wholegrain foods, nuts, pulses).
Iodine	Ensure an adequate dietary supply (sources include milk and dairy food, fish, eggs).
Vitamin A	Avoid foods with a potentially high vitamin A content, such as liver and liver products (e.g. pâté), supplements containing vitamin A, and fish liver oils that contain high levels of vitamin A.
Alcohol	The safest approach is not to drink alcohol at all, to keep risks to a minimum.
Smoking	Do not smoke.
Physical activity	Ensure regular activity by aiming for at least 150 min (2.5 h) of moderate intensity activity per week (one way to approach this is to do 30 min on at least 5 days a week).

Table 10.15 Pregnancy: diet and lifestyle messages.

Diet and lifestyle aspect	Key messages
Weight gain	In the UK, at present, there are no formal, evidence-based guidelines from the UK Government or professional bodies on what constitutes appropriate weight gain during pregnancy. But avoid poor weight gain and excessive weight gain. Never diet to lose weight when pregnant because this could lead to growth restriction and developmental abnormalities in the baby.
Energy	An additional 0.8 MJ/day (800 kJ/day or 191 kcal/day) is required during the third trimester only. This should be added to energy requirements calculated according to pre-pregnancy body weight.
Protein	Include protein-containing foods such as lean meat, poultry, fish and shellfish, eggs, milk, cheese and other dairy products, beans, nuts, pulses and soya foods (there is a small increase in protein requirements from 45 to 51 g/day).
Fibre	Include plenty of high-fibre foods (e.g. fruit, vegetables and starchy foods, particularly wholegrain varieties and other higher fibre choices, such as potatoes in skins).
Folate/folic acid	Take a 400 μg folic acid supplement daily for the first 12 weeks and eat folate-containing foods on a daily basis (e.g. green leafy vegetables, brown rice, some breads, peas, beans, oranges, berries, fortified breakfast cereals, wholegrain products, nuts). Larger supplements are needed by women who have already had an NTD-affected pregnancy and possibly by obese women.
Vitamin D	Take a 10 μg vitamin D supplement daily and include vitamin-D-containing foods in the diet (e.g. oily fish, eggs, fortified foods) and enable skin synthesis whilst avoiding sunburn.
Iron	Consume plenty of iron-containing foods (e.g. red meat, pulses, fish, wholemeal bread, dried fruit nuts, seeds, fortified foods), preferably with foods or drinks containing vitamin C (such as fruit or vegetables, or a glass of fruit juice) for enhancing iron absorption from non-haem sources.
Zinc	Ensure adequate supply (e.g. from meat, cheese, shellfish, wholegrain foods, nuts, pulses).
Iodine	Ensure adequate supply (sources include milk and dairy products, fish, eggs).
Vitamin A	Avoid foods with potentially high vitamin A content, such as liver and liver products (e.g. pâté), supplements containing vitamin A and fish liver oils that contain high levels of vitamin A. The recommended intake is 700 μg/day.
Vitamin B$_{12}$	No increment from pre-pregnancy requirement, but if vegan or vegetarian it may be necessary to take a supplement.
Calcium	There is no increment in calcium requirement during pregnancy, but an adequate intake must be maintained. Calcium is found in dairy foods, calcium-fortified soya products, canned oily fish, some dark green vegetables, breads, and some nuts and seeds.
n-3 fatty acids	In the UK, 450 mg/day of DHA and EPA combined is recommended for adults and pregnant women; this equates to the consumption of two servings of fish a week, one of which is oil rich. Advice to limit consumption of some types of fish is also relevant (see Section 10.6: 'Foods to limit or avoid during pregnancy').
n-6 fatty acids	Seeds and vegetable oils and spreads are rich sources of the n-6 essential fatty acid linoleic acid.
Foods to avoid	Certain foods should be avoided to reduce risk of exposure to food pathogens (e.g. unpasteurised milk, some types of cheese, pâté, raw or partially cooked eggs, raw or undercooked meat, undercooked ready meals, raw shellfish). Liver products and supplements containing vitamin A or fish liver oils should be avoided owing to risk from high intakes as well as fish more likely to be contaminated with methylmercury (shark, swordfish and marlin). Intake of tuna should be limited to no more than two tuna steaks a week or four medium-size cans of tuna a week.
Allergens	No specific advice.
Dental health	Attend routine dental check-ups and brush regularly with a fluoride toothpaste. Oral health may require closer attention during pregnancy; for example, gums bleed more easily. Do not consume high-sugar foods and drinks too frequently (to protect against dental caries) or acidic foods and drinks (to prevent dental erosion). Caffeine intake should be kept below 200 mg/day (2 cups of instant coffee or 3 cups of tea).
Fluid	Ensure adequate fluid intake (at least six to eight glasses per day).
Alcohol	The safest approach is not to drink alcohol at all, to keep risks to a minimum.
Smoking	Do not smoke.
Physical activity	Continue to be active in pregnancy via low-impact and low-risk activities (e.g. walking and swimming), as it can assist weight control.

However, as nutritional status is cumulative over time, focusing on prenatal nutrition alone will have limited affects. What is needed are strategies to improve women's nutrition throughout the life cycle, beginning as early as possible.

Acknowledgements

I am grateful to Dr Emma Williams, Nutrition Scientist, at the British Nutrition Foundation for her help in preparing this chapter.

References

Ars, C.L., Nijs, I.M., Marroun, H.E. *et al.* (2016) Prenatal folate, homocysteine and vitamin B$_{12}$ levels and child brain volumes, cognitive development and psychological functioning: the Generation R Study. *British Journal of Nutrition*, in press. doi: https://doi.org/10.1017/S0007114515002081.

Baker, P.N., Wheeler, S.J., Sanders, T.A. *et al.* (2009) A prospective study of micronutrient status in adolescent pregnancy. *The American Journal of Clinical Nutrition*, **89**(4), 1114–1124.

Bates, B., Lennox, A., Prentice, A. *et al.* (eds) (2014) National Diet and Nutrition Survey: Results from Years 1, 2, 3 and 4 (Combined) of the Rolling Programme (2008/2009-2011/2012). Public Health England, London. https://www.gov.uk/government/uploads/system/uploads/attachment_data/file/310995/NDNS_Y1_to_4_UK_report.pdf (accessed 6 December 2016).

Bates, B., Prentice, A., Bates, C. *et al.* (eds) (2015) National Diet and Nutrition Survey Rolling Programme (NDNS RP): Supplementary Report: Blood Folate Results for the UK as a Whole, Scotland, Northern Ireland (Years 1 to 4 Combined) and Wales (Years 2 to 5 Combined). Public Health England, London. https://www.gov.uk/government/uploads/system/uploads/attachment_data/file/414745/NDNS_Y1_4_Folate_report.pdf (accessed 6 December 2016).

Bath, S.C., Steer, C.D., Golding, J. *et al.* (2013) Effect of inadequate iodine status in UK pregnant women on cognitive outcomes in their children: results from the Avon Longitudinal Study of Parents and Children (ALSPAC). *The Lancet*, **382**(9889), 331–337.

Berti, C., Decsi, T., Dykes, F. *et al.* (2010) Critical issues in setting micronutrient recommendations for pregnant women: an insight. *Maternal & Child Nutrition*, **6** (Suppl 2), 5–22.

Best, K.P., Gold, M., Kennedy, D. *et al.* (2016) Omega-3 long-chain PUFA intake during pregnancy and allergic disease outcomes in the offspring: a systematic review and meta-analysis of observational studies and randomized controlled trials. *The American Journal of Clinical Nutrition*, **103**, 128–143.

Black, R.E., Victora, C.G., Walker, S.P. *et al.* (2013) Maternal and child undernutrition and overweight in low-income and middle-income countries. *The Lancet*, **382**, 427–451.

British Nutrition Foundation (ed.) (2013) *Nutrition and Development: Short- and Long-term Consequences for Health*, 1st edn. Wiley-Blackwell, Chichester.

Centre for Maternal and Child Enquiries (2010) *Maternal Obesity in the UK: Findings from a National Project*. CMACE, London.

Cole, Z.A., Gale, C.R., Javaid, M.K. *et al.* (2009) Maternal dietary patterns during pregnancy and childhood bone mass: a longitudinal study. *Journal of Bone Mineral Research*, **24**(4), 663–668.

Committee on Medical Aspects of Food Policy (1991) *Dietary Reference Values for Food Energy and Nutrients for the United Kingdom. Report of the Panel on Dietary Reference Values of the Committee on Medical Aspects of Food Policy*. HMSO, London.

Cooper, C., Harvey, N.C., Bishop, N.J. *et al.* (2016) Maternal gestational vitamin D supplementation and offspring bone health (MAVIDOS): a multicentre, double-blind, randomised placebo-controlled trial. *Lancet Diabetes Endocrinology*, **4**(5), 393–402.

Craig, R. and Mindell, J. (eds) (2012) Health Survey for England – 2011. Volume 1. Health, Social Care and Lifestyles. http://content.digital.nhs.uk/catalogue/PUB09300/HSE2011-All-Chapters.pdf (accessed 5 January 2017).

Darling, A.L., Hart, K.H., MacDonald, H.M. *et al.* (2013) Vitamin D deficiency in UK South Asian women of childbearing age: a comparative longitudinal investigation with UK Caucasian women. *Osteoporosis International*, **24**, 477–488.

Department of Health, Physical Activity, Health Improvement and Protection (2011) Start Active, Stay Active: A Report on Physical Activity from the Four Home Countries' Chief Medical Officers. https://www.gov.uk/government/uploads/system/uploads/attachment_data/file/216370/dh_128210.pdf (accessed 6 December 2016).

EFSA Panel on Dietetic Products, Nutrition and Allergies (NDA) (2010a). Scientific Opinion on dietary reference values for fats, including saturated fatty acids, polyunsaturated fatty acids, monounsaturated fatty acids, trans fatty acids, and cholesterol. *EFSA Journal*, **8**, 1461.

EFSA Panel on Dietetic Products, Nutrition and Allergies (NDA) (2010b) Scientific Opinion on dietary reference values for water. *EFSA Journal*, **8**(3), 1459.

EFSA Panel on Dietetic Products, Nutrition and Allergies (NDA) (2015) Scientific Opinion on the safety of caffeine. *EFSA Journal*, **13**(5), 4102.

Emmett, P.M., Jones, L.R. and Golding, J. (2015) Pregnancy diet and associated outcomes in the Avon Longitudinal Study of Parents and Children. *Nutrition Reviews*, **73**, 154–174.

FAO/WHO/UNU (2007) Protein and Amino Acid Requirements in Human Nutrition. Report of a Joint FAO/WHO/UNU Expert Consultation. WHO Technical Report Series 935. World Health Organization, Geneva. http://apps.who.int/iris/bitstream/10665/43411/1/WHO_TRS_935_eng.pdf?ua=1 (accessed 6 December 2016).

FAO/WHO/UNU Committee (2004) Human Energy Requirements. Report of a Joint FAO/WHO/UNU Expert Consultation. FAO Food and Nutrition Technical Report Series 1. FAO, Rome.

Food Standards Agency (2008) Food Standards Agency Publishes New Caffeine Advice for Pregnant Women. http://tna.europarchive.org/20111116080332/http://www.food.gov.uk/news/pressreleases/2008/nov/caffeineadvice (accessed 6 December 2016).

Geissler, C. and Singh, M. (2011) Iron, meat and health. *Nutrients*, **3**(3), 283–316.

Grieger, J.A., Grzeskowiak, L.E. and Clifton, V.L. (2014) Pre-conception dietary patterns in human pregnancies are associated with preterm delivery. *Journal of Nutrition*, **144**, 1075–1080.

Hermoso, M., Vollhardt, C., Bergmann, K.J. and Koletzko, B. (2011) Critical micronutrients in pregnancy, lactation and infancy. *Annals of Nutrition and Metabolism*, **59**(1), 5–9.

Howard, G. and Bartram, J. (2003) *Domestic Water Quantity, Service Level and Health*. WHO/SDE/WSH/3.02. World Health Organization, Geneva.

Huxley, R., Owen, C.G., Whincup, P.H. *et al.* (2007) Is birth weight a risk factor for ischemic heart disease in later life? *The American Journal of Clinical Nutrition*, **85**, 1244–1250.

Institute of Medicine of the National Academies (2004) *Dietary Reference Intakes for Water, Potassium, Sodium, Chloride and Sulfate*. The National Academies Press, Washington, DC.

Institute of Medicine (US) Panel on Micronutrients (2001) *Dietary Reference Intakes for Vitamin A, Vitamin K, Arsenic, Boron, Chromium, Copper, Iodine, Manganese, Molybdenum, Nickel, Silicon, Vanadium and Zinc*. National Acadmy Press, Washington, DC.

McAndrew, F., Thompson, J., Fellows, L. *et al.* (2012) Infant Feeding Survey 2010. Health and Social Care Information Centre. http://content.digital.nhs.uk/catalogue/PUB08694/Infant-Feeding-Survey-2010-Consolidated-Report.pdf (accessed 6 December 2016).

MRC, Vitamin Study Research Group (1991) Prevention of neural tube defects: results of the Medical Research Council Vitamin Study. *The Lancet*, **338**, 131–137.

NHMRC (2006) Nutrient Reference Values for Australia and New Zealand: Including Recommended Dietary Intakes. http://www.nhmrc.gov.au/_files_nhmrc/publications/attachments/n35.pdf (accessed 5 December 2016).

NICE (2008) Antenatal Care for Uncomplicated Pregnancies. Clinical guideline CG62. https://www.nice.org.uk/guidance/cg62 (accessed 6 December 2016).

NICE (2010) Weight Management Before, During and After Pregnancy. Public health guideline PH27. http://www.nice.org.uk/guidance/ph27 (accessed 6 December 2016).

Osmond, C., Barker, D.J., Winter, P.D. *et al.* (1993) Early growth and death from cardiovascular disease in women. *BMJ*, **307**, 1519–1524.

Ota, E., Hori, H., Mori, R. *et al.* (2015) Antenatal dietary education and supplementation to increase energy and protein intake. *The Cochrane Database of Systematic Reviews*, (6) CD000032.

Peña-Rosas, J.P., De-Regil, L.M., Dowswell, T. and Viteri, F.E. (2012) Daily oral iron supplementation during pregnancy. *The Cochrane Database of Systematic Reviews*, (12) CD004736.

Prentice, A.M., Mendoza, Y.A., Pereira, D. *et al.* (2017) Dietary strategies for improving iron status: balancing safety and efficacy. *Nutrition Reviews*, **75**(1), 49–60.

Public Health England (2016) *Maternal Obesity*. http://www.noo.org.uk/NOO_about_obesity/maternal_obesity (accessed 6 December 2016).

Rasmussen, K.M. and Yaktine, A.I. (eds) (2009) *Weight Gain During Pregnancy: Reexamining the Guidelines*. National Academies Press, Washington, DC.

Ross, A.C., Taylor, C.L., Yaktine, A.L. and Del Valle, H.B. (eds) (2011) *Dietary Reference Intakes for Calcium and Vitamin D*. The National Academies Press, Washington, DC. https://www.nap.edu/catalog/13050/dietary-reference-intakes-for-calcium-and-vitamin-d (accessed 6 December 2016).

SACN (2004) *Advice on Fish Consumption: Benefits & Risks*. The Stationery Office, London.

SACN (2011) *The Influence of Maternal, Fetal and Child Nutrition on the Development of Chronic Disease in Later Life*. TSO, London. https://www.gov.uk/government/uploads/system/uploads/attachment_data/file/339325/SACN_Early_Life_Nutrition_Report.pdf (accessed 6 December 2016).

SACN (2016) Vitamin D and Health. https://www.gov.uk/government/uploads/system/uploads/attachment_data/file/537616/SACN_Vitamin_D_and_Health_report.pdf (accessed 29 November 2016).

Schoenaker, D.A., Soedamah-Muthu, S.S., Callaway, L.K. and Mishra, G.D. (2015) Prepregnancy dietary patterns and risk of developing hypertensive disorders of pregnancy: results from the Australian Longitudinal Study on Women's Health. *The American Journal of Clinical Nutrition*, **102**(1), 94–101.

Spiro, A. and Buttriss, J.L. (2014) Vitamin D: an overview of vitamin D status and intake in Europe. *Nutrition Bulletin*, **39**(4), 322–350.

Tennant, P.W., Rankin, J. and Bell, R. (2011) Maternal body mass index and the risk of fetal and infant death: a cohort study from the North of England. *Human Reproduction*, **26**, 1501–1511.

Van der Meer, I.M., Karamali, N.S., Boeke, A.J.P. *et al.* (2006) High prevalence of vitamin D deficiency in pregnant non-Western women in The Hague, Netherlands. *The American Journal of Clinical Nutrition*, **84**, 350–353.

Wald, N.J., Law, M.R., Morris, J.K. and Wald, D.S. (2001) Quantifying the effect of folic acid. *The Lancet*, **358**(9298), 2069–2073.

Whincup, P.H., Kaye, S.J., Owen, C.G. *et al.* (2008) Birth weight and risk of type 2 diabetes: a systematic review. *Journal of the Americal Medical Association*, **300**, 2886–2897.

WHO (2010) *Global Recommendations on Physical Activity for Health*. World Health Organization, Geneva, Switzerland http://apps.who.int/iris/bitstream/10665/44399/1/9789241599979_eng.pdf (accessed 6 December 2016).

WHO (2016a) *Obesity and Overweight*. Fact sheet no. 311. http://www.who.int/mediacentre/factsheets/fs311/en/ (accessed 13/02/2016).

WHO (2016b) *Daily Iron and Folic Acid Supplementation during Pregnancy*. e-Library of Evidence for Nutrition Actions (eLENA). http://www.who.int/elena/titles/daily_iron_pregnancy/en/ (accessed 6 December 2016).

WHO/FAO (2004) *Vitamin and Mineral Requirements in Human Nutrition*, 2nd edn. World Health Organization, Geneva. http://whqlibdoc.who.int/publications/2004/9241546123.pdf (accessed 6 December 2016).

WHO/FAO (2010) *Fats and Fatty Acids in Human Nutrition. Report of an Expert Consultation*. Food and Agriculture Organization, Rome.

WHO, UNICEF and ICCIDD (2007) *Assessment of Iodine Deficiency Disorders and Monitoring their Elimination: A Guide for Programme Managers*, 3rd edn. World Health Organization, Geneva. http://whqlibdoc.who.int/publications/2007/9789241595827_eng.pdf (accessed 6 December 2016).

11
Nutrition and Infant/Child Development

Alison M Lennox

Key messages

- National survey and longitudinal studies, particularly birth cohorts, are the most useful resources for examining the dietary intakes of infants and young children and the impact these have on health and disease.
- Breastfeeding protects against weight gain in later childhood and adulthood, with the greater the protection the longer breastfeeding is continued.
- Breastfeeding may be related to cognitive development and IQ. Both long-chain fatty acids and iodine may play a role in the relationship between breastfeeding and cognitive function.
- Breastfeeding protects against a number of other conditions, such as otitis media (ear infection), gastrointestinal and respiratory tract infections, allergic conditions, asthma and wheeze.
- Exclusive breastfeeding for 6 months is recommended in the UK, following the recommendation by the World Health Organization.
- The percentage of mothers who begin breastfeeding has risen in the UK in recent decades, but the duration of breastfeeding remains short, with only a small proportion continuing for several months. Age, education and ethnic background influence the likelihood of breastfeeding.
- Long-chain fatty acids, iron and vitamin D are the major nutrients of concern in relation to infant feeding in the UK. Both intakes and status of iron and vitamin D status are poorer in breastfed infants than formula fed because these nutrients are added to infant formula. Parents are recommended to give vitamin drops to infants, but the proportion doing so remains low.
- Recommendations for the timing of introduction of peanuts to the diet has changed recently to indicate that 4–6 months is the optimum period for exposure to peanuts in infants at higher risk of allergy, and in some countries this timing is recommended for all infants. A timing of 4–6 months has also been recommended for introduction of gluten, alongside continued breastfeeding, but this recommendation remains under discussion in the UK because it is at odds with the recommendation for exclusive breastfeeding until 6 months of age.

- The feeding of various foods is avoided by some parents of young children, most commonly nuts, meat, poultry, fish, seafood and offal, spicy foods, sweets/chocolate, eggs and dairy products, and processed foods. The reasons for avoidance range from allergy or fear of allergy, fear of choking, family behaviours and religion, and general health concerns.
- A number of longitudinal studies have shown that early diet can impact later health and development. Healthy dietary patterns, characterised by higher intakes of fruit and vegetables, are associated with lower body weight in older childhood and better cognitive performance and IQ. The impact of picky eating is mixed and may depend on the specific behaviours of the children concerned.
- The dietary intakes of children 1.5–3 years and 4–10 years of age, as assessed in the National Diet and Nutrition Survey, are satisfactory in many aspects, but there are concerns about intakes of iron and vitamin D, since substantial proportions had intakes that were too low, with considerable numbers having blood status markers below the cut-offs for deficiency. Intake of non-milk extrinsic sugars decreased markedly since the previous NDNS surveys of these age groups, but remained higher than the new recommendation of 5% of energy. Fruit and vegetable consumption increased substantially since the previous surveys, but evidence indicates greater consumption outside the home, such as at day-care and school, with friends, rather than at home with parents.
- There is a need for continued vigilance in relation to the diets of infants and young children in the UK and an ongoing need to promote healthy eating in the youngest of the population. Setting good food habits at these early stages of life will lead to healthier adolescents and adults in the future.

Public Health Nutrition, Second Edition. Edited by Judith L Buttriss, Ailsa A Welch, John M Kearney and Susan A Lanham-New.
© 2018 by The Nutrition Society. Published 2018 by John Wiley & Sons, Ltd.
Companion website: www.wiley.com/go/buttriss/publichealth

11.1 Introduction

The first years are a key stage of life in relation to dietary intake. The way the infant and young child is fed can have a lasting effect on later health and development, and yet this is a period where there is much confusion about the best ways to proceed to achieve an optimum intake. While there is uniformity in recommendations regarding breast-feeding, the advice for complementary feeding, in what should be fed, how much, at what stages and in what manner, is still conflicting and varies widely around the world. New mothers, keen to follow best practice and do the best for their young children can often be confused by the different information provided to them. This chapter aims to summarise existing knowledge about dietary intakes in infancy and young childhood and the impact that different dietary practices and nutrient intakes can have on the health and future well-being of children.

11.2 Sources of information about infants and young children

The primary source of information about the usual feeding practices and dietary intakes of infants and young children are national surveys and national or regional birth cohorts where children have been followed since birth. The UK is fortunate in having a number of large birth cohorts which can be used to examine the effect of diet on health and well-being as well as a regular programme of assessment of infant feeding. It also conducted a detailed survey of the dietary intakes of infants and young children in 2011. Very few other countries conduct large detailed surveys of infants, but where these exist they provide useful comparisons for intakes in the UK. Some of the most useful resources are as follows.

- *Infant Feeding Survey* The Infant Feeding Survey has been carried out every 5 years since 1975, funded by the Department of Health. The survey is conducted through recruitment of about 10 000 mothers from birth registration records. The mothers complete a questionnaire at three time points in the first year of their child's life. Since the majority of questions in the questionnaire have been the same at each 5-year time point, trends in feeding practices over the last three decades can be examined.
- *Diet and Nutrition Survey of Infants and Young Children (DNSIYC)* The Infant Feeding Survey assesses intakes through questionnaires and it is not possible to determine energy or nutrient intakes from these. To find out this information, the Department of Health funded DNSYIC in 2011. This survey examined dietary intakes through a record of 4 days of consumption of

2683 infants aged from 4 to 18 months from around the UK, recruited through the Child Benefit Register. DNSIYC provides a detailed picture of the eating habits and nutrient intakes of the youngest of the UK population.

- *National Diet and Nutrition Survey (NDNS)* For children older than 18 months of age, the NDNS rolling programme provides detailed information about current dietary intakes, also collected using a 4-day dietary record. Until the NDNS rolling programme began in 2008, the NDNS of children aged 1.5 to 4.5 years, conducted in 1992–1993, and the NDNS survey of young people aged 4–18 years, in 1997, were the major resources for this age group and provide useful data from the past to examine changes in intake over time. Four years of results from the rolling programme (2008–2012) are currently available and the programme will continue to provide information on increasing numbers of young children as the years progress.
- *Feeding Infant and Toddlers Study (FITS)* FITS was conducted in 2002 and repeated in 2007 on about 3000 mothers of children aged 4–24 months around the USA, sampled through a commercial database. The survey used the 24-h dietary assessment method, which is that most frequently used for detailed dietary information in the USA. FITS provides nutrient intake information that is useful to compare with DNSIYC, particularly to assess the impact of different fortification practices between the two countries.
- *National Health and Nutrition Examination Survey (NHANES)* NHANES is the largest cross-sectional nutrition survey in the world, established in 1975 and now a continuous programme, studying 7000 individuals of all ages from age 2 months upwards each year across the USA, with oversampling of infants, older adults, and black and Mexican Americans to obtain adequate numbers. The dietary assessment method is two repeated 24-h recalls.

A number of European countries also conduct dietary surveys on a regular basis with inclusion of younger children, but in other countries such surveys often begin at age 6 years, leaving the youngest in the population unstudied.

All of the surveys described so far are cross-sectional and cannot be used for assessing relationships between diet in early life and later disease. For this purpose, longitudinal studies are the studies of choice. There are now longitudinal cohorts, many studied from birth onwards, which provide unique opportunities to investigate how early nutritional practices and nutrient intakes impact on later health and disease. Some of these cohorts are now long established, the oldest being the 1946 British Birth cohort or National Survey of Health and Development, where a cohort of individuals born in one week in March in 1946 have been followed throughout life and are now in the sixth decade. Other studies are more recent:

- *Millennium Cohort Study (MCS)* The MCS follows around 19 000 children born in the UK in 2000–2001. The MCS studies parenting, child behaviour and cognitive development, child and parental health, and social capital and ethnicity. In relation to nutrition, there is considerable information on breastfeeding practices, but there has been limited nutrition information included since infancy.
- *Avon Longitudinal Study of Parents and Children (ALSPAC)* ALSPAC, also known as the Children of the 90s, began in the early 1990s, when over 14 000 pregnant women in Bristol and the surrounding area, known as Avon, were recruited to take part. These women and their families have been studied since and now include the children themselves, their mothers and fathers, their grandparents and their brothers and sisters. Since the children are now in their 20s, their own children are now going to be studied. Nutrition has been a major part of ALSPAC from the beginning, with dietary information collected from the mothers when they were pregnant, and of the children using questionnaires and diet diaries at various time points up to the age of 15 years. With considerable health information about the children to the current time, ALSPAC provides a valuable resource for examining the relationship between dietary factors in infancy and young childhood and later health.

- *Southampton Women's Survey (SWS)* The SWS recruited over 3000 women in the Southampton area of Hampshire who had an infant between 1998 and 2007, having followed these through their pregnancy. The children were followed up at 6 months, 1 year, 2 and 3 years. A sample of over 1000 children was seen at 4 years of age, more than 2000 have been seen so far at 6–7 years, and more than 1000 at 8–9 years. Food intake information has been collected by food frequency questionnaires, as well as a 24-h recall at 6 months and a food diary at 3 years on about half the cohort.
- *Western Australian Pregnancy Cohort (Raine) Study* The Raine cohort was established between 1989 and 1991, when 2900 pregnant women entered the study, resulting in 2868 live births. The infants born in the study have been followed up at 1, 2, 3, 5, 8, 10, 13, 16, 18 and 20 years of age. Many researchers utilise the Raine study for their investigations of childhood and later health, in areas including asthma and atopy, cardiovascular and metabolic heath, childhood growth and development, diabetes, infection and immunity, mental health and musculoskeletal development. Dietary information was collected by food frequency questionnaires.

Figure 11.1 outlines the longitudinal study resource in the UK. The studies shown are very useful for relating

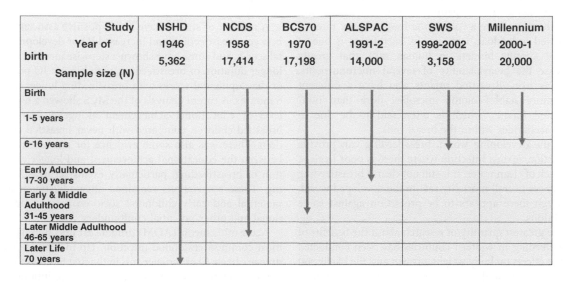

Study Year of birth Sample size (N)	NSHD 1946 5,362	NCDS 1958 17,414	BCS70 1970 17,198	ALSPAC 1991-2 14,000	SWS 1998-2002 3,158	Millennium 2000-1 20,000
Birth						
1-5 years						
6-16 years						
Early Adulthood 17-30 years						
Early & Middle Adulthood 31-45 years						
Later Middle Adulthood 46-65 years						
Later Life 70 years						

↓ **Data collection period**   NCDS = National Child Development Study   BCS = British Cohort Study

Figure 11.1 UK longitudinal studies.

early life practices to health in later life, but unfortunately many of the birth cohorts did not collect detailed dietary information. Finding out how infant diet affects later health is therefore drawn from a number of different types of studies with varying strengths. Much of the information given in this chapter is drawn from research using the studies listed in this section.

11.3 Feeding the infant: breastfeeding

Benefits of breastfeeding

Breast milk provides all the nutrients required for the infant in a form that is hygienic and easy to digest. The protein, carbohydrate and fat profiles in human breast milk are different from the milks of other species, and they also vary from woman to woman, the composition altering in response to the age and requirements of each infant. Breast milk contains a range of compounds, including antimicrobial and anti-inflammatory factors, digestive enzymes, hormones and growth factors. Antimicrobial agents in milk include leucocytes, secretory immunoglobulin antibodies, oligosaccharides, lysozyme, lactoferrin, lipids, fatty acids and mucins. Colostrum, produced during the first few days of life, is particularly high in antimicrobial factors. Growth factors such as insulin-like growth factor and epidermal growth factor are also present and are thought to be important for the maturation of the gastrointestinal tract. Leptin in breast milk may be important in the development of both adipose tissue and appetite regulatory systems, and may therefore have a role in the lower obesity rates of breastfed individuals later in life. Lactoferrin is one of several specific binders in human milk that greatly increase the bioavailability of several micronutrients, such as iron. Breastfed infants also have a different and more stable colonic microbial flora than non-breastfed infants, which is often said to be due to oligosaccharides within the breast milk.

In the developing world, breastfeeding can provide protection against infection where there is poor hygiene and lack of clean water. It is still not clear if breastfeeding influences overall mortality rate in the developed world, although there appears to be protection against some conditions.

The greatest quantity of research about the benefits of breastfeeding in western countries has been conducted on the effects on body weight, growth and the likelihood of overweight and obesity. There is now substantial evidence that rapid weight gain in infancy can result in higher body weight in later childhood, adolescence and adulthood, and it is therefore important to know if breastfeeding affects weight gain. There are now many

studies which have shown slower growth in infancy the longer breastfeeding has continued, and slower growth in infancy is now known to lead to lower weight in later years. The Raine study, for example, showed a significantly higher frequency of overweight and obesity at age 14 years when breastfeeding was stopped before 4 months of age compared with a longer period of time. In ALSPAC, breastfeeding was also associated with lower weight gain, particularly if continued for more than 6 months. From these and other studies showing similar results, the World Health Organization (WHO) has concluded that infants who are breastfed are less likely to be obese in childhood and adolescence.

Another area of interest currently is whether or not breastfeeding has an effect on cognitive development and IQ. The long-chain polyunsaturated fatty acids in breast milk, particularly eicosapentanoic acid (C20:5) and docosahexanoic acid (C22:6), are the main components of interest in relation to cognitive function. These play a role in cellular development in the maturing brain and retina and can accumulate in the brain through consumption of breast milk. The fatty acids in breast milk derive from both the mother's diet and her body stores. Results from ALSPAC have shown that higher consumption of fish, which contains these important fatty acids, in pregnancy is associated with better cognitive performance in children at 8 years of age. Another possible influence on cognitive development that has been gaining interest is iodine, which is also present in fish. Iodine status of pregnant women has also been found to be related to the cognitive status of children at age 8 years in ALSPAC.

A number of studies have found positive associations between breastfeeding and increased IQ or developmental scores, and some have shown a stepwise increase with longer duration of breastfeeding, with highest IQ points or developmental scores with breastfeeding longer than 6 months. A recent analysis of the MCS showed a higher level of educational achievement at age 5 years in breastfed children compared with never breastfed children. There was also some evidence for an association between the educational achievement and longer duration of breastfeeding, particularly exclusive breastfeeding. These associations remained after adjustment for maternal and early childhood socio-economic, educational and other potential confounders.

Acute otitis media (AOM) (middle ear infection) is the most common childhood infection. Up to 75% of children are likely to experience this in the first 5 years of life, and it is the major reason for antibiotic prescriptions for young children, presenting a substantial medical and economic burden. Young children are prone to AOM because the Eustachian tube is shorter, more flexible and horizontal than in older children and adults, allowing pathogens from the nose and throat to enter the middle ear relatively easily. In children who experience repeated attacks of AOM, the Eustachian tube has been shown to be particularly short. There is now convincing evidence that breastfeeding protects infants against AOM, possibly because the pressure gradients of suck and swallow are distinct from those of bottle feeding, providing for aeration of the Eustachian tube during feeding.

There is also good evidence that breastfeeding protects against gastrointestinal and respiratory tract infections. This is thought to be due to the presence of secretory immunoglobulin A antibodies, which contribute to an anti-inflammatory response, or protective factors like lactoferrin and oligosaccharides, which attach to microbial receptors to prevent microbes from attaching to the gastrointestinal mucosa, or the transfer of cytokines and growth factors from breast milk may help stimulate the infant's immune system. A combination of all these factors may play a part in the protection conferred by breastfeeding.

For other conditions and diseases, the protective effect of breastfeeding is less well established or results are conflicting. For example, evidence from various studies has indicated no demonstrable benefit of breastfeeding on blood pressure in childhood, but a small but significant reduction in blood pressure in later life. Similarly, infants who were breastfed appear to have slightly lower total serum cholesterol concentrations in adult life. There is evidence for breastfeeding having a protective effect against type 1 and type 2 diabetes mellitus, although it is unclear whether the positive effects seen for breastfeeding depend on the breast milk itself or avoidance of other foods given to infants, or other factors such as lower prevalence of infections in the breastfed child. In relation to cancer, there is some evidence for a reduced risk of childhood leukaemia and possibly other childhood cancers with breastfeeding, but there is still too little solid research to judge associations between breastfeeding and cancers in adulthood. There is also very little evidence that breastfeeding is related to allergies, asthma and wheeze. Future longitudinal studies may clarify the role of breastfeeding in these conditions.

There is some evidence that breastfeeding is protective against coeliac disease, if gluten is introduced in small amounts while still breastfeeding. There is also evidence that breastfeeding provides protection against inflammatory bowel disease. For both these conditions, well-performed prospective studies with reliable, well-defined breastfeeding data are still needed.

Recommendations for breastfeeding

The positive benefits shown between breastfeeding and its effects on body weight, cognitive function, infection and a number of common conditions have led to the development of recommendations for the public, both by individual countries and by international organisations. Recommendations relate to any breastfeeding and also exclusive breastfeeding, which means that no other liquids or foods are consumed, except for water. Prior to 1991, the global recommendation by the WHO was that infants should be exclusively breastfed for between 4 and 6 months before the introduction of complementary foods. In 2001, an Expert Consultation met to discuss the scientific evidence to that date, which was mainly drawn from observational studies. The evidence suggested that exclusive breast feeding for 6 months had protective effects, particularly against gastrointestinal infection, and hence the WHO recommended exclusive breastfeeding up to this age, with complementary feeding and continued breastfeeding from then on. The UK adopted this recommendation, as have most western countries, although there continue to be debates about the appropriateness of the recommendation for developed countries, with concerns about the ability of exclusive breastfeeding to meet the energy needs of many infants at 6 months of age. In the USA there is a statement within the recommendation about individualising the feeding of those 4–6 months depending on the dietary requirement and feeding patterns of the infant.

Current practice in breastfeeding

Figure 11.2 shows the rates of breastfeeding in four UK birth cohorts, those with births in 1946, 1958, 1970 and 2000–2001, and demonstrates the changes in proportions of infants who were breastfed at various times during the 20th century. The increasing proportion who were never breastfed, from 24–25% in 1946 to 30–31% in 1958 to 62% in 1970 reflects the attitudes to breastfeeding at the various times; studies from the 1930s to the 1950s suggested that there were few differences in growth or health between breastfed and bottle-fed infants, and this view persisted until the 1970s, when the health benefits of breastfeeding began to be recognised, initially in relation to infectious disease, but later in relation to obesity and other conditions. The post-war declines were also partly due to increased proportions of mothers returning to work in the first year after giving birth.

With active promotion of breastfeeding, rates have increased in most developed countries, and the results from the MCS, with only 30% never trying, indicate this awareness in the UK. Results from the Infant Feeding Surveys show the rates over time in the UK for those breastfeeding initially, from 62% in 1990 to 81% in 2010 (Figure 11.3). The survey examined a number of factors which influence breastfeeding rates, such as age and education of the mother. As shown in Figure 11.4 for

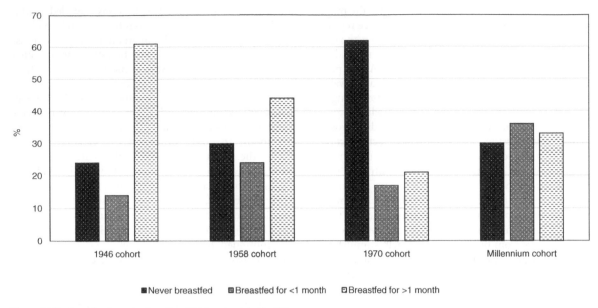

Figure 11.2 Breastfeeding rates in national birth cohorts in the UK.

the 2010 survey, age and country within the UK have marked influences on the rates, with older mothers more likely to breastfeed than younger mothers, and those in England more likely to start breastfeeding than in Wales, Scotland and Northern Ireland. For women under 20 years of age, 61% start breastfeeding in England, while in Northern Ireland, this figure is only 34% and in Scotland

39%. Mothers from Asian, Black and Chinese or other ethnic groups were more likely to breastfeed initially than white mothers.

Although breastfeeding rates have increased, which is a positive development, the proportion of mothers who continue to breastfeed for several months remains low. Some countries, such as Sweden, Norway and Finland,

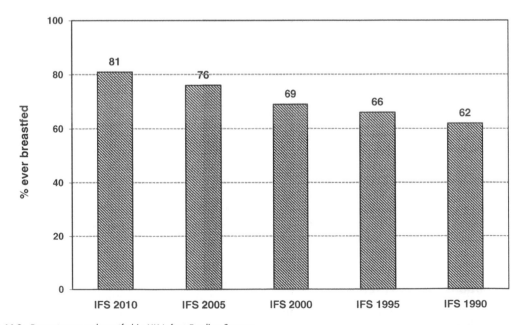

Figure 11.3 Percentage ever breastfed in UK Infant Feeding Surveys.

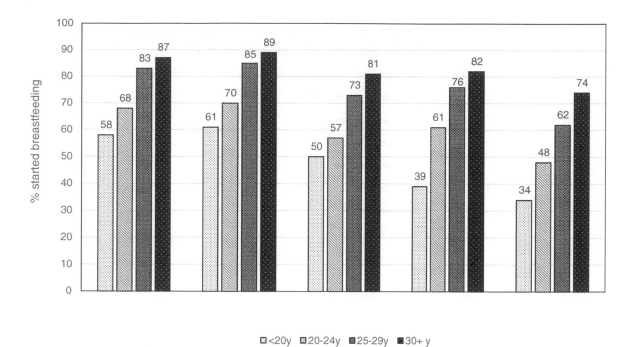

Figure 11.4 Incidence of breastfeeding in the UK by age and country for the Infant Feeding Survey 2010.

have much higher rates of continuing than others, such as Italy, Netherlands and the UK. In DNSIYC, the proportion continuing beyond 3 months was only about 40%. In the 2010 Infant Feeding Survey, the prevalence of breastfeeding fell from 81% at birth to 69% at 1 week, and to 55% at 6 weeks. At 6 months, only 34% of mothers were still breastfeeding, and just 1% exclusively.

Reasons for not breastfeeding

Why do some mothers breastfeed and others not? Pregnant women who intended to breastfeed in the 2010 Infant Feeding Survey were asked their reasons. A total of 83% of mothers believed that breastfeeding was best for the child's health. Other reasons included: convenience (22%), health benefits for the mother (17%), closer bond between mother and baby (16%), breastfeeding was free, or cheaper than infant formula (15%), breastfed previously (12%), breastfeeding was natural (11%) and expectation that weight loss would be easier (6%).

Those who did not want to breastfeed said that they did not like the idea of breastfeeding (20%); bottle feeding meant other people could feed the baby (17%); fed earlier children with infant formula (21%); more convenient/due to mother's lifestyle (19%), breastfeeding previous children had not been successful (11%); medical reasons (10%); embarrassed to breastfeed (10%);

domestic reasons, coping with other children (3%); allowed them to see how much the baby had consumed (5%); expected to return to work soon (1%); feeding with infant formula was less tiring (1%).

Reasons for stopping breastfeeding are shown in Figure 11.5 for the 2010 Infant Feeding Survey. It can be seen that the most common reason for stopping is the perception of insufficient milk, and this remains the main reason that exclusive breastfeeding to 6 months is not followed: that the infant is not receiving enough.

Promoting breastfeeding

Debates about the appropriateness of the 6 months exclusive breastfeeding recommendations have tended to overshadow efforts and recommendations to promote breastfeeding in western countries. However, since the 1990s there have been considerable efforts to encourage mothers to breastfeed their infants in most countries. In 1990, the WHO and the United Nations Children's Fund (UNICEF) developed the Declaration on the Protection, Promotion and Support of Breastfeeding, which was signed by over 30 countries. This had four operational targets for each country, to:

- appoint a breastfeeding coordinator and establish a multisector breastfeeding committee;

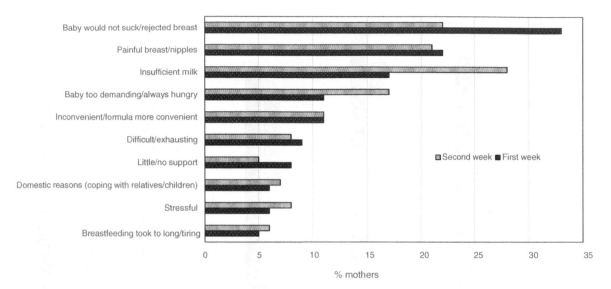

Figure 11.5 Reasons for stopping breastfeeding in the Infant Feeding Survey 2010.

- practise 10 steps to successful breastfeeding in maternity facilities;
- put into effect the International Code of Marketing of Breast Milk Substitutes;
- enact legislation to protect the breastfeeding rights of working women.

UNICEF and the WHO also launched the Baby Friendly initiative, to ensure facilities providing care to new mothers would support breastfeeding. Over 10 000 centres have now earned the Baby Friendly award. An investigation from the MCS found that mothers who had their babies in Baby-Friendly-accredited maternity units were more likely to start breastfeeding than those delivering in other units but were not more likely to still be breastfeeding at 1 month. This suggests that while high initiation rates can be maintained, other efforts are needed to encourage mothers to continue breastfeeding when they leave hospital.

11.4 Feeding the infant: infant formula

For those who chose not to breastfeed or cannot breastfeed, infant formula is the recommended mode of feeding infants until the age of 1 year. Increased knowledge and understanding of the composition and molecular structure of breast milk has led to improvements in the composition of formula to make it as similar to breast milk as possible. The protein, fat and carbohydrate content of formula milks are similar to breast milk, and the position of the various fatty acids on the triglycerides have also been matched to their position in the fats of breast milk. In recent years, infant formulas have

also been fortified with prebiotics, which has resulted in the gut microflora of formula-fed infants being more similar to those of breastfed infants. With new technologies, changes to formula are likely to continue to make it as close to breast milk as possible.

Most milks available in the UK are based on cows' milk and can be either 'whey based' or 'casein based'. Whey-based milks are the preferred alternative to breast milk because the protein is adjusted so that the casein to whey ratio is similar to breast milk (40:60) and also have a lower mineral content (in particular, sodium and potassium), which is important for the newborn, who have immature kidneys. Soy-based formulas are also available; although not commonly used, they are the only choice available for those seeking non-animal sources of protein, and are the only vegan option.

In the UK, nearly all infants are given infant formula at some point in the first year of life. The Infant Feeding Survey indicated that 75% of infants were receiving formula at 2 months of age; at 9 months this was 95%. After 1 year, use of formula diminishes rapidly as cows' milk is given instead. In DNSIYC, only 38% of infants 12–18 months had formula.

11.5 Feeding the infant: complementary foods

Timing of introduction of complementary food

In the developing world, the infant traditionally moved abruptly from exclusive breastfeeding to family foods, often when the next child arrived. In many societies, this pattern still holds, although many countries have moved to patterns closer to those of the developed world, where the infant has an elongated period of mixed feeding, passing by degrees from a diet largely of breast milk to one eventually without breast milk. The age at which solid food should be introduced to the infant has changed dramatically in the last 100 years. In past times, solid food might be introduced in the second or third month of life. Up until 2003, the age recommended was from 4 to 6 months, but following the advice from the WHO about exclusive breastfeeding until 6 months, from 2003, the UK Department of Health has recommended that complementary feeding should start at around 6 months. Breastfeeding and/or formula should continue beyond the first 6 months, supplemented with appropriate types and amounts of solid foods. Solid foods should be tried when a baby can sit up, wants to chew and is putting toys and other objects in its mouth, and reaches and grabs accurately. In industrialised countries, the WHO advises that the additional energy the infants need from complementary foods is approximately 130 kcal/day at 6–8 months of age, 310 kcal/day at 9–11 months, and 580 kcal/day at 12–23 months.

In spite of the recommendation to breastfeed exclusively until 6 months or beyond, virtually all mothers in the UK report introducing other foods before 6 months, often because they consider their babies to be hungry and not satisfied on breast milk alone. Mother's age was a factor, with only 19% of mothers aged 35 or over having introduced solids by 4 months, while 57% of infants of teenage mothers had been given them. By 5 months, only 5% of infants of teenage mothers had yet to receive solids. In spite of the advice to exclusively breastfeed until 6 months of age, the reality is that most infants are introduced to solid food before this age, and it is therefore important that parents have access to sound advice on introduction of complementary foods should they decide to commence earlier than 6 months.

Providing solid foods

The introduction of solid foods has to be in the context of neuromuscular development and the infant's willingness to try new tastes and textures. Young infants have poor head control, and before about 3 months it is difficult to hold a baby in a position that allows them to swallow semisolid food. Newborn babies suck at food, and before 3 months a baby cannot easily form a bolus of food in the mouth and move the bolus from the front to the back of the mouth. They are not eager to experiment with foods of different flavour, texture or consistency at this age. By 4 months most babies can maintain posture if supported, by 5 months they can usually move soft puréed food from

the front of the mouth and swallow it, and by 6 months they are able to chew. There may be critical developmental stages when these skills are learned, and teaching older infants to chew can be difficult if the opportunity is missed. There are also critical periods for exposure to different textures during weaning.

The Department of Health advice is that a gradual transition is made from spoon-fed puréed foods and baby rice to foods prepared with a coarser texture, finger foods and eventually consumption of family foods by 12 months of age. Feeding difficulties later in life have been associated with a delay in the introduction of food that contains lumps. This has been studied in ALSPAC, where it was found that children at 15 months were more likely to reject lumpy solids and chewy foods when these were introduced at or after 10 months of age, compared with being given lumpy foods at 8 or 9 months. These feeding problems were also present at age 7 years.

The introduction of solid foods should therefore begin around 6 months of age, not later, because the gradual changes are important in helping the baby learn to accept different tastes and textures, and to learn to move food around the mouth and to chew. As the introduction of solids progresses, the foods provided should gradually be increased in amount and variety so that, by 12 months, solid foods are the main part of the diet, with breast or formula milk making up the balance.

Baby-led weaning

In recent years, a new approach to complementary food introduction, known as baby-led weaning, has been growing in popularity in the UK and other countries. The baby-led weaning approach is one where the usual practice of spoon-feeding puréed foods or baby rice is bypassed in favour of introducing foods in their whole form as finger foods rather than puréed, and where infants self-feed as opposed to being spoon-fed by adults, with reliance on breast milk until the infant has the skills to take in enough energy.

A recent cross-sectional study of 655 mothers in the Swansea area in Wales found that baby-led weaning was associated with a later introduction of complementary foods, a higher number of milk feeds, increased participation in family mealtimes and fewer maternal concerns about the weaning process. Mothers found the approach to be a natural and enjoyable way to introduce complementary food to their infants, convenient and fitting well into family mealtimes. There were some concerns about choking, and with mess and waste. The success of baby-led weaning depends on the ability of the infant to reach out, pick up and hold food, and put it into the mouth, and many infants can do this by the age of 6 months and most by 8 months. A pragmatic approach to weaning seems the most sensible advice, with the weaning method based on the child's development. Baby-led weaning may be feasible for the majority of infants but might lead to problems for more delayed infants. There is currently insufficient research on the outcomes of baby-led weaning compared with standard weaning methods, although studies to date suggest that baby-led infants are more likely to be underweight and spoon-fed more likely to be overweight. There is currently a large randomised trial in progress in New Zealand which may provide more definitive conclusions about the benefits and drawbacks of the baby-led approach.

Complementary foods: what to feed

In the UK, current advice is that whole cows' milk is not appropriate as the main drink for infants less than 1 year of age, although it can be used in foods prepared for babies over 6 months of age. Cows' milk does not contain enough iron and other nutrients to be the main drink for infants in the first year. After the age of 1 year, formula or follow-on milk can be replaced with cows' milk or mothers can continue to breastfeed. Once the introduction of solids is under way, whole milk and full-fat dairy products are advised until the child is 2 years old; semi-skimmed milk can be introduced once the child is 2 years old. Milks other than cow's milk, such as goats' and sheep's milks, should be avoided until the child is 1 year old, because, like cows' milk, they do not provide enough iron and other nutrients that the infant needs. Goats' and sheep's milk should always be pasteurised. In DNSIYC, 36% of infants over 12 months were given cows' milk as their most common drink, while the percentage below 12 months was very low, indicating compliance with the recommendation regarding cows' milk.

For other beverages, fruit juice, squashes and soft drinks should be limited and, if provided, should be artificially sweetened. Tea and coffee should also be avoided, since they contain caffeine and may reduce iron absorption.

Nutrients of concern

Long-chain fatty acids
There are a number of key nutrients that should be included in the infant diet in adequate amounts through the appropriate choice of foods. The long-chain fatty acids eicosapentaenoic acid and docosahexaenoic acid, present in fish, are important for development of the brain and other neural tissue like the retina. Inclusion of fish in the infant diet twice a week should supply an adequate amount.

Iron
Iron can be lacking in the infant diet, particularly in breastfed infants since it is low in breast milk. Lack of iron can lead to anaemia, which can delay both physical and mental development. Dietary iron is found in two forms, as haem, as in meat and fish, which is easily absorbed by the body, and non-haem iron, as found in plant foods, such as grains and vegetables, from which it is absorbed much less well. Since very young children do not eat very much meat, having adequate iron can be a problem. It is for this reason that iron is added to infant cereals and some other infant foods in some countries, although this is not the case in the UK. It is felt that the form of the iron in the fortified foods is not readily available and the added iron would make little difference to iron status. A small amount of meat or fish in the child's diet is therefore advised, as are foods or drinks that are rich in vitamin C at mealtimes, as vitamin C aids the absorption of non-haem iron from non-meat sources.

With the detailed dietary information in DNSIYC, it is possible to examine sources of iron and compare these with countries where iron is added to infant foods. Figure 11.6a shows the iron intakes of the children in DNSIYC subdivided by age (4–6, 7–9, 10–11, 12–18 months) and, the percentage of children with intakes below the lower reference nutrient intake (LRNI) for each age group are shown in Figure 11.6b. Average intake was about 6–7 mg/day, and 10–14% of children had intakes below the lowest recommended intake. These intakes compare with those in the USA as found in NHANES and FITS of about 16 mg/day. These results can be subdivided by socio-economic position and ethnic group, as shown in Figure 11.7. In those over 1 year of age, the percentage with intakes below the LRNI rose to 23% for the lowest socioeconomic group and 28% of those of South Asian origin, indicating that the problem is greater in some specific groups in the UK. In those less than 1 year of age, the major sources of iron in DNSIYC were infant formula (42–56%), commercial infant foods (16–21%) and cereal products (5% for 4–6 months, rising to 21% for 10–11 months). For those over 12 months, the main sources were cereal products (41%), infant formula (17%), vegetables and potatoes (10%), commercial infant foods (9%) and meat (9%).

Iron status was also measured in DNSIYC and is shown in Figure 11.8. The percentages of children with iron status markers (ferritin, transferrin receptors or haemoglobin) below the cut-off for deficiency were as high as 15% for those over 1 year of age. To classify as iron-deficiency anaemia, all the status markers must be below the cut-off. The percentage of children with anaemia was 2–3% in DNSIYC.

Zinc
Zinc is important for making new cells and enzymes, healing wounds and helping the body to process carbohydrate, fat and protein from food. Like iron, zinc is in

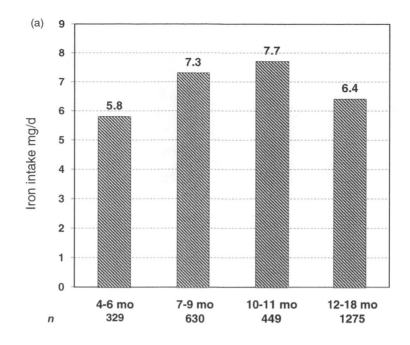

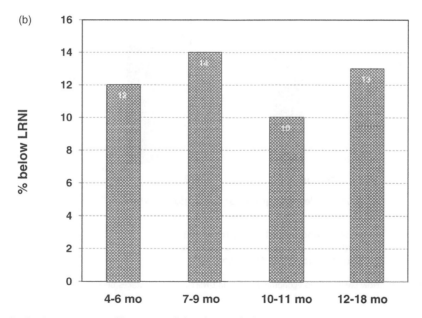

Figure 11.6 (a) Iron intakes in DNSIYC 2011. (b) Percentage below the LRNI for iron in DNSIYC 2011.

low amounts in breast milk, and infants therefore depend on complementary foods to meet their needs. Although zinc can be low, results from DNSIYC indicate that it is not such a problem as iron in terms of intakes, since only 3–5% of children were below the LNRI for zinc.

Vitamin D

Vitamin D is important for laying down of bone during development of the skeleton; low vitamin D status can lead to rickets, resulting in bending of the bones, particularly of the legs, a condition that remains for life (see

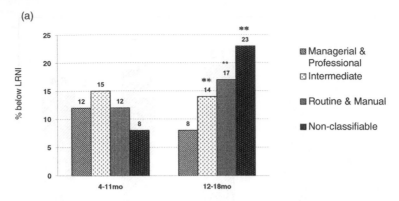

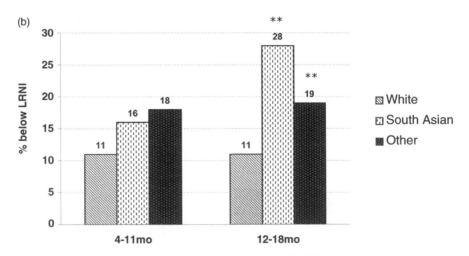

Figure 11.7 (a) Iron intakes below LRNI by socio-economic position in DNSIYC. (b) Iron intakes below LRNI by ethnic group in DNSIYC.

Chapter 20). Long thought to be a disease of Victorian times, rickets began to reappear in the UK in the 1970s, particularly among those of Asian background. A recent survey in one hospital in Glasgow recorded 160 cases between 2002 and 2008, all but three of these being in children of South Asian, Middle Eastern or sub-Saharan ethnic background.

Vitamin D is obtained both from foods and from the action of sunlight on the skin. Breast milk contains little vitamin D, and in food it is naturally present in only a few foods, such as oily fish. Since fish is consumed infrequently by young children, supplements of vitamin D are recommended in the UK, especially since its latitude means very little exposure to ultraviolet light for many months of the year. Vitamin drops are recommended starting at 1 month and continuing until 5 years of age. These can be purchased or are provided free of charge for those on low income and eligible for 'Healthy Start'

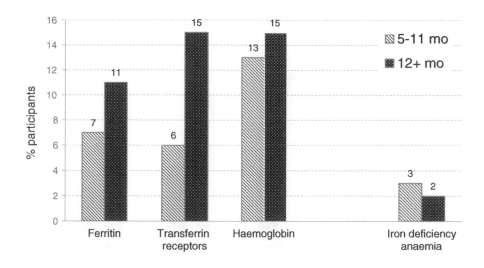

n 5-11 mo= 171, 12+ mo 325

Figure 11.8 Percentage below cut-offs for iron status measures in DNSIYC 2011.

vouchers. Healthy Start vitamin drops contain vitamin A, vitamin C and vitamin D. In DNSIYC, the proportion of infants given vitamin-containing supplements in the previous year was only 4% for those aged 4–6 months, 11% for 7–11 months and 13% for those over 12 months, indicating very little compliance with the current recommendation.

Because of concerns about vitamin D adequacy, this nutrient was studied in detail in DNSIYC. Intakes are shown in Figure 11.9 for breastfed and non-breastfed infants. The difference can clearly be seen and is a result of the addition of vitamin D to infant formula. Once formula is no longer being consumed, vitamin D intakes drop to less than 3 μg/day. For those over 12 months, the average intakes of under 3 μg/day can be compared with those from FITS in the USA, where average intake for those aged 12–24 months was about 6 μg/day. Over 80% of this came from cows' milk, to which vitamin D is added in the USA, as it is in other countries like Canada and Finland. A recent Scientific Committee of Nutrition (SACN) report proposes a 'safe intake' of vitamin D of 8.5 μg/day up to the age of 6 months and 10 μg/day over 6 months. These recommendations are for both formula-fed and breastfed infants and, based on available information, are considered to cover the needs of ethnic groups in the UK.

Vitamin D status was measured in DNSIYC. There is considerable debate about the appropriate cut-off for adequacy – that level in the blood which would mean an

increased risk of poor musculoskeletal health, which in the case of young children means increased risk of rickets. In the UK, 25 nmol/L of 25-hydroxyvitamin D (25(OH)D) is used, whereas in other countries, such as the USA and Germany, 50 nmol/L is the cut-off for a sufficient intake. In DNSIYC, 6% of infants aged 5–11 months had serum 25(OH)D below 25 nmol/L, while 2% of those over 12 months were below this cut-off. For 50 nmol/L, 16% of infants 5–11 months were below this concentration, while the percentage for those over 12 months was 29%. For those 5–11 months, all the infants below the 25 nmol/L cut-off were breastfed. Blood samples were taken in DNSIYC from February to August. In other studies in the UK on other age groups where samples have been taken over the entire year, adequate 25(OH)D concentrations are seen for the summer months, with the higher percentages of low concentrations for samples taken in the winter.

Complementary feeding: first foods

The first foods traditionally given to infants vary from country to country, even within Europe. In 11 participating countries in a study examining this, called the Euro-Growth study, fruit (73%) and cereals (51%) were the first foods given to most infants. In the All Babies in Southwest Sweden study of over 10 000 infants, the most common first foods were vegetables, specifically potatoes, carrots and sweetcorn or products containing these.

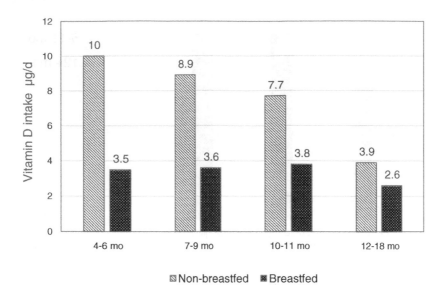

- Vitamin D intakes from all sources except breast milk
- Breastfeeding status denoted by the inclusion of breast milk in the diet diary
- Exclusively breastfed *n*=2.

Figure 11.9 Vitamin D intakes by age: breastfed and non-breastfed infants in DNSIYC.

Most of the infants in a study from Bavaria in Germany received a mash of vegetable, meat and potato as their first solid food.

There are few studies from the UK which report the first type of food introduced. In the Glasgow Longitudinal Infant Growth Study, commercially prepared cereals were the most commonly used first weaning foods, used by 82% of mothers, the most common type being baby rice. In the 2010 Infant Feeding Survey the most common foods given to infants aged 4–6 months were fruit or vegetables, usually as purées (66%), which were as likely to be commercially prepared as homemade. By 8–10 months, mothers used commercial brands less often and offered home-prepared foods more often.

DNSIYC provides detailed information about the food and nutrient intakes of infants and young children in the UK. The major sources of energy, protein, fat, non-milk extrinsic sugars (NMES), vitamin D and iron for children over 12 months of age are listed in Table 11.1. For infants in the first year of life, intake was dominated by breast or formula milk, with small contributions from other food groups, such as commercial infant products, mainly cereal or meat based, as well as non-infant-specific groups like cereal products, milk and milk products, fruit and vegetables, amounts increasing with increasing age. After 1 year, the diet was more similar to that of the other members of the family but still dominated by cereal products and milk and milk products.

In establishing a healthy diet in young children, it is important to introduce new tastes and textures at the appropriate periods, and there is evidence of a 'window' from about 5 to 7 months when infants are most receptive to new flavours. One of the areas of emphasis is to encourage consumption of fruit and vegetables. Total consumption of fruit and vegetables in DNSIYC is shown in Figure 11.10a. This includes all fruit and vegetables in mixed dishes as well as on their own. These intakes are substantial and are similar to those of older children and teenagers seen in NDNS. Figure 11.10b shows that the proportion of infants consuming both fruit and vegetables increases with age such that after the age of 1 year over 90% of children consumed both some fruit and some vegetables in the 4-day period of the diet record in DNSIYC. These are increases over an earlier survey conducted in 1986–1987 and indicates awareness by the public of the advice to consume more fruit and vegetables. However, consumption was higher in those of higher socio-economic status and by white children compared with those of other ethnic groups, indicating the need for more targeted efforts to increase consumption.

Table 11.1 Contribution of various food groups to intakes of energy, protein, fat, NMES, vitamin D and iron in children aged 12–18 months in DNSIYC.

Food group	Contribution (%)					
	Energy	Protein	Fat	NMES	Vitamin D	Iron
Non-infant-specific foods						
Cereals and cereal products	24	18	12	23	7	41
Milk and milk products	27	35	37	27	16	2
Eggs and egg dishes	1	2	3	0	7	2
Fat spreads	2	0	7	0	11	0
Meat and meat products and dishes	8	17	10	1	13	9
Fish and fish dishes	2	4	2	0	5	2
Vegetables, potatoes	7	6	4	3	1	10
Fruit	6	2	1	7	0	5
Sugar, preserves and confectionery	2	1	2	12	0	1
Beverages	1	0	0	10	0	1
Infant-specific foods						
Infant formula	10	7	12	2	29	17
Breast milk	2	1	3	0	n.a.	1
Commercial infant foods	6	5	4	11	9	9

In terms of nutrients, DNSIYC showed that infants and young children in the UK are largely meeting recommendations, apart from a number of specific nutrients, such as iron and vitamin D. They are consuming sufficient energy with substantial proportions above the recommendation for energy for age and sex, and adequate protein is being consumed by the majority. The proportions of macronutrients change as the children mature and begin to move away from a purely milk-based diet to include more complementary foods. The percentage energy for protein increased from about 10% of energy at 4–6 months to nearer 16% after 1 year, while fat decreased from about 40% energy at 4–6 months to 35% after 1 year of age. The type of carbohydrate changed, with lower intakes of milk sugars and higher intakes of starch and NMES. NMES intakes increased steadily with age to be about 8% of energy after 1 year.

Avoiding certain foods

Advice is given about specific foods or ingredients that should be avoided in the diets of infants and young children. Salt should not be added to food, and high-salt foods, such as cheese, bacon and sausages, should be limited. Sugar should be added to food sparingly and only when necessary, while whole and chopped nuts should be avoided because of fear of choking. Eggs should only be given after the age of 6 months to safeguard against allergic responses and should be well cooked when given to older infants.

Allergy has been defined as 'an adverse health effect arising from a specific immune response that occurs reproducibly on exposure to a given food'. The food component causing the response is termed an allergen, and is usually a water-soluble protein of molecular weight between 5 and 50 kDa present in specific foods to which the body reacts. Normally when food is eaten, the gastrointestinal tract blocks allergens from entering the body. In young infants, however, many of the immunological and mechanical barriers involved in this blocking are immature, allowing allergens to enter the bloodstream. In most infants, the immune system develops a tolerance to the allergens and there are no symptoms. However, in some infants there is a failure to develop tolerance and an excessive production of immunoglobulin E (IgE) antibodies occurs, a process known as sensitisation. When the food containing the allergen is next eaten and the allergen reaches these IgE antibodies, which are bound to mast cells, a number of chemicals, including histamine, are released, leading to symptoms, mainly affecting the skin, nose, lungs and/or the heart and circulation.

The mechanisms of developing tolerance are still not fully understood, but the timing of the introduction of foods may be important for normal tolerance development. There may be critical windows of time when the presence of an allergen can induce tolerance rather than induce an adverse response. It is also unclear why most childhood allergies, such as milk and egg allergy, disappear after 12–24 months while others, such as peanut allergy, are usually present for life. The commonest

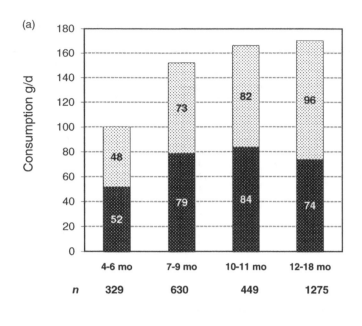

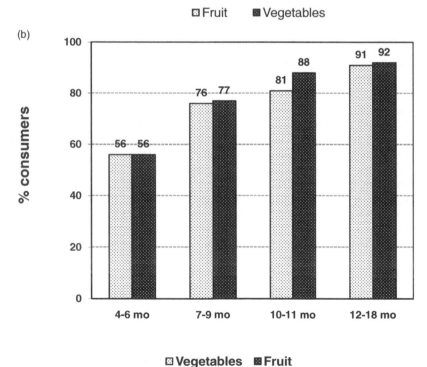

Figure 11.10   (a) Fruit and vegetable consumption in the DNSIYC. (b) Percentage consumers of fruit and vegetables in the DNSIYC.

allergies are to cows' milk protein, egg, soya, wheat, nuts and shellfish. Diagnosis is based on history, skin-prick testing, the measurement of food-specific IgE antibodies, patch tests and food challenge testing.

Peanut allergy

Children with allergic reactions to peanuts become sensitised to peanuts early in life, perhaps through breastfeeding, via skin lesions or via the respiratory system following exposure to peanut allergen in their immediate environment. Factors that can predispose an individual to peanut allergy include family and personal history, age and dietary exposure at a vulnerable stage. Children with asthma seem to be at increased risk of developing severe food allergy reactions. In the past, advice has been to avoid exposure of infants to peanuts too early, but this has recently changed with the results of a study called Learning Early About Peanut Allergy, which tested the introduction of peanut products, including peanut butter and foods with peanut flour, for 5 years to infants with previous allergic symptoms (high risk) aged 4–11 months at the outset. Infants who had these early introductions had a much reduced risk of peanut allergy compared with those who avoided peanuts. Early exposure to peanuts is therefore recommended for such infants.

Gluten sensitivity and coeliac disease
Coeliac disease is a permanent autoimmune condition, triggered in susceptible individuals by the presence in the diet of gluten, derived from wheat, rye or barley. Results from a mass screening project carried out in Finland, Germany, Italy and the UK showed that around 1% of the general population are affected by this disorder, most being asymptomatic or having mild signs and symptoms. Recent evidence suggests that the timing of the introduction of gluten to the diet and the pattern of breastfeeding may play a role in the development of coeliac disease in susceptible individuals. A systematic review found that longer duration of breastfeeding, and breastfeeding at the time of introduction of gluten-containing foods, protected against the development of coeliac disease. Another contributory factor may be the amount of gluten introduced. The European Society for Paediatric Gastroenterology, Hepatology and Nutrition recommends avoidance of both early (less than 4 months) and late (greater than 7 months) introduction of gluten and that small amounts should be introduced while the child is still being breastfed. This timing has been agreed by the European Food Safety Authority, but to date has not been approved in the UK since it is inconsistent with the recommendation to exclusively breastfeed until 6 months of age. In a statement, the Committee on Toxicology and SACN concluded that the currently available evidence is insufficient to change the recommendation about the introduction of gluten into the infant diet. The topic remains under discussion.

Current practice in food avoidance
In DNSIYC, 83% of parents said they never added salt to their child's food, although this proportion was lower for those over 1 year than under, with 8% of parents of children over 1 year indicating that they often added salt and 17% sometimes. Of foods parents avoided giving

their children, the most common were nuts (40%), meat, poultry, fish, seafood and offal (33%), spicy foods (27%), sweets/chocolate (24%), eggs and dairy (22%) and processed foods (21%). Of those not giving these foods, the major reason for not giving nuts was fear of choking (54%) and allergic/adverse reaction (42%), for avoiding meat, poultry and fish it was that it was not cooked in the household (49%), and for not giving sweets and chocolate it was health reasons (73%).

11.6 Feeding the child over the age of 18 months

Childhood diet and later health
Unlike the wealth of research about the effects of breastfeeding and the timing of the introduction of solid foods on later health, there is much less information on the effects on health of the composition of the diet of children once they move to family foods. This is largely because there are few cohorts which have collected dietary intake data in enough detail to be able to investigate the variations in diet among populations sufficiently and to then have disease prevalence in later childhood or adulthood to enable such relationships to be explored.

Traditional nutrition has examined the relationship between specific nutrients and later health outcomes, but in recent years there has been a move to examine the diet as a whole, using 'dietary patterns', combinations of foods that exist together in foods. Various methods are used to capture the variety of foods in an overall pattern of consumption, and within each pattern there are a number of foods that stand out as characterising that pattern. One of the first studies to examine dietary patterns in relation to health outcomes in childhood used a group of 241 children from the SWS whose diet had been assessed at 6 and 12 months and who were then followed through childhood. Cognitive tests were performed at age 4 years. A pattern characterised by consumption of fruit, vegetables and home-prepared foods at 6 and 12 months was found to be associated with higher verbal IQ and better memory at age 4 years than other types of diets.

In ALSPAC, diet from an early age has also been found to be associated with cognitive function, based on appropriate tests for each age studied. Higher scores of a dietary pattern characterised by biscuits, chocolate, sweets, soft drinks and crisps at ages 6, 15 and 24 months were associated with a lower IQ at age 8 years, while a pattern characterised by legumes, cheese, raw fruit and vegetables was associated with a higher IQ.

The Raine study has also examined early diet and later cognitive function. Developing an 'eating assessment in toddlers' score for diet quality from the 24-h recalls collected, they showed that higher diet quality at 1 year was associated with better cognitive function at 10 years and at 17 years of age. At age 10 years, increased fruit consumption was independently associated with higher cognitive scores, while higher soft drink consumption was associated with lower scores. Dairy consumption at ages 2 and 3 years was also associated with better cognitive scores at 10 years of age.

Early diet has also been examined in relation to weight gain in ALSPAC and the SWS. In ALSPAC, energy density of the diet has shown some relationship with later weight gain, but this was not seen at each age investigated. No relationship between soft drink consumption and later weight gain has been found, nor with milk or dairy foods overall. Dietary pattern analysis at age 7, 10 and 13 years has shown that high scores on an 'energy-dense, high-fat, low-fibre' diet is associated with increasing adiposity between 11 and 15 years of age. Such a dietary pattern is one low in fruits and vegetables and high in white bread, cakes/biscuits, confectionery and crisps and is one associated with poorer nutrient intake.

In the SWS, a diet quality index was developed, based on consumption of key foods, including fruits, vegetables and fish, and was calculated for dietary intakes at ages 6 months, 12 months, 3 years and 6 years. A consistently low score on the index, representing low consumption of these foods and hence poor diet quality at each age, was associated with a higher fat mass score at 6 years of age.

'Picky' or fussy eating, generally defined as an unwillingness to eat unfamiliar foods or try new foods, is beginning to be explored in longitudinal studies. In ALSPAC, the prevalence of picky eating has been found to be about 10–15%, with a peak prevalence at 38 months of age. Picky eaters generally have a diet with lower intakes of fruit and vegetables than non-picky eaters. The impact of picky eating on body weight in children can vary, with some studies showing lower body weight and height in such children, while others suggest a greater risk of overweight, since those rejecting foods like fruit and vegetables tend to have lower diet quality. The specific behaviours and the extent of pickiness may impact the effect of such dietary habits on health. By measuring pickiness at various ages, the ALSPAC study has shown that pickiness persists from early life (24 months) to later childhood (11 years).

The results from the largest cohorts in the UK with longitudinal diet and health data indicate that instituting good dietary habits at the time of complementary feeding and maintaining these patterns throughout childhood are important for later health and development.

Food consumption of children in the UK

The NDNS provides the most comprehensive information about food consumption and nutrient intakes of children in the UK. Since 2008, the NDNS has been a rolling programme, assessing the dietary intakes of the population from the age of 18 months and over on a continuing basis. The data from the first 4 years of the rolling programme from 2008 to 2012 were published in 2014.

Table 11.2 indicates the contribution of the major food groups to intakes of energy, protein, fat, NMES, vitamin D and iron in children aged 1.5–3 and 4–10 years. The importance of cereal products and milk and milk products in the diets of children can be seen, and the changing pattern from the toddler years to school age, with less emphasis on milk and milk products and moves to greater importance of meat and meat products in providing major nutrients. For fat and vitamin D, fat spreads are major sources, although these contribute little to other major nutrients. Vegetables and potatoes are major sources of iron, this being mainly derived from green vegetables, and alongside cereal products and fruit these are also major sources of dietary fibre (not shown here).

One of the major areas of interest currently is in consumption of free sugars, particularly with the revised recommendation to reduce consumption to 5% of energy. Figure 11.11 shows the intake of NMES in NDNS for children 1.5–3 and 4–10 years in 2008–2012 compared with the previous NDNS survey for each of these age groups, 1992–1993 for 2.5–3 years and 1997 for 4–10 years. This shows a decrease in intake of NMES from over 17% of energy to under 12% for toddlers and 14–15% for children 4–10 years over about a 20-year period and suggests changes to eating behaviour. One of these is in terms of soft drinks, as shown in Figure 11.12, where percentage consumers of soft drinks (not low calorie) is seen to decrease from over 80% of children to lower proportions 20 years later, particularly in the toddlers, where less than half are consuming these over a 4-day period.

As with infants, the two nutrients where there is the greatest concern regarding whether children aged 4–10 years are obtaining enough are iron and vitamin D. In NDNS 2008–2012, iron intakes seemed adequate for most, with 6% of those aged 1.5–3 years and only 1% of those 4–10 years below the LRNI. However, when iron status was measured, nearly 13% of those aged 1.5–3 years were below the cut-off for increased risk for haemoglobin and 35% below the cut-off for ferritin, indicating that iron stores are depleted. For those aged 4–10 years, 3% were below the cut-off for haemoglobin

Table 11.2 Contribution of various food groups to intakes of energy, protein, fat, NMES, vitamin D and iron in children aged 1.5–3 and 4–10 years in NDNS 2008–2012.

Food group	Contribution (%)											
	Energy		Protein		Fat		NMES		Vitamin D		Iron	
	1.5–3 years	4–10 years	1.5–3 years	4–10 years	1.5–3 years	4–10 years	1.5–3 years	4–10 years	1.5–3 years	4–10 years	1.5–3 years	4–10 years
Cereals and cereal products	31	36	24	28	19	24	25	29	14	20	53	55
Milk and milk products	25	15	34	21	34	20	18	12	24	13	6	2
Eggs and egg dishes	1	1	2	2	3	2	0	0	2	3	3	2
Fat spreads	3	3	0	0	10	9	0	0	20	21	0	0
Meat and meat products and dishes	11	13	22	29	15	19	1	1	21	25	11	13
Fish and fish dishes	2	2	5	5	3	3	0	0	8	8	2	2
Vegetables, potatoes	8	9	6	8	6	8	3	2	1	1	12	13
Fruit	6	4	2	1	1	0	3	1	0	0	5	3
Sugar, preserves and confectionery	4	6	1	2	4	5	19	22	0	0	2	2
Beverages	4	5	1	1	0	0	27	30	0	0	2	2

and 11% of boys and 20% of girls were below the cut-off for ferritin. When both markers were considered, 5% of those aged 1.5–3 years and 1% of those 4–10 years were below both lower limits, indicating deficiency. For vitamin D, intakes for both age groups were only about 2 µg/day, whereas the new recommendation being by SACN for this age group is 10 µg/day. When status was measured, about 8% of those aged 1.5–3 years were below the cut-off of 25 nmol/L 25(OH)D. The proportion was even higher for children aged 4–10 years, with 12% of boys

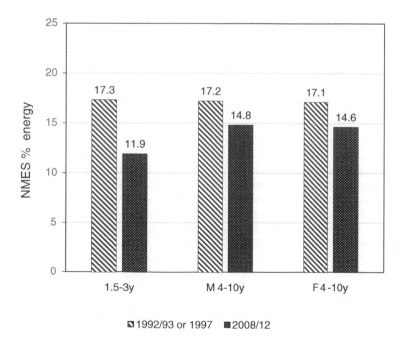

Figure 11.11 Intake of NMES in children 1.5–3 and 4–10 years in NDNS 2008–2012 compared with earlier NDNS surveys.

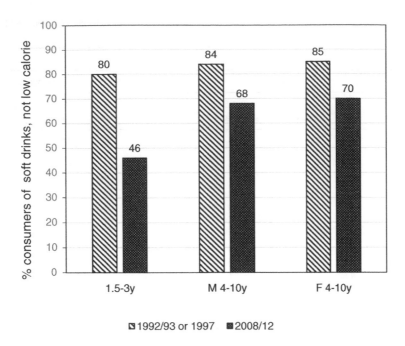

NDNS of children 4–18 years in 1997 was a 7-day survey.
Percentage consumers over 7 days has been recalculated for 4 days of consumption.

Figure 11.12 Percentage consumers of soft drinks, not low calorie in children 1.5–3 and 4–10 years in NDNS 2008–2012 compared with earlier NDNS surveys.

and 16% of girls below this cut-off. These are higher proportions than for infants, indicating that the problem persists as children are growing and eating family foods. These results for iron and vitamin D point to the need for education of parents about optimal diets for their children and possibly for other interventions, such as fortification or supplementation to improve the status of these two key nutrients.

Consumption of fruit and vegetables in children has shown a marked increase compared with the previous NDNS, as shown in Figure 11.13 for boys and girls aged 4–10 years. NDNS food records include *where* and *with whom* each food item has been eaten, and analysis of these in relation to fruit and vegetables has shown that children are more likely to consume fruit and vegetables and to consume larger portions outside the home, such as at day-care and at school, than at home. They are more likely to consume these with friends, rather than with parents. These results suggest that much of the increase in fruit and vegetable consumption may be the result of initiatives to improve offerings to children in structured environments outside the home, such as the free fruit scheme and in school meals. There remains a need to encourage parents to feed healthier foods to their children.

11.7 Conclusions

National nutrition surveys and prospective cohort studies which have included dietary assessment in infancy and young childhood provide the most complete information about the dietary intakes of infants and young children and the impact these have on health and disease later in life. Evidence from these sources indicates that in many respects infants and children in the UK are eating a satisfactory diet, but there remain a number of areas where improvements could be made. Breastfeeding has been shown to be beneficial for an appropriate rate of weight gain and to protect against a number of disorders, but the compliance with the recommendation to breastfeed and to continue for 6 months is poor. While there have been improvements in the proportion of mothers beginning to breastfeed their infants, the majority do not continue beyond 3 months of age. The timing of introduction of complementary feeding remains controversial, and only about 1% of infants in the UK are exclusively breastfed to 6 months. New evidence suggests that introduction of some allergenic foods earlier than 6 months may be beneficial, and feeding difficulties are seen if introduction of more complex textures, such as lumpy foods, is later than 6 months. For infants over the

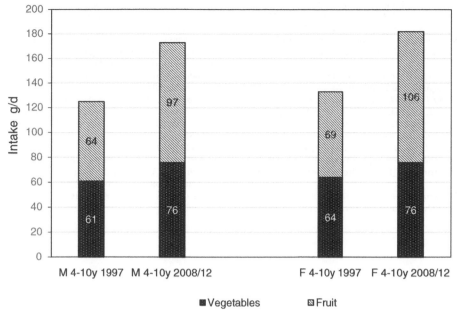

Figure 11.13 Consumption of fruit and vegetables (not including those in mixed dishes) in children 4–10 years old in NDNS 2008–2012 compared with NDNS in 1997.

age of 12 months and for older children (1.5–10 years), diets are largely satisfactory and consumption of fruit and vegetables is good, but intakes and status of iron and vitamin D are a cause for concern. New research has shown that the higher intakes of fruit and vegetables are more likely to take place in environments outside the home with friends, rather than at home with parents. There is scope for improvement of the diets of infants and young children, and encouragement of parents to provide healthy diets for their children continues to be worthwhile.

Further reading

Bates, B., Lennox, A., Prentice, A. *et al.* (eds) (2014) *National Diet and Nutrition Survey. Results from Years 1, 2, 3 and 4 (Combined) of the Rolling Programme (2008/2009–2011/2012). A Survey Carried Out on Behalf of Public Health England and the Food Standards Agency.* Public Health England, London. https://www.gov.uk/government/uploads/system/uploads/attachment_data/file/310995/NDNS_Y1_to_4_UK_report.pdf (accessed 6 December 2016).

British Medical Association (2009) *Early Life Nutrition and Lifelong Health.* British Medical Association, London.

British Nutrition Foundation (2013) *Nutrition and Development: Short and Long Term Consequences for Health.* Wiley-Blackwell, Chichester.

Butte, N.F., Fox, M.K., Briefel, R.R. *et al.* (2010) Nutrient intakes of US infants, toddlers, and preschoolers meet or exceed dietary reference intakes. *Journal of the American Dietetic Association,* **110,** S27–S37.

Daniels, L., Heath, A.L., Williams, S.M. *et al.* (2015) Baby-Led Introduction to SolidS (BLISS) study: a randomised controlled trial of a baby-led approach to complementary feeding. *BMC Pediatrics,* **15,** 179–194.

Emmett, P.M. and Jones, L.R. (2015) Diet, growth, and obesity development throughout childhood in the Avon Longitudinal Study of Parents and Children. *Nutrition Reviews,* **73** (Suppl 3), 175–206.

Emmett, P.M., Jones, L.R. and Northstone, K. (2015) Dietary patterns in the Avon Longitudinal Study of Parents and Children. *Nutrition Reviews,* **73** (Suppl 3), 207–230.

Fleischer, D.M., Sicherer, S., Greenhawt, M. *et al.* (2015) Consensus communication on early peanut introduction and the prevention of peanut allergy in high-risk infants. *Pediatrics,* **31,** 2015–2394.

Heikkilä, K., Kelly, Y., Renfrew, M.J. *et al.* (2014) Breastfeeding and educational achievement at age 5. *Maternal and Child Nutrition,* **10,** 92–101.

Kramer, M.S. and Kakuma, R. (2001) *The Optimal Duration of Exclusive Breastfeeding: A Systematic Review.* World Health Organization, Geneva.

Lennox, A., Sommerville, J., Ong, K. *et al.* (eds) (2013) *Diet and Nutrition Survey of Infants and Young Children, 2011.* Department of Health/Food Standards Agency, London. https://www.gov.uk/government/uploads/system/uploads/attachment_data/file/139572/DNSIYC_UK_report_ALL_chapters_DH_V10.0.pdf (accessed 6 December 2016).

McAndrew, F., Thompson, J., Fellows, L. *et al.* (2012) *Infant Feeding Survey – 2010.* NHS Information Centre. http://data.gov.uk/dataset/infant-feeding-survey-2010 (accessed 6 December 2016).

Mak, T.N., Prynne, C.J., Cole, D. *et al.* (2012) Assessing eating context and fruit and vegetable consumption in children: new methods using food diaries in the UK National Diet and

Nutrition Survey Rolling Programme. *The International Journal of Behavioral Nutrition and Physical Activity*, **9**, 126–141.

Nyaradi, A., Foster, J.K., Hickling, S. *et al.* (2014) Prospective associations between dietary patterns and cognitive performance during adolescence. *Journal of Child Psychology and Psychiatry*, **55**, 1017–1024.

Nyaradi, A., Li, J., Hickling, S. *et al.* (2013) Diet in the early years of life influences cognitive outcomes at 10 years: a prospective cohort study. *Acta Paediatrica*, **102**, 1165–1173.

Oddy, W.H., Mori, T.A., Huang, R.C. *et al.* (2014) Early infant feeding and adiposity risk: from infancy to adulthood. *Annals of Nutrition and Metabolism*, **64**, 262–270.

SACN (2010) *Iron and Health*. TSO, London. https://www.gov.uk/government/uploads/system/uploads/attachment_data/file/339309/SACN_Iron_and_Health_Report.pdf (accessed 6 December 2016).

SACN (2016) *Vitamin D and Health*. Public Health England, London. https://www.gov.uk/government/uploads/system/uploads/attachment_data/file/537616/SACN_Vitamin_D_and_Health_report.pdf (accessed 6 January 2017).

SACN/Committee on Toxicology (2011) Joint Statement. Timing of introduction of gluten into the infant diet. Department of Health, London. https://www.gov.uk/government/uploads/system/uploads/attachment_data/file/339407/SACN_COT_Timing_of_the_Introduction_of_Gluten_into_the_Infant_Diet_2011.pdf (accessed 6 December 2016).

Siega-Riz, A.M., Deming, D.M., Reidy, K.C. *et al.* (2010) Food consumption patterns of infants and toddlers: where are we now? *Journal of the American Dietetic Association*, **110**, S38–S51.

WHO (2001) *The Optimal Duration of Exclusive Breastfeeding. Report of an Expert Consultation, Geneva, Switzerland 28–30 March 2001*. World Health Organization, Geneva. http://apps.who.int/iris/bitstream/10665/67219/1/WHO_NHD_01.09.pdf?ua=1 (accessed 6 December 2016).

12
Nutrition and Teenagers/Young Adults

Elisabeth Weichselbaum

Key messages

- The transition from childhood into teenage and young adolescence is characterised by a number of physical changes and rapid growth.
- Energy and nutrient requirements are particularly high during this time of rapid growth, yet dietary habits of young people tend to deteriorate as they become more independent, increasing the possibility of inadequate nutrient intakes.
- For females, a healthy diet with a good supply of essential nutrients not only affects their own development and health, but possibly also that of another life if they become pregnant.
- Factors influencing dietary choices of adolescents include socio-economic background, peer influence, advertising, the physical environment and body image.
- Physical activity, which is crucial for development of a healthy musculoskeletal system and helps with weight control, declines to a large degree as girls enter adolescence, whereas in boys, such a decline is less obvious. Young males are generally more active than young females, who have physical activity levels far below recommended levels.
- Overweight and obesity rates have already reached epidemic proportions in young people. Childhood obesity is associated with cardiovascular changes and risk of type 2 diabetes at a young age. Young people who are overweight or obese are also more likely to carry excess weight in adulthood.

- Adolescence and young adulthood are crucial periods for growth and development of the musculoskeletal system, yet calcium intakes are often low and vitamin D status insufficient. Low vitamin D levels are particularly found among some ethnic minorities living in the UK and elsewhere in Europe.
- Low iron status is relatively common in young females due to high demands for iron with the onset of menstruation coupled with low intakes. Around one-third of adolescent girls in the UK have low plasma ferritin levels, a marker for long-term iron intake, and almost 1 in 10 young females has haemoglobin levels indicative of iron-deficiency anaemia. Boys are less affected by low iron levels and anaemia.
- Dietary choices in adolescents and young adults also influence cognitive function and performance. Skipping breakfast adversely affects cognitive performance throughout the morning, yet is common among young people.
- Body image can adversely affect dietary choices, with young people being particularly vulnerable. Attempts to achieve a certain body shape can lead to practices including smoking, meal skipping, severely reduced intake of foods deemed fattening (including nutrient-dense foods such as meat and milk) and the adoption of very low energy (and therefore nutrient) diets.

12.1 Introduction

As children transition into adolescence and young adulthood, they experience a number of physiological and psychological changes. A healthy diet is particularly crucial during this stage of life to meet the higher nutrient demands and ensure healthy growth and development. This chapter discusses physiological changes and how they affect dietary requirements, and looks at how actual dietary habits compare with requirements. Several

developmental and health issues are covered, with particular reference to this critical stage in human development.

12.2 Puberty: a time of transition into adulthood

During adolescence the human body undergoes a large number of changes as a result of puberty, a time of hormonal changes and sexual maturation. The onset of

Public Health Nutrition, Second Edition. Edited by Judith L Buttriss, Ailsa A Welch, John M Kearney and Susan A Lanham-New.
© 2018 by The Nutrition Society. Published 2018 by John Wiley & Sons, Ltd.
Companion website: www.wiley.com/go/buttriss/publichealth

puberty is characteristically earlier in females than it is in males. Girls reach puberty at around 10.5–11 years of age, whereas onset in boys is at around 12.5–13 years. As males reach puberty later than females, they experience on average two more years of pre-pubertal growth than females, resulting in typically higher stature at the onset of puberty for males.

Bodily changes during puberty

With the onset of puberty, the growth rate accelerates over a period of 1–3 years. After the peak velocity of growth in puberty has been attained, the growth rate slows considerably until growth in height ceases at around 16 years of age in girls and 18 years in boys. Before puberty, boys and girls are of similar average height, but significant skeletal differences become obvious during the adolescent growth spurt. During this growth spurt boys gain approximately 20 cm and girls approximately 15 cm in height. A physiologically driven rapid increase in bone mass accompanies increased deposition of calcium and phosphate. Although linear growth levels off at around 16–18 years, bone development continues into young adulthood, with peak bone mass being achieved sometime between 18 and 35 years.

Growth and development in adolescents is also associated with changes in body composition, which affects the proportion of body fat and lean tissue. Lean body mass (i.e. muscle mass) increases to a much greater extent in males than in females, whereas girls experience a much larger increase in body fat.

12.3 Diet in teenagers and young adults

Role of a healthy diet in adolescence and young adulthood

Adolescence is a time of particularly rapid growth, some aspects of which continue into early adulthood. The demands for most nutrients during adolescence are high compared with the needs of younger children, and are also high compared with the needs of adults. Boys generally have higher needs of protein and energy to support their later growth spurt. During this period of transition, it is particularly important to follow a healthy and balanced diet, based on the Eatwell Guide (or other national or international dietary guidelines), in order to meet demands during this time of rapid growth and to ensure optimal physical and mental development, tissue maintenance and to support healthy levels of physical activity.

For females, a healthy diet with a good supply of essential nutrients not only affects their own development and health, but possibly also that of another life if they become pregnant. A low status of one or more nutrients can have adverse effects on the pregnancy outcome and the baby. For example, an adequate folate status is essential to protect against neural tube defects, including cleft palate, spina bifida and brain damage. This is particularly important during the first few weeks of pregnancy, when many are not yet aware that they are pregnant, in particular when the pregnancy was unplanned. A poor vitamin D status during pregnancy can affect the bone development of a baby, whereas a poor iron status is associated with increased risk of low birth weight and perinatal mortality.

In the longer term, food patterns during childhood, adolescence and young adulthood can set the scene for future dietary preferences and eating behaviour in adult life. There is also substantial evidence that poor diet and poor physical activity patterns in childhood can lead to problems that manifest later in life, particularly in relation to cardiovascular disease (CVD), obesity, type 2 diabetes, osteoporosis and some forms of cancer.

Dietary patterns

To meet increasing demands for nutrients during this critical developmental stage, a nutrient-dense diet should be consumed. However, eating habits seem to deteriorate in the transition from childhood to adolescence, making it less likely that high nutrient demands are readily met. In the UK, data from the National Diet and Nutrition Survey highlights some of the dietary differences between children aged 4–10 years and young people aged 11–18 years (see Figure 12.1). For example, milk intake decreases by around 30% in boys and by around 40% in girls. Milk and dairy products are a major source of calcium, which is particularly important for bone development during puberty and adolescence. Such drastic decreases in milk consumption are therefore likely to have a negative effect on bone development and health. Intakes of fruit are also lower in older compared with younger boys and girls, whereas vegetable intake (excluding potatoes) remains fairly stable. Intakes of sugar-sweetened soft drinks are significantly higher in older boys and girls, possibly replacing milk from the diet. Changes towards a more unfavourable dietary pattern while nutrient requirements are increasing result in a large proportion of adolescents having inadequate nutrient intakes. Data from the National Diet and Nutrition Survey show that, in particular, adolescent girls have inadequate intakes of several nutrients.

Data from the Health Behaviour in School-aged Children (HBSC) survey carried out in 2005–2006 across

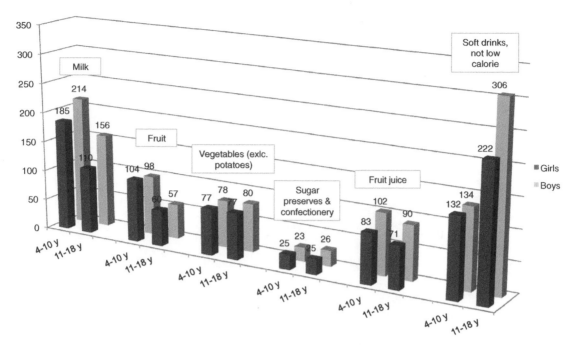

Figure 12.1 Average daily intakes of selected foods in UK children and adolescents. *Source*: Bates *et al*. (2012). Reproduced under OGL.

Europe (and selected non-European countries, including the USA, the Russian Federation and Israel) show similar unfavourable patterns across the continent. The proportion of boys and girls who eat fruit daily decreases from an average of 37% and 45% in 11-year-old boys and girls respectively, to 25% and 34% in 15-year-old boys and girls respectively. The proportion of those drinking soft drinks daily increases from 24% and 20% in 11-year-old boys and girls respectively, to 32% and 25% in 15-year-old boys and girls respectively.

Skipping breakfast also becomes more frequent as children develop into adolescents. Data from the HBSC survey show that 15-year-olds in the UK and in the rest of Europe, are less likely to regularly eat breakfast on school days compared with 11-year olds (see Figure 12.2). Regularly eating breakfast is associated with several benefits for health, including higher intakes of several micronutrients and lower risk of obesity, and better cognitive performance throughout the morning. Skipping breakfast at a time of rapid growth and development and of high nutrient requirements may be particularly detrimental.

Factors influencing dietary choices

When children enter adolescence they not only experience bodily changes, but also social changes, which can markedly affect eating behaviours. Adolescents become more independent, and the parental influence decreases, in particular on food choices made outside the home. Parental influence is still critical while young people still live and eat at home, but diminishes when young people live independently.

Socio-economic status (SES) of the family has been suggested to impact upon the dietary and lifestyle habits of people within the UK. Data from the 1997 National Diet and Nutrition Survey found that the energy, protein, total carbohydrate, and non-starch polysaccharides intakes of boys whose parents were in receipt of benefits, was lower than that of boys whose parents were not. Intakes of some micronutrients, including vitamin C, calcium and magnesium, have also been found to be lower in children from households in receipt of benefits. However, data from the Low Income Diet and Nutrition Survey (LIDNS) suggest nutrient intake levels in children and young people from families with low SES are similar to those of young people in the general population, although there are some differences in consumption of certain foods. For example, lower intakes of wholemeal bread, semi-skimmed milk, fruits and vegetables, and higher intakes of whole milk, processed meat and non-diet soft drinks were found in the LIDNS. The HBSC survey also found associations between family income and indicators of dietary behaviour. Eating breakfast daily is significantly associated with family affluence in the majority of countries, in particular for boys. Those who are from more affluent families are more likely to regularly eat breakfast, particularly in western and

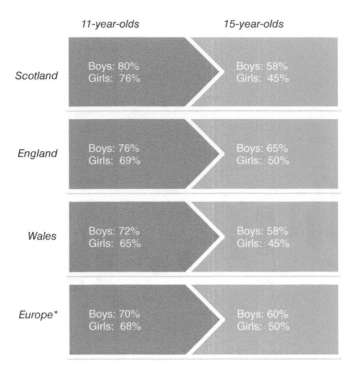

Figure 12.2 Proportion of young people eating breakfast every school day. Asterisk indicates including selected non-European countries (including USA, Russian Federation, Turkey and Israel). *Source*: Currie *et al*. (2008). Reproduced with permission of WHO.

northern Europe. Fruit consumption is also significantly associated with family affluence, with those from less affluent families having lower levels of fruit intake. Soft drink consumption is also associated with family affluence in many countries. An inverse relationship between family affluence and soft drink consumption is particularly found in western and northern Europe, while the reverse pattern is seen in eastern Europe and the Baltic states.

Peers also exert a major influence on overall adolescent behaviour. Adolescents spend a substantial amount of time with friends, and eating is an important form of socialisation and recreation. Because adolescents seek peer approval and social identity, it is assumed that peer influence and group conformity are important determinants in food acceptability and selection. However, the role of the peer group in influencing food choices is not well studied, and the few studies published have not found a strong association. A lack of association may be due to difficulties in assessing social influences by simply asking young people to rate the perceived influence of others, as adolescents, like adults, may not be aware of the social influences on their eating behaviour.

The physical environment influences eating behaviour. Adolescents still attending school can be influenced by the school food environment. Throughout the UK, food-based and/or nutrient-based school food standards are in place, which have improved the quality of school lunches and other food and drink offered at school. These improvements seem to increase the quality of the overall diet of young people, although more so in young children than in older children or adolescents. The availability of vending machines, convenience stores or fast-food outlets at or close to schools, universities or the work place can also influence dietary choices.

Advertising of food can influence dietary behaviour of young people. Bans on advertising foods that are high in fat and/or sugar on children's TV channels in the UK have led to less exposure of children to such advertisements. However, exposure to advertising is more difficult to control in adolescents and young people, who watch a larger array of TV channels and have access to many other types of media, and generally have more freedom to choose when and what they watch and read. The extent to which advertising influences dietary choices in adolescents and young people remains unknown and is difficult to assess.

Concerns and aspirations about body shape and image also influence dietary habits. In particular, the desire to be slim in young females can lead to unhealthy eating practices in an effort to lose weight. This topic is discussed further in Section 12.8: 'Body image'.

12.4 Physical activity in teenagers and young adults

Role of physical activity in teenage and young adulthood

Physical activity together with the time spent being sedentary have a major impact on health at all stages of life, and play a particularly important role during growth and development (also see Section 12.6: 'Physical activity and bone/muscle health'). Being physically active when young affects not only current health status but can also influence health in later life. The many benefits for young people of being physically active include helping to maintain energy balance, and therefore a healthy body weight; aiding bone and musculoskeletal development; reducing the risk of diabetes and hypertension; as well as numerous psychological and social benefits (including improved psychological well-being, and higher self-confidence and self-esteem).

The UK physical activity recommendations, which also include recommendations to reduce time spent sitting, are presented in Table 12.1.

Variety in the type of activity undertaken is important during growth and development: moderate to vigorous bouts of activity will benefit the cardio-respiratory system; activities to support healthy bone development are those which produce high physical stress on the bones, and include running, jumping and skipping; active play (e.g. climbing, carrying and 'rough and tumble') helps to improve muscle strength and flexibility.

Sedentary behaviour

Sedentary behaviour refers to activities that do not increase energy expenditure substantially above the resting level; these include screen-based behaviours such as TV viewing and playing computer games, as well as activities such as reading and listening to music, and sitting and lying down. Studies suggest there is a link between sedentary behaviour and body weight in young people, although the evidence is not conclusive, with a small number of studies finding no association when sedentary behaviour was measured objectively. More studies with objectively measured levels of sedentary behaviour are needed to improve understanding of this relationship. The association between sedentary behaviour and obesity may be complex and may not be as simple as sedentary behaviours directly displacing physically active ones. An increase in sedentary behaviour may not just mean fewer calories are expended; evidence indicates that activities such as TV viewing are often associated with negative eating habits, including the consumption of energy-dense food and drinks, thereby exacerbating the problem.

Changes in levels of physical activity from childhood to teenager

Physical activity levels tend to decrease in both boys and girls during adolescence. This was highlighted in findings from the *Health Survey for England – 2008* (Craig *et al.*, 2009), where physical activity levels were measured objectively with an accelerometer (see Figure 12.3). While a third of girls age 4–10 years met the target to be active for 60 min/day and 39% showed low activity levels (less than 30 min/day), almost all girls age

---

Table 12.1 Recommendations for physical activity in the UK.

Children and young people (5–18 years)

All children and young people should engage in moderate to vigorous-intensity physical activity for at least 60 min and up to several hours every day.
Vigorous-intensity activities, including those that strengthen the muscle and bone, should be incorporated at least 3 days a week.
All children and young people should minimise the amount of time spent being sedentary (sitting) for extended periods.

Adults (19–64 years)

Adults should aim to be active daily. Over a week, activity should add up to at least 150 min (2.5 h) of moderate-intensity activity in bouts of 10 min or more – one way to approach this is to do 30 min on at least 5 days a week.
Alternatively, comparable benefits can be achieved through 75 min of vigorous-intensity activity spread across the week or combinations of moderate and vigorous-intensity activity.
Adults should also undertake physical activity to improve muscle strength on at least 2 days a week.
All adults should minimise the amount of time spent being sedentary (sitting) for extended periods.

Source: Department of Health, Physical Activity, Health Improvement and Protection (2011).

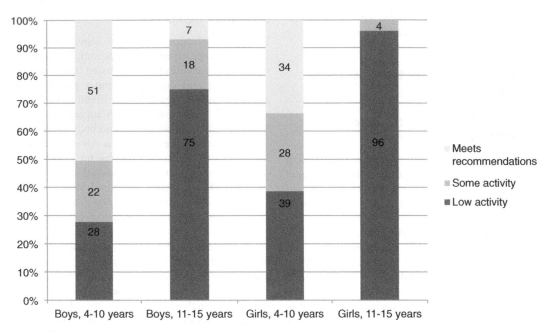

Figure 12.3 Objectively measured activity levels of boys and girls age 4–10 and 11–15 years in England. Meets recommendations: 60 min or more at least moderate activity on all 7 days; some activity: 30–59 min on all 7 days; low activity: lower levels of activity. *Source*: Craig *et al*. (2009).

11–15 years were found to have low activity levels. Similar trends were found in boys, although boys generally are more active than girls.

Decreasing levels of activity have also been confirmed in other studies; for example, in the Health Behaviour in Teenagers Study, which explored physical activity levels in schoolchildren (age 11–12 years at baseline) from 36 London schools over a period of 5 years. The number of days of vigorous physical activity per week fell over the 5-year study period, and more so in girls than in boys. In contrast, hours of sedentary behaviour increased over the study period by an average of 2.5 h per week in boys and 2.8 h per week in girls (Brodersen *et al.*, 2007). Overall, there seems to be a consistent decrease in physical activity in girls with increasing age, whereas in boys the physical activity levels seem to vary to a lesser extent. These decreasing activity levels with increasing age, in particular in females, are worrying, as adolescence and young adulthood are periods where growth is still ongoing and physical activity supports the development of bone and muscle.

Factors influencing physical activity levels

Many factors influence young people's physical activity habits, and understanding these, is the key to helping them achieve physical activity recommendations. This is particularly important as research indicates that physical activity behaviours in childhood and adolescence may track into adulthood.

As discussed earlier, age has a significant effect on physical activity levels. Gender also has a considerable effect on physical activity levels in young people, starting in childhood and continuing until young adulthood, whereas differences become less obvious later in adulthood. Also, the types of activity differ between boys and girls, and often reflect gender stereotypes (e.g. boys play more football and cricket, whereas girls spend more time being active with pets, skipping and dancing). Boys spend more time doing vigorous activities than girls, in particular during out-of-school time.

Ethnicity also influences physical activity levels. In the UK, young people of Asian descent are generally less active than white or black boys and girls. Differences between ethnic groups can also be seen with sedentary behaviour, with one study finding that black students of both sexes reported higher levels of sedentary behaviour than their white peers, the difference being greater in girls. Trends in sedentary behaviour also differ between white and Asian girls, with increasing sedentary behaviour occurring at younger age in Asian girls.

Whether SES influences physical activity levels remains unclear as studies have come to different conclusions, with some studies suggesting lower SES is associated with lower activity levels, whereas other studies (e.g. the 2008 Health Survey for England and Scottish

National Health Survey 2009) have found either no association or that young people with lower SES are more active. It is unclear why there are discrepancies in the data, but methodological differences are likely to have contributed to these variations. It has been suggested that the type of activity may also differ, with children from a lower socio-economic background tending to participate in unstructured activities or free play, whereas children from higher SES groups are more likely to take part in structured activities or belong to sports clubs.

Physical activity levels in young people may also be influenced by their peers, suggesting that promoting physical activity via friendship groups may be one way to increase physical activity levels.

The environment in which we live has received increasing attention over recent years in terms of the role it plays in influencing physical activity levels of individuals. The characteristics of the built environment are often cited as a cause of inactivity. In particular, an increasing reliance on car use in place of walking and cycling, concerns over safety, and a lack of green space are commonly cited as barriers to being physically active. However, a systematic review comparing the physical activity levels of 5- to 18-year-olds living in different built environments did not find major differences between children from rural and urban areas (Sandercock *et al.*, 2010). Mode of travel also plays a role in physical activity levels and is suggested to be associated with physical fitness in schoolchildren.

12.5 Overweight and obesity in teenagers and young adults

The prevalence of overweight and obesity is a major issue among young people, and according to the World Health Organization this has reached epidemic proportions in most industrialised countries. A high body mass index (BMI) at a young age is associated with an increased risk of obesity in adulthood and premature mortality.

Prevalence of overweight and obesity

The prevalence of overweight and obesity is high in the UK, including in children, adolescents and young adults (see Chapters 17 and 19). Data from the HBSC shows that overweight and obesity in young people is a Europe-wide problem (see Figure 12.4).

There is a clear difference between boys and girls in this European dataset, with girls being less likely to be overweight or obese than boys, although the use of self-reported data means the findings have to be interpreted with caution. In the UK, obesity also seems to be more prevalent in boys than girls, although prevalence of overweight is generally similar between boys and girls. Young people from Mediterranean countries seem most likely to be overweight or obese, whereas low prevalence rates are found in eastern European regions. Family affluence is also significantly inversely associated with overweight and obesity in around half of countries, mainly in western European countries, with those from lower affluence families being more likely to be overweight or obese.

Health implications of overweight and obesity

Overweight and obesity are associated with an increased risk of various conditions, including CVD, type 2 diabetes, high blood pressure and some cancers, typically occurring in adulthood. However, obese children and young people often display many of the changes associated with vascular disease in adults. Obesity and in particular excess weight around the waist are major risk factors for the development of insulin resistance in young people. Considered previously to be a disease of adults, type 2 diabetes has become a far more common occurrence in children and adolescents over the last decade. Depending on the ethnic composition of the population, between 8 and 50% of newly diagnosed adolescent diabetic patients have type 2 diabetes, the remainder being type 1 and other forms of diabetes. Adolescents with evidence of insulin resistance are also more likely to have an abnormal lipid profile.

Obese young people also have a higher risk of impaired endothelial function, lower arterial compliance and elasticity, and increased intima-media thickness, which are measures of vascular health and associated with adverse cardiovascular events in adulthood. Autopsy studies in children and adolescents have also shown that the extent of early atherosclerosis of the aorta and coronary arteries is directly associated with levels of lipids, blood pressure and obesity. Obesity is also a well-established risk factor for hypertension in children.

In addition to the negative impact of obesity on factors associated with CVD, multiple studies have suggested that childhood overweight and obesity track into adulthood. Overweight children are more prone to becoming overweight adults, especially at higher BMIs or if they have an obese parent. Important evidence for this comes from a US study (the Bogalusa Heart Study) that began in 1972 and has followed many participants from childhood into adulthood; the outcomes of this study show that children who were overweight at age 2–5 years were over four times more likely to become obese than those with a BMI <50th percentile. Data from a UK cohort (Thousand Families Cohort Study, comprising 1142 children born in 1947 and followed up into adulthood) showed a moderate, statistically significant correlation between

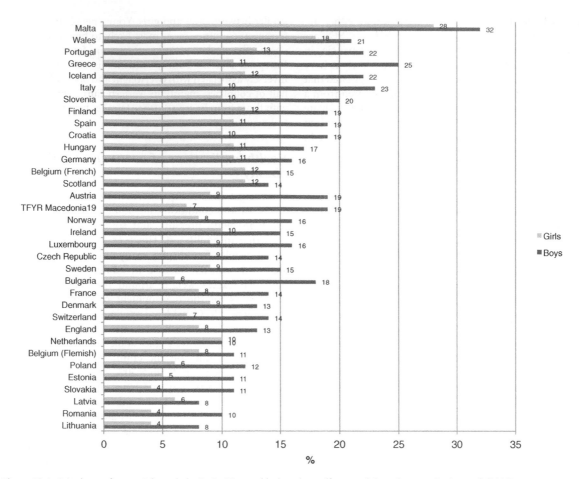

Figure 12.4 Prevalence of overweight and obesity in 15-year-olds, based on self-reported data. *Source:* Currie *et al.* (2008).

childhood and adult BMI. At age 50, those who had been above the 90th percentile for BMI at age 9 or 13 years were between five and nine times more likely to be obese than those in the thinnest quartile in childhood. However, most of those in the top quartile for body fat aged 50 years had not been overweight as children, which indicates that although those who are overweight or obese in childhood have an increased risk of being overweight and obese as adults, thinness in childhood does not protect against overweight and obesity in adulthood.

Although there is consistent evidence to suggest that childhood obesity is associated with risk factors for CVD in adulthood, there is little evidence that overweight and obesity in childhood are *independently* associated with CVD risk factors, CVD morbidity or CVD mortality in adulthood, suggesting that increased risk is mainly due to overweight and obesity tracking into adulthood. Findings of the Thousand Families Cohort Study suggest that those thinnest in childhood but overweight in adulthood have the highest overall risk of adult disease.

Factors involved in development of overweight and obesity

Obesity is a complex condition, and biology, eating and physical activity behaviours, people's beliefs and attitudes, and broader economic and social drivers all have a role to play (see chapter 24 for more detail). To tackle obesity levels in children and adolescents, the various contributing factors need to be taken into account rather than simply addressing one factor. Evidence on the influence of selected nutritional factors is discussed here; however, the list is by no means exhaustive.

Breakfast

Evidence from cross-sectional and cohort studies suggests a protective effect of eating breakfast against becoming overweight or obese. However, owing to most of the evidence coming from observational studies, causality cannot be assumed. Factors other than having breakfast per se may be responsible for observed associations. Some studies show a protective effect despite those eating breakfast having higher average daily energy intakes. This could suggest that children who regularly consume breakfast cereals may be more physically active than those who consume breakfast cereals less frequently. There is also the possibility that a low consumption of breakfast is a result of skipping breakfast in order to lose weight, which would mean the low consumption could be a result of the higher body weight rather than vice versa.

Snacking

Snacking between meals is commonly believed to be contributing to the increased incidence of overweight and obesity within populations. However, the evidence linking snacking and bodyweight remains inconsistent, with some studies showing positive, some negative and some no associations between snacking and body weight. Overall, evidence points towards a lower risk of being overweight or obese in those eating more frequently, although some studies do not adequately control for other diet and lifestyle factors that may have contributed to any observed association. For example, individuals who snack more frequently may do so in association with a more active lifestyle and, therefore, the potential increase in energy intake would be offset by, or in response to, greater energy expenditure.

Portion size

It has been shown that presenting children with larger portions leads to an increased intake of the respective food, but also to an increased food and energy intake overall. Energy density does not seem to influence the total amount of food consumed during a meal, which suggests that children do not compensate for the higher energy density by eating a smaller portion, which in turn can lead to an overall higher energy intake if energy-dense foods are consumed regularly. Research so far does not suggest that the tendency to overeat when large portions are presented is specific to overweight children. Research in adolescents and young adults is lacking.

Sugar-sweetened beverages

Evidence from observational studies suggests there is a possible link between consumption of sugar-sweetened beverages and overweight, although the evidence remains conflicting. Evidence from randomised controlled trials suggests that consuming sugar-sweetened beverages, compared with non-calorically sweetened beverages, leads to an increase in energy intake. It has been suggested that energy-containing liquids could lead to excess energy consumption because they fail to trigger satiety compared with equivalent energy intakes from solid food. However, studies comparing the effects of equivalent amounts of liquid or solid energy on satiety have yielded inconsistent results and do not consistently support the hypothesis that liquid calories go undetected by appetite control systems. Studies are also often short term, making it difficult to draw conclusions on long-term impact.

Most of the evidence on the association between sugar-sweetened beverage consumption and risk of overweight and obesity comes from observational studies, which means no 'cause–effect' relationships can be established, and it is possible that other factors that may have contributed to any associations (or lack of association) may not have been adequately considered. Interesting findings come from the European Energy Balance Research to Prevent Excessive Weight Gain among Youth project, a pan-European, EU-funded project. In the course of this project, a school-based survey was carried out among schoolchildren aged 10–12 years from seven European countries (Belgium, Greece, Hungary, Netherlands, Norway, Slovenia, and Spain). The country with the highest prevalence of overweight and obesity (Greece) had the lowest soft drink consumption, whereas the country with the highest consumption of soft drinks (Netherlands) had only the fourth highest prevalence of overweight and obesity, even though consumption of soft drinks was about five to six times as high as in Greece. Although no analyses were carried out to identify possible associations and such associations are purely cross-sectional, these findings highlight that obesity is the result of a variety of factors and not solely one single factor. Further studies in this area will hopefully shed more light on whether consuming sugar-sweetened beverages is associated with an increased risk of being overweight or obese.

Prevention and treatment of overweight and obesity

Treatment of established obesity can prove difficult, and therefore much more effort should be put into obesity prevention. However, evidence does not consistently demonstrate that diet and exercise interventions are effective in preventing weight gain and obesity in children, although they can be effective in promoting a healthy diet and increased physical activity levels. Interventions that were effective are generally those that are longer, with a focus on younger children and including settings other than just the community. In particular, interventions that include a school component and focus on both diet and physical activity may be more effective in preventing overweight or obesity. However, some evidence suggests that, when implemented alone, school-based diet and physical activity related policies appear insufficient to prevent or treat overweight or obesity in children, but that they do appear to have an effect when developed and implemented as part of a more extensive intervention programme that aims to influence behaviour at multiple levels (e.g. home, school, neighbourhood). Evidence in young adults suggests that behavioural/motivational interventions and interventions that combine diet, exercise and motivational skills lead to weight loss. However, limitations in study design make it difficult drawing firm conclusions, and evidence from long-term studies for this age group is lacking.

For management of obesity in young people, the National Institute for Clinical Excellence (NICE) suggests that multicomponent interventions are the treatment of choice; weight management programmes (either for weight maintenance of loss, depending on age and stage of growth) should include behaviour change strategies to increase physical activity levels or decrease inactivity, improve eating behaviour and diet quality, and reduce energy intake. Interventions should address lifestyle within the family and also social settings; that is, encourage other family members to also adjust their eating and lifestyle habits. The guidelines for management of obesity in children from the Scottish Intercollegiate Guidelines Network (SIGN) are similar to those from NICE. SIGN also suggests that, for most obese children, weight maintenance is an acceptable treatment goal. Orlistat should only be prescribed for severely obese adolescents with co-morbidities or those with very severe to extreme obesity attending a specialist clinic, whereas bariatric surgery can be considered for post-pubertal adolescents with very severe to extreme obesity and severe co-morbidities.

12.6 Bone and muscle development during teenage and young adulthood

Optimising bone development in childhood and adolescence is crucial in order to decrease the risk of osteoporosis later in adult life. Most of the skeletal mass is laid down during that early stage of life, and it is estimated that by post-puberty (16 years onwards) approximately 80–90% of peak bone mass is achieved. Throughout early childhood, bone mass increases linearly with skeletal growth, whereas during the pubertal years a rapid increase in bone mass and density can be observed. In girls this is between the ages of 11 and 14 years, and in boys between 13 and 17 years as puberty starts later in males. Bone density continues to increase for several years after the cessation of growth until peak bone mass is achieved. The exact age at which this occurs remains controversial but is between 18 and 35 years of age. Besides genetic factors that influence peak bone mass and

account for roughly 70–75% of the variance seen, nutrition and physical activity play an important role in bone development. A healthy development of muscle mass is also important for bone health. Studies have shown that muscle mass is a major determinant for bone mass and density.

Adolescence is a crucial time in bone and muscle development, but it is also a time where eating habits tend to deteriorate and girls become less physically active. This may lead to less than optimal bone and muscle development, with potentially significant consequences later in life.

Dietary factors influencing bone and muscle development

Calcium
Calcium is essential for bone growth as it is required for the mineralisation of bone (see Chapter 21). An adequate intake of calcium during adolescence and young adulthood is one of a number of factors that are important for acquiring and attaining optimum peak bone mass. Diets containing insufficient calcium may lead to a low bone mineral density and contribute to impaired bone development, with implications for bone health in later life. Whereas the daily amount of calcium deposited in the skeleton during childhood is about 150–200 mg on average, during times of rapid growth, for example during puberty, this increases and peaks at around 400 mg per day. Therefore, total calcium needs are greater during adolescence than at any other time of life. A good proportion of adolescents (especially girls) and young women in the UK have intakes that fall below the lower reference nutrient intake and so are likely to be inadequate.

Whether calcium supplementation in early life helps bone development remains controversial, with effects generally being modest at best and usually only seen when baseline intakes are low. Regularly including calcium-rich foods in the diet of adolescents and young adults is a preferable approach to increase the calcium intake in the diet due to these foods also providing other nutrients that are associated with bone health.

Vitamin D
Vitamin D is critical for bone development and health as it is required for calcium absorption (see Chapter 20). There has been some debate around concentrations of plasma 25-hydroxyvitamin D, a marker of vitamin D status, that may be regarded as optimal. In the UK, 25 nmol/L of 25-hydroxyvitamin D has been used for some time as the lower threshold for vitamin D adequacy, below which there is an increased risk of rickets

and osteomalacia. However, more recently the US Institute of Medicine and others have introduced some higher cut-off levels (e.g. >50 nmol/L) to define vitamin D sufficiency. While the debate among scientists continues, the most commonly used cut-off level in the UK to define vitamin D deficiency has been <25 nmol/L. This topic was one of the aspects of the review undertaken in the UK by SACN; the final report was published in 2016 (SACN, 2016) (see chapter 20 for details).

According to the latest National Diet and Nutrition Survey around one in five 11- to 18-year-old boys and one in four girls living in the UK has blood vitamin D levels below 25 nmol/L. Vitamin D levels decrease progressively with age in both boys and girls, and are around 7 nmol/L lower in 11- to 18-year-olds than in 4- to 10-year-olds. Time spent exercising and playing outdoors has been associated with vitamin D status, whereas spending more time watching TV was associated with lower vitamin D levels (Absoud et al., 2011). Lower vitamin D levels in adolescents are likely to be the result of changes in lifestyle habits from childhood to adolescences, with less time spent being physically active outside and more time spent inside. A higher risk of vitamin D in some ethnic groups living in the UK was also apparent, with 85% of non-white children and adolescents having 25-hydroxyvitamin D levels below 50 nmol/L (the level considered as sufficient by some authorities), compared with 30% of white children and adolescents. There also seem to be socio-economic differences, with children and adolescents from families receiving income support having significantly lower vitamin D levels (56.2 nmol/L) compared with those not in receipt of benefits (62.9 nmol/L). Around half of young people from families on income support, as opposed to a third of those from families not eligible for support, have vitamin D levels below 50 nmol/L.

Protein

Dietary protein intake is also important for bone development, with positive associations between total protein intake, bone mineral content and bone size being reported in children and adolescents. There has been some controversy about the relationship between dietary protein, in particular that derived from animal sources, and calcium metabolism. In adults, excess dietary protein can result in increased urinary calcium losses, and therefore the potential for increased bone loss. More recently it has been argued that increased urinary calcium excretion associated with higher protein intakes may be a consequence of increased gut calcium absorption. It has been suggested that dietary protein is most beneficial for the bone in the presence of calcium sufficiency and adequate fruit and vegetable intakes, which will reduce the acidity of the diet as a whole.

Adequate levels of protein in the diet during adolescence and young adulthood are not only important for bone but also for muscle development, which in turn affects bone development. For older adults there is evidence that an even distribution of protein intake throughout the day is beneficial for muscle mass, whereas in young, growing people, the timing of intake does not seem to play a significant role.

Fruit and vegetables

A high intake of fruit and vegetables has been found to be associated with better bone mineral status in adolescents, with some studies suggesting the association is mainly explained by fruit intake. Although the specific mechanisms remain to be determined, it has been suggested that vitamin C and other fruit-specific antioxidants may play a role. It has also been argued that vegetables and fruit, as a good source of alkaline-forming components, could neutralise the calciuric effects of acids derived from the diet, or that alkaline-forming cations may have an independent impact on improving calcium balance and bone health.

Young people aged 11–24 years living in the UK only consume on average around three portions of fruit and vegetables a day, which is clearly below the recommended five daily portions (see chapter 8 for more on poor dietary patterns).

Other dietary factors

Vitamin K is also important for the skeleton, and deficiency of vitamin K may lead to a reduction in bone formation and decreased bone strength. High sodium intake and caffeine consumption have both been suggested to negatively influence calcium balance, although the evidence is inconsistent. There has also been concern that carbonated drinks may negatively impact on bone development through a contribution to acid load. However, purported associations between high intakes of carbonated drinks and bone development may be due to the displacement of milk from the diet rather than negative effects of carbonated drinks per se, which is particularly relevant for adolescents and young adults as these tend to be the highest consumers of soft drinks. Boys aged 11–18 years consume around 500 mL and girls around 400 mL of soft drinks (standard and low calorie combined) per day, compared with only around 150 mL and 110 mL of milk in boys and girls of younger age groups respectively.

Physical activity and bone/muscle health

Physical activity is crucial for bone development, particularly high-impact activities that include hopping, jumping and skipping, as well as weight training. For optimal bone development, young people are advised to follow the UK guidelines for physical activity (see Section 12.4). Physical activity levels significantly decrease in girls entering adolescence to levels that are less than adequate for optimal bone development, whereas adolescent boys and young men are generally more active.

While weight-bearing exercise is known to have a positive effect on bone mineral density, paradoxically bone health is a cause for concern in some girls who are engaged in competitive sports, such as gymnastics or distance running, in particular when combined with low energy intakes. This may be due to the combination of intensive training and low energy intakes interfering with growth and development, and efforts to control weight in sports where minimal body fat is perceived desirable. This combination often also results in late onset of menstruation or amenorrhoea. These factors can lead to some highly trained female athletes and ballet dancers having poor bone density. Therefore, for those who engage in competitive sports, an adequate supply of energy (as well as nutrients) is crucial.

Other lifestyle factors affecting bone and muscle development

Alcohol consumption has been linked to bone health, although most of the data available are from studies in adults. The effects of alcohol consumption on bone are linked to the dose ingested and the duration of consumption. Low alcohol consumption (one drink per day for women or two drinks for men) has not been associated with deleterious effects, with some studies even finding beneficial effects. However, chronically higher alcohol consumption has deleterious effects on the bone. A more common form of drinking among adolescents and young adults is binge drinking. Evidence from human studies on binge drinking and its effect on bone health is lacking, but data from animal studies suggests that it may trigger both short-term and long-term damage to the skeleton. Studies in rats showed that, in particular, impairment of the bone micro-architecture and bone mineral density, via a change in bone remodelling (increased resorption and decreased formation), occurs with binge drinking. These findings suggest that young people who regularly engage in binge drinking may decrease their peak bone mass and be at risk for later skeletal problems.

In adults, cigarette smoking is associated with lower bone mineral density and increased fracture risk. Evidence from several observational studies in adolescents and young adults suggests that associations with smoking are already evident early in life. This suggests that smoking in adolescence and young adulthood negatively impacts on peak bone mass, which in turn has implications for bone health later in life.

12.7 Iron deficiency in teenagers and young adults

Iron deficiency is the primary cause of anaemia, a public health problem that affects populations in both rich and poor countries. It is estimated that around 25% of the world's population has anaemia, around half of which is iron-deficiency anaemia. The main risk factors for iron deficiency and iron-deficiency anaemia are low intake of iron, poor iron absorption (from diets high in phytate or phenolic compounds, or low in ascorbic acid and meat/fish), periods of life when iron requirements are especially high (e.g. growth and pregnancy), heavy blood loss as a result of menstruation, and acute and chronic infections.

Anaemia carries implications for both mental and physical performance. Symptoms include fatigue, lassitude and breathlessness on exertion, and evidence from observational studies suggests that iron-deficiency anaemia is associated with poor cognition. However, iron-deficiency anaemia is also associated with a number of socio-economic and biomedical disadvantages that can affect young people's development.

Prevalence of iron deficiency and iron-deficiency anaemia

The highest prevalence of anaemia is in pre-school children (<5 years), with an estimated 43% being affected worldwide (11% in high-income regions, 26% in central and eastern Europe), whereas the worldwide prevalence of anaemia in older children and adolescents is estimated to be approximately 25% according to the World Health Organization. Iron requirements rise once menstruation starts, and in the UK, iron intakes are particularly poor in young females. Iron intakes below the lower reference nutrient intake are found in 44% of girls aged 11–15 years and 40% of those aged 16–24 years.

Almost a third of 11- to 18-year-old girls have low plasma ferritin levels (below 15 µg/L), a marker for long-term iron intake, and 9% have low haemoglobin levels (below 120 g/L), indicating iron-deficiency anaemia. The prevalence of low haemoglobin levels is similar in women aged 19–34 years with 7–8% being affected, whereas the prevalence of low plasma ferritin levels decreases with age and is around 16% in 19- to 24-year-old women and 8% in 25- to 34-year-olds. Low haemoglobin and plasma ferritin levels are less common among adolescent boys and young men. It is estimated that around 5% of 15- to 18-year-old girls have iron-deficiency anaemia; prevalence is lower in young women. Iron-deficiency anaemia has been shown to be particularly common in girls who have tried to lose weight and among vegetarians.

Role of diet in preventing iron deficiency

Although there is no clear association between levels of iron in the diet and iron status, low iron intakes over an extended period of time are likely to lead to depletion of body stores. Around 90% of iron in the UK diet is present as non-haem iron. The remainder exists as haem iron, which is found almost entirely in foods of animal origin. Haem iron is generally well absorbed in the intestines. The extent to which non-haem iron is absorbed is principally influenced by systemic iron needs; more iron is absorbed from the diet in a state of iron deficiency and less is absorbed when iron stores are replete. Evidence, mainly from single meal studies, suggests that iron absorption is also influenced by the presence of other components in the diet (e.g. vitamin C and meat enhance absorption, phytates and phenolic compounds inhibit absorption). Evidence from whole diet studies over a number of days or weeks suggests that the overall effect of enhancers and inhibitors on iron absorption is considerably less than predicted from single meal studies (see Chapter 10 for more details).

There is some evidence to suggest that iron supplementation may improve attention and concentration in adolescents irrespective of baseline iron status, and improves intelligence quotient in anaemic children. Data from studies in children suggest there is evidence for a beneficial effect of iron treatment on cognitive development in anaemic children, but none of the trials reported long-term follow-up of children to determine whether any benefits were sustained.

12.8 Cognitive function and mental health

Dietary factors influencing cognitive function and performance

Various dietary factors have been studied in relation to cognitive function and performance. Most studies have been carried out in children or adolescents as the school setting provides a unique opportunity to study the effect of diet on cognitive performance, or in older people with regard to cognitive decline.

Breakfast

Eating breakfast as opposed to skipping breakfast has been found to have a positive effect on cognitive performance, which is more obvious later in the morning. Evidence suggests breakfast has beneficial effects for on-task behaviour in the classroom, mainly in younger children (<13 years). For school performance outcomes, there may be a positive association between habitual breakfast frequency/quality and school grades/achievement test scores. However, research on breakfast and educational outcomes is prone to confounding, not least because breakfast consumption levels vary by socio-economic background, which some studies fail to account for.

Several studies in young people have considered the glycaemic index (GI) of breakfast, finding that consuming a lower GI breakfast is associated with beneficial effects on cognitive performance, including memory, attention, response time and accuracy. Beneficial effects of a low-GI compared with a high-GI breakfast or breakfast omission were mainly observed later in the morning. However, there is insufficient evidence to demonstrate a consistent directional effect of the glycaemic load (GL) of breakfast (a measure that combines both the GI and the amount of carbohydrate present) on short-term cognitive performance. This may be because GL can be lowered in two ways: by lowering the GI of a food, or by lowering the carbohydrate content. If the amount of carbohydrate eaten at breakfast is low, even if it is released into the bloodstream slowly, it will only affect blood sugar levels for a small amount of time. Evidence to date suggests that more studies in this area may be warranted.

Snacking

Although there is a limited amount of research in this area, some studies hint that increased eating frequency and snacking appears to be beneficial for cognitive function (especially memory) and mood, by counteracting the decline in cognitive function sometimes experienced between meals. More research is needed to confirm these findings and to understand if the timing of intake and/or snack composition modifies any potential effects.

Omega-3 fatty acids

Early studies on the effects of the long-chain omega-3 fatty acids, eicosapentaenoic acid (EPA) and docosahexaenoic acid (DHA), suggested that DHA and EPA may improve cognitive performance, although these studies were carried out in children and adolescents with symptoms of neurodevelopmental disorders (dyspraxia and attention deficit hyperactivity disorder). However, the findings of two subsequent UK studies did not support this proposition, and it is unlikely that taking fish oil supplements will improve cognitive function or performance in young people. No health claims relating to DHA intake in children, adolescents or adults and cognitive function are as yet permitted in the EU.

Vitamins and minerals

There is evidence that deficiency of some nutrients (e.g. iron-deficiency anaemia) can lead to impaired cognitive function. Vitamins and minerals suggested to be linked to cognitive processes in children are iodine, iron, zinc and vitamin B_{12}. Although evidence for a potential benefit of supplementation of single nutrients is missing, data from clinical trials in children and adolescents aged 5–16 years suggest that supplementation with preparations providing at least three micronutrients given for a minimum duration of 4 weeks is associated with an increase in non-verbal intelligence and academic performance. However, observed increases are marginal and more research is needed before public health recommendations can be given.

Eating disorders in teenage and young adulthood

The illnesses anorexia nervosa, bulimia nervosa, binge eating disorder and their variants are characterised by a serious disturbance in eating, as well as distress or excessive concern about body shape or weight. In addition to their impact on psychological well-being, they can have a devastating effect on health through the physiological consequences of altered nutritional status and/or purging. The epidemiology of eating disorders has gradually changed. Eating disorders have typically been seen in girls and young women, but there is now an increasing prevalence in males. Of particular concern is the increasing prevalence of eating disorders at progressively younger ages.

Anorexia nervosa is a serious illness in which people keep their body weight abnormally low by dieting, vomiting or exercising excessively, leading to prolonged and extreme weight loss. A major factor in the development of this disease is anxiety about body shape and weight that originates from a fear of being fat or from wanting to be thin. Factors associated with the onset of anorexia nervosa include perceived pressure from the family and the environment, obsessive desires to be in control of the body, as well as media obsession with thinness and the media's 'bullying' of fatness (e.g. celebrities being gibed for gaining weight). The effects of anorexia nervosa include loss of muscle and bone strength, cessation of periods and, if prolonged and severe, it can lead to death. Anorexia nervosa in young people is similar to that in adults in terms of its psychological characteristics, but young people who are still growing may, in addition to being underweight, also have stunted growth.

People who suffer from bulimia nervosa feel that they have lost control over their eating, as opposed to obsession with control in anorexic people. Bulimia nervosa is characterised by a cycle of eating large quantities of food (binge eating) and then vomiting, taking laxatives and diuretics (purging), or excessive exercising and fasting in order to prevent weight gain. In contrast to anorexia nervosa, the body weight of people with bulimia nervosa is often normal. Bulimia nervosa can lead to tiredness, feeling bloated, constipation, abdominal pain, irregular periods, or occasional swelling of the hands and feet. Excessive vomiting can cause erosion of teeth, while laxative misuse can seriously affect the heart.

A large number of people with eating disorders do not meet the strict criteria for anorexia nervosa and bulimia nervosa. These eating disorders are often labelled as 'eating disorder not otherwise specified', and their prevalence is estimated to be higher than the prevalence of anorexia and bulimia nervosa. Patients with eating disorders not otherwise specified often experience the same physical and psychological consequences as do those who reach the threshold for diagnosis of anorexia or bulimia nervosa. Athletes and performers, particularly those who participate in sports and activities that reward a lean body (e.g. gymnastics, running, wrestling, dance, modelling) may be at particular risk of developing partial-syndrome eating disorders.

Although the manifestations of these disorders are via the diet, they are in fact psychological disorders and underlying problems need to be treated by trained and expert multidisciplinary teams.

Body image

Body image has an important role in self-evaluation, mental health and psychological well-being. Young people experience many bodily changes throughout adolescence, and pubertal development is often associated with poorer body image among girls but with more positive body attitudes among boys. Although being 'slim' is greatly valued in society, particularly among females, and the stigmatisation of overweight and obesity is high, body image seems to act independently of actual body weight. Rather, the perception of being overweight is the strongest predictor of attempts to lose weight, with consequent dieting that can pose health risks. Figure 12.5 shows that, across Europe, more girls than boys think they are a bit or much too fat, which is in contrast to data showing a higher prevalence of overweight and obesity in boys than in girls (see Section 12.5: 'Prevalence of overweight and obesity').

Popular media are thought to have a large influence on young people's body image, and although for young girls this typically 'slim' look is often unobtainable, the adoption of unhealthy practices may occur in a bid to try to conform. These practices may include smoking, meal skipping (notably breakfast), as well as severely reducing

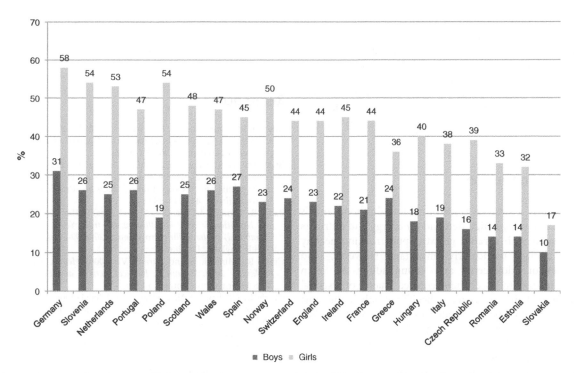

Figure 12.5 Proportion of 15-year-olds from selected European countries who think they are a bit or much too fat. *Source*: Currie *et al.* (2008). Reproduced with permission of WHO.

intake of foods deemed fattening (often red meat and dairy foods, which are sources of protein, iron, zinc and calcium, among other nutrients) and the adoption of very low energy (and therefore nutrient) diets. Girls tend to be more dissatisfied with their appearance than boys; however, data from the 1997 National Diet and Nutrition Survey, which found 16% of girls and 3% of boys aged 15–18 years reported being on some form of diet, suggests boys also feel such social pressures.

High levels of body dissatisfaction and body image disturbances are also predictive of depressive mood and psychosomatic complaints. They also can lead to inappropriate eating behaviours or eating disorders such as anorexia.

Adopting a healthy attitude to diet and physical activity has become increasingly difficult in a society where obesity is endemic and body fat is stigmatised. Young people's eating habits are strongly influenced by the world around them, including the attitudes and habits of family, in particular of the mother, and friends. It is therefore important that those involved in young people's development and upbringing try to instil in youngsters the need to develop healthy dietary and physical activity habits, in the hope that such behaviours will track through into the adult years.

12.9 Pregnancy in teenage and young adulthood

The UK has one of the highest teenage pregnancy rates in western Europe. Teenage pregnancy has profound consequences for those affected, and is 'strongly associated with the most deprived and socially excluded young people' in society (DfES, 2006). Pregnancy during the teenage years will affect both the emotional and physiological status of the mother. Nutritional demands increase to meet the needs of a growing fetus, at a time when the maternal body still requires extra nutrients for growth and development. The situation is compounded by the fact that a considerable percentage of young girls and women have suboptimal intakes of some nutrients (see earlier in this chapter and Chapter 17 for more information). Iron is one such nutrient that is particularly important during pregnancy, but for which intakes are generally low in young women. Epidemiological studies suggest that a low haemoglobin concentration during pregnancy is a marker of increased risk of low birth weight and perinatal mortality, although a causal relationship with iron supply has not been established. Folate intake is also of particular concern – an adequate intake of folate is essential before and during the first 3 months of pregnancy, to help reduce the risk of neural tube defects in the developing fetus. It is for this reason that the Department of Health recommends women of childbearing age to take a folic acid supplement daily. However, as the majority of teenage pregnancies are unplanned, consumption of folic acid supplements prior to conception and during the first trimester of pregnancy is unlikely.

12.10 Conclusions

Teenage is a time of transition into adulthood and is characterised by a high demand for energy and nutrients associated with a rapid growth spurt, making healthy food choices particularly important. However, food choices of adolescents and young adults are often poor, leading to lower than required intakes of essential nutrients. This can impact on health not only in the short term, but can have consequences for health later in life. For example, insufficient intakes of calcium coupled with low vitamin D status can have implications for bone health in later adulthood. Dietary choices not only affect physical development, but also cognitive function and performance. This is particularly relevant for young people who attend school or university, as unhealthy food choices may limit their cognitive capacity. For example, eating breakfast is associated positively with cognitive performance, but is regularly skipped by adolescents and young adults. Owing to the importance of a healthy diet during a time of rapid growth and possible implications of dietary shortcomings during this life stage for health in later life, dietary and lifestyle interventions focused at this age group are of particular importance. However, owing to increased independence of adolescents and young adults, it may be difficult to target this age group, as opposed to younger children who can generally still be more easily reached through school-based interventions.

References

Absoud, M., Cummins, C., Lim, M.J. et al. (2011) Prevalence and predictors of vitamin D insufficiency in children: a Great Britain population based study. PLoS One, 6(7), e22179.

Brodersen, H.N., Steptoe, A., Boniface, D.R. and Wardle, J. (2007) Trends in physical activity and sedentary behaviour in adolescence: ethnic and socioeconomic differences. British Journal of Sports Medicine, 41, 140–144.

Bates, B., Lennox, A., Prentice, A. et al. (eds) (2012) National Diet and Nutrition Survey. Headline results from Years 1, 2 and 3 (Combined) of the Rolling Programme (2008/09-2010/11) Public Health England, London.

Craig, R., Mindell, J. and Hirani, V. (2009) Health Survey for England – 2008. Volume 1: Physical Activity and Fitness. The NHS Information Centre, London.

Currie, C., Gabhainn, S.N., Godeau, E. et al. (eds) (2008) Inequalities in Young People's Health. Health Behaviour in School-aged Children International Report from the 2005/2006 Survey. WHO Regional Office for Europe, Copenhagen.

Department of Health, Physical Activity, Health Improvement and Protection (2011) Start Active, Stay Active: A Report on Physical Activity from the Four Home Countries' Chief Medical Officers. https://www.gov.uk/government/uploads/system/uploads/attachment_data/file/216370/dh_128210.pdf (accessed 6 December 2016).

DfES (2006) Teenage Pregnancy: Accelerating the Strategy to 2010. Department for Education and Skills. http://webarchive.nationalarchives.gov.uk/20130401151715/http://www.education.gov.uk/publications/eOrderingDownload/DFES-03905-2006.pdf (accessed 9 January 2017).

SACN (2016) Vitamin D and Health. https://www.gov.uk/government/uploads/system/uploads/attachment_data/file/537616/SACN_Vitamin_D_and_Health_report.pdf (accessed 9 January 2017).

Sandercock, G., Angus, C. and Barton, J. (2010) Physical activity levels of children living in different built environments. Preventive Medicine, 50, 193–198.

13
Nutrition in Older Adults

Ashley T LaBrier, Clare A Corish, and Johanna T Dwyer

Key messages

- Globally, the demographic profile is shifting towards a more elderly population.
- Although individuals of industrialised nations who are over 65 years of age are healthier than ever before, chronic degenerative diseases and other illnesses still affect older adults increasingly with advancing age.
- Changes that often accompany the ageing process, such as hearing and vision loss and anthropometric changes, create challenges to nutritional assessment in the older adult population. Determining the most appropriate outcome measures, such as longevity or quality of life, is also challenging with this age group.

- Nutrition screening and assessment using biological and social determinants of nutritional status are critical to implementing effective nutritional or other interventions to ameliorate diet-related health complications.
- Nutritional interventions vary from medical nutritional therapy to social meal programmes and exist both at the individual and community levels.
- Challenges remain for public health nutrition in older adults, including the development of stronger evidence-based dietary reference standards, nutritional interventions and means for maintaining functional status and quality of life.

13.1 Introduction

The ageing population

The simultaneous decline in birth rate and the rise in life expectancy both at birth and age 65 years in many countries are creating a worldwide demographic shift in which older adults constitute a greater and greater proportion of the population than at any other time in history. In 2000, approximately 7% of the world population was aged 65 years or older – which represented an increase of 5% from 1950. This trend is expected to continue, and the proportion of older adults is expected to reach nearly 16% by the year 2050 (Figure 13.1) (United Nations, 2013). In contrast, the share of the population worldwide made up of persons under age 15 years is anticipated to drop from 26% in 2013 to 21% in 2050. This demographic process, in which the proportion of older persons in the population increases and that of the younger persons lessens, is known as population ageing.

Although, historically, it was the highly industrialised nations that had the greatest proportion of older adults in their population, and the proportion continues to grow, today the most rapid increase in the number of older adults is occurring in the developing world. Europe is the 'oldest' region in the world and it is expected to maintain this title well into the twenty-first century, as it has had the highest population proportion of adults aged 65 years and over for several decades. The proportion of older individuals in the USA also continues to rise. From 2005 to 2030, the number of older adults in the USA is predicted to nearly double, so that it will then constitute 20% of the country's residents (Figure 13.1) (United Nations, 2013). Worldwide population ageing makes the public health challenge to increase the number of older adults who lead high-quality, productive and independent lives globally relevant to all.

Conditions and diseases affecting the health of older adults

In Europe, the USA and highly industrialised countries elsewhere in the world, advances in modern medicine and public health have largely eliminated the infectious

Public Health Nutrition, Second Edition. Edited by Judith L Buttriss, Ailsa A Welch, John M Kearney and Susan A Lanham-New.
© 2018 by The Nutrition Society. Published 2018 by John Wiley & Sons, Ltd.
Companion website: www.wiley.com/go/buttriss/publichealth

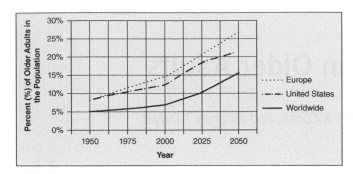

Figure 13.1 The percentage of adults 65 years old or older in the total population of Europe, the USA and worldwide from 1950–2050. *Source*: adapted from United Nations (2013).

diseases of childhood and many communicable diseases in adults, such as tuberculosis. As a result, in Europe, people reaching the age of 65 years are expected to live an average of 15.5 years more, while life expectancy at birth of the typical American has increased by 30 years in the last century. Although the decline in infectious diseases and acute illnesses has allowed more individuals to live longer, the prevalence of age-related chronic degenerative diseases and illnesses is rising, simply because life expectancy has increased so much and in spite of the fact that at least until the eighties, people at any given age are healthier than ever before. Heart disease and cancers are now the major killers of those living in the highly industrialised world, along with other chronic degenerative diseases such as chronic obstructive lung disease, stroke, Alzheimer's disease and diabetes mellitus – some of which are exacerbated by or contribute to poor nutrition (Figure 13.2). These chronic diseases have caused the number of healthy life years (HLYs) to remain unchanged in recent years despite the increase in average

life expectancy of approximately 0.25 years annually; unfortunately, because the number of HLYs remains unchanged, Europeans still spend 20–25% of their lives in poor health.

Chronic degenerative diseases and conditions have a great and long-lasting negative impact on the quality of life of older people. For example, approximately 80% of older US adults are living with at least one chronic condition, and 50% are living with at least two. Within the World Health Organization (WHO) European region, the proportion of disease burden due to chronic disease reaches about 95% in people aged 60 years and older. These individuals are at a greater risk for having a lower quality life than their healthy counterparts since chronic disease is so often associated with a decline in functional ability and mental status, and greater likelihood of limitations in performing usual activities. The lessening of physical capabilities creates challenges in performing normal tasks of self-care in daily life that are measured with a scale called the activities of daily living (ADLs), such as self-feeding,

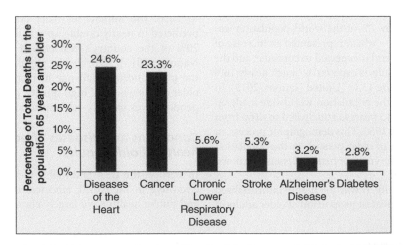

Figure 13.2 Percentage of total deaths from various chronic conditions in adults 65 years and older in the USA, 2008–2009. *Source*: adapted from Heron (2012).

Table 13.1 Percentage of persons 18 years and older having limitation in ADLs, instrumental ADLs (IADLs), and percentage of those who are limited as a result of one or more chronic conditions, USA, 2010.

Age group (years)	Limited in ADLs (%)	Limited in IADLs (%)	Limited in usual activities due to one or more chronic conditions (%)
18–44	0.6	1.4	5.8
45–64	1.9	3.7	16.5
65–74	3.7	6.5	25
≥75	11	18.8	42.5

Source: Adams *et al.* (2011).

toileting and managing personal hygiene (Table 13.1). The presence of these limitations can mean a loss in independence and a need for institutionalised care. In addition to the decline in physical functional status, emotional and mental problems may affect an individual's performance of the IADLs. Although IADLs are not necessary for physical functioning, they represent important activities that must be carried out if the individual is to be able to live independently. IADLs include an individual's ability to complete household chores, take medications, manage basic finances, use various mechanisms for communication and transport his/herself within the community. Chronic disease can also restrict an individual's engagement in life, social interactions and enjoyment with family and friends.

The WHO quantifies the burden of disease using disability-adjusted life years (DALYs), a metric that calculates the number of years of healthy life by considering years lost due to poor health, disability and premature death. When the measure is summed across a population, it indicates the difference between current health status and an ideal scenario in which the average population lives free of disability and disease to an advanced age. DALYs provide a means to compare between countries, and, if the effects of interventions on these parameters are known, to evaluate their relative significance on public health.

Prevalence of morbidity and functional limitations in older adults

Since adults are living longer than ever before, it is important that morbidity and functional limitations be avoided or compressed into the fewest number of years possible, so that quality of life is maintained to the greatest extent. However, US and European health statistics show that some debilitating conditions, many of which have a dietary component, are on the rise within the older population. For example, in Europe, it is estimated that 18.5 million people aged 60–79 years in

the EU27 have diabetes, while the prevalence of diagnosed diabetes in US adults over 65 years of age has increased by almost 10% in only 30 years. Currently, approximately 30% of older US adults are diagnosed with diabetes, and it is estimated that nearly another 10% of this population remains undiagnosed, and thus unmanaged, setting them up for a higher likelihood of experiencing diabetes-related health complications later in life. The current disability measures are particularly discouraging for the older population, as approximately two-thirds of older adults report that they are limited in their ability to complete at least one basic or complex activity. Physical limitations and disease increase the risk of a variety of poor health outcomes, including poor nutritional status, which may result in a downward cycle of health and quality of life.

Dietary standards for the older adult population

Health Canada and the National Academy's Institute of Medicine (IOM) in the USA provide nutrient requirements in the dietary reference intakes (DRIs), a compilation of nutrient reference standards by life stage and gender and their rationales. Table 13.2 provides relevant

Table 13.2 The DRIs and their definitions from the US IOM

DRI reference value	Definition
Estimated average requirement (EAR)	The average daily nutrient intake level that is estimated to meet the requirements of half of the healthy individuals in a particular life stage and gender group.
Recommended dietary allowance (RDA)	The average daily dietary nutrient intake level that is sufficient to meet the nutrient requirements of nearly all (97–98%) healthy individuals in a particular life stage and gender group
Adequate intake (AI)	The recommended average daily intake level based on observed or experimentally determined approximations of nutrient intake by a group (or groups) of apparently healthy people that are assumed to be adequate; used when RDA cannot be determined.
Tolerable upper intake level (UL)	The highest average daily nutrient intake level that is likely to pose no risk of adverse health effects to almost all individuals in the general population. As intake increases above the UL, the potential risk of adverse effects increases.

Source: Otten *et al.* (2006).

Table 13.3 DRIs from the IOM of the National Academies in the USA. RDAs and AIs for macronutrients for adults aged 51 years and older.

Gender and age (years)	Carbohydrate (g/day)	Total fibre (g/day)	Fat (g/day)	Linoleic acid (g/day)	α-Linolenic acid (g/day)	Protein (g/day)
Men						
51–70	130	30[a]	ND	14[a]	1.6[a]	56[b]
>70	130	30[a]	ND	14[a]	1.6[a]	56[b]
Women						
51–70	130	21[a]	ND	11[a]	1.1[a]	46[b]
>70	130	21[a]	ND	11[a]	1.1[a]	46[b]

Source: The Institute of Medicine of the National Academies (2002/2005).
ND: not determined.
[a] AIs are shown when the information to determine an RDA is insufficient.
[b] Based 0.8 g per kilogram body weight per day for the reference body weight.

definitions. The recommendations provide a scientific foundation for the development of food guides and nutrition education to meet the needs of healthy individuals at all life stages, including old age. Worldwide, similar dietary standards exist; the EU produced population reference intakes in 1993, which have been undergoing review since 2010. In the UK, the series of dietary reference values (established in 1991) are used. In 2003 the WHO European region published its *Food Based Dietary Guidelines* (WHO, 2003), while Australia and New Zealand produced nutrient reference values in 2006. In the USA, the RDA is one of the DRI standards that represents the average daily intake of a nutrient that is sufficient to meet the nutritional requirement for 97–98% of healthy individuals within the specific reference population. The equivalent reference value in the UK is the reference nutrient intake. When data are insufficient to determine an RDA on the functional criterion of interest, an AI is suggested by the IOM. The specific US RDAs and AIs for men and women aged 51 years and older are given in Tables 13.3, 13.4 and 13.5.

The corresponding UK values are listed in this book's Appendix.

As ageing occurs, the body undergoes physiological changes, and the requirements for some nutrients alter as a result. Within the population of older adults there are specific concerns about intakes of several macronutrients (including energy, protein and alcohol) and micronutrients (including vitamin B_{12}, vitamin D and calcium).

Energy

With ageing, energy requirements usually decrease due both to a reduced resting metabolic rate (which is due chiefly to the decline in lean body mass) and reduced energy expenditure (because of declines in physical activity). In 2011, the UK Scientific Advisory Committee on Nutrition (SACN) revised its dietary reference values for energy for all population groups including for those aged 65–74 years and ≥75 years (Scientific Advisory Committee on Nutrition, 2011). The SACN noted that age-related changes in lifestyle and activity are very variable, and that in mobile older adults the energy

Table 13.4 DRIs from the IOM of the National Academies in the USA. RDAs and AIs for selected vitamins for adults 51 years old and older.

Gender and age (years)	Vitamin A (µg/day)	Vitamin C (mg/day)	Vitamin D (IU/day)	Vitamin E (mg/day)	Vitamin K (µg/day)	Thiamin (mg/day)	Riboflavin (mg/day)	Niacin (mg/day)	Vitamin B_6 (mg/day)	Folate (µg/day)	Vitamin B_{12} (µg/day)
Men											
51–70	900	90	600	15	120[a]	1.2	1.3	16	1.7	400	2.4
>70	900	90	800	15	120[a]	1.2	1.3	16	1.7	400	2.4
Women											
51–70	700	75	600	15	90[a]	1.1	1.1	14	1.5	400	2.4
>70	700	75	800	15	90[a]	1.1	1.1	14	1.5	400	2.4

Sources: Institute of Medicine (US) Standing Committee on the Scientific Evaluation of Dietary Reference Intakes (1997), Institute of Medicine (US) Standing Committee on the Scientific Evaluation of Dietary Reference Intakes and its Panel on Folate, Other B Vitamins, and Choline (1998), Institute of Medicine (US) Panel on Dietary Antioxidants and Related Compounds (2000), Institute of Medicine (US) Panel on Micronutrients (2001) and Ross *et al.* (2011).
[a] AIs are shown when the information to determine an RDA is insufficient.

Table 13.5 DRIs from the IOM of the National Academies in the USA. RDAs and AIs for selected elements for adults 51 years old and older.

Gender and age (years)	Calcium (mg/day)	Chromium (μg/day)	Copper (μg/day)	Fluoride (mg/day)	Iodine (μg/day)	Iron (mg/day)	Magnesium (mg/day)	Selenium (μg/day)	Zinc (mg/day)
Men									
51–70	1000	30[a]	900	4[a]	150	8	420	55	11
>70	1200	30[a]	900	4[a]	150	8	420	55	11
Women									
51–70	1200	20[a]	900	3[a]	150	8	320	55	8
>70	1200	20[a]	900	3[a]	150	8	320	55	8

Sources: Institute of Medicine (US) Standing Committee on the Scientific Evaluation of Dietary Reference Intakes (1997), Institute of Medicine (US) Panel on Dietary Antioxidants and Related Compounds (2000), Institute of Medicine (US) Panel on Micronutrient (2001) and Ross *et al.* (2011).
* AIs are shown when the information to determine an RDA is insufficient.

requirements are unlikely to differ substantially from younger adults; thus, reference values can be described in the same way. For individuals with reduced mobility and older people who are not in good health, energy requirements can be based on the less active 25th centile physical activity level (PAL) value of 1.49, recognising that for some groups of older people with specific diseases or disabilities and for patient groups who are bed-bound or confined to a wheelchair, the PAL value may be consistently lower than this. For older adults as a group, US national survey data show that the decline in energy need roughly parallels a decline in energy consumption. In the population-based US National Health and Nutrition Examination Survey (NHANES), the average adult aged at least 60 years consumes approximately 25% less energy than the population of 20- to 39-year-olds, in which energy intake is the highest.

Unfortunately for many older individuals, with ageing, the energy intakes do not decline as much as do energy outputs, and elevated energy intakes contribute to overweight and obesity with their attendant health risks. In the NHANES time series, among the 60–74 years age group, despite declining intake with age, average energy consumption rose over the last few decades. From the early 1970s to 2000 in the USA, the mean daily energy intake of men and women increased by11% and 20% respectively, correlating with the rise in prevalence of obesity in this age group. Indeed, from the early 1970s to the year 2000, the prevalence of obesity in US men increased by 25% and in women by 16%. In Europe, studies such as the Scottish Health Survey 1999–2008, the French ObEpi survey 1997–2006 and the Spanish ENRICA study 2008–2010 predicted that the prevalence of obesity among older people in Europe would reach 20–30% by 2015 (Mathus-Vliegen *et al.*, 2012). The recently published UK National Diet and Nutrition Survey provides evidence for the predicted increase in bodyweight with 29% of all older UK adults now classified as obese (Bates *et al.*, 2014).

Although a somewhat higher body mass index (BMI) in elderly people may have some protective health effects in populations with some diseases and conditions, such as end-stage renal disease, overweight and obesity are typically associated with significant impairments in health-related quality of life, and therefore weight control is desirable. Overweight and obesity also contribute to the severity of several chronic diseases including, type 2 diabetes, hypertension, osteoarthritis and certain cancers (breast, prostate, colon and endometrial). Therefore, it is important to achieve energy balance as energy needs decrease with age. Recently, however, a specific condition in the elderly has been described; the term 'sarcopenic obesity' was used to characterise the confluence of excess fat coexisting with low lean body mass (Roubenoff, 2004). In sarcopenic obesity, muscle mass is low relative to the total weight. Loss of muscle quantity and quality is observed with decreased number and size of muscle fibres, reduced mitochondrial function and decreased synthesis of muscle protein. These changes result in decreased functional capacity and quality of life, increased risk of disability, morbidity and mortality, and increased risk of frailty, falls and loss of independency. Thus, obesity and sarcopenia in the elderly may potentiate each other, maximising their effects on disability and morbidity.

In addition to overweight and obesity, some older persons are underweight with very low BMIs, and underweight may be so marked that it is associated with protein–energy undernutrition. This condition is linked with multiple poor outcomes, including increasing frailty and liability to infection, a greater risk of institutional placement and an increased risk of morbidity and mortality. The decline in energy intake is often associated with deteriorating intakes of essential nutrients. This is particularly true when energy-dense but nutrient-poor high-fat foods with added sugar are plentiful and replace nutrient-dense foods in an older person's diet. Dietary guidelines in highly industrialised countries that provide recommendations for promoting health and preventing diet-related disease encourage consumption of nutrient-dense foods, which provide vitamins and minerals with relatively few calories to meet nutrient needs within energy needs. Public health professionals need to be alert to signs of excessive as well as deficient energy intakes and take steps to correct them whenever possible.

Protein

As is the case with energy intakes, in cross-sectional studies, protein consumption is highest in middle-aged adults and lower in older adults. NHANES data from 2009–2010 show that average protein intake was lower than the highest intakes by 31% (74 g/day) in men and 14% (60 g/day) in women older than 70 years. Since NHANES is a cross-sectional survey, and not a longitudinal study of the same individuals, this does not imply that all older individuals have lower protein intakes than younger adults. However, it does suggest that decreases in intakes are likely with advancing age, although it should be noted that mean intakes are still adequate. The current IOM recommendations for protein are for an RDA of 0.8 g of protein per kilogram body weight per day for non-pregnant, non-lactating adults 19 years or older, or 56 g of protein for men and 46 g for the average woman. IOM recommendations do not suggest that higher intakes are needed for older persons. The UK Committee on Medical Aspects of Food and Nutrition Policy 1991 recommendations are similar to those of the IOM with the reference nutrient intake set at 0.75 g of protein per kilogram body weight per day, equating to approximately 56 g/day and 45 g/day for men and women respectively. The European Food Safety Authority recommends a population reference intake of 0.83 g of protein per kilogram body weight per day for adults of all ages applicable both to high-quality protein and to protein in mixed diets. The most recent nitrogen balance studies do not indicate that requirements are increased in healthy older adults, or that the timing of protein intake throughout the day may be important to maximise utilisation, but further research is needed with more sophisticated measures of protein metabolism before the issue can be definitively resolved (Volpi *et al.*, 2013). Moreover, not all elderly adults are healthy. Thus, there is currently much controversy about appropriate protein intakes for older individuals and whether in fact recommendations should be higher to maximise parameters other than nitrogen balance, the criterion used in the DRI. The rationale for suggesting that a higher intake may be appropriate for elderly adults is based on a large longitudinal study, the ABC study, in the USA in older adults that showed better function among those with higher protein intakes as measured with a food frequency questionnaire. Some also claim that

higher intakes will help maintain muscle mass and avoid sarcopenia. With pronounced sarcopenia, mobility may be impaired and the risk of falls and fall-related fractures rises. Although the pathophysiology of sarcopenia is not well understood, it may be associated with catabolic responses to illness. Furthermore, the anabolic response of muscle to dietary protein requires more protein with increasing age. Dietary protein also positively affects hormone levels and calcium absorption, both of which may facilitate muscle and bone synthesis. Studies using isotopic tracers suggest that needs may be higher than those estimated by nitrogen balance studies to maintain homeostasis. However, it remains to be seen if the increased intakes are linked to improvements in functional status. On the basis of these considerations, some experts now recommend intakes in the range of 1.0–1.2 g of protein per kilogram body weight per day for healthy individuals aged 65 years or more (Bauer *et al.*, 2013). Protein quality, timing of intake and amino acid supplementation may be considered so as to achieve the greatest benefits from protein intake, but further studies are needed to make explicit recommendations. Even higher protein intakes are suggested for individuals with moderate to severe acute or chronic disease, and for any older person exhibiting protein–energy malnutrition. The notable exception to these recommendations is older persons with severe chronic kidney disease, not undergoing regular dialysis, who cannot tolerate such protein loads (Bauer *et al.*, 2013).

The findings on protein requirements in older people remain tantalising hypotheses until more experimental data on requirements and outcomes in terms of functional status are available to resolve the issue. In the meantime, it is important to remember that the vast majority of healthy older people living in highly industrialised countries, including the USA and Europe, have protein intakes that far surpass the RDA. Nevertheless, there may be some frail and ill individuals whose energy and protein intakes are so low they are catabolic, and metabolise dietary protein for energy. These individuals need to be identified and treated by provision of adequate amounts of energy and protein to prevent sarcopenia and frailty. It may not be possible to reverse the catabolic process by nutritional interventions among older persons who are suffering from wasting or other disease processes, but adequate dietary intake may help to ameliorate the secondary malnutrition.

Alcohol

Although age does not dramatically affect the rate of absorption or elimination of alcohol from the body, other age-associated changes may cause adverse events at a relatively low level of alcohol consumption in older adults. The decrease in lean body mass and increase in adipose tissue that are associated with ageing correspond to a decrease in total body water. Since alcohol is water soluble and distributes throughout total body water, the volume of distribution is less, and alcohol concentration higher, in elderly individuals. Thus, an equivalent amount of alcohol administered to an older and a younger individual of similar size and of the same gender produces a higher blood alcohol concentration in the older individual. Moreover, many older adults take medications that may interact with alcohol and alter cognition. Finally, illness, death of loved ones and other adverse life events may lead to heavy drinking or binges to deal with the crises.

The 2012 US National Survey on Drug Use and Health (NSDUH) found that approximately 41% of older adults reported at least one incident of alcohol use in the month prior to survey completion; this is nearly 12% less than the population aged 55–65 years and 28% less than among those 21- to 25-year-olds whose alcohol use is the highest. The NSDUH also found the reported prevalence of 'binge' and 'heavy' alcohol use was lower in older adults than all other adult age groups. The European VINTAGE (Good Health into Older Age) study highlighted that older Europeans generally drink less than their younger counterparts, drink less hazardously and suffer less harm, but that within their drinking volumes the older persons' drinking patterns, determinants and associations appear no different from the younger population. This study confirmed the paucity of data on the topic and the need for more specific research. It was also noted that older persons seem to respond equally well to alcohol policy, screening instruments and brief interventions, as do younger people.

However, alcohol abuse remains a problem in a substantial minority of older adults. The US National Institute on Alcohol Abuse and Alcoholism has targeted older adults as a distinct group in which alcohol consumption, especially binge and heavy drinking, presents increased risks of health problems. Heavy alcohol intake is associated with a poor diet, and this is a particular concern in elderly adults whose age-associated decline in energy intake already makes adequate consumption of micronutrients difficult (Breslow et al., 2013). Additionally, many chronic diseases, including diabetes, chronic obstructive pulmonary disease, hypertension, heart failure, stroke, Alzheimer disease and other types of dementia, and mood disorders like depression, become more difficult to treat or are worsened by alcohol consumption. Public health professionals need to encourage primary care providers and those staffing emergency rooms to be alert for signs of alcohol abuse and treat it when it occurs, and to routinely screen for alcohol-related behavioural pathology.

Vitamin B$_{12}$

There is little evidence to suggest that vitamin B$_{12}$ intakes decrease with age, and yet low serum levels are more common in old age than in younger adults. One reason for this is malabsorption of vitamin B$_{12}$ due to atrophic gastritis, a condition that decreases secretion of gastric acid, which is an increasingly common phenomenon with ageing. Since naturally occurring vitamin B$_{12}$ is mainly found bound to the proteins of animal products, low secretion of gastric acid that occurs with ageing may result in an inability of the body to release vitamin B$_{12}$ from food proteins, making it unavailable for absorption. Decreased hydrochloric acid levels may also cause an overgrowth of intestinal bacteria that use vitamin B$_{12}$ in the stomach, further reducing the nutrient's availability to the body. Another cause of vitamin B$_{12}$ deficiency in ageing can be the excess use of proton pump inhibitors for gastroesophageal reflux, which neutralise gastric acid. Additionally, the prevalence of pernicious anaemia, a rare autoimmune disease that causes the destruction of parietal cells in the stomach whose secretion of intrinsic factor is required for the absorption of vitamin B$_{12}$, increases with age.

Vitamin B$_{12}$ status is important because the nutrient is a cofactor for enzymatic processes and is critical for blood formation and cognitive function; an inadequate supply may result in neuropathy, including numbness and tingling in the hands and feet, confusion, dementia, megaloblastic anaemia and gastrointestinal symptoms such as constipation. Prevention of poor vitamin B$_{12}$ status is particularly important because the reversibility of these neurological complications depends on the duration of deficiency before receiving treatment. To avoid insufficient vitamin B$_{12}$ levels, older persons are advised to consume fortified foods, such as vitamin-B$_{12}$-fortified cereals, as well as vitamin B$_{12}$ supplements, in addition to naturally occurring sources of vitamin B$_{12}$. Intake of sources where vitamin B$_{12}$ is not protein bound (as it is in naturally occurring sources) is more likely to prevent deficiency in older adults where the prevalence of atrophic gastritis is high. Individuals with pernicious anaemia need medical therapy with pharmacologic doses of vitamin B$_{12}$, but for other individuals this is not necessary. Periodic screening and early intervention to correct inadequate vitamin B$_{12}$ status in older adults has also been suggested as a mechanism to reduce deficiency in the population.

Vitamin D

About 80% of the body's vitamin D is synthesised de novo when skin is exposed to ultraviolet light, and remaining stores are obtained from dietary intake and supplements. Vitamin D (see Chapter 20) originating from food and supplements is biologically inert and must undergo subsequent activation by the liver and then the kidneys. Older adults are commonly deficient in vitamin D because both the skin conversion from irradiation and the kidneys' ability to convert the nutrient into the active hormone form decrease with age. Additional common risk factors for vitamin D deficiency in older adults include a decrease in dietary intake of vitamin-D-containing foods, impaired intestinal absorption, reduced sun exposure and the use of sunscreen. The recent review by Cashman and Kiely (2014) provides evidence for the prevalence of vitamin D deficiency across Europe.

Vitamin D promotes bone mineralisation through its role in intestinal absorption of calcium and phosphorus and their uptake into bone. Without adequate levels of vitamin D, individuals are at a higher risk of osteomalacia, osteoporosis and osteoporotic fractures. Thus, vitamin D is especially critical in ageing since bone mineralisation decreases with age. Muscle function in older adults may also decrease with inadequate vitamin D intake. Supplementation of vitamin D to adequate levels appears to improve muscle strength, walking distance, and overall functional ability in the elderly (Cashman and Kiely, 2014). Over the last decade, the scientific community has had an elevated interest in vitamin D's potential to prevent or ameliorate chronic degenerative diseases other than those related to bone. Researchers have suggested a relationship between the vitamin and health outcomes, such as increased immunity and prevention of colon or other cancers and diabetes. At present, these relationships are based largely on epidemiological data, and causal inference is difficult. The IOM in 2010 noted that current evidence supports the role of vitamin D in bone health, but that more research was needed to determine the role (if any) of vitamin D in other health conditions. The review by Cashman and Kiely (2014) summarises the US and European recommendations for vitamin D and suggests dietary strategies for increasing vitamin D intake and status. From the public health standpoint, it is important for all elderly individuals to achieve RDA levels from foods, fortified foods and dietary supplements. This strategy, combined with moderate exposure to sunlight, will help ensure adequate vitamin D status and contribute to bone health and, if these other health outcomes prove to be linked to vitamin D status, to them as well.

Calcium

Over 99% of calcium in the body is found in bone or teeth, where it provides strength to these hard tissues. Maintaining an AI of calcium can reduce the rate of age-related bone loss, although this is challenged by a decrease in calcium absorption with increased ageing. Evidence suggests that in postmenopausal women with low dietary calcium intake, calcium supplementation reduces the rate of bone loss. Other research has shown calcium and vitamin D supplementation given to deficient institutionalised elderly patients helps to preserve bone mineral density and reduce the risk of hip fracture.

Bone loss begins in adulthood, at around 30–40 years of age and is more severe in women than men due to the decade period of rapid bone loss that occurs with the onset of menopause, typically when women are in their early to mid fifties. In the seventh decade of life, this accelerated rate of bone loss declines, and from then on individuals of both sexes undergo continuous age-associated loss through the rest of their lifespans. Advancing age and its associated loss of bone result in a decrease in bone density that increases risk of fractures. The difference in men's and women's rate of bone loss correlates with an 11.5% lower lifetime risk of hip fracture at age 50 years in men than in women. Older persons who have fractures are often hospitalised and usually require a long convalescence, and full independence may never be regained. Fractures in the elderly are also linked with a shortened life expectancy, and have an overall negative socio-economic impact on the population.

In order to accommodate the age-related changes surrounding calcium and its role in bone health, the IOM recently reviewed the evidence for re-establishing calcium's DRIs, and set the RDA at 1000 mg/day for men aged 51–70 years old and 1200 mg/day for women 51–70 years old. The RDA was established at 1200 mg of calcium per day for all individuals above the age of 70, when the effect of ageing on bone loss appears to be similar in both men and women. From the public health standpoint, it is important to ensure that relatively inexpensive dietary sources of calcium, both naturally occurring and fortified, are available, and if needs are not met by food alone, to use calcium supplements. Also, although risks of fracture increase with poor calcium and vitamin D status, and thus intakes should be optimised, it is also important to remember environmental measures to prevent falls and broken bones.

13.2 Associations between diet and disease in older adults

Challenges to dietary intake assessment in older adults

One problem in dietary assessment of older adults is that their health is often poor due to decreases in mobility, sensory processes and cognitive function. These same changes often make dietary assessment of older persons difficult. For example, sensory impairments are quite common in the elderly population. In US adults over 65 years old, approximately 15% of individuals report difficulty seeing. Cataracts, which cause cloudy vision, are a common cause of faulty eyesight in the elderly. Of adults who live to 80 years, half will have cataracts that impact their vision. Auditory problems are even more frequent in older adults. Almost 50% of men and over 30% of women over 65 years note having some difficulty hearing. Vision and hearing impairments may impede an older person's ability to understand assessment questions, read materials and communicate with health practitioners.

Cognitive changes are also associated with ageing. Dementia, a syndrome involving impairments in memory, thinking and judgment to the extent that normal cognitive function may be interrupted, is more prevalent in adults of older age. The UK Alzheimer Society estimates that 1 in 14 people over the age of 65 years in the UK suffer from dementia. This estimate increases to one in six people for those who are over 80 years old. Alzheimer patients face a higher risk of poor nutritional intake, so it is important to circumvent memory deficits to assess dietary intake and avoid falsely low intakes. Successful interviews with those who have issues with memory may require probing, additional time and extra information or diet records kept by a caregiver.

Appropriate dietary standards for older adults

A second set of problems in dietary assessment of the elderly involves determining appropriate anthropometric, biochemical and clinical standards to use. The measurement of height, and thus the derivation of BMI, is difficult in ageing persons who suffer from scoliosis and loss of height. For this reason, measured rather than reported height is to be preferred. Also, measured weight is more accurate than reported weight. The current consensus on anthropometric standards is that some, such as BMI, remain approximately the same for older and younger adults, although a slightly increased weight may be advantageous in those with certain diseases. Overweight and obesity, which can be identified by BMI over $25\,kg/m^2$ and $30\,kg/m^2$ respectively, are associated with an increased risk of disease and premature mortality in younger adults, and it is generally agreed that the relationship exists in most older adults as well. Guidelines to categorise the weight status of all adults use the same BMI cut-offs (Table 13.6). However, the most favourable weight for optimal longevity may be higher for the elderly who are affected by chronic conditions, such as end-stage kidney disease, heart failure and obstructive lung diseases. This phenomenon of higher BMI categories associated with improved survival in specific populations is sometimes referred to the 'obesity paradox' or a 'reverse epidemiologic event'. Although the

Table 13.6 The standard weight status categories associated with BMI ranges for all adults.

BMI (kg/m²)	Weight status
<18.5	Underweight
18.5–24.9	Normal
25.0–29.9	Overweight
≥30	Obese

Source: CDC (2015).

phenomenon was first described in dialysis patients in the early 1980s and it has been observed in multiple populations since, the association is not yet well understood and remains controversial, creating challenges for determining appropriate anthropometric guidelines in these diseased groups (Flegal and Kalantar-Zade, 2013). Standards for other anthropometric measures, such as skinfolds, are even more difficult to interpret in the elderly.

Nutritional status is evaluated using a variety of tools, including biomarkers. Biochemical indices of nutritional status may be altered by medications and disease and thus may be nonspecific, reflecting poor health, medication usage or hydration status, as well as poor nutritional status, in older adults. For example, serum proteins, such as albumin, prealbumin and transferrin, are commonly measured as indicators of protein nutriture, but results can be difficult to interpret since they decrease with acute illness even in the face of good protein nutritional status. Chronic disease is a risk factor for protein–energy malnutrition, and low serum protein levels often indicate its presence rather than low protein intakes. Many chronic conditions, such as those of the liver and kidney, may independently lower serum protein levels even among persons in good nutritional status, making it challenging to distinguish the root cause of the biochemical alteration. Medication use, which is common in older people, is another example of how biochemical indices may be altered in the elderly. According to the US Centers for Disease Control (CDC), 9 out of 10 elderly people reported using at least one prescription drug in the last 30 days and nearly 7 out of 10 had used three or more. In Europe, use of potentially inappropriate medications among frail, community-dwelling elderly persons appears to be common, and the negative effects can be observed on dietary intake and nutritional status.

Medication use can also increase the risks of dehydration in the elderly. Dehydration makes the interpretation of biochemical data challenging because indicators become more concentrated within the body fluids. Excessive hydration and haemodilution as well as abnormal hydration of the lean body mass may occur with some renal diseases and congestive heart failure, both common among the elderly (Mentes, 2013).

Challenges to outcomes assessment in older adults

A final challenge in assessing the nutritional status of older adults is determining the most appropriate measures for judging health- and nutrition-related outcomes. Traditionally, health outcomes have been measured in terms of age-specific morbidity and mortality rates, but these have little meaning to individuals. Longevity alone is a futile criterion if quality of life and functional status are poor. Although DALYs, as discussed previously, take into account some of these factors on a wide scale, more outcome assessment measures should reflect the natural human desire to maintain well-being and quality of life in old age. Frailty, which may result from poor nutrition or other pathological processes, is a specific example of a clinical outcome linked to disability, and that may be a useful concept to consider for outcomes.

Quality of life and well-being

In addition to longevity, maintaining a positive sense of well-being, which subjectively incorporates social, mental and physical health, is a significant outcome from the perspective of the elderly population. Aside from meeting basic needs and having good health, being included and involved socially and having positive personal relationships are among the strongest positive influences on maintaining a sense of well-being and quality of life. For example, older individuals who experience exclusion in social situations are more likely to have a lower quality of life and less likely to feel empowered and satisfied with life. In order for the older adult to live a long life with vitality, rather than just a long life, western society needs to acknowledge and care for all the components of an individual's well-being in a collective manner. Measures of well-being and quality of life are starting to gain recognition for their value as statistics that provide a more holistic impression of older adults' health. For example, in public health surveillance, the CDC in the USA uses a variety of self-report surveys to capture statistics on the population's well-being. However, converting the information gathered from assessment techniques into cost-effective public health interventions to improve elderly well-being remains a challenge.

Frailty and the 'frailty phenotype'

Frailty is a particularly problematic clinical outcome in the elderly population because it increases vulnerability to many negative health outcomes. Although there is consensus that treating frailty is important for both the

individual and from a public health angle, a well-established tool is not available to define and identify the condition. The concept of frailty is recognised in advanced care facilities, like hospitals and nursing homes, where patients had possibly arrived as a result of a frailty-related consequence, such as a fall. Recently, the 'frailty phenotype' has been developed, which provides an operational definition of frailty to improve screening for the condition and prevent such outcomes. The phenotype consists of five clinically measurable components, and an individual is determined to be frail if three or more of these criteria are met. They include: 'shrinking' (indicated by weight loss), 'weakness' (indicated by grip strength), poor endurance and energy (indicated by self-report), slowness (indicated by walking speed) and low physical activity level (indicated by a weighted score of kilocalories expended per week). The public health realm will benefit from greater use of additional outcome measure assessments in older people, such as of the 'frailty phenotype', that help to distinguish individuals that need a targeted intervention to improve their health status.

13.3 Approaches to nutritional screening and assessment

Older adults bear a disproportionately higher nutritional risk – which is the risk of poor health as a result of nutritional problems – than do the younger population. This is because the ageing process tends to give rise to characteristics such as a greater disease burden that are associated with an increased likelihood of poor nutritional status. Limitations to an older adult's access to food or ability to prepare or consume food, as well as changes in appetite, absorption or metabolism of nutrients, may increase their chances of malnutrition (Table 13.7) (White *et al.*, 1991; Bernstein and Luggen, 2010). Many poor outcomes are associated with malnutrition in older adults, including a loss of lean muscle mass resulting in frailty, pressure ulcers with delayed wound healing, diminished immunity, infection and sepsis, respiratory and cardiac complications, and ultimately death. Between half and two-thirds of malnourished elderly patients are unrecognised as such. Therefore, tools to identify malnutrition and avoid these complications are important components of elderly health care (Elia *et al.*, 2005).

Nutrition screening

Nutrition screening quickly differentiates those who have characteristics known to increase the risk of nutritional problems to determine whether a detailed

Table 13.7 Risk factors associated with poor nutritional status, including elements by which risk is assessed, in the ageing population.

Characteristic or problem associated with poor nutritional status	Example
Inappropriate, inadequate or excessive food intake	• Quantity, quality or both with respect to intake of dairy products, meat/meat substitutes, fruits and vegetables, breads and cereals, fats, sweets and alcohol • Dietary modifications (prescribed or self-imposed) • Alcohol abuse
Poverty	• Low income • Low food expenditures or inadequate food resources • Reliance on economic assistance programme for food or other basic needs
Social isolation	• Reduced social contact • Isolate or inadequate (relative to cooking, food storage or transportation) living arrangements
Chronic medication use	• Prescribed/self-administered • Polypharmacy • Nutritional supplements
Dependency/ disability	• Functional status, ADLs, IADLs • Disabling conditions, lack of manual dexterity, use of assistive devices
Acute/chronic diseases or conditions	• Abnormalities of body weight • Alcohol abuse • Cognitive or emotional impairment, depression, dementias • Oral health problems • Pressure sores • Sensory impairment • Others
Advanced age	

Source: White *et al.* (1991).

assessment of nutritional status is necessary (Mueller *et al.*, 2011). A problem with screening for malnutrition in older individuals is that it is difficult to separate changes in nutritional status that are preventable or treatable by nutritional means from those that are due to underlying pathological processes. Also, screening is crude because it identifies individuals at risk of nutritional complications as well as those who have already developed malnutrition. When a nutrition screen reveals that an individual has few risk factors, then additional effort is unnecessary at that time, although a follow-up for re-screening may be advisable, particularly in older populations where age itself is a risk. Conversely, when a screen flags an individual as being nutritionally vulnerable, that person can then be referred into the nutrition

care process for a full nutrition assessment and intervention to correct nutritional inadequacy, if necessary. Screening and assessment are worthless if there is no follow-up. Therefore, public health programmes need to include all components: screening, assessment, diagnosis, intervention and monitoring or follow-up.

Tools to screen and inform groups about possible nutritional risks

The Nutrition Screening Initiative
The Nutrition Screening Initiative (NSI) was developed in the USA in 1990 as part of a national effort to improve nutritional care of older Americans. This collaboration between the American Academy of Family Physicians, the American Dietetic Association and the National Council on Aging resulted in a two-tiered tool for nutrition screening and assessment.

The 'Determine Your Nutritional Health' checklist and the level I (LI) screen make up the first tier of NSI. Older individuals or their carers answer simple questions cued from the mnemonic 'DETERMINE', which is based on some common nutrition risk factors in older adults:

Disease
Eating poorly
Tooth loss or oral pain
Economic hardship
Reduced social contact
Multiple medications or drugs
Involuntary weight loss or gain
Needs assistance with self-care
Elderly person is older than age 80.

Mini Nutritional Assessment
The Mini Nutrition Assessment (MNA) is a nutrition screening tool designed for older adults that can be completed in the community by the patient, a loved one or caretaker. Health-care professionals can also incorporate the screen into encounters with older patients. Completion of the screen yields a score derived from answers to diet and health related questions, none of which requires laboratory data.

The MNA is similar to the NSI, in that it has two tiers: the MNA short form (MNA-SF) and the more complex 'full' MNA. The MNA-SF consists of six questions, requires a height and weight, and takes about 3 min to administer. The maximum score is 14 points, with a score of 11 or more providing strong evidence that malnutrition is not present. Any score below 11 indicates a risk of undernutrition. In a recent review of 10 nutrition screens, this one was deemed the most reliable and valid in evaluating the nutritional status in community-dwelling older adults (Phillips *et al.*, 2010).

If the MNA-SF score is less than 11, then nutrition risk may be present and it is recommended that the full version of MNA be completed for further evaluation. Theoretically, MNA is good at identifying at-risk frail elderly because it considers both the physical and mental aspects of health that may have an impact on nutritional status. It focuses chiefly on identifying undernutrition and protein–energy malnutrition and has predictive validity for adverse health outcomes, length of hospital stay and mortality.

Malnutrition Universal Screening Tool

The Malnutrition Universal Screening Tool (MUST) was developed in 2003 to screen all adults, using surrogate measures of height and weight when actual measures are unavailable. Supported by the British Association of Parenteral and Enteral Nutrition, the British Dietetic Association and other European health organisations, MUST is frequently used in Europe, especially in the UK. Although it was originally developed for community-dwelling older adults, it has predictive validity in the hospital environment as well, where it has proved to be convenient and faster to administer than most screens, taking only 3–5 min to complete. The MUST consists of five easy steps that classify malnutrition risk as low, medium or high on the basis of BMI, history of unexplained weight loss and acute illness. When screening patients 65 years or older, MUST has been shown to have 'good' agreement with full dietetic assessment for detecting malnutrition while also correlating with other nutrition screening tools, including MNA (Stratton *et al.*, 2006).

Nutrition assessment

Nutrition assessment is a comprehensive review of nutritional status that employs medical, nutritional, and medicinal history, physical examination, and anthropometric and laboratory data to diagnosis nutritional problems (Mueller *et al.*, 2011). Currently, there is no 'gold standard' for assessing and diagnosing nutritional depletion of older adults.

Tools to assess older adults

Nutrition Screening Initiative level I and II screens

The NSI LI screen, to be administered by a health or social service professional, provides information on possible signs of nutritional risk. If it indicates possible risk, then a physician or qualified health professional performs a level I (LII) screen in a clinical setting by completing a comprehensive review of the patient's nutritional status, including diagnostic material. Although this portion of NSI is termed the 'LI and LII

screen', the detailed nature of tier 2 actually qualifies it as a nutrition assessment tool. To date neither tier has been validated; until they are, other methods may be more appropriate.

Subjective Global Assessment

The Subjective Global Assessment (SGA) tool was first developed in 1982 as a tool for clinicians to assess a patient's nutritional status, particularly wasting and protein–energy malnutrition, at the bedside without need to have detailed information on body composition. Components of the assessment include a history and physical examination. The section on history considers weight and dietary intake changes, gastrointestinal symptoms, functional capacity or energy level and disease as it relates to nutritional status. The physical examination notes the presence of oedema, ascites, muscle wasting and the loss of subcutaneous fat. All information from the assessment is combined to provide a letter grade of A (well nourished), B (suspicion of malnutrition) or C (severely malnourished) being assigned to the patient.

Assessment Lexicon: ABCDEF

Another tool for individual nutritional assessment is the mnemonic 'ABCDEF' that cues the clinician to indicators that comprise the core elements of nutrition assessment. The included elements are anthropometry, biochemical data, clinical observations, dietary intake (and use of drugs/medications), extra information (such as exercise and physical activity patterns, socioeconomic, family and cultural issues) and functional status (Dwyer, 2001).

- *Anthropometry* Certain anthropometric measures are simple, non-invasive and inexpensive methods for assessing and monitoring nutrition status. Weight and height are two measurements to obtain that provide useful information. When available, measured weight and height should be used to calculate BMI. With ageing, height tends to decline by 0.5 to 1.5 cm per decade because the vertebrae compact, so the measure may be somewhat imprecise, but nevertheless indicates grossly deviant values. A dramatic and unintentional weight loss is a predictor of risk and may indicate malnutrition. A change in BMI by more than one unit in either direction is cause for concern and should be investigated further. It may be associated with oedema or ascites as well as with excess fat. Very high and very low BMIs are associated with an increased mortality risk.

  Complications may arise when evaluating many other aspects of body composition in older adults because age-related changes in body composition make the reference standards that are derived from younger adult populations inappropriate. Other standards, such as fat folds, are more difficult to interpret. For example, relative to younger adults, individuals of the older population tend to have less fat-free mass and more fat, resulting in a decrease in total body water, and adipose tissue redistributed to the trunk from the extremities. Mid-arm muscle circumference and triceps skin-fold measures can also be used, but for the aforementioned reasons they may be less reliable in older adults. Standards have been published for elderly adults, and they should be used.

- *Biochemical data* Biomarkers such as serum or urine levels of nutrients can often be measured to provide indicators of nutritional status. Biomarkers are somewhat more objective than subjectively reported dietary intakes, and can often provide accurate measures that reflect nutritional status.

  Since micronutrient deficiencies may not produce clinical signs or tell-tale and specific symptoms until they are severe, biochemical tests using these biomarkers allow for earlier detection. However, as discussed previously, it is important to evaluate biochemical data in older individuals critically because it may be affected by medication usage, acute illness and chronic disease, as well as hydration status.

- *Clinical assessment* Clinical assessment of the elderly individual should include a brief review of medical history and physical examination to develop a more complete picture of factors that may affect nutritional status. The medical history is important to review because certain chronic diseases may affect nutritional status through physiological mechanisms or by influencing an individual's dietary choices. Further, older adults managing chronic disease may take one or more medications that have the capacity to alter nutrient absorption or metabolism.

  The physical examination for clinical signs and history of symptoms of malnutrition can reveal dietary excess, such as obesity, and also the classical signs of malnutrition. The classical signs may be seen in a patient's hair, eyes, skin and mouth, but these can be rare and difficult to recognise in elders, and are therefore often missed. The oral cavity may provide an indication of nutritional status, and poorly fitting dentures or a lack of teeth can alter food intake.

- *Dietary and drug history* All older patients should be asked about their food intake, patterns of consumption and usage of dietary supplements, such as multivitamins, as well as any prescribed or over-the-counter medications taken on a regular basis. Food records, 24-h dietary recalls and food frequency questionnaires may be utilised to develop an understanding of the eating habits of older people. The diet history may make risk factors for malnutrition apparent, such as

regular meal skipping or poor variety of food intake. Some medications, such as digitalis, are associated with decreased food intake, and these should be noted and changed if possible to others that do not do so. The physiological changes in taste and smell that occur with ageing should also be considered, as well as the effects that some medications can have on taste sensations and olfactory function.

- *Extra information* Extra information obtained in the interview focuses on important factors that influence energy and nutrient intakes, such as exercise and physical activity, as well as aspects such as socio-economic status and social, family or other cultural or religious beliefs that may affect food intakes (see Table 13.7). For example, with respect to exercise and physical activity in the USA, Canada and Europe, declines in physical activity and intake are usually associated with ageing. However, physical activity levels vary dramatically in the older population, so it is important to gain an understanding of the amount and intensity of activity, as well as the strength of each individual. It is also important to note a downward trend in physical activity and exercise, if it is present, as a decrease may reflect a health status change. Age- and condition-appropriate activities should be encouraged if this is possible. Likewise, changes in socio-economic status, such as reduced/loss of pension funds, or changes in the living situation, such as death of a spouse, can have major implications for energy and nutrient intakes. Health- and nutrition-related beliefs as well as the effects of advertising can be powerful influencers of dietary intake and should be considered in undertaking a comprehensive nutritional assessment (Bernstein and Munoz, 2012).

- *Functional status* Assessment of functional status is important to ascertain whether or not an older adult needs assistance or services. Functional status can be assessed by an elderly individual's ability to complete ADLs, like bathing, dressing and feeding oneself, and IADLs, such as meal preparation, house cleaning and handling money. If an older individual struggles with these activities, it is possible that functional impairments also challenge that individual's ability to obtain and prepare food.

Nutrition Care Process Model

The US Academy of Nutrition and Dietetics has developed a framework for the provision of nutritional care that incorporates four components; nutritional assessment, nutritional diagnosis, nutritional intervention and monitoring. The purpose of the nutritional assessment is to obtain, verify and interpret data needed to identify nutrition-related problems, their causes and significance. It is comprised of five categories of data, which can come directly from the patient/client through interview, observation and measurements, a medical record, and the referring health-care provider.

- *Food- and nutrition-related history* This domain examines food and nutrient intake (composition and adequacy of food and nutrient intake, meal and snack patterns, current and previous diets and/or food modifications, and eating environment), food and nutrient administration (current and previous diets and/or food modifications, eating environment, and enteral and parenteral nutrition administration), medication and complementary/alternative medication use (prescription and over-the-counter medications, including herbal preparations and complementary/alternative products used), knowledge, beliefs and attitudes (understanding of nutrition-related concepts and readiness to change nutrition-related behaviours), behaviour, food and supply availability, physical activity and function, nutrition-related patient/client-centred measures (patient's/client's perception of impact of nutrition intervention on life).
- *Anthropometric measures* This domain includes measures of height, weight, weight change, BMI and body compartment estimates.
- *Biochemical data, medical tests and procedures* These include assessment of blood and urine biochemical tests (acid–base balance, electrolytes, etc.), metabolic rate, inflammatory status, review of major systems (endocrine, gastrointestinal, renal profiles) and clinical signs and symptoms of malnutrition, such as anaemia.
- *Nutrition-focused physical findings* The findings from this domain include the evaluation of body systems, muscle and subcutaneous fat wasting, functional status, oral health, suck/swallow/breathe ability, appetite and affect.
- *Client history* Includes current and past information related to personal, medical, family and social history.

The nutrition assessment data are compared with criteria, relevant norms and standards for interpretation and decision-making. Nutrition assessment findings are documented in nutrition diagnosis statements and nutrition intervention goal setting. While the nutrition assessment component of the Nutrition Care Process Model (NCPM) has considerable overlap with the ABCDEF model of nutrition assessment, the NCPM is increasingly being used in the USA, Australia and Europe as a standardised method of nutritional care.

Tools for screening and assessing groups of older persons in the community

Demographics and vital statistics
Certain demographic characteristics of older adults are known to be associated with a higher risk for nutritional

problems. National, state and local-level statistics on mortality, morbidity and altered functional status often have nutritional implications. These serve as community-level nutritional screens by indicating vulnerable subpopulations that may have modifiable risk factors for poor nutritional status. Although chronological age and functional ability do not necessarily correspond precisely, the oldest old are often at highest nutritional risk because progressive disability and functional impairments contribute significantly to malnutrition in the elderly. The identification of high-risk groups who have high rates of diet-related problems provides the evidence-based need for targeted community-based nutrition programmes and policies.

Free-living older adults
Although the prevalence of malnutrition within free-living older adults is thought to be lower than in older populations living in residential facilities or nursing homes, some malnutrition nevertheless exists. The high rates of malnutrition on admission to hospital indicate that nutritional problems leading to malnutrition can and do occur in the community setting. For this reason, it is important that health and social care professionals and carers should routinely monitor for malnutrition using the screening tools and information described above, even with patients who seem to be relatively well off economically.

Older adults in sheltered housing
Although older people who reside in sheltered housing have more support than community-dwelling adults, this population is not exempt from nutritional risk. In most US states and in Europe, clear standards on food and nutrition quality within sheltered-housing facilities do not yet exist, and only the most basic nutrition aspects of care, such as food safety, are regulated and enforced with high priority. Many important aspects of nutritional care, such as menu nutrient analysis and nutrition assessment, are often only loosely regulated. Food quality is extremely important in this setting because most residents depend virtually completely on their facility to meet their nutritional requirements.

Another problem with sheltered-housing facilities is that many elderly prefer living in these rather than a nursing home or hospital, even if they are ill, because of the greater freedom that these facilities provide. Thus, many older people who are actually quite ill and incapacitated are living in sheltered housing and they can be missed if nutritional screening is not performed. There is often little monitoring done by the operators of these facilities to identify such persons who are slipping into malnutrition. More regulation of sheltered-housing facilities is clearly in order.

Residential care and nursing homes

Relative to free-living and sheltered-housing facilities, rates of malnutrition are higher among elderly individuals living in residential care and nursing homes. Estimates, using a variety of methods, suggest that between 17 and 97% of residents in long-term care facilities in Europe are at risk or already malnourished. Data collected by the British Association of Parenteral and Enteral Nutrition indicate that over 40% of residents in residential care homes are at nutritional risk. However, much of the malnutrition is the result of disease processes and it cannot be reversed by diet alone. Guidance documents on nutritional recommendations also exist; for example, guidance produced by the National Institute for Health and Care Excellence in the UK in 2006 and reviewed in 2011.

In both the USA and UK, residential care facilities, nursing homes and hospitals have clear standards set down for them by governmental regulatory authorities (e.g. the Care Quality Commission in the UK), and these settings are also better monitored than sheltered-housing facilities. Such regulations specify that these facilities are required to provide residents with meals that meet the age- and gender-specific RDAs. These must be prepared so that the nutritional value is preserved and that they are 'palatable' and 'attractive' to the consumer. Specifications protect more vulnerable patients by requiring that a feeding assistant, special utensils or other feeding devices be provided to any individual who requires such support. If the patient's nutritional requirements are still not met, the regulations note that further assessment is necessary to determine the next appropriate intervention, such as a naso-gastric feeding tube. In the USA, in order to verify that nutritional needs are being met, nursing home residents are also to be assessed for appropriate biochemical and anthropometric status.

Nutritional interventions and management

Goals: USA and Europe

Healthy People 2020 is the federal blueprint for preventive health services in the USA. The goal for older adults is to improve their function and quality of life. It provides specific objectives for the behavioural-, social- and health-services-related determinants of health in older adults, and includes many nutrition-related objectives. The entire report is web based at http://www. healthypeople.gov/2020/. In Europe, the WHO provides recommendations for the 53 countries of the European region in its policy framework and strategy document *Health 2020*. These recommendations support those of the EU to increase the number of HLYs by 2 years by 2020 (World Health Organization, 2013).

Nutrition interventions for older adults

Nutrition screening and assessment tools are worthwhile only if subsequent actions are taken to improve the status of those identified with nutritional risk. In many developed countries, a variety of specific nutrition interventions exist, from nutrition education to inform older adults about healthy eating to community-level programmes, such as free or subsidised home-delivery meal services (known as meals-on-wheels in the UK), which are often geared to low-income or frail individuals. However, provision is often determined by local authority policy. Interventions are most effective when they are focused and personalised towards groups with the highest need.

- *Individual nutrition education* Theoretically, nutrition education for older adults should make it possible to improve their health and quality of life. However, some believe that nutrition education is not useful because they believe older adults will refuse to change their well-established behaviours; but this may be a false assumption. Many older people are highly motivated to alter their diets in more healthful directions, and age is not necessarily a limiting factor for nutrition education. However, it is true that behaviour changes and health outcomes resulting from nutrition education vary between individuals. The most positive nutrition education outcomes are thought to occur when messages are limited to one or two central ideas that are simple, practical and targeted to meet the older person's specific needs, combined with behaviour modification techniques to make better food choices for healthful ageing. The Age UK 'Fit as a Fiddle' programme showed demonstrable benefits in terms of improvements in healthy eating, physical activity and mental well-being in a large cohort of older adults (http://www.ageuk.org.uk/health-wellbeing/fit-as-a-fiddle/about-fit-as-a-fiddle/), and the initiatives developed have now been funded to continue in a new programme 'Fit for the Future' (http://www.ageuk.org.uk/health-wellbeing/fit-as-a-fiddle/fit-for-the-future/).

- *Community nutrition intervention programmes* In the USA, the Older Americans Act includes provisions for several community nutrition intervention programmes; for example, the Supplemental Nutrition Assistance Program, which provides eligible low-income participants with monetary benefits to purchase qualified nutritious food. Part of the Older Americans Act also includes home-delivered meal services that bring nutritionally adequate meals to home-bound frail older adults, while also checking on elder health status, and providing social support. In both the USA and UK, meals-on-wheels agencies serve communities across the country, targeting older adults with some of the highest nutritional risk. Priority is given to individuals who are low income and home-bound or disabled, making the alternative of institutionalisation likely if such a service is not provided. Although such community meal services are available throughout most developed countries, the legislation supporting their nutritional quality varies greatly between countries (O'Dwyer *et al.*, 2009). In the UK, the Malnutrition Task Force provides good examples of shared learning and good practice in hospital, community (including care homes) and food and beverage providers (http://www.malnutritiontaskforce. org.uk).

13.4 Challenges to nutrition in older adults

The increasing population of very old and very frail

While the population of older adults grows, those over 85 years – known as the 'oldest old' – constitute the most rapidly increasing group within the population. Although frailty can occur in younger adults, it is concentrated in this age group. Frail adults are among the most vulnerable groups in society, and therefore require a disproportionately high amount of care within the health system. Frailty is linked with a higher risk for falls, disability, hospitalisation and mortality. Minimising nutritional and other health risks of frail older adults may have a significant impact on improvement of their health-related quality of life. Studies are ongoing to assess this. Improvements in health promotion programmes that encourage a healthy lifestyle, including healthy nutrition, as well as advancements in medical care that incorporate frequent nutrition screening and assessment, will help to decrease the risks that these individuals face. Thus, nutrition will continue to be vital component of care as more individuals age past 85 years. The health system will be increasingly faced with providing services that minimise disability, such as frailty, and maximise healthful ageing in a cost-effective fashion. Such a health system needs to be highly organised and have a comprehensive infrastructure which supports older people living in their own homes and allows for transition between levels of care that accounts not only for the physical and mental needs of older people, but also their social and emotional needs.

Generational investment strategies favour the young

Public health and social welfare programmes other than social security and other old age cash distribution programmes tend to favour the young over older adults in most western countries. As described earlier, with the ageing of populations worldwide, there is a global need for a more comprehensive investment strategy to assure the quality of life and health of older people, and a more extensive infrastructure to encourage 'ageing in place' in one's own home, rather than institutionalisation.

Applying emerging science in ageing

There is much interest in the significance of the microbiota on human health, and studies on the effects of ageing, disease, diet and medications, both over the counter and prescribed, upon the microbiome of the elderly are only now beginning. Another topic of great interest is whether there is a place for functional foods or ingredients that have potentially beneficial effects on health beyond those of nutrients alone. In the EU, several studies addressing this issue are being covered in the NU-AGE project under the direction of the European Commission (see http://www.nu-age.eu). Some similar projects are also getting under way in the USA and Canada.

13.5 Conclusion

Older people are a nutritionally vulnerable group and they have some nutritional needs that are unique from those in the general population that must be dealt with on a public health basis. Many older adults are afflicted with chronic and acute diseases and conditions that may alter their nutritional status, and changes in their functional status may impair their ability to live and eat independently and look after their health needs. The associations between diet and disease in the elderly clearly exist. Dealing with increasing frailty and other nutritional complications that result from disease through nutritional and other means is a major challenge in all countries. Methods for screening and assessing older people as individuals or on a community basis must be put into place and used more routinely to identify those in need of special nutritional care and interventions.

Disclaimer

The use of trade, firm, or corporation names in these methods is for the information and convenience of the reader. Such use does not constitute an official endorsement or approval by the U.S.D.A. Agricultural Research Service, of any product or service to the exclusion of others that may be suitable. In addition, The USDA-ARS makes no warranties as to the merchantability or fitness of the methodologies described on these pages for any particular purpose, or any other warranties expressed or implied. These methodologies provide a guide and do not replace published work. The USDA-ARS is not liable for any damages resulting from the use or misuse of these methodologies.

References

Adams, P.E., Martinez, M.E., Vickerie, J.L. and Kirzinger, W.K. (2011) Summary health statistics for the U.S. population: National Health Interview Survey, 2010. *Vital and Health Statistics. Series 10, Data from the National Health Survey*, (251), 1–117.

Bates, B., Lennox, A., Prentice, A. et al. (2014) National Diet and Nutrition Survey: Results from Years 1, 2, 3 and 4 (Combined) of the Rolling Programme (2008/2009-2011/2012). A Survey Carried Out on Behalf of Public Health England and the Food Standards Agency. Public Health England, London. https://www.gov.uk/government/uploads/system/uploads/attachment_data/file/310995/NDNS_Y1_to_4_UK_report.pdf (accessed 6 December 2016).

Bauer, J., Biolo, G., Cederholm, T. et al. (2013) Evidence-based recommendations for optimal dietary protein intake in older people: a position paper from the PROT-AGE Study Group. *Journal of the American Medical Directors*, **14** (8), 542–559.

Bernstein, M.A. and Luggen, A.S. (2010) *Nutrition for Older Adults*. Jones & Bartlett Learning, Sudbury, MA.

Bernstein, M. and Munoz, N. (2012) Position of the Academy of Nutrition and Dietetics: food and nutrition for older adults: promoting health and wellness. *Journal of the Academy of Nutrition and Dietetics*, **112** (8), 1255–1277.

Breslow, R.A., Chen, C.M., Graubard, B.I. et al. (2013) Diets of drinkers on drinking and nondrinking days: NHANES 2003–2008. *The American Journal of Clinical Nutrition*, **97** (5), 1068–1075.

Cashman, K.D. and Kiely, M. (2014) Recommended dietary intakes for vitamin D: where do they come from, what do they achieve and how can we meet them? *Journal of Human Nutrition and Dietetics*, **27** (5), 434–442.

CDC (2015) *About Adult BMI.* http://www.cdc.gov/healthyweight/assessing/bmi/adult_bmi/index.html (accessed 9 December 2016).

Dwyer, J.T. (2001) An assessment lexicon: assessment of dietary trends, physical activity patterns and nutritional status in the elderly. *The Journal of Nutrition, Health, & Aging*, **5** (2), 108–112.

Elia, M., Zellipour, L. and Stratton, R.J. (2005) To screen or not to screen for adult malnutrition. *Clinical Nutrition*, **24** (6), 867–884.

Flegal, K.M. and Kalantar-Zadeh, K. (2013) Overweight, mortality and survival. *Obesity*, **21** (9), 1744–1745.

Heron, M. (2012) Deaths: leading causes for 2009. *National Vital Statistics Reports*, **61** (7).

Institute of Medicine (US) Panel on Dietary Antioxidants and Related Compounds (2000) *Dietary Reference Intakes for Vitamin C, Vitamin E, Selenium, and Carotenoids*. National Academies Press, Washington, DC.

Institute of Medicine (US) Panel on Micronutrients (2001) Dietary Reference Intakes for Vitamin A, Vitamin K, Arsenic, Boron, Chromium, Copper, Iodine, Iron, Manganese, Molybdenum, Nickel, Silicon, Vanadium, and Zinc. National Academies Press, Washington, DC.

Institute of Medicine (US) Standing Committee on the Scientific Evaluation of Dietary Reference Intakes (1997) *Dietary Reference Intakes for Calcium, Phosphorous, Magnesium, Vitamin D, and Fluoride*. National Academies Press, Washington, DC.

Institute of Medicine (US) Standing Committee on the Scientific Evaluation of Dietary Reference Intakes and its Panel on Folate, Other B Vitamins, and Choline (1998) *Dietary Reference Intakes for Thiamin, Riboflavin, Niacin, Vitamin B6, Folate, Vitamin B$_{12}$, Pantothenic Acid, Biotin, and Choline*. National Academies Press, Washington, DC.

Mathus-Vliegen, E.M., Basdevant, A., Finer, N. et al. (2012) Prevalence, pathophysiology, health consequences and treatment options of obesity in the elderly: a guideline. *Obesity Facts*, **5** (3), 460–483.

Mentes, J.C. (2013) The complexities of hydration issues in the elderly. *Nutrition Today*, **48** (3S), S1–S3.

Mueller, C., Compher, C., Ellen, D.M. et al. (2011) A. S. P. E. N. Clinical Guidelines: nutrition screening, assessment, and intervention in adults. *Journal of Parenteral and Enteral Nutrition*, **35** (1), 16–24.

O'Dwyer, C., Corish, C.A. and Timonen, V. (2009) Nutritional status of Irish older people in receipt of meals-on-wheels and the nutritional content of meals provided. *Journal of Human Nutrition and Dietetics*, **22** (6), 521–527.

Otten, J.J., Hellwig, J.P. and Meyers, L.D. (eds) (2006) *Introduction to the dietary reference intakes. In Dietary Reference Intakes: The Essential Guide to Nutrient Requirements*. The National Academies Press, Washington, DC.

Phillips, M.B., Foley, A.L., Barnard, R. et al. (2010) Nutritional screening in community-dwelling older adults: a systematic literature review. *Asia Pacific Journal of Clinical Nutrition*, **19** (3), 440–449.

Ross, A.C., Taylor, C.L. Yaktine, A.L. and Del Valle, H.B. (eds) (2011) *Dietary Reference Intakes for Calcium and Vitamin D*. National Academies Press, Washington, DC.

Roubenoff, R. (2004) Sarcopenic obesity: the confluence of two epidemics. *Obesity Research*, **12** (6), 887–888.

Scientific Advisory Committee on Nutrition (2011) *Dietary Reference Values for Energy*. TSO, London. https://www.gov.uk/government/uploads/system/uploads/attachment_data/file/339317/SACN_Dietary_Reference_Values_for_Energy.pdf (accessed 8 December 2016).

Stratton, R.J., King, C.L., Stroud, M.A. et al. (2006) 'Malnutrition Universal Screening Tool' predicts mortality and length of hospital stay in acutely ill elderly. *British Journal of Nutrition*, **95** (2), 325–330.

The Institute of Medicine of the National Academies (2002/2005) Dietary Reference Intakes for Energy, Carbohydrate, Fiber, Fat, Fatty Acids, Cholesterol, Protein, and Amino Acids. The National Academies Press, Washington, DC.

United Nations (2013) World Population Prospects, the 2012 Revision. http://www.un.org/en/development/desa/publications/world-population-prospects-the-2012-revision.html (accessed 8 December 2016).

Volpi, E., Campbell, W.W., Dwyer, J.T. et al. (2013) Is the optimal level of protein intake for older adults greater than the recommended dietary allowance? *The Journals of Gerontology Series A: Biological Sciences and Medical Sciences*, **68** (6), 677–681.

White, J.V., Ham, R.J., Lipschitz, D.A. et al. (1991) Consensus of the Nutrition Screening Initiative: risk factors and indicators of poor nutritional status in older Americans. *Journal of the American Dietetic Association*, **91** (7), 783–787.

WHO (2003) Food Based Dietary Guidelines in the WHO European Region. WHO Regional Office for Europe, Copenhagen. http://www.euro.who.int/__data/assets/pdf_file/0017/150083/E79832.pdf (accessed 3 January 2017).

World Health Organization (2013) *Health 2020. A European Policy Framework and Strategy for the 21st Century*. WHO Regional Office for Europe, Copenhagen.

Part Three

Diet and Disease

14
Obesity: Maternal

Debbie M Smith, Tracey A Mills, and Christine Furber

Key messages

- Increasing numbers of women of reproductive age are now obese – body mass index (BMI) $\geq 30\,\text{kg/m}^2$. Therefore, maternal obesity (a BMI $\geq 30\,\text{kg/m}^2$ during pregnancy) is a new and emerging threat to public health.
- While the impact of obesity for public health is widely acknowledged, the adverse effects of maternal obesity on maternal, fetal and infant health during pregnancy, labour and after birth are less well recognised.
- The concept of 'fetal programming' provides evidence to support a relationship between suboptimal nutrition *in utero* and increased risk of ill-health in later life. Therefore, provision of effective information and support surrounding healthy weight and diet to pregnant women should be a key public health priority.

- There is a lack of consensus about routine weighing and what constitutes 'excessive weight gain' in pregnancy. In particular, health professionals are unsure of what to advise pregnant obese women about gestational weight gain, which can lead to confusion for the women. Thus, more research and training are needed on this issue.
- Antenatal intervention has been suggested as ideal due to women's increased motivation during this time. However, there is little agreement on what is the optimal intervention for pregnant woman with a BMI $\geq 30\,\text{kg/m}^2$.
- Health professionals must be aware that women's pregnancy expectations and experiences are influenced by ethnicity and country of birth. Thus, psychosocial and cultural influences on women's maternity needs must be better understood to ensure good communication.

14.1 Introduction

This chapter presents a summary of the issues raised by the rising prevalence of maternal obesity. The main public health challenges are addressed with reference to current UK maternity care: routine weighing, excessive weight gain and the role of the health professional, the optimal antenatal interventions for maternal obesity and ethnicity and maternal obesity. The chapter closes with recommendations for future research and clinical practice to support health professionals caring for pregnant women with a body mass index (BMI) $\geq 30\,\text{kg/m}^2$.

Prevalence of maternal obesity

Given the acknowledged worldwide 'obesity epidemic' in high–, mid– and, increasingly, low-resource settings, it is not surprising that increasing numbers of women of reproductive age are now obese – body mass index (BMI) $\geq 30\,\text{kg/m}^2$. The Health Survey for England reported that

the prevalence of obesity among women aged 15–44 years had increased from 12.0% in 1993 to 18% in 2006 (NHS Information Centre, 2008). In the USA in 2009–2010, an estimated 31.9% of women aged 20–39 years were obese (Flegal *et al.*, 2012). This rise accounts directly for the increased numbers of women entering pregnancy with a BMI $\geq 30\,\text{kg/m}^2$. A recent study of 619 323 births in 34 maternity units in England reported that first-trimester obesity had more than doubled from 7.6% of pregnant women in 1989 to 15.6% in 2007 (Heslehurst *et al.*, 2010). Similarly, in the USA, over 50% of pregnant women were overweight or obese in 2009–2010 (Flegal *et al.*, 2012).

Risks associated with maternal obesity

Adverse pregnancy outcomes
The public health effects of the obesity epidemic, including the rapid rise in the incidence of type 2 diabetes, are widely acknowledged. However, the significant negative

Public Health Nutrition, Second Edition. Edited by Judith L Buttriss, Ailsa A Welch, John M Kearney and Susan A Lanham-New.
© 2018 by The Nutrition Society. Published 2018 by John Wiley & Sons, Ltd.
Companion website: www.wiley.com/go/buttriss/publichealth

impacts on women's reproductive health are generally less well recognised. The Confidential Enquiry into Maternal Deaths (CEMD), which assesses causes and contributing factors to deaths during or after pregnancy in the UK, has identified an excess risk of mortality associated with obesity (CMACE, 2011). In the last triennial report (2006–2008), 27% of the women who died were obese; specific associated conditions included thromboembolism (78% of those who died were overweight or obese) and cardiac disease (61% overweight or obese) (CMACE, 2011). In addition to mortality, a plethora of complications and adverse outcomes are increased in the presence of high maternal BMI. Obese women are significantly more likely to experience miscarriage, gestational diabetes (Ehrenberg et al., 2004), hypertensive disorders of pregnancy, including pre-eclampsia (Bodnar et al., 2005), and thromboembolism in pregnancy or postnatally (Larsen et al., 2007). Obesity also increases the risk of complications during labour and birth and the need for instrumental and Caesarean delivery (Heslehurst et al., 2008). Intrapartum interventions contribute to increased postpartum morbidity with a greater risk of postpartum haemorrhage, puerperal infection and longer hospital stay, compared with women with a healthy BMI (18.5–24.9; Heslehurst et al., 2008). In addition to the negative impacts on the mother, maternal obesity is also recognised as a significant risk factor for adverse fetal outcomes, notably stillbirth. A recent meta-analysis identified overweight and obesity as the most important modifiable factor in reducing late-gestation stillbirths in high-resource countries (Flenady et al., 2011).

In utero programming of adult obesity

In addition to the immediate obstetric, fetal and neonatal risks, described above, there is accumulating evidence that the rise in maternal obesity could have longer term negative public health implications. Observational studies consistently demonstrate an association between maternal obesity and large for gestational-age infants (birth weight >95th centile or over 4000 g; Heslehurst et al., 2008). Infants of obese women are also more likely to be overweight or obese in childhood, adolescence and as adults (Drake and Reynolds, 2010). The factors underlying the increased risk of obesity in the offspring of obese women are not fully elucidated, although genetic inheritance is often cited. Children born after their mothers had undergone bariatric surgery were three times less likely to develop severe obesity than siblings born prior to surgery being performed (Smith et al., 2009). This suggests that other factors, such as the high-energy/poor-quality diet associated with pre-pregnancy obesity, are likely to contribute and that maternal obesity/overnutrition 'programmes' obesity in the offspring (Parlee and MacDougald, 2014).

The concept of 'fetal programming' was first proposed by Barker and colleagues during the 1980s to explain the observed increase in risk of coronary heart disease in adult men of low birth weight (Barker et al., 1989). Barker contended that adult diseases could result from a maladaptation of developmental plasticity. This describes the process by which the mammalian embryo/fetus is able to adapt its metabolism and physiology in response to environmental stimulus or insult, protecting the growth of crucial organs, particularly the brain, at the expense of others, including the liver. Developmental plasticity is thought to have evolved particularly in response to the threat of nutritional restriction, resulting from frequent periods of food shortage which affected long periods of human history. According to Barker, the increased risk arises when there is a mismatch between the prenatal and postnatal environment; for example, if food is more abundant after birth. In this situation, the adaptations which promoted survival under hostile conditions in utero cause metabolic dysfunction affecting food intake and fat storage, increasing the risk of metabolic disorders, notably obesity (Barker et al., 2007). This theory is supported by studies in animal models: rats exposed to nutrient restriction in utero were more likely to have increased body fat and abnormal metabolic profiles in adulthood, if weaned onto a richer diet (i.e. higher in calories, fat and/or sugar) than that of the mother (Desai et al., 2005).

Based on the evidence for a role for nutrient restriction in pregnancy in programming obesity, it might be assumed that maternal obesity and/or overnutrition in pregnancy would protect against development of obesity in the offspring, due to the similarity of diets in the pre/postnatal period. However, evidence from animal models indicates that maternal obesity and high fat/sugar/salt diet are associated with high birth weight, abnormal metabolic profile and adult obesity (Samuelsson et al., 2008). Rat pups born to mothers fed on a 'junk food' diet in pregnancy also tend to consume more calories and exhibit greater preference for high-fat/sugar foods compared with controls (Bayol et al., 2008). The underlying mechanisms are incompletely understood; evidence suggests that maternal obesity is associated with placental dysfunction, particularly inflammation and upregulated expression and activity of the glucose and system A amino acid transporters, which may contribute to incidence of high birth weight (Jones et al., 2009; Zhu et al., 2010). In a recent review of the literature, Parlee and MacDougald (2014) suggested that evolution has not influenced development of a response to protect the offspring from the effects of maternal overnutrition because of nutritional surpluses rarely occurred in evolutionary history. Primate studies suggest that placental inflammation associated with maternal obesity might lead to restricted transfer of nutrients (McCurdy *et al.*, 2009). In this scenario, the fetus might experience nutritional restriction leading to programming and a mismatched pre/postnatal environment as suggested by Barker. Findings from human epidemiological studies provide further support for the association between excessive maternal weight gain in pregnancy and childhood obesity (Alfaradhi and Ozanne, 2011). A recent US study of 42 133 women and 91 045 children demonstrated that maternal weight gain predicted BMI at age 12 years and the likelihood of being overweight or obese (Ludwig *et al.*, 2013). The *within-family* design utilising data from biological siblings minimised the influence of variable environmental and genetic factors. The findings suggested limiting excessive weight gain in pregnancy might reduce childhood obesity; but as inadequate nutritional intake is known to negatively impact fetal development, further research is needed to define optimal weight gain related to pre-pregnancy BMI.

Maternal obesity is a significant and escalating threat to public health. Not only do obese women face increased risks of major adverse outcomes throughout the pregnancy continuum, but accumulating evidence also suggests long-term negative impacts, including increased adult obesity, in the offspring. Further research is needed to understand mechanisms underlying increased incidence of pregnancy complications associated with maternal overnutrition and the long-term consequences. This knowledge will allow for the development of effective therapeutic interventions to prevent maternal obesity and to improve health for obese women and their children.

14.2 Challenges

The main public health challenges associated with maternal obesity and nutrition are addressed in this section and summarised in the conclusion with some recommendations for future research and clinical practice.

Routine weighing, excessive weight gain and the role of the health professional

The absence of robust evidence-based guidance on acceptable pregnancy weight gain has contributed to the confusion and subsequent lack of advice and support on weight management. In the USA, over the last two decades, recommendations from the Institute of Medicine have been used to guide advice on gestational weight gain (Institute of Medicine, 1990; Rasmussen and Yaktine, 2009). Gestational weight gain within the Institute of Medicine recommendations is associated with the best outcomes of pregnancy for mothers (e.g. Cedergren,

2006), and low weight gain has been suggested as beneficial for obese women (Dodd *et al.*, 2008). However, these recommendations are based on observational studies, not well-designed experimental trials (Abrams *et al.*, 2000; Artal *et al.*, 2010), and despite implementation in several other countries they are not currently accepted by the National Institute for Health and Care Excellence (NICE) in the UK (Amorim *et al.*, 2008). Moreover, there is no international agreement on weight management and pregnancy policies (Scott *et al.*, 2014). Despite the publication of over 30 documents/reports that are related to obesity in pregnancy in the UK over the last 10 years or so, clear evidence-based guidance on weight management in pregnancy for health professionals does not exist (Heslehurst, 2011). Indeed, it was only in 2008 that the threshold of BMI criteria for risk of pregnancy complications reduced from $35 \, kg/m^2$ to $30 \, kg/m^2$ in England (National Collaborating Centre for Women's and Children's Health, 2008).

Although pre-pregnancy BMI as opposed to excessive gestational weight gain is more clearly associated with adverse outcomes (e.g. Fleten *et al.*, 2010), excessive gestational weight gain is also associated with increased risk and complication in pregnancy, birth and the postnatal period (e.g. Butte *et al.*, 2004). For example, a matched case–control study indicated that high weight gain before 24 weeks' gestation in overweight/obese women may precipitate gestational diabetes mellitus (Gibson *et al.*, 2012). Monitoring pregnancy weight and identifying when the weight gained makes the woman susceptible to obesity-related complications is a challenge for health professionals. Although the UK NICE guidance recommends all women should have BMI calculated at the first antenatal contact (ideally by 10 weeks' gestation), so that those who are obese are referred for gestational diabetes screening and provided with advice on nutrition and suitable exercise (National Collaborating Centre for Women's and Children's Health, 2008), there is no guidance that suggests weight gain should be routinely monitored during the rest of the pregnancy in order to identify subsequent risk associated with maternal obesity. Evidence indicates that UK-based health professionals follow this guidance (Brown and Avery, 2012; personal communication with community midwife, Alexandra Hawkins-Drew, 1 October 2014).

Consequently, some women are in danger of being overlooked for specialised care if they fall short of the obesity category at booking but gain weight at a later stage (National Collaborating Centre for Women's and Children's Health, 2008; NICE, 2008). Pregnancy naturally involves weight gain with the increase of blood volume and development of the fetus and reproductive organs (Coad and Tunstall, 2012). High weight gain in pregnancy in women of all weight categories is not unusual, and is frequently reported (Abrams *et al.*, 2000; DiPietro *et al.*, 2003; Rodrigues *et al.*, 2010; Wilkinson and Tolcher, 2010; Herring *et al.*, 2012; Ferrari and Siega-Riz, 2013; Heslehurst *et al.*, 2013). Waring *et al.* (2013) found that excessive weight gain tends to recur with successive pregnancies, especially for obese women. Furthermore, pregnant women have also reported a carefree attitude to eating in pregnancy (Olander *et al.*, 2011), and a lack of concern and knowledge of the impact of weight gain in pregnancy (Weir *et al.*, 2010; Keely *et al.*, 2011; Herring *et al.*, 2012).

Research conducted with a range of UK-based health professionals indicates that midwives, obstetricians and other community service providers have limited knowledge about pregnancy weight management (Ellison and Holliday, 1997; Oteng-Nitim *et al.*, 2010; Khazaezadeh *et al.*, 2011; Olander *et al.*, 2011; Smith *et al.*, 2011; Heslehurst *et al.*, 2013; Basu *et al.*, 2014). In the USA, pregnant women have a limited understanding of the guidelines for gestational weight gain and report gaining information about these from non-health-care sources such as the internet (Downs *et al.*, 2014). Even dietitians have questioned the value of their input when obese women are referred to them for additional dietary advice and support (Heslehurst *et al.*, 2011) in accordance with NICE (2008) guidance. Furthermore, a systematic review of quantitative and qualitative literature from developed countries indicates that advice given by health professionals to women focuses on healthy eating rather than weight management (Campbell *et al.*, 2011). This highlights the need for collaboration between health professionals in maternity care, and the development of close partnership working. For example, midwives are the main point of contact for pregnant women but they are not experts in dietary advice, so they may need to refer women to dietitians or work with dietitians to provide women with suitable advice, knowledge and skills.

Obese pregnant women have corroborated the findings of studies with health professionals when they have taken part in research exploring their experiences of childbearing (Weir *et al.*, 2010; Keely *et al.*, 2011; Olander *et al.*, 2011; Wennberg *et al.*, 2013). Worryingly, health professionals are reported as providing advice that is inconsistent, and unsafe. For example, although there is no evidence supporting weight loss to be safe in obese pregnant women (Furber *et al.*, 2013), Heslehurst *et al.* (2011) found that some health professionals advocated weight loss in obese pregnant women as acceptable after adopting a healthy lifestyle.

Regular weighing of pregnant women began in the 1940s to assess maternal nutrition and later was associated with the detection of adverse maternal and fetal outcomes, including pre-eclampsia and low birth weight

(Ellison and Holliday, 1997). Until the early 1990s, all pregnant women were routinely weighed during the antenatal period in the UK (Olander *et al.*, 2011), and other countries such as Sweden (Schmied *et al.*, 2011). However, debate over this practice, especially the lack of rationale for this screening test, meant that routine maternal weighing practices ceased (Hytten, 1990; Dawes *et al.*, 1992). However, the obesity epidemic is a recent phenomenon, and monitoring obesity was not part of the initial motive to weigh pregnant women (Hytten, 1990). Currently, antenatal weighing practices vary across maternity services in the UK (Heslehurst *et al.*, 2013) and weighing after the booking interview appears to be motivated to provide safe care such as calculation of safe medication dosages and the need for bariatric equipment at birth (CMACE/RCOG, 2010). There appears to be a dearth of information about weight management practice of other health professionals internationally in the literature; however, Australian midwives have also reported variable practices with obesity management (Biro *et al.*, 2013).

The current lack of emphasis on monitoring weight in pregnancy reinforces the message that gestational weight gain is unimportant (Olander *et al.*, 2011; Schmied *et al.*, 2011; Heslehurst *et al.*, 2013). Women who misperceive their pre-pregnancy weight are more likely to gain excessive amounts of gestational weight (Herring *et al.*, 2008) and thus need to be informed about their weight and the risk associated with it. Several studies highlight that health professionals feel inhibited about broaching obesity with pregnant women (Furber and McGowan, 2011; Keely *et al.*, 2011; Heslehurst *et al.*, 2013) and thus require more training (Smith *et al.*, 2012). However, women want information about weight in pregnancy (Wilkinson and Tolcher, 2010), to be weighed (Mollart, 1999; Heslehurst *et al.*, 2013) and are accepting of weight gain in pregnancy (e.g. Smith and Lavender, 2011). Caution is needed in terms of the words health professionals use to discuss weight, as individual differences are evident in preferences (Gray *et al.*, 2011). Although some women report feeling anxious about pregnancy weighing (Nyman *et al.*, 2010; Olander *et al.*, 2011; Johnson *et al.*, 2013; Chang *et al.*, 2014), and believe that the practice is part of the submission demanded of women during antenatal care (Warriner, 2000; Nyman *et al.*, 2010), the reintroduction of weighing is recommended by many as there is potential to discuss healthy lifestyles in relation to diet and exercise during the weighing process, and an opportunity to develop a rapport about obesity that may be followed up in the postnatal period (Smith *et al.*, 2011). The role of self-weighing in pregnancy as a weight management method needs further research and has been found to help limit gestational and postnatal weight gain if used in collaboration with an antenatal lifestyle intervention (Harrison *et al.*, 2014).

Apart from the controversy over optimal gestational weight gain for women based on pre-pregnancy BMI, the practical challenge of assessing weight needs consideration. Maternal weight, and subsequent weight increase during pregnancy, can vary according to time of initial assessment, clothing worn, presence of oedema and scales used (Amorim *et al.*, 2008), thus outlining the important role of the initial weighing conducted by midwives and recommended by NICE to occur as early in pregnancy as possible. However, Rees *et al.* (2012) audited one maternity service in the UK and found that 9% of records had no BMI recorded, more than 50% had either no height or weight documented, and some records were noted in imperial format (stones/pounds rather than kilograms). A review of health care for women with BMI >40 kg/m^2 in Australia also found that almost half of the sample had not had BMI documented (Slavin *et al.*, 2013). Furthermore, Rees *et al.* (2012) observed that some BMIs had been calculated by maternal self-reported height and weight. Objective measures of BMI must be used, and self-report cannot be relied upon as research has found that self-reported weight and height may lead to underestimation of BMI (Gorber *et al.*, 2007).

In summary, health professionals must ensure the relevant resources are available to record BMI for each woman at their initial appointment. Evidence indicating the importance of gestational weight gain as a contributing factor to poor outcomes suggests that monitoring maternal weight during pregnancy should be reconsidered. This might allow advice and support surrounding weight management to be initiated earlier, with the possibility of minimising some of the adverse maternal and fetal outcomes outlined.

The optimal antenatal intervention for maternal obesity

It has already been established in this chapter that women want to receive advice about weight management in pregnancy and that health professionals discuss weight at the earliest opportunity with women. However, there is still a lot of debate internationally surrounding the optimal antenatal weight management intervention for women who have a BMI ≥30 kg/m^2, and this presents a challenge to health professionals and service providers.

One reason that health professionals, such as midwives, report not wanting to discuss weight management is that they are not aware of what advice to offer or where to refer women if they do request help. Guidelines such as NICE (2010) and CMACE/RCOG (2010) suggest that weight management advice should be provided to women early in pregnancy by midwives. However, there is little guidance on what advice or interventions should be provided to women, and 'inconsistent and inconclusive evidence' of suitable antenatal interventions has been reported (Campbell *et al.*, 2009: 12). The NICE guideline suggests that any intervention should contain behaviour change components. Behaviour change techniques (BCTs) are widely used in complex interventions and should be included in antenatal interventions to help women make health changes to their behaviours – for more information on BCTs, see Michie *et al.* (2013). A recent systematic review and meta-analysis of weight management interventions for women before and during pregnancy highlighted a number of BCTs present in the successful studies (including feedback and weight monitoring). Research such as this is vital to further our understanding of why behavioural interventions impact on gestational weight gain (Agha *et al.*, 2014).

Pregnancy is a transitional point in a woman's life in which they review the past and plan for the future (NICE, 2007) and has been labelled by some as a 'teachable moment' (Phelan, 2010). This presents health professionals with an ideal opportunity to intervene with weight management advice that may have short– and long-term impacts on women, their families and their children. This is especially true for those women who have a BMI ≥30 kg/m^2 who are reported to be more accepting of their weight gain than outside of pregnancy (Smith and Lavender, 2011) and women from vulnerable groups for whom maternity care may be their first contact with the health professionals.

Over the last few years, there has been a surge of research interest in antenatal interventions aiming to manage weight gain for women with a BMI ≥30 kg/m^2. Most intervention studies are still in the early pilot stages (e.g. Adamo *et al.*, 2013; Poston *et al.*, 2013), and mixed findings have been reported from completed research (e.g. Vinter *et al.*, 2011). For example, one Australian study found a reduction in the birth weight of the babies born to overweight and obese women attending their antenatal lifestyle intervention but did not impact on the gestational weight gain of the women (Dodd *et al.*, 2014). Current evidence suggests that the dietary components play a crucial role in successful interventions (Tanentsapf *et al.*, 2011; Thangaratinam *et al.*, 2012). However, these reviews need to be interpreted with caution as the studies included are low to medium quality (Oteng-Ntim *et al.*, 2012). It has been suggested that dietary interventions should focus on highlighting the possible positive outcomes for both the mother and baby if they are to be successful (Gardner *et al.*, 2012). Furthermore, women's perspectives should be included in the design of interventions as their needs can then be addressed (Heslehurst *et al.*, 2015).

It is clear that more research that includes randomised controlled trials with long-term follow-ups and qualitative work is needed to increase our knowledge of the most suitable and appropriate antenatal intervention for pregnant women with a BMI $\geq 30\,\text{kg/m}^2$. The use of technology in providing these interventions also requires more research attention, as a recent systematic review suggests a possible role for 'technology-supported' antenatal lifestyle interventions (O'Brien et al., 2014). Thus, service providers and researchers must explore the delivery modes of these interventions in addition to innovative technology such as social networking (Palmén and Kouri, 2012).

Ethnicity and maternal obesity

Differences in ethnic background in the pregnant population inevitably cause further challenges for health professionals, as obesity prevalence varies according to ethnicity. For example, adults of black African, Caribbean and Pakistani backgrounds tend to have higher obesity prevalence than other ethnic groups (NHS Information Centre, 2006). Evidence indicates that South Asian groups have increased risk of developing type 2 diabetes mellitus and cardiovascular disease (WHO Expert Consultation, 2004; Heslehurst et al., 2012). As a result, NICE (2013) recommended that a lower BMI threshold of $27.5\,\text{kg/m}^2$ be used in South Asian populations for identification of those who may go on to develop metabolic complications. This guidance was timely; the UK population has become more culturally mixed over the last decade due to both immigration and the birth of children in families of already established ethnic groups (Jivraj, 2012). Although the largest minority ethnic group in England and Wales is South Asian (Office for National Statistics, 2012), over the last 20 years the African ethnic group has also significantly increased (Jivraj, 2012).

These recent demographic changes in the UK have important implications for health professionals delivering maternity care. CMACE (2011) identified that black women and those from minority ethnic groups, particularly recently arrived immigrants, are more likely to experience serious pregnancy complications, including those related to maternal obesity, resulting in increased maternal death compared whith white women. New immigrants may also find that the health professionals that they encounter may have differing views on maternal size than they hold;, for example, being overweight or obese is preferable for some African cultures (Rguibi and Belahsen, 2006; Oteng-Nitim et al., 2010; Herring et al., 2012). This may cause confusion and upset in the dynamic of the relationship between health professionals and pregnant women if their views on maternal size conflict.

Beliefs about food may also differ (Lindsay et al., 2012). Extended families are reported to encourage eating more in pregnancy, and larger portions than normal are more frequent (Herring et al., 2012). In Somalian culture, fruit and vegetables are the main diet of poor people, so meat is preferred as a symbol of affluence (McEwen et al., 2009). In pregnancy, Somalian women are forbidden some vegetables and dairy products (Esegbone-Adeigbe, 2011). Therefore, advice received about eating healthily and incorporating more fruit and vegetables into the diet may not be readily understood by these women. Furthermore, research with other new immigrants suggests that lack of skills in preparation and cooking of western foods, little time due to working long hours, and increased purchasing power and access to fast food has led to an increased consumption of highly processed food, high in fat and sugar, rather than a diet considered to be more healthy (Tovar et al., 2010; Agne et al., 2012; Lindberg et al., 2012; Garnweidner et al., 2012, 2013). New immigrants also report that the lack of a social network and missing friends from home, and restrictions on taking exercise, because of a lack of safe walking environment, leads to isolation and depression which may precipitate weight gain (Agne et al., 2012). It should not be forgotten that many immigrants may have other underlying health problems and also suffer from psychological trauma; for example, Nigerian women may have vitamin and mineral deficiencies (Lindsay et al., 2012).

Other factors that health professionals who manage the care of obese women from differing cultures need to be aware of is that vitamin D status tends to be lower when obese (Vimaleswaran et al., 2013). Women from cultures who cover their skin are therefore at higher risk of vitamin D deficiency as natural vitamin D synthesis in the skin is limited (Denison and Chiswick, 2011). To offset this risk, it has been suggested that all obese pregnant women should be recommended to take $10\,\mu\text{g/day}$ vitamin D supplementation (CMACE/RCOG, 2010).

In conclusion, health professionals involved with the care of obese pregnant women from outside the UK should recognise that their care needs to reflect sociocultural factors in order to provide support and advice that is acceptable and suitable. Women want dietary advice that is congruent with their beliefs (Garnweidner et al., 2012) as well as practical support, such as help reading food labels and cooking on a budget (Khazaezadeh et al., 2011). Health professionals should be cognisant of the fact that many immigrants are less likely to be obese on arrival to the host country (De Maio, 2010; Elo and Culhane, 2010), but often adopt western food practices with dietary acculturation (Gilbert and Khokhar, 2008). Choudhry and Wallace (2010) found that South Asian mothers who were highly acculturated were more aware of formula feeding practices. Dietary advice from health professionals that reflects cultural expectations and the dilemmas of living in a new environment is required to support practices that may minimise both maternal and infant health complications related to obesity in the future. Further training is required to ensure that culture-specific maternity care is provided to such women. This should include advice about culturally specific food preferences, cooking skills needed to prepare western foods and the problems that can occur with diets reliant on fast foods. Advice should be tailored to local communities and relate to the resources available and individual needs and expectations.

14.3 Conclusion and recommendations

Maternal obesity is a key area of concern in public health nutrition due to the increasing rates and association with risks and complications for mother and baby. Several challenges to addressing maternal obesity have been discussed, with the following recommendations being made:

- A greater understanding of the mechanisms by which maternal obesity impacts on pregnancy and the health of the offspring is required.
- More research is needed to examine the use of routine weighing in pregnancy.
- Health professionals' training must include dietary and nutritional information to increase their knowledge and confidence in their ability to discuss this with women.
- Diet and physical activity must be included in interventions to reduce weight gain in pregnancy as they are found to be active ingredients.
- Psychosocial and cultural influences on women's maternity needs must be understood to ensure good communication.

References

Abrams, B., Altman, S.L. and Pickett, K.E. (2000) Pregnancy weight gain: still controversial. *The American Journal of Clinical Nutrition*, 71(Suppl), 1233S–1241S.

Adamo, K.B., Ferraro, Z.M., Goldfield, G. *et al.* (2013) The Maternal Obesity Management (MOM) trial protocol: a lifestyle intervention during pregnancy to minimize downstream obesity. *Contemporary Clinical Trials*, 35, 87–96.

Agha, M., Agha, R.A. and Sandell, J. (2014) Interventions to reduce and prevent obesity in pre-conceptual and pregnant women: a systematic review and meta-analysis. *PLoS One*, 9(5), e65132.

Agne, A.A., Daubert, R., Munoz, M.L. *et al.* (2012) The cultural context of obesity: exploring perceptions of obesity and weight loss among Latina immigrants. *Journal of Immigrant Minority Health*, 14, 1063–1070.

Alfaradhi, M.Z. and Ozanne, S.E. (2011) Developmental programming in response to maternal overnutrition. *Frontiers in Genetics*, 2(27), 1–13.

Amorim, A., Linne, Y., Kac, G. and Lourenco, P.M. (2008) Assessment of weight changes during and after pregnancy: practical approaches. *Maternal & Child Nutrition*, 4, 1–13.

Artal, R., Lockwood, C.J. and Brown, H.L. (2010) Weight gain recommendations in pregnancy and the obesity epidemic. *Obstetrics & Gynecology*, 115(1), 152–155.

Barker, D.J., Winter, P.D., Osmond, C. *et al.* (1989) Weight in infancy and death from ischaemic heart disease. *Lancet*, 2(8663), 577–580.

Barker, D.J., Osmond, C., Forsen, T.J. *et al.* (2007) Maternal and social origins of hypertension. *Hypertension*, 50(3), 565–571.

Basu, A., Kennedy, L., Tocque, K. and Jones, S. (2014) Eating for 1, healthy and active for 2; feasibility of delivering novel, compact training for midwives to build knowledge and confidence in giving nutrition, physical activity and weight management advice during pregnancy. *BMC Pregnancy and Childbirth*, 14, 218.

Bayol, S.A., Simbi, B.H., Bertrand, J.A. and Stickland, N.C. (2008) Offspring from mothers fed a 'junk food' diet in pregnancy and lactation exhibit exacerbated adiposity that is more pronounced in females. *Journal of Physiology*, 586(13), 3219–3230.

Biro, M.A., Cant, R., Hall, H. *et al.* (2013) How effectively do midwives manage the care of obese pregnant women? A cross-sectional survey of Australian midwives. *Women and Birth*, 26, 119–124.

Bodnar, L.M., Ness, R.B., Markovic, N. and Roberts, J.M. (2005) The risk of preeclampsia rises with increasing prepregnancy body mass index. *Annals of Epidemiology*, 15(7), 475–482.

Brown, A. and Avery, A. (2012) Healthy weight management during pregnancy: what advice and information is being provided. *Journal of Human Nutrition and Dietetics*, 25, 378–388.

Butte, N.G., Wong, W.K., Treuth, M. *et al.* (2004) Energy requirements during pregnancy based on total energy expenditure and energy deposition. *The American Journal of Clinical Nutrition*, 79(6), 1078–1087.

Campbell, F., Messina, J., Johnson, M. *et al.* (2009) Systematic review of dietary and/or physical activity interventions for weight management in pregnancy. Report, ScHARR Public Health Collaboration Centre, The University of Sheffield.

Campbell, F., Johnson, M., Messina, J. *et al.* (2011) Behavioural interventions for weight management in pregnancy: a systematic review of quantitative and qualitative data. *BMC Public Health*, 11, 491.

Cedergren, M. (2006) Effects of gestational weight gain and body mass index in obstetric outcome in Sweden. *International Journal of Gynecology & Obstetrics*, 93, 269–274.

Chang, M.W., Nitzke, S., Buist, D. *et al.* (2014) I am pregnant and want to do better but I can't: focus groups with low-income overweight and obese pregnant women. *Maternal and Child Health Journal*, 19(5), 1060–1070.

Choudhry, K. and Wallace, L.M. (2012) 'Breast is not always best': South Asian women's experiences of infant feeding in the UK within an acculturation framework. *Maternal & Child Nutrition*, 8, 72–87.

CMACE (2011) Saving Mothers' Lives: reviewing maternal deaths to make motherhood safer: 2006–2008. The Eighth Report of the Confidential Enquiries into Maternal Deaths in the United Kingdom. *BJOG*, 118 (Suppl 1), 1–203.

CMACE/RCOG (2010) *CMACE/RCOG Joint Guideline: Management of Women with Obesity in Pregnancy*. Centre for Maternal and Child Enquiries/Royal College of Obstetricians and Gynaecologists, London.

Coad, J. and Tunstall, M. (2012) *Anatomy and Physiology for Midwives*, 3rd edn. Churchill Livingstone, Edinburgh.

Dawes, M.G., Green, J. and Ashurst, H. (1992) Routine weighing in pregnancy. *British Medical Journal*, 304, 487–489.

De Maio, F.G. (2010) Immigration as pathogenic: a systematic review of the health of immigrants in Canada. *International Journal for Equity in Health*, 9, 27.

Denison, F.C. and Chiswick, C. (2011) Improving pregnancy outcome in obese women. *Proceedings of the Nutrition Society*, 70, 457–464.

Desai, M., Gayle, D., Babu, J. and Ross, M.G. (2005) Programmed obesity in intrauterine growth-restricted newborns: modulation by newborn nutrition. *American Journal of Physiology: Regulatory, Integrative and Comparative Physiology*, 288(1), R91–R96.

DiPietro, J.A., Millett, S., Costigan, K.A. *et al.* (2003) Psychosocial influences on weight gain attitudes and behaviors during pregnancy. *Journal of the American Dietetic Association*, 103(10), 1314–1319.

Dodd, J.M., Crowther, C.A. and Robinson, J.S. (2008) Dietary and lifestyle interventions to limit weight gain during pregnancy for obese or overweight women: a systematic review. *Acta Obstetricia et Gynecologica*, 87, 702–706.

Dodd, J.M., Grivell, R.A. and Ownes, J.A. (2014) Antenatal dietary and lifestyle interventions for women who are overweight or obese: outcomes from the LIMIT randomised trial. *Current Nutritional Reports*, 3, 392.

Downs, D.S., Savage, J.S. and Rauff, E.L. (2014) Falling short of guidelines? Nutrition and weight gain knowledge in pregnancy. *Journal of Women's Health Care*, 3, 184.

Drake, A.J. and Reynolds, R.M. (2010) Impact of maternal obesity on offspring obesity and cardiometabolic disease risk. *Reproduction*, 140(3), 387–398.

Ehrenberg, H.M., Mercer, B.M. and Catalano, P.M. (2004) The influence of obesity and diabetes on the prevalence of macrosomia. *American Journal of Obstetrics and Gynaecology*, 191(3), 964–968.

Ellison, G.T.H. and Holliday, M. (1997) The use of maternal weight measurements during antenatal care. A national survey of midwifery practice through the United Kingdom. *Journal of Evaluation in Clinical Practice*, 3(4), 303–317.

Elo, I.T. and Culhane, J.F. (2010) Variations in health and health behaviours by nativity among pregnant black women in Philadelphia. *Research and Practice*, 100(11), 2185–2192.

Esegbone-Adeigbe, S. (2011) Acquiring cultural competency in caring for black African women. *British Journal of Midwifery*, 19(8), 489–496.

Ferrari, R.M. and Siega-Riz, A.M. (2013) Provider advice about pregnancy weight gain and adequacy of weight gain. *Maternal and Child Health Journal*, 17, 256–264.

Flegal, K.M., Carroll, M.D., Kit, B.K. and Ogden, C.L. (2012) Prevalence of obesity and trends in the distribution of body mass index among US adults, 1999–2010. *JAMA*, 307, 491–497.

Flenady, V., Koopmans, L., Middleton, P. *et al.* (2011) Major risk factors for stillbirth in high-income countries: a systematic review and meta-analysis. *Lancet*, 377(9774), 1331–1340.

Fleten, C., Stigum, H., Magnus, P. and Nystad, W. (2010) Exercise during pregnancy, maternal prepregnancy body mass index, and birth weight. *Obstetrics & Gynecology*, 115(2), 331–337.

Furber, C. and McGowan, L. (2011) A qualitative study of the experiences of women who are obese and pregnant in the UK. *Midwifery*, 27, 437–444.

Furber, C., McGowan, L., Quenby, S. *et al.* (2013) Antenatal interventions for reducing weight in obese women for improving pregnancy outcome. *The Cochrane Database of Systematic Reviews*, (1), CD009334.

Gardner, B., Croker, H., Barr, S. *et al.* (2012) Psychological predictors of dietary intentions in pregnancy. *Journal of Human Nutrition and Dietetics*, 25, 345–353.

Garnweidner, L.M., Terragni, L. and Pettersen, K.S. (2012) Perceptions of the host country's food culture among female immigrants from Africa and Asia: aspects relevant for cultural sensitivity in nutrition communication. *Journal of Nutrition Education and Behaviour*, 44(4), 335–342.

Garnweidner, L.M., Pettersen, K.S. and Mosdol, A. (2013) Experiences with nutrition-related information during antenatal care of pregnant women of different ethnic backgrounds residing in the area of Oslo, Norway. *Midwifery*, 29(12), e130–e137.

Gibson, K.S., Waters, T.P. and Catalano, P.M. (2012) Maternal weight gain in women who develop gestational diabetes mellitus. *Obstetrics & Gynecology*, 119(3), 560–565.

Gilbert, P.A. and Khokar, S. (2008) Changing dietary habits of ethnic groups in Europe and implications for health. *Nutrition Reviews*, 66(4), 203–215.

Gorber, S.C., Tremblay, M., Moher, D. and Gorber, B. (2007) A comparison of direct vs. self-report measures for assessing height, weight and body mass index: a systematic review. *Obesity Reviews*, 8, 307–326.

Gray, C.M., Hunt, K., Lorimer, K. *et al.* (2011) Words matter: a qualitative investigation of which weight status terms are acceptable and motivate weight loss when used by health professionals. *BMC Public Health*, 11, 513.

Harrison, C.L., Teede, H.J. and Lombard, C.B. (2014) How effective is self-weighing in the setting of a lifestyle intervention to reduce gestational weight gain and postpartum weight retention? *Australian and New Zealand Journal of Obststrics and Gynaecology*, 54(4), 382–385.

Herring, S.J., Oken, E., Haines, J. *et al.* (2008) Misperceived prepregnancy body weight status predicts excessive gestational weight gain: findings from a US cohort study. *Pregnancy and Childbirth*, 8, 54–63.

Herring, S.J., Henry, T.Q., Klotz, A.A. *et al.* (2012) Perceptions of low-income African-American mothers about excessive gestational weight gain. *Maternal and Child Health Journal*, 16, 1837–1843.

Heslehurst, N. (2011) Identifying 'at risk' women and the impact of maternal obesity of National Health Service maternity services. *Proceedings of the Nutrition Society*, 70, 439–449.

Heslehurst, N., Simpson, H., Ells, L.J. *et al.* (2008) The impact of maternal BMI status on pregnancy outcomes with immediate short-term obstetric resource implications: a meta-analysis. *Obesity Reviews*, 9(6), 635–683.

Heslehurst, N., Rankin, J., Wilkinson, J.R. and Summerbell, C.D. (2010) A nationally representative study of maternal obesity in England, UK: trends in incidence and demographic inequalities in 619 323 births, 1989–2007. *International Journal of Obesity (London)*, 34(3), 420–428.

Heslehurst, N., Moore, H., Rankin, J. *et al.* (2011) How can maternity services be developed to effectively address maternal obesity? A qualitative study. *Midwifery*, 27, e170–e177.

Heslehurst, N., Sattar, N., Rajasingam, D. *et al.* (2012) Existing maternal obesity guidelines may increase inequalities between ethnic groups: a national epidemiological study of 502, 474 births in England. *BMC Pregnancy and Childbirth*, 12, 156.

Heslehurst, N., Russell, S., McCormack, S. *et al.* (2013) Midwives perspectives of their training and education requirements in maternal obesity: a qualitative study. *Midwifery*, 29, 736–744.

Heslehurst, N., Russell, S., Brandon, H. *et al.* (2015) Women's perspectives are required to inform the development of maternal obesity services: a qualitative study of obese pregnant women's experiences. *Health Expectations*, 18, 969–981.

Hytten, F. (1990) Is it important or even useful to measure weight gain in pregnancy? *Midwifery*, 6, 28–32.

Institute of Medicine (1990) *Nutrition during Pregnancy. Part I: Weight Gain*. National Academy Press, Washington, DC.

Jivraj, S. (2012) How Has Ethnic Diversity Grown 1991–2001–2011? The Dynamics of Diversity: Evidence from the 2011 Census. Centre of Dynamics of Ethnicity, The University of Manchester. http://www.ethnicity.ac.uk/medialibrary/briefings/dynamicsofdiversity/how-has-ethnic-diversity-grown-1991-2001-2011.pdf (accessed 10 December 2016).

Johnson, M., Campbell, F., Messina, J. et al. (2013) Weight management during pregnancy: a systematic review of qualitative evidence. Midwifery, 29(12), 1287–1296.

Jones, H.N., Woollett, L.A., Barbour, N. et al. (2009) High-fat diet before and during pregnancy causes marked up-regulation of placental nutrient transport and fetal overgrowth in C57/BL6 mice. FASEB Journal, 23(1), 271–278.

Keely, A., Gunning, M. and Denison, F. (2011) Maternal obesity in pregnancy: women's understanding of risks. British Journal of Midwifery, 19(6), 364–369.

Khazaezadeh, N., Pheasant, H., Bewley, S. et al. (2011) Using services-users' views to design a maternal obesity intervention. British Journal of Midwifery, 19(1), 49–56.

Larsen, T.B., Sørensen, H.T., Gislum, M. and Johnsen, S.P. (2007) Maternal smoking, obesity, and risk of venous thromboembolism during pregnancy and the puerperium: a population-based nested case-control study. Thrombosis Research, 120(4), 505–509.

Lindberg, N.M., Stevens, V.J., Vega-Lopez, S. et al. (2012) A weight-loss intervention progam designed for Mexican-American women: cultural adaptations and results. Journal of Immigrant Minority Health, 14, 1030–1039.

Lindsay, K.J., Gubney, E.R. and McAuliffe, F.M. (2012) Maternal nutrition among women from sub-Saharan Africa, with a focus on Nigeria, and potential implications for pregnancy outcomes among immigrant populations in developed countries. Journal of Human Nutrition and Dietetics, 25, 534–546.

Ludwig, D.S., Rouse, H.L. and Currie, J. (2013) Pregnancy weight gain and childhood body weight: a within family comparison. PLOS Medicine, 10(10), e1001521.

McCurdy, C.E., Bishop, J.M., Williams, S.M. et al. (2009) Maternal high-fat diet triggers lipotoxicity in the fetal livers of nonhuman primates. Journal of Clinical Investigation, 119(2), 323–335.

McEwen, A., Straus, L. and Croker, H. (2009) Dietary beliefs and behaviour of a UK Somali population. Journal of Human Nutrition and Dietetics, 22, 116–121.

Michie, S., Richardson, M., Johnston, M. et al. (2013) The behavior change technique taxonomy (v1) of 93 hierarchically-clustered techniques: building an international consensus for the reporting of behavior change interventions. Annals of Behavioral Medicine, 46(1), 81–95

Mollart, L. (1999) A weight off my mind: the abandonment of routine antenatal weighing a change of practice research. Australian College of Midwives Incorporated Journal, 12(3), 26–31.

National Collaborating Centre for Women's and Children's Health (2008) Antenatal Care: Routine Care for the Healthy Pregnant Woman. NICE Clinical Guidelines, No. 62. RCOG Press, London.

NHS Information Centre (2006) Health Survey for England 2004: Health of Minority Ethnic Groups. NHS Information Centre, London.

NHS Information Centre (2008) Health Survey for England 2006: Latest Trends. Office for National Statistics, London.

NICE (2007) Behaviour Change at Population, Community and Individual Levels. NICE Public Health Guidance 6. National Institute for Health and Clinical Excellence, London.

NICE (2008) Maternal and Child Nutrition. Public Health Guideline PH11. National Institute for Health and Care Excellence, London. https://www.nice.org.uk/guidance/ph11 (accessed 9 December 2016).

NICE (2013) BMI: Preventing Ill Health and Premature Death in Black, Asian and Other Minority Ethnic Groups. Public Health Guideline PH46. National Institute for Health and Clinical Excellence, London. https://www.nice.org.uk/guidance/ph46 (accessed 4 January 2017).

Nyman, V.M.K., Prebensen, A.K. and Flensner, G.E.M. (2010) Obese women's experiences of encounters with midwives and physicians during pregnancy and childbirth. Midwifery, 26(4), 424–429.

O'Brien, O.A., McCarthy, M., Gibney, E.R. and McAuliffe, F.M. (2014) Technology-supported dietary and lifestyle intervention in healthy pregnant women: a systematic review. European Journal of Clinical Nutrition, 68(7), 760–766.

Office for National Statistics (2012) Ethnicity and National Identity in England 2011. Office for National Statistics, London. http://www.ons.gov.uk/ons/dcp171776_290558.pdf (accessed 10 December 2016).

Olander, E.K., Atkinson, L., Edmunds, J.K. and French, D.P. (2011) The views of pre– and post-natal women and health professionals regarding gestational weight gain: an exploratory study. Sexual & Reproductive Healthcare, 2, 43–48.

Oteng-Ntim, E., Pheasant, H., Khazaezadeh, N. et al. (2010) Developing a community-based maternal obesity intervention: a qualitative study of service providers' views. BJOG, 117, 1651–1655.

Oteng-Ntim, E., Varma, R., Croker, H. et al. (2012) Lifestyle interventions for overweight and obese pregnant women to improve pregnancy outcome: systematic review and meta-analysis. BMC Medicine, 10, 47.

Palmén, M. and Kouri, P. (2012) Maternity clinic going online: mothers' experience of social media and online health information for parental support in Finland. Journal of Communication in Healthcare, 5, 190–198.

Parlee, S.D. and MacDougald, O.A. (2014) Maternal nutrition and risk of obesity in offspring: the Trojan horse of developmental plasticity. Biochimica et Biophysica Acta, 1842(3), 495–506.

Phelan, S. (2010) Pregnancy: a 'teachable moment' for weight control and obesity prevention. American Journal of Obstetrics & Gynecology, 202, 135.e1-135. e8.

Poston, L., Briley, A.L., Barr, S. et al. (2013) Developing a complex intervention for diet and activity behaviour change in obese pregnant women (the UPBEAT trial): assessment of behavioural change and process evaluation in a pilot randomised controlled trial. BMC Pregnancy and Childbirth, 13, 148.

Rasmussen, K. and Yaktine, A.L. (eds) (2009) Weight Gain During Pregnancy: Reexamining the Guidelines. National Academies Press, Washington, DC.

Rees, G.A., Porter, J., Bennett, S. et al. (2012) The validity and reliability of weight and height measurements and body mass index calculations in early pregnancy. Journal of Human Nutrition and Dietetics, 25, 117–120.

Rguibi, M. and Belahsen, R. (2006) Body size and sociocultural influences on attitudes towards obesity among Moroccan Sahraoui women. Body Image, 3, 395–400.

Rodrigues, P.L., de Oliveira, L.C., dos Santos, A. and Kac, G. (2010) Determinant factors of insufficient and excessive gestational weight gain and maternal–child adverse outcomes. Nutrition, 26, 617–623.

Samuelsson, A.M., Matthews, P.A., Argenton, M. et al. (2008) Diet-induced obesity in female mice leads to offspring hyperphagia, adiposity, hypertension, and insulin resistance: a novel murine model of developmental programming. Hypertension, 51(2), 383–392.

Schmied, V.A., Duff, M., Dahlen, H.G. et al. (2011) 'Not waving but drowning': a study of the experiences and concerns of midwives and other health professionals caring for obese childbearing women. Midwifery, 27, 424–430.

Scott, C., Anderson, C.T., Valdez, N. *et al.* (2014) No global consensus: a cross-sectional survey of maternal weight policies. *BMC Pregnancy and Childbirth*, **14**, 167.

Slavin, V.J., Fenwick, J. and Gamble, J. (2013) Pregnancy care and birth outcomes for women with moderate to super-extreme obesity. *Women and Birth*, **26**(3), 179–184.

Smith, D. and Lavender, T. (2011) The pregnancy experience for women with a body mass index ≥30 kg/m^2; a meta-synthesis. *British Journal of Obstetrics and Gynaecology*, **118**, 779–789.

Smith, D.M., Cooke, A. and Lavender, T. (2012) Maternal obesity is the new challenge; a qualitative study of health professionals' views towards an antenatal lifestyle intervention for pregnant women with a body mass index (BMI) ≥30 kg/m^2. *BMC Pregnancy and Childbirth*, **12**, 157.

Smith, J., Cianflone, K., Biron, S. *et al.* (2009) Effects of maternal surgical weight loss in mothers on intergenerational transmission of obesity. *Journal of Clinical Endocrinology and Metabolism*, **94**(11), 4275–4283.

Smith, S.A., Heslehurst, N., Ells, L.J. and Wilkinson, J.R. (2011) Community-based service provision for the prevention and management of maternal obesity in the North East of England: a qualitative study. *Public Health*, **125**, 518–524.

Tanentsapf, I., Heitmann, B.L. and Adegboye, A.R.A. (2011) Systematic review of clinical trials on dietary intervention to prevent excessive weight gain during pregnancy among normal weight, overweight and obese women. *BMC Pregnancy and Childbirth*, **11**, 81.

Thangaratinam, S., Rogozinska, E., Jolly, K. *et al.* (2012) Effects of interventions in pregnancy on maternal weight and obstetric outcomes: meta-analysis of randomised evidence. *BMJ*, **344**, e2088.

Tovar, A., Chasen-Taber, L., Bermudez, O.I. *et al.* (2010) Knowledge, attitudes, and beliefs regarding weight gain during pregnancy among Hispanic women. *Maternal and Child Health Journal*, **14**, 938–949.

Vimaleswaran, K.S., Berry, D.J., Lu, C. *et al.* (2013) Causal relationship between obesity and vitamin D status: bi-directional Mendelian randomization analysis of multiple cohorts. *PLoS Medicine*, **10**(2), e1001383.

Vinter, C.A., Beck-Nielsen, H., Jensen, D.M. *et al.* (2011) The LIP (Lifestyle in Pregnancy) study: a randomised controlled trial of lifestyle intervention in 360 obese pregnant women. *Diabetes Care*, **34**, 2502–2507.

Waring, M., Moore Simas, T.A. and Liao, X. (2013) Gestational weight gain within recommended ranges in consecutive pregnancies: a retrospective cohort study. *Midwifery*, **29**, 550–556.

Warriner, S. (2000) Women's views on being weighed during pregnancy. *British Journal of Midwifery*, **8**(10), 620–623.

Weir, Z., Bush, J., Robson, S.C. *et al.* (2010) Physical activity ion pregnancy: a qualitative study of the beliefs of overweight and obese pregnant women. *BMC Pregnancy and Childbirth*, **10**, 18.

Wennberg, A.L., Lundqvist, A., Hogberg, U. *et al.* (2013) Women's experiences of dietary advice and dietary changes during pregnancy. *Midwifery*, **29**, 1027–1034.

WHO, Expert Consultation (2004) Appropriate body-mass index for Asian populations and its implications for policy and intervention strategies. *Lancet*, **363**(9403), 157–163.

Wilkinson, S.A. and Tolcher, D. (2010) Nutrition and maternal health: what women want and can we provide it? *Nutrition & Dietetics*, **67**, 18–25.

Zhu, M.J., Ma, Y., Long, N.M. *et al.* (2010) Maternal obesity markedly increases placental fatty acid transporter expression and fetal blood triglycerides at midgestation in the ewe. *American Journal of Physiology: Regulatory, Integrative and Comparative Physiology*, **299**(5), R1224–R1231.

15
Obesity: Childhood

Laura Stewart, Jenny Gillespie, and Taryn Young

Key messages

- Prevalence of childhood overweight and obesity has trebled in some countries in the last three decades.
- The term 'obesogenic environment' describes a societal environment which encourages intake of high--energy foods and drinks, combined with decreased physical activity and increased screen time (sedentary behaviours).
- Parents do not easily recognise unhealthy weight in their own child.
- Childhood overweight and obesity can only be diagnosed when body mass index (BMI) is calculated and then plotted on the appropriate BMI centile chart. Interpretation of the BMI centile requires the use of agreed clinical or epidemiological cut-offs.

- It is recognised that there are a number of medical and social consequences of childhood obesity, including cardiovascular disease risk factors and lower quality of life.
- Prevention of childhood obesity requires interventions targeting changes in social norms and behavioural changes at personal, community and national levels – with schools being a key environment to influence these changes.
- Treatment programmes must aim to manipulate energy balance by decreasing total energy intake, increasing physical activity levels, decreasing time spent in sedentary behaviours and making use of a range of behavioural change tools. The outcome is for BMI to decrease.

15.1 Introduction

Childhood obesity is one of the most important global public health issues, described by the World Health Organization (WHO) as being one of the most serious health challenges of the 21st century (WHO, 2012).

The importance of obesity as a major public health issue is due to the increased risk of disease and ill health associated with high levels of body fat. The body will store excess fat when there is a long-term energy imbalance; that is, when more energy is taken through food and drink than is expended through activity. However, the Foresight (2007) report illustrates the complex, intertwined determinants and relationships between social norms, environment, physiology and personal behaviours which can lead to this individual energy imbalance.

Prevalence

The WHO estimates that across the world there are 170 million children under the age of 18 years classified as overweight, with the prevalence in some countries having trebled in the past 30 years (WHO, 2012). While adult obesity continues to increase globally, there is some indication that childhood and adolescent obesity prevalence in some countries is flattening (Swinburn et al., 2011). Table 15.1 shows the prevalence of childhood obesity across Europe.

Social deprivation

There would appear to be a tendency towards higher levels of childhood obesity in families living in deprivation. In an English study of 20 973 children, there was a significant trend for higher rates of obesity related to increasing deprivation in both boys and girls (Kinra et al., 2000). Similar results were found with socio-economic gradient and body mass index (BMI) in an Australian study involving almost 5000 4– to 5-year-olds (Wake et al., 2007).

However, an inverse relationship between childhood obesity and deprived groups should not be assumed in all countries (Griffiths et al., 2013). Various studies have also shown that, in ethnic minority groups, this

Public Health Nutrition, Second Edition. Edited by Judith L Buttriss, Ailsa A Welch, John M Kearney and Susan A Lanham-New.
© 2018 by The Nutrition Society. Published 2018 by John Wiley & Sons, Ltd.
Companion website: www.wiley.com/go/buttriss/publichealth

Table 15.1 Percentage of childhood overweight in the EU member states, using measured heights and weights.[a]

Country	Collection year	Age (years)	Overweight (%)		Cut-off used
			Boys	Girls	
Austria	2003	8–12	22.5	16.7	90th centile
Belgium	2010	10–12	16.9	13.5	IOTF
Bulgaria	2004	5–17	22	17.9	IOTF
Cyprus	2010	10–12	37.5	34.1	Country-specific cut-off
Czech Republic	2005	6–17	24.6	16.9	IOFT
England	2010	5–17	21.9	23.1	IOFT
Estonia	2007/8	2–9	13.6	14.9	IOFT
France	2006-7	3–17	13.1	14.9	IOFT
Germany	2008	4–16	22.6	17.6	IOFT
Greece	2010	10–12	44.4	37.7	IOFT
Hungary	2010	10–12	27.7	22.6	IOFT
Republic of Ireland	2003/4	5–12	19.4	28.9	IOFT
Italy	2008	8	37.2	34.7	IOFT
Latvia	2008	7	15.3	15.1	IOFT
Lithuania	2008	7	16.1	16.2	IOFT
Malta	2012	10–11	38.9	30.1	IOFT
Netherlands	2010	10–12	16.8	15.4	IOFT
Poland	2000	7–17	16.3	12.4	IOFT
Portugal	2008	6–8	30	26.1	IOFT
Scotland	2010	12–15	32.7	34.3	85 th centile
Slovakia	2001	7–17	17.5	16.2	IOFT
Slovenia	2010	10–12	31.7	22.5	IOFT
Spain	2012	8–17	32.3	29.5	IOFT
Sweden	2000	10	17	19.5	IOFT

Source: http://www.worldobesity.org/resources/.
IOFT: International Obesity TaskForce.
[a] Data from Denmark, Finland, Luxembourg and Romania were produced from self-reported data and so are not listed here.

association is not consistent with weight-related behaviours or BMI status (Griffiths *et al.*, 2013).

Ethnic variation

Variations in obesity between ethnic groups and white populations in the UK and internationally have been previously documented. In studies undertaken in the UK, results have shown that British African-Caribbean and Pakistani girls have higher levels of obesity than girls in the general population in England (Lakshim *et al.*, 2012). It has been suggested that social factors rather than ethnicity may mediate obesity risk (Smith *et al.*, 2011).

The composition of some metabolic markers in ethnic groups has been found to differ when compared with white or Caucasian children. Research has shown that whilst Indian children have a lower BMI, narrower waist circumference and less subcutaneous fat than white UK children, overall percentage body fat is higher, which suggests that a large proportion of body fat in Indian children is located outside the subcutaneous compartment, and likely to be within the abdominal cavity (Lakshim *et al.*, 2012).

15.2 The obesogenic environment

The term obesogenic environment (see Chapter 23) has been coined to describe a societal environment that encourages the intake of high-energy (and often low-nutrient) food and drink in combination with decreasing physical activity and increasing sedentary behaviours (discussed in this chapter as screen time). Swinburn *et al.* (2011) comment that global food systems and the reduction in 'time-cost' of food are major drivers of the obesogenic environment. They postulated that the second half of the 20th century saw an energy balance 'flipping point' when mechanisation combined with increased food energy supply led to increased individual energy intake and thus population weight (Swinburn *et al.*, 2011).

Risk factors

A 2012 systematic review of environmental factors that may influence obesity development in young children aged up to 8 years identified availability of sweetened drinks, portion sizes and food promotion as having the most impact on developing obesity (Osei-Assibey *et al.*, 2012). A further systematic review of risk factors for obesity development in the first year of life highlighted early rapid weight gain, high birth weight, maternal pre-pregnancy overweight and maternal smoking in pregnancy. Intake of infant formula feeds and the early introduction of solids were seen as moderate risk factors influencing obesity development (Weng *et al.*, 2012).

The Avon Longitudinal Study of Parents and Children Study, a UK birth cohort study, looked at data from over 8000 children at age 7 years and noted eight risk factors from early childhood (Reilly *et al.*, 2005):

- parental obesity;
- very early BMI or adiposity rebound;
- more than 8 h watching TV per week at age 3 years;
- weight at 8 and 18 months;
- catch-up growth;
- weight gain in the first year;
- birth weight;
- short sleeping duration at age 3 years.

The strength of the evidence around these risk factors in pregnancy and early years highlights this as an important area for public health messages and interventions.

15.3 Genetics

The knowledge around genetics and obesity is growing and shows a complex picture:

- *Monogenic causes* – although extremely rare, the mutation of one particular gene, such as mutations in leptin production, leptin receptors, propeptide pro-opiomelanocortin and the melanocortin 4 receptor, can lead to extreme obesity, particularly noted in early life (Farooqi and O'Rahilly, 2006).
- *Polygenic causes* – where no single gene has been identified as predisposing obesity. Instead, it would appear that there are a number of genes which can act on appetite, food preferences and activity levels (Farooqi and O'Rahilly, 2006).

However, the genetic component to obesity alone cannot explain the global increase in the prevalence of childhood obesity since the 1980s. Therefore, family lifestyle in combination with the obesogenic environment remain the major area for public health attention (Swinburn *et al.*, 2011).

Underlying medical causes

There are a number of known endocrine and metabolic causes of childhood obesity. Although these are rare, they should be considered, particularly in young children with extreme obesity and in obese children who appear to be short for stature (Lobstein *et al.*, 2004; NICE, 2006; SIGN, 2010). Dysfunction of hormones produced by the endocrine glands can lead to hypothyroidism, growth hormone insufficiency, hypopituitarism, hypogonado-tropic hypogonadism, hypogonadism, excessive cortico-steroid administration, pseudohypoparathyroidism and craniopharyngioma. A number of inherited disorders where learning disabilities and dysmorphic features are common, such as Down's syndrome, Prader–Willi syndrome and Fragile X, are also associated with obesity (Lobstein *et al.*, 2004).

15.4 Parental influences

Parental weight is known to be associated with the development of obesity in children; Whitaker *et al.* (1997) reported that for both obese and non-obese children under 10 years the risk of developing obesity more than doubled if they have an obese parent. Whitaker *et al.* (2010) showed that children of two obese parents had an odds risk (OR) of becoming obese of 12.0 (95% confidence interval (CI): 7.2, 20.1), while children of two severely obese parents had an OR of 22.3 (95% CI: 10.3, 48.4). A significantly stronger association was found with maternal–child BMI in comparison with paternal–child BMI, regardless of the child's sex (Whitaker *et al.*, 2010).

Recognising unhealthy weight

There is a strong body of evidence to show that parents struggle to recognise unhealthy weight in their own children, which can in turn create parental resistance to entering programmes. Carnell *et al.* (2005) reported that in parents of children classified as overweight or obese, only 6% described their child as 'overweight' and none as 'very overweight'. Interestingly, parents in this study could recognise obesity in other children but not in their own (Carnell *et al.*, 2005). Jeffery *et al.* (2005) reported that only 25% of parents could correctly recognise overweight in their own child, while more could recognise obesity in their own child (Jeffery *et al.*, 2005). Stewart *et al.* (2008a) gave typologies to parents of overweight children:

- *avoiders* – those who were aware their child had a weight problem but did not wish to raise the subject with them;
- *deniers* – those who did not recognise a weight concern with their child;
- *seekers* – those who were actively seeking help for their child's weight.

Reporting on how to engage parents in treatment programmes, Reid (2009) reported that parents reacted more positively to the issue when handled sensitively. The parents found discussion around physical activity levels of their children less threatening and judgemental than being interrogated on their children's dietary habits (Reid, 2009).

15.5 Diagnosis of childhood obesity

As with adult obesity, BMI is considered the most appropriate method for diagnosing and grading levels of overweight and obesity in children (see Chapter 12), as a proxy for measuring body fat (NICE, 2006; SIGN, 2010):

$$BMI = \frac{weight(kg)}{height^2(m^2)}$$

In childhood, BMI should be plotted on centile charts to give meaningful information. In the UK, UK–WHO BMI charts should be used (available in the UK from Harlow Printing). Centile lines on the charts are used as cut-off points for diagnosis of healthy weight, overweight and obesity. Internationally, discussions on the most appropriate cut-off points have been ongoing for many years; however, in the UK, both Scottish Intercollegiate Guideline Network (SIGN) and National Institute for Health and Clinical Excellence (NICE) recommend the cut-offs given in Table 15.2 for clinical use and epidemiological studies (NICE, 2006; SIGN, 2010).

It has now become historical in the UK to have these two sets of cut-off points which differ for clinical diagnosis and epidemiological use. However, these cut-off points are shown to have a high correlation with body fat in children, greater correlation with co-morbidities and, importantly, a low rate of false diagnosis (Reilly, 2010).

When reporting on the outcome of studies and programmes, BMI, SD or Z scores are considered the most meaningful method for reporting outcomes in childhood obesity management.

Table 15.2 UK grading for overweight and obesity

Weight grading	Clinical cut-offs	Epidemiological cut-offs
Overweight	91st centile (1.34 SD)	85th centile (1.04 SD)
Obese	98th centile (2.06 SD)	95th centile (1.65 SD)

Source: NICE (2006) and SIGN (2010).
SD: standard deviation.

15.6 Consequences

The medical and social consequences of childhood obesity are well documented (NICE, 2006; SIGN, 2010). These comprise cardiovascular disease risk factors, seen in children and adulthood, such as high blood pressure, dyslipidaemia, abnormalities in ventricular mass and/or function, abnormalities in endothelial cells and hyperinsulinaemia with or without insulin resistance (Reilly, 2005). Type 2 diabetes, non-alcoholic liver disease, respiratory problems (such as sleep apnoea) and cancers (including colorectal, kidney and oesophageal) are also possible consequences (WHO, 2012). Viner *et al.* (2005) assessed the prevalence of the metabolic syndrome (insulin resistance syndrome) in a UK paediatric obesity clinic and reported that in 103 obese children, aged 2–18 years, 40% had hyperinsulinism, 32% hypertension, 30% dyslipidaemia and 11% impaired fasting glucose. It was also found that 30% of children under 12 years of age from their clinical sample had the metabolic syndrome (Viner *et al.*, 2005).

Lower levels of quality of life have been reported in overweight and obese children, with low self-esteem associated with bullying, name calling and social isolation (Lobstein *et al.*, 2004). Long-term consequences of social and economic effects, such as achieving a lower income, have been particularly reported in women (Reilly, 2005).

The evidence supports that obesity in childhood, particularly for teenagers, persists (or tracks) into adulthood (Reilly, 2005).

15.7 Prevention

Prevention of childhood obesity requires interventions on a number of fronts, which target changes in social norms and behavioural changes at national, community and personal levels. In the WHO (2004) report *Global Strategy on Diet, Physical Activity and Health* a strategic approach to improving global diet and physical activity patterns, particularly in children and adolescents, with four overriding objectives is suggested:

- Encourage public health action and interventions to reduce the risk factors resulting from unhealthy diet and physical inactivity.
- Recognition of the implications of unhealthy diet and inadequate physical activity levels and knowledge of preventative measures.
- Promote policies and action plans at all levels to address diet and physical activity behaviours.
- Increase knowledge of preventative initiatives including monitoring, evaluation and research (WHO, 2012).

Swinburn *et al.* (2011) stress that to tackle obesity, a reverse in the obesogenic environment is needed that requires Government leadership and funding. Their framework for policy development suggests that upstream interventions promoting changes in the environment and behaviours are necessary for a large positive effect at population level (Swinburn *et al.*, 2011).

Community interventions

The ANGELO (analysis grid for environments linked to obesity) model views the environment as macro-environmental sectors (e.g. media, food production, food marketing, urban/rural development and health systems) and micro-environmental settings (e.g. homes, schools, workplaces, food retailers, neighbourhoods and transport service centres). This gives a conceptual construct for scoping obesogenic elements of environmental settings and sectors, helping the decision process by identifying necessary changes and informing policy decisions (Swinburn *et al.*, 1999).

The *Ensemble Prévenons l'Obésité Des Enfants* (EPODE – *Together Let's Prevent Childhood Obesity*) is a very interesting model that has shown positive changes in a population weight can be made when the whole community is involved in taking responsibility. The programme first started in 2004 in 10 French communities. An overview of the EPODE approach by Borys *et al.* (2012) noted that the EPODE methods were being implemented in over 500 communities across six different countries. EPODE is described as 'a coordinated, capacity building approach' which aims to influence social norms and environment to help facilitate positive lifestyle changes around healthy eating and physical activity which in turn influences weight (Borys *et al.*, 2012). The approach attempts to include everyone from policy makers through to individuals, such as:

- schools
- preschools
- extracurricular activities
- media
- local sports and leisure associations
- parent associations
- catering
- health
- elected representatives
- the private sector (e.g. shop owners, local producers).

This multi-stakeholder approach is fundamental and drives development of local sustainable policies and strategies, localising the 'right' message and incorporating monitoring and evaluation of the local programme (Borys *et al.*, 2012).

Evaluation of eight of the French pilot communities included annual weight and height measurements from over 23 000 children aged from 4 to 12 years old between 2005 and 2009. These EPODE pilot communities showed a significant decrease in overweight and obesity, from 20.6% in 2005 to 18.8% in 2009 ($p < 0.0001$). During the same period, the prevalence of childhood overweight and obesity in France remained static (http://www.epode-european-network.com/een-news/154-encouraging-results-in-french-epode-pilot-towns.html).

The most recent Cochrane review on preventing obesity in childhood described strong evidence on the effect of prevention, particularly in the 6–12 years age group. Although noting heterogeneity in the studies and the need for further high-quality studies, the review gives a very useful list of promising areas for policy decisions and strategies (Waters *et al.*, 2011):

- including healthy eating, physical activity and body image in school curriculums;
- increased physical activity and the development of basic movement skills in schools;
- improved nutritional quality of food in schools;
- environments and cultural practices that support children to eat healthier foods and be active daily;
- support for school teachers and other staff to implement health promotion strategies and activities;
- parental support including home activities that encourage children to be more active, eat nutritious foods and reduce screen-based activities.

Of the 55 studies, eight looked at adverse effects with no evidence of increase in health inequalities, body image sensitivities, poor eating habits nor increased prevalence of underweight (Waters *et al.*, 2011). The lack of evidence of these possible adverse effects will be important to many who have concerns that interventions, particularly those within schools, may be doing harm.

Marketing to children

The 'Sydney Principles', developed by the International Obesity Taskforce (IOTF), aim to decrease the effect of direct advertising of high-energy (often low in nutrient) foods and drinks to children. It specifically addresses eliminating advertising in childhood environs such as schools, with an international curb on advertising across borders, on the internet, satellite, cable and free-to-view TV.

However, a review of regulatory and self-regulatory restrictions on marketing unhealthier foods to children by Galbraith-Emani and Lobstein (2013) found that there was mixed evidence of a decline in advertising. Data from scientific and peer reviewed journals show that these types of advertising remain high compared with evidence from food-industry-sponsored reports showing good adherence to voluntary codes (Galbraith-Emani and Lobstein, 2013).

15.8 Treatment management

Worldwide guidelines suggest that family involvement is essential to managing childhood obesity and, indeed, that treatment should only be commenced with parents who are motivated to change (NICE, 2006; SIGN, 2010). One of the challenges of childhood obesity is delivering a message that is meaningful to the age of the child. Figure 15.1 gives a suggestion on the level of interaction with children and parents in treatment programmes based on best practice.

Indeed, there are programmes which are aimed directly at the parents: results from the Australian study HIKCUPS (Hunter Illawarra Kids Challenge Using Parent Support) showed that there was a greater change in BMI SD from the parent-centred intervention group compared with parent and child groups (Collins et al., 2011).

Groups or individual sessions

Most childhood weight management programmes are community-based groups (Savoye et al., 2007; Sacher et al., 2010), although there are also programmes for individual families (Stewart et al., 2005). However, there are no comparison studies which look at whether groups or individual sessions are more effective. In the UK, weight management camps have shown positive outcomes with Gately et al. (2005) reporting a mean weight loss of 6.0 kg and decrease in BMI SD scores by 0.28. While these results are very positive, any lifestyle changes made during the camp programme need to be supported once the young person returns to their home environment.

There is room to postulate that community groups are more successful with those children in the lower obesity

levels, while individual sessions perhaps benefit those with more complex medical and social needs and those in the extreme obesity range. Therefore, the best programmes to be used may depend on:

- age of the children/young people;
- population social demographics;
- geography.

Treatment messages

Although the causes of childhood obesity as discussed earlier are very complex and multifactorial, the evidence leads treatment programmes to give three main messages for manipulating energy balance (NICE, 2006; SIGN, 2010):

- decrease total energy intake;
- increase total physical activity levels;
- decrease time spent in sedentary behaviours.

Dietary
Collins et al. (2006) have shown that total energy decrease is the most important aim of dietary change and that manipulation of specific macronutrients (e.g. low fat, high protein, low carbohydrate regimes) is no more successful. The most commonly seen method of helping families to consider energy reduction is the use of a traffic light regimen, mainly based on the regimen used by Epstein et al. (1985) in the USA (Collins et al., 2006).

A traffic light regimen categorises food and drink as:

- Red – high in sugar and fat; to be restricted.
- Amber – mainly protein, starchy and dairy foods; portion sizes to be controlled.
- Green – mainly fruit and vegetables; to use as snacks.

Physical activity
The physical activity message is to increase activity to at least 1 h per day. In the UK, it is recommended for children under 3 years of age (who can move independently) to be physically active for a minimum of 3 h per

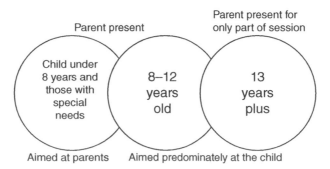

Figure 15.1 Suggested age interaction with children and parents.

day (Department of Health, Physical Activity, Health Improvement and Protection, 2011). This time can be split up over the day and does not necessarily need to be in one episode. Importantly, evidence suggests that the intensity of the activity is important, and this should be at a moderate to vigorous level. Moderate level can be described as getting hot and red in the face, whilst a vigorous level is not being able to hold a conversation.

Screen time

Work from the USA originally showed the emergence of an association with TV watching and childhood obesity, Epstein *et al.* (2000) showed that a reduction of sedentary behaviours to no more than 2 h per day or 14 h a week could have a positive effect in managing childhood obesity. Within childhood obesity weight management, there is an acceptance of the message of no more than 2 h of screen time a day, with screen time including TV watching, computer/table use, phone texting/gaming and playing video games (NICE, 2006; SIGN, 2010).

Behavioural change tools

The SIGN and NICE guidelines state that behavioural change tools should be used in all childhood obesity programmes. They recommend that the following should be used:

- stimulus control
- self monitoring
- goal setting
- rewards for setting goals
- problem solving.

Parents should also be encouraged to give praise and to be positive behavioural role models (NICE, 2006; SIGN, 2010).

A systematic review by Sahota *et al.* (2010) showed that no particular behavioural change tool could be identified as being most effective in the treatment of childhood obesity. What was important was the combination of tools used. It was also interestingly noted that an important factor appeared to be the development of rapport between the child/family and the health practitioner (Sahota *et al.*, 2010). This builds on work by Stewart *et al.* (2008b), which found that parents saw the non-judgemental attitude of the health practitioner and their ability to build rapport with the child and family as important to perceiving a positive outcome.

Drugs

Currently, orlistat is the only anti-obesity drug that is available in the UK, with SIGN and NICE guidelines recommending that it can be used for adolescents (those over 12 years of age) with regular review (NICE, 2006; SIGN, 2010). The main study on the use of orlistat with teenagers (aged 12–16 years) is by Chanoine *et al.* (2005), which showed that those adolescents taking the drug for a year, plus a lifestyle intervention, had a decrease in BMI while the placebo group had an increase in BMI.

Surgery

Bariatric surgery in adolescents is still controversial for some but is certainly increasing and is recommended by both SIGN and NICE for extremely obese adolescents (NICE, 2006; SIGN, 2010). A major study by O'Brien *et al.* (2010) has shown that, in young people aged 14–18 years, having gastric banding resulted in a significant decrease in weight, with a loss of 50% of their excess weight, as well as positive benefits to health outcomes and quality of life.

Treatment outcomes

The main outcome in childhood obesity treatment programmes is for BMI to decrease. Owing to the fact that children are growing in height, this can be achieved without a weight loss. The younger a child is, the faster the BMI can be decreased through weight staying the same and height increasing. SIGN (2010) and NICE (2006) recommend that weight maintenance should be the main weight outcome.

In adult obesity, there is well-accepted evidence that a weight loss of 5–10% can lead to positive health outcomes. In childhood obesity it is still unclear what change in BMI SD would lead to a significant clinical positive outcome. However, the evidence is growing, but the answer still remains unclear with age and puberty status possible confounding factors. Kolsgaard *et al.* (2011) suggest a modest reduction in BMI SD score of −0.1 shows improvement in health outcomes, with Hunt *et al.* (2007) suggesting a reduction of −0.25 and Reinehr and Andler (2004) suggesting a reduction of −0.5. What does seem clear is that significant changes in BMI SD are more likely to be seen in interventions with younger children compared with older children (Reinehr *et al.*, 2010).

References

Borys, J.M., Le Bodo, Y., Jebb, S.A. *et al.* (2012) EPODE approach for childhood obesity prevention: methods, progress and international development. *Obesity Reviews*, **13**, 299–315.

Carnell, S., Edwards, C., Croker, H. *et al.* (2005) Parental perceptions of overweight in 3–5 y olds. *International Journal of Obesity*, **29**, 353–355.

Chanoine, J.P., Hampl, S., Jensen, C. *et al.* (2005) Effect of orlistat on weight and body composition in obese adolescents. *JAMA*, **293** (23), 2873–2883.

Collins, C.E., Warren, J., McCoy, P. and Stokes, B.J. (2006) Measuring effectiveness of dietetic interventions in child obesity: a systematic review of randomized trials. *Archives of Pediatric & Adolescent Medicine*, **160** (9), 906–922.

Collins, C.E., Okely, A.D., Morgan, P.J. *et al.* (2011) Parent diet modification, child activity or both in obese children: an RCT. *Paediatrics*, **127**, 619–627.

Department of Health, Physical Activity, Health Improvement and Protection (2011) Start Active, Stay Active. A Report on Physical Activity for Health from the Four Home Countries' Chief Medical Officers. https://www.gov.uk/government/uploads/system/uploads/attachment_data/file/216370/dh_128210.pdf (accessed 10 December 2016).

Epstein, L.H., Wing, R.R. and Valoski, A.M. (1985) Childhood obesity. *Pediatric Clinics of North America*, **32** (2), 363–379.

Epstein, L.H., Paluch, R.A., Gordy, C.C. and Dorn, J. (2000) Decreasing sedentary behaviors in treating pediatric obesity. *Archives of Pediatric & Adolescent Medicine*, **154** (3), 220–226.

Farooqi, I.S. and O'Rahilly, S. (2006) Genetics of obesity in humans. *Endocrine Reviews*, **27** (7), 710–718.

Foresight (2007) *Tackling Obesity: Future Choices – Project Report*. Government Office for Science, London.

Galbraith-Emani, S. and Lobstein, T. (2013) The impact of initiatives to limit the advertising of food and beverage products to children: a systematic review. *Obesity Reviews*, **14** (12), 960–974.

Gately, P.J., Cooke, C.B., Barth, J.H. *et al.* (2005) *Children's residential weight loss camps can work*, Pediatrics, **116**, 73–77.

Griffiths, G., Gately, P.J., Marchant, P. and Cooke, C.B. (2013) Area-level deprivation and adiposity in children: is the relationship linear? *International Journal of Obesity*, **37** (4), 486–492.

Hunt, L.P., Ford, A., Sabin, M.A. *et al.* (2007) Clinical measures of adiposity and percentage fat loss: which measure most accurately reflects fat loss and what should we aim for? *Archives of Disease in Childhood*, **92**, 399–403.

IOTF (n.d.) *The Sydney Principles*. http://www.worldobesity.org/iotf/obesity/childhoodobesity/sydneyprinciples/ (accessed 10 December 2016).

Jeffery, A.N., Voss, L.D., Metcalf, B.S. *et al.* (2005) Parents' awareness of overweight in themselves and their children: cross sectional study within a cohort (EarlyBird 21). *BMJ*, **330**, 23–24.

Kinra, S., Nelder, R.P. and Lewendon, G.J. (2000) Deprivation and childhood obesity: a cross sectional study of 20 973 children in Plymouth, United Kingdom. *Journal of Epidemiology and Community Health*, **54** (6), 456–460.

Kolsgaard, M.L.P., Joner, G., Brunborg, C. *et al.* (2011) Reduction in BMI z-score and improvement in cardiometabolic risk factors in obese children and adolescents. The Oslo Adiposity Intervention Study – a hospital/public health nurse combined treatment. *BMC Pediatrics*, **11**, 47.

Lakshim, S., Metcalf, B.S., Joglekar, C. *et al.* (2012) Differences in body composition and metabolic status between white UK and Asian Indian children (EarlyBird 24 and the Pune Maternal Nutrition Study). *Pediatric Obesity*, **7**, 347–354.

Lobstein, T., Baur, L. and Uauy, R. (2004) Obesity in children and young people: a crisis in public health. *Obesity Review*, **5** (Suppl 1), 4–85.

NICE (2006) *Obesity Guidance on the Prevention, Identification, Assessment and Management of Overweight and Obesity in Adults and Children*. NICE Clinical Guideline CG43. National Institute for Health and Clinical Excellence, London.

O'Brien, P.E., Sawyer, S.M., Laurie, C. *et al.* (2010) Laparoscopic adjustable gastric banding in severely obese adolescents. *JAMA*, **303** (6), 519–526.

Osei-Assibey, G., Dick, S., MacDiarmid, J. *et al.* (2012) The influence of the food environment on overweight and obesity in young children: a systematic review. *BMJ Open*, **2**, e001538.

Reid, M. (2009) *Debrief of a Study to Identify and Explore Parental, Young People's and Health Professionals' Attitudes, Awareness and Knowledge of Child Healthy Weight*. Report 2008/2009 RE036. NHS Health Scotland, Edinburgh. http://www.healthscotland.com/uploads/documents/10002-RE036Final Report0809.pdf (accessed 10 December 2016).

Reilly, J.J. (2005) Descriptive epidemiology and health consequences of childhood obesity. *Best Practice and Research Clinical Endocrinology and Metabolism*, **19** (3), 327–341.

Reilly, J.J. (2010) Assessment of obesity in children and adolescents: synthesis of recent systematic reviews and clinical guidelines. *Journal of Human Nutrition and Dietetics*, **23**, 205–211.

Reilly, J.J., Armstrong, J., Dorosty, A.R. *et al.* (2005) Early life risk factors for childhood obesity: cohort study. *BMJ*, **330**, 1357–1359.

Reinehr, T. and Andler, W. (2004) Changes in the atherogenic risk factor profile according to degree of weight loss. *Archives of Disease in Childhood*, **89**, 419–422.

Reinehr, T., Schaefer, A., Winkel, K. *et al.* (2010) An effective lifestyle intervention in overweight children: findings from a randomized controlled trial on 'Obeldicks light'. *Clinical Nutrition*, **29**, 331–336.

Sacher, P.M., Kalotourou, M., Chadwick, P. *et al.* (2010) Randomised controlled trial of the MEND program: a family community intervention for childhood obesity. *Obesity*, **18** (S2), S1–S7.

Sahota, P., Wordley, J. and Woodward, J. (2010) *Health Behaviour Change Models and Approaches for Families and Young People to Support HEAT 3: Child Healthy Weight Programmes*. NHS Health Scotland, Woodburn House, Edinburgh.

Savoye, M., Shaw, M., Dziura, J. *et al.* (2007) Effects of a weight management program on body composition and metabolic parameters in overweight children. *JAMA*, **297** (24), 2697–2704.

SIGN (2010) *Management of Obesity: A National Clinical Guideline*. SIGN Guideline 115. Scottish Intercollegiate Guideline Network, Edinburgh.

Smith, N., Kelly, Y. and Nazroo, J. (2011) The effects of acculturation on obesity rates in ethnic minorities in England: evidence from the Health Survey for England. *European Journal of Public Health*, **22** (4), 508–513.

Stewart, L., Chapple, J., Hughes, A.R. *et al.* (2008a) Parents' journey through treatment for their child's obesity: qualitative study. *Archives of Disease in Childhood*, **93**, 35–39.

Stewart, L., Chapple, J., Hughes, A.R. *et al.* (2008b) The use of behavioural change techniques in the treatment of paediatric obesity: qualitative evaluation of parental perspectives on treatment. *Journal of Human Nutrition and Dietetics*, **21** (5), 464–473.

Stewart, L., Houghton, J., Hughes, A.R., Pearson, D., Reilly, J.J. (2005) Dietetic management of pediatric overweight: Development of a practical and evidence-based behavioral approach. *Journal of the American Dietetic Association*, **105** (Nov), 1810–1815.

Swinburn, B., Egger, G. and Raza, F. (1999) Dissecting obesogenic environments: the development and application of a framework for identifying and prioritizing environmental interventions for obesity. *Preventive Medicine*, **29**, 563–570.

Swinburn, B., Sacks, G., Hall, K.D. *et al.* (2011) The global pandemic: shaped by global drivers and local environments. *Lancet*, **378**, 804–814.

Viner, R.M., Segal, T.Y., Lichtarowicz-Krynska, E. and Hindmarsh, P. (2005) Prevalence of the insulin resistance syndrome in obesity. *Archives of Disease in Childhood*, **90**, 10–14.

Wake, M., Hard, P., Canterford, L. *et al.* (2007) Overweight, obesity and girth of Australian preschoolers: prevalence and socio-economic correlates. *International Journal of Obesity*, **31** (7), 1044–1051.

Waters, E., de Silva-Sanigorski, A., Hall, B.J. *et al.* (2011) Interventions for preventing obesity in children. *Cochrane Database of Systematic Reviews*, (12), CD001871.

Weng, S.F., Redsell, S.A., Swift, J.A. *et al.* (2012) Systematic review and meta-analyses of risk factors for childhood overweight identifiable during infancy. *Archives of Disease in Childhood*, **97** (12), 1019–1026.

Whitaker, R.C., Wright, J.A., Pepe, M.S. *et al.* (1997) Predicting obesity in young adulthood from childhood and parental obesity. *The New England Journal of Medicine*, **337** (13), 869–873.

Whitaker, K.L., Jarvis, M.J., Beeken, R.J. *et al.* (2010) Comparing maternal and paternal intergenerational transmission of obesity risk in a large population-based sample. *The American Journal of Clinical Nutrition*, **91**, 1560–1567.

WHO (2004) *Global Strategy on Diet, Physical Activity and Health*. World Health Organization, Geneva. http://www.who.int/dietphysicalactivity/strategy/eb11344/strategy_english_web.pdf (accessed 4 January 2017).

WHO (2012) *Prioritizing Areas for Action in the Field of Population-based Prevention of Childhood Obesity. A Set of Tools for Member States to Determine and Identify Priority Areas for Action*. World Health Organization, Geneva.

16
Cardiovascular Diseases: Sodium and Blood Pressure

Linda M Oude Griep and Paul Elliott

Key messages

- Collection of 24 h urinary excretion is an objective, but relatively burdensome method for measurement of sodium intake. Casual urine collection is a less burdensome and low-cost alternative to estimate population sodium intakes, but is less suitable to estimate individuals' sodium intakes.
- The vast majority of adult populations across the world have high average sodium intakes of more than 100 mmol/day, with some countries showing intakes of over 200 mmol/day, mainly in Asian countries.
- In western diets, major sodium sources are manufactured and restaurant-prepared foods. In Asian diets, discretionary sodium use as salt or soy sauce added during cooking contributes to high sodium intakes.
- The evidence for an adverse effect of sodium intake on blood pressure is strong and well established.

- Evidence on the relationship between higher sodium intake and the development of cardiovascular diseases is less consistent due to problems of sodium intake assessment and reverse causality.
- Blood pressure during childhood may be related to long-term development of high blood pressure and cardiovascular diseases later in life.
- A reduction in blood pressure by lowering sodium intakes through population-wide public health strategies has important public health benefits.
- Most effective strategies are reduction in sodium levels of manufactured foods and improving food labelling in western countries. Sodium substitutes to reduce discretionary sodium use in Asian countries may also be beneficial.

16.1 Introduction

Sodium is an essential nutrient for the human body. It has an important role in complex physiologic processes, including maintenance of extracellular volume and plasma osmolality, cellular membrane potential and functioning of transport systems. About 95% of the total sodium content in the body is found in extracellular fluid and the rest within cells. The kidneys normally excrete more than 90% of ingested sodium in the urine within 24–48 h, unless sweating is excessive.

Salt, sodium chloride, is the most important sodium source, providing over 90% of dietary sodium. Though salt comprises 40% sodium and 60% chloride, the terms salt and sodium are often used interchangeably. The amount of dietary sodium needed to maintain physiologic function is estimated to be no more than 10–20 mmol/day

(200–500 mg/day). Diets across the world are high in sodium. The majority of sodium comes from packaged and restaurant foods and condiments (e.g. soy sauces). Average sodium consumption in adults in many countries is far above the World Health Organization (WHO) defined recommended levels of <85 mmol/day (<2 g/day sodium, <5 g/day salt) (WHO, 2012).

High sodium intake has an important role in the pathogenesis of elevated blood pressure, one of the most important modifiable risk factors for cardiovascular diseases. It is estimated that systolic blood pressure higher than 110 mmHg contributes to over 50% of coronary heart disease disability-adjusted life-years attributed to sub-optimal blood pressure levels (Lim *et al.*, 2012). Hypertension currently affects nearly half of adults globally, with larger numbers experiencing elevated blood pressure. In this chapter, we look at ways to measure sodium intakes in

Public Health Nutrition, Second Edition. Edited by Judith L Buttriss, Ailsa A Welch, John M Kearney and Susan A Lanham-New.
© 2018 by The Nutrition Society. Published 2018 by John Wiley & Sons, Ltd.
Companion website: www.wiley.com/go/buttriss/publichealth

the population, summarise the evidence relating sodium intake to elevated blood pressure and cardiovascular diseases, and examine approaches to lower sodium intakes in populations for the benefit of public health.

16.2 Dietary sodium intake

Assessment of sodium intake

The accurate measurement of sodium intake is complicated by high variations in daily sodium intakes. Dietary surveys and urine collections are two commonly used approaches to assess sodium intake, each with its own strengths and limitations. Dietary surveys use food frequency questionnaires, food diaries, weighed records or 24 h dietary recalls to estimate an individual's food intake over a set time period. To convert reported food intake data to nutrient intakes, standardised food composition tables are used. These methods have limitations, such as underreporting of food intake, inaccurate or incomplete food composition tables, and coding errors. Other problems include quantifying the amount of salt added during cooking or at the table, the proportion of salt left behind on the plate, and variability in the sodium content of manufactured foods, and the sodium concentration of local water supplies (James et al., 1987). These dietary assessment methods generally underestimate sodium intakes compared with sodium intake estimated from 24 h urine collections.

Collection of 24 h urinary excretion is not prone to reporting biases in food intakes, nor reliance on food composition tables, and is therefore a more objective and preferred method to estimate sodium intakes. A 24 h period captures more than 95% of consumed sodium, excreted in the urine, and is not affected by diurnal variations in urinary excretion of sodium, other electrolytes or water. The highest electrolyte excretion rates in healthy individuals are found around midday, with lowest excretion at night towards the end of sleep. The 24 h urinary excretion method takes no account of electrolyte loss other than via the kidney and thus tends to underestimate true intake. Urine collections must be complete or near complete to prevent biased excretion estimates. There are no absolute checks on completeness, though urinary excretion of biomarkers such as ingested para-amino benzoic acid has been advocated in this context. Accurate timing, as used for example in the INTERMAP study (Stamler et al., 2003), avoids undercollection and enables correction for minor deviations from a 24 h collection period. Single-day urine collection is valuable in characterising group intake, but is imprecise for estimating an individual's usual sodium intake; usually two or more 24 h urine collections are required to give more precise estimates of a person's true habitual sodium intake, but these are rarely done in population surveys.

The 24 h urine collections are relatively burdensome to individuals, so casual (spot) urine collections are more often used instead. Casual urine excretion compared with 24 h sodium excretion among over 5000 participants from the INTERSALT study showed modest correlations for individuals but high validity at the mean level for populations. Casual urine may therefore be a useful, low-burden, and low-cost alternative to 24 h collections to estimate population sodium intakes, but is less suitable to estimate individuals' sodium intakes (Brown et al., 2013).

Sodium intakes across populations

Louis Dahl was the first to publish data, over 50 years ago, showing large variations in sodium intakes and levels of hypertension across populations. He found the lowest daily sodium intakes among Alaskan Eskimos (68 mmol/day) and the highest among people from the northeast of Japan (462 mmol/day). Subsequently, many observational and intervention studies have published data on sodium intake or urinary sodium excretion among populations around the world (Brown et al., 2009). The INTERSALT study collected the most extensive standardised data on 24 h urinary sodium excretion patterns of over 10 000 men and women aged 20–59 years from 52 population samples in 32 countries between 1985 and 1987 (INTERSALT Cooperative Research Group, 1988). Four isolated populations — Yanomamo Indians of Brazil, Xingu Indians of Brazil, Papua New Guinea Highlanders and the Luo in rural Kenya — had sodium intakes of less than 50 mmol/day. All other population samples had mean sodium intakes of more than 100 mmol/day, with the highest found in Tianjin, People's Republic of China. The INTERMAP study collected standardised data on sodium intakes between 1996 and 1999 from dietary and 24 h urinary collections among 17 population samples in Japan, People's Republic of China, UK and USA (Stamler et al., 2003). The vast majority of INTERMAP participants had urinary sodium excretions of over 100 mmol/day and only few participants had values less than 70 mmol/day. A review of all available data on sodium intakes concluded that the majority of the adult populations across the world have average sodium intakes over 100 mmol/day with intakes of over 200 mmol/day found particularly in Asian countries (Brown et al., 2009).

Only few data are available on sodium intakes in children, mainly from western countries (Australia, Europe and North America) (Brown et al., 2009). Sodium intake in children is also high, with reported intake levels of >100 mmol/day in children over 5 years old in nearly all countries. It has been estimated that sodium intake increases per year of age by 4.3 mmol/day, reflecting higher total food consumption at older ages (rather than differences in food choices with age).

Food sources of sodium

The addition of sodium to the human diet is a relatively new phenomenon. Humans evolved on a low-sodium diet of no more than 20–40 mmol/day, since natural foods contain only small amounts of sodium (Anderson *et al.*, 2010). Sodium intakes increased substantially since the Chinese discovered ~5000 years ago that salt can be used to preserve foods. Although salt was no longer required as preservative after the invention of the refrigerator and freezer, salt intakes remain high due to high sodium levels in processed foods among industrialised populations. In western diets, around 75% of sodium intake comes from manufactured or restaurant-prepared foods, while discretionary use at home or at the table has only modest contribution to total sodium intake (James *et al.*, 1987). Results from

the INTERMAP study showed that manufactured foods, including bread, grain, cereal, soup, sauces and cured meat, accounted for the vast majority of sodium consumed in the UK and the USA (Figure 16.1) (Anderson *et al.*, 2010). Discretionary sodium use as salt or soy sauce added during cooking, miso, salted vegetables and fruits, and fresh and salted fish accounted for most sodium consumption in Japan and the People's Republic of China. There are only limited data available on sodium sources in children. In the UK, the National Diet and Nutrition Survey 2011 surveyed children and adolescents aged 4–18 years old (NDNS, 2011). Cereals and cereal products were the largest sodium sources, contributing 37% of daily sodium intake, and comprised mainly white bread (11–13%) and pasta, rice and pizza (8–11%). Other important sources of sodium intake were meat and meat products (23–27%) and milk products (8–11%). It is important to identify dietary sources of sodium so that effective population-wide sodium reduction strategies can be designed and implemented.

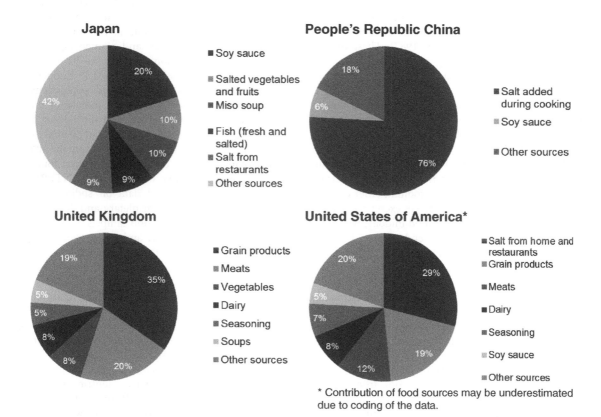

Figure 16.1 Food sources of sodium in Japan, People's Republic China, UK and USA. Data from the INTERMAP study. *Source*: Anderson *et al.* (2010). Reproduced with permission of Elsevier.

16.3 The evidence on sodium intake, blood pressure and cardiovascular health

Sodium intake and blood pressure

The aetiological relationship between excessive sodium intake and elevated blood pressure is well established. Some of the first reports about the importance of sodium intake on blood pressure came from studies among isolated, undeveloped populations without access to salt. They showed low blood pressure levels and no rise in blood pressure with age compared with developed populations. Migration from rural to urban areas in Kenya, for example, was accompanied by increased sodium intakes and a significant rise in blood pressure (Poulter *et al.*, 1990). Besides 24 h urinary sodium excretion patterns, the INTERSALT study also collected individual measurements of blood pressure. INTERSALT found a consistent significant positive relationship of sodium with blood pressure differences with age among populations. A 6 g/day higher urinary excretion of salt (100 mmol sodium) was associated with 9–11 mmHg greater rise in systolic blood pressure over a 30-year period (Figure 16.2) (INTERSALT Cooperative Research

Group, 1988; Elliott *et al.*, 1996). These results were mirrored by experimental studies in chimpanzees, who have 98.8% of their genes in common with humans. Chimpanzees with salt intake of up to 15 g/day added to their usual low-sodium diet over 20 months had a 33/10 mmHg higher systolic/diastolic blood pressure compared with a control group consuming their normal diet (Denton *et al.*, 1995). As salt was removed from their diet, blood pressure showed rapid reversal towards baseline values. More modest reductions in sodium intake of chimpanzees within the range of sodium intakes commonly found among human populations were also associated with reductions in blood pressure (Elliott *et al.*, 2007).

During the last decades, many controlled intervention studies in humans assessed the effect of sodium reduction on blood pressure. Regardless of methodological differences, meta-analyses showed significant reduction in systolic and diastolic blood pressure with lower sodium intake in individuals with or without hypertension (Aburto *et al.*, 2013; He *et al.*, 2013). Because participants in individual trials experienced difficulties complying with a lower sodium diet, especially in the long term, meta-analyses tend to underestimate the blood pressure effect of sodium reduction. Strong evidence comes particularly from the Dietary Approaches to Stop Hypertension-Sodium (DASH-sodium) study that achieved dietary compliance by providing all foods for 3 months (Sacks *et al.*, 2001). Participants received three levels of salt intake (8, 6 and 4 g/day) for 4 weeks each in a crossover design comparing a typical American diet or DASH dietary pattern high in plant foods and low in meat, high-fat and sugary foods. The DASH-sodium trial showed a clear dose–response relationship between sodium reduction and blood pressure (Figure 16.3),

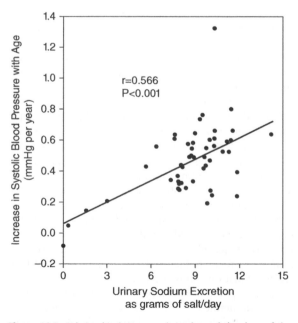

Figure 16.2 Relationship between salt intake and the slope of the rise in systolic blood pressure with age across 52 population samples in the INTERSALT study. *Sources:* INTERSALT Cooperative Research Group (1988) and Elliott *et al.* (1996). Reproduced with permission of BMJ Publishing Ltd.

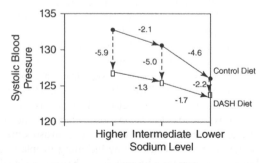

Figure 16.3 The effect on systolic blood pressure of reduced sodium intake and the DASH diet. The mean changes in blood pressure are shown for various sodium levels of control and DASH diets (solid lines). Mean changes in blood pressure between the two diets at each level of sodium intake are shown by the dotted lines. *Source:* Sacks *et al.* (2001). Reproduced with permission of Massachusetts Medical Society.

evident for both pre-hypertensive and hypertensive individuals; the fall in blood pressure was greater from 6 to 4 g/day (intermediate to lower levels of salt) compared with 8 to 6 g/day (higher to intermediate). Only two intervention studies are published with duration over 1 year (He *et al.*, 2013), partly reflecting the difficulty of adhering to a lower salt diet over the longer term when most sodium comes from processed and restaurant food.

With regard to children, meta-analysis of controlled trials found that modest reduction in sodium intake showed a small but significant reduction in systolic and diastolic blood pressure (Aburto *et al.*, 2013). Dietary patterns of lower sodium intakes adopted during childhood may continue during adulthood. Since blood pressure early in life may be related to the risk of hypertension during adulthood, lowering sodium intake in childhood may be an important public health approach to the early prevention of hypertension and risk of cardiovascular diseases in later life.

Sodium intake and cardiovascular health

The relationship between blood pressure and cardiovascular diseases is strong and independent of other risk factors for all age, ethnic and socio-economic groups. For individuals aged 40–70 years, each 20 mmHg increment in systolic blood pressure or 10 mmHg in diastolic blood pressure doubles the risk of cardiovascular diseases (Lewington *et al.*, 2002). Risk increases across the range of blood pressure levels, from lowest to highest (Lewington *et al.*, 2002). Several studies have examined the risk of cardiovascular diseases in relation to salt intake. A meta-analysis of 13 prospective cohort studies showed a positive and direct relationship between higher sodium intake and stroke (hazard ratio (HR) comparing highest versus lowest categories of intake: 1.23; 95% confidence interval (CI): 1.06–1.43), but found a borderline significant positive association for total cardiovascular events (HR: 1.14; CI: 0.99–1.31) (Strazzullo *et al.*, 2009). A meta-analysis for WHO including nine cohort studies reported HR 1.24 (CI: 1.08–1.43) for stroke comparing highest versus lowest categories of salt intake, but no significant association for fatal coronary heart disease (HR: 1.12; CI: 0.93–1.34) (WHO, 2012; Aburto *et al.*, 2013). The quality of this evidence was graded as low to very low, reflecting concerns about study design, systematic error in sodium assessment and potential reverse causality by including people with cardiovascular diseases who may have changed their salt intakes (Cobb *et al.*, 2014). Findings from the large-scale Prospective Urban Rural Epidemiology (PURE) study showed a J-shaped relationship of sodium intakes estimated from single casual fasting urine samples on all-cause mortality and cardiovascular events, with higher risks of CVD at lower and higher sodium intakes

(O'Donnell *et al.*, 2014; Mente *et al.*, 2016). The findings of these studies, however, have been strongly criticised for methodological limitations including invalid measurement of sodium intake and other potential biases (Cogswell *et al.*, 2016). This emphasises the importance of careful study designs and accurate measurement to identify true associations of sodium intakes with cardiovascular diseases.

Only a few randomised controlled trials have examined the effects of lowered sodium intake on cardiovascular diseases, but these were mainly designed to investigate effects on blood pressure and were underpowered to show meaningful results for cardiovascular diseases (He and MacGregor, 2011; Taylor *et al.*, 2011; Aburto *et al.*, 2013). A large-scale randomised trial is under way to determine the effect of a salt substitute-based sodium reduction strategy in the prevention of stroke in rural China.

16.4 Public health strategies to reduce population-wide sodium intake

The evidence for a beneficial effect of sodium reduction on population health has led the WHO to set a global goal to reduce daily sodium intake to less than 2 g (85 mmol sodium, 5 g salt) per person by 2025. This would result in a shift of the population's blood pressure distribution downwards, leading to worldwide reductions in cardiovascular diseases and premature deaths (Lewington *et al.*, 2002). Reduction in salt consumption will potentially have greater effects in the long term, as reduced intakes would attenuate the rise in blood pressure associated with age.

A public health approach is needed to achieve population-wide reductions in sodium intake. In western countries, because most sodium consumed is added in food manufacturing, population-wide reductions in sodium intakes require action by the food industry to remove added sodium from their products. This can be done in a gradual, stepwise fashion that may go unnoticed by consumers, but which could lead to major public health benefits. This should be accompanied by improvements in food labelling to allow consumers informed choices about the food they eat. Though several countries aim to reduce sodium intakes as per WHO recommendations, only a few countries have currently set specific public health targets. The majority of countries with defined public health strategies focus on increasing public awareness through educational campaigns, food labelling and promotion of foods with reduced salt content. Only a minority of countries have set targeted sodium reduction strategies aimed at the food industry. Moreover, monitoring population

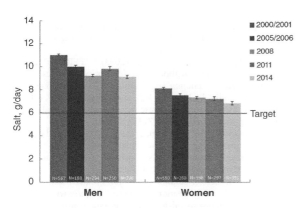

Figure 16.4 The 10-year trend in salt intake (grams per day, estimated by 24 h urine collections) in the UK, 2001–2014. *Source:* NDNS (2011 and 2014).

sodium intakes and changes over time in the whole population and among subgroups is important to evaluate the effectiveness of public health strategies.

A population-wide strategy to reduce population salt intake was introduced in the UK in 2004. This national strategy comprised a combined approach of voluntary agreements with the food industry to lower salt content in 85 categories of processed foods, improved food labelling and increasing public awareness by media campaigns. Sodium intake was monitored by repeated national surveys using 24 h urine collections. The average sodium intake fell from 3.80 g/day (9.5 g salt) in 2001 to 3.44 g/day (8.6 g salt) in 2008 and to 3.13 g/day (8.0 g salt) in 2014 (Figure 16.4). In 2014, the estimated salt intake of adult men (8.6 g/day) was on average higher than of adult women (6.2 g/day). This public health strategy showed that lowering the sodium content of foods by 5–15% is possible without noticeable changes in flavour, taste or sales. The current UK's salt reduction goals aim for a maximum intake of 6 g/day by 2017 through continued product reformation; intervention studies show that further reduction to 3 g/day salt will have greater effects on blood pressure (He *et al.*, 2013). To encourage the food industry to continue their efforts, Consensus Action on Salt and Health (CASH) monitors and published salt levels in popular household foods as well as in foods eaten out of home and in children's meals of family friendly restaurants. In some Asian country settings (e.g. rural China) use of sodium substitutes and reducing discretionary sodium use by increasing public awareness may be beneficial given the importance of sodium added in cooking and use of condiments (e.g. soy sauce) in these countries.

As sodium intakes among children are high, the adverse effects of high sodium intake on long-term development of raised blood pressure and cardiovascular diseases already start in childhood. This emphasises the need for early introduction of public health strategies to reduce sodium intakes starting in childhood and thus prevent or attenuate the rise of blood pressure with age for major long-term cardiovascular health benefit.

References

Aburto, N.J., Ziolkovska, A., Hooper, L. *et al.* (2013) Effect of lower sodium intake on health: systematic review and meta-analyses. *BMJ*, **346**, f1326.

Anderson, C.A., Appel, L.J., Okuda, N. *et al.* (2010) Dietary sources of sodium in China, Japan, the United Kingdom, and the United States, women and men aged 40 to 59 years: the INTERMAP study. *Journal of the American Dietetic Association*, **110** (5), 736–745.

Brown, I.J., Tzoulaki, I., Candeias, V. and Elliott, P. (2009) Salt intakes around the world: implications for public health. *International Journal of Epidemiology*, **38** (3), 791–813.

Brown, I.J., Dyer, A.R., Chan, Q. *et al.* (2013) Estimating 24-hour urinary sodium excretion from casual urinary sodium concentrations in western populations: the INTERSALT study. *American Journal of Epidemiology*, **177** (11), 1180–1192.

Cobb, L.K., Anderson, C.A.M., Elliott, P. *et al.* (2014) Methodological issues in cohort studies that relate sodium intake to cardiovascular disease outcomes. *Circulation*, **129** (10), 1173–1186.

Cogswell, M.E., Mugavero K., Bowman B.A., *et al.* (2016) Dietary sodium and cardiovascular disease risk: measurement matters. *New England Journal of Medicine*. **375** (6), 580–586.

Denton, D., Weisinger, R., Mundy, N.I. *et al.* (1995) The effect of increased salt intake on blood pressure of chimpanzees. *Nature Medicine*, **1** (10), 1009–1016.

Elliott, P., Stamler, J., Nichols, R. *et al.* (1996) Intersalt revisited: further analyses of 24 hour sodium excretion and blood pressure within and across populations. *British Medical Journal*, **312** (7041), 1249–1253.

Elliott, P., Walker, L.L., Little, M.P. *et al.* (2007) Change in salt intake affects blood pressure of chimpanzees – implications for human populations. *Circulation*, **116** (14), 1563–1568.

He, F.J. and MacGregor, G.A. (2011) Salt reduction lowers cardiovascular risk: meta-analysis of outcome trials. *The Lancet*, **378** (9789), 380–382.

He, F.J., Li, J.F. and MacGregor, G.A. (2013) Effect of longer term modest salt reduction on blood pressure: Cochrane systematic review and meta-analysis of randomised trials. *BMJ*, **346**, f1325.

INTERSALT Cooperative Research Group (1988) An international study of electrolyte excretion and blood pressure. Results for 24 hour urinary sodium and potassium excretion. *BMJ*, **297** (6644), 319–328.

James, W.P., Ralph, A. and Sanchez-Castillo, C.P. (1987) The dominance of salt in manufactured food in the sodium intake of affluent societies. *The Lancet*, **1** (8530), 426–429.

Lewington, S., Clarke, R., Qizilbash, N. *et al.* (2002) Age-specific relevance of usual blood pressure to vascular mortality: a meta-analysis of individual data for one million adults in 61 prospective studies. *The Lancet*, **360** (9349), 1903–1913.

Lim, S.S., Vos, T., Flaxman, A.D. *et al.* (2012) A comparative risk assessment of burden of disease and injury attributable to 67 risk factors and risk factor clusters in 21 regions, 1990–2010: a systematic analysis for the Global Burden of Disease Study 2010. *The Lancet*, **380** (9859), 2224–2260.

Mente, A., O'Donnell, M., Rangarajan, S., *et al.* (2016) Associations of urinary sodium excretion with cardiovascular events in individuals with and without hypertension: a pooled analysis of data from four studies. *Lancet,* **388** (10043), 465–475.

NDNS (2011) *National Diet and Nutrition Survey. Headline Results from Years 1 and 2 (Combined) Tables.* https://www.gov.uk/government/uploads/system/uploads/attachment_data/file/216485/dh_128556.pdf (accessed 10 December 2016).

NDNS (2014) *National Diet and Nutrition Survey Assessment of dietary sodium in adults in England.* https://www.gov.uk/government/statistics/national-diet-and-nutrition-survey-assessment-of-dietary-sodium-in-adults-in-england-2014 (accessed 10 December 2016).

O'Donnell, M., Mente, A., Rangarajan, S., *et al.* (2014) Urinary sodium and potassium excretion, mortality, and cardiovascular events. *New England Journal of Medicine,* **371** (7), 612–623.

Poulter, N.R., Khaw, K.T., Hopwood, B.E. *et al.* (1990) The Kenyan Luo migration study: observations on the initiation of a rise in blood pressure. *BMJ,* **300** (6730), 967–972.

Sacks, F.M., Svetkey, L.P., Vollmer, W.M. *et al.* (2001) Effects on blood pressure of reduced dietary sodium and the Dietary Approaches to Stop Hypertension (DASH) diet. *The New England Journal of Medicine,* **344** (1), 3–10.

Stamler, J., Elliott, P., Dennis, B. *et al.* (2003) INTERMAP: background, aims, design, methods, and descriptive statistics (non-dietary). *Journal of Human Hypertension,* **17** (9), 591–608.

Strazzullo, P., D'Elia, L., Kandala, N.B. and Cappuccio, F.P. (2009) Salt intake, stroke, and cardiovascular disease: meta-analysis of prospective studies. *BMJ,* **339** (7733), 1296.

Taylor, R.S., Ashton, K.E., Moxham, T. *et al.* (2011) Reduced dietary salt for the prevention of cardiovascular disease: a meta-analysis of randomized controlled trials (Cochrane review). *American Journal of Hypertension,* **24** (8), 843–853.

WHO (2012) *Guideline: Sodium Intake for Children and Adults.* World Health Organization, Geneva. http://www.who.int/nutrition/publications/guidelines/sodium_intake_printversion.pdf (accessed 10 December 2016).

17
Carbohydrates and Metabolic Health

Judith L Buttriss

Key messages

- Recent interest in the topic of carbohydrates and health has been driven by concerns about increasing global prevalence of obesity and developments in understanding of the relationships between carbohydrates and metabolic disease.
- Several major reviews on the topic of carbohydrates and health have recently been published. This chapter summarises the findings and implications of the report from the UK's Scientific Advisory Committee on Nutrition (SACN).
- Carbohydrates comprise digestible carbohydrates, in the form of starches and sugars, and non-digestible carbohydrates, collectively known as dietary fibre.
- SACN concluded that the dietary reference value for total carbohydrate should remain at an intake of around 50% of dietary energy, with emphasis on high-fibre starchy carbohydrate sources, and sugars contained within the cellular structure of fruits and vegetables and in milk; no evidence was found to warrant a change from the dietary reference value set in 1991. Average intakes in UK adults fall slightly short of this recommendation.
- SACN reported that the quality of evidence for dietary fibre in relation to cardiovascular disease and type 2 diabetes mellitus (and also colorectal cancer) has strengthened considerably. Although there is a lack of randomised controlled trials with hard endpoints, SACN recommended that fibre intakes should increase to 30 g/day AOAC fibre. The previous recommendation equated to 23–24 g/

day, and current intakes in adults average 18 g/day, meaning that substantial increases in intake will be required to achieve the new recommendation. The main dietary sources are cereals and cereal products, vegetables, potatoes and fruit.
- SACN concluded that free sugars intake is a dietary factor that increases energy intake in situations where food intake is unrestricted. Based on the relationship between sugars intake and total energy intake, SACN recommended that population intakes of free sugars should be reduced to below 5% of total energy intake for all groups over the age of 2 years. Current intakes in the UK are two to three times this level, being especially high in teenagers, among whom soft drinks provide 40% of free sugars consumption.
- No association was found between the incidence of type 2 diabetes mellitus and total or individual sugars intake. But prospective cohort studies associate greater consumption of sugars-sweetened drinks with increased risk of type 2 diabetes mellitus. Based on this, SACN advised that the consumption of sugars-sweetened drinks should be minimised in children and adults.
- The new recommendations for dietary fibre and free sugars have been adopted by the UK Department of Health and sit within a broader framework of dietary reference values. Achievement of the recommendations will require substantial dietary change across the UK population.

17.1 Introduction

Interest in the topic of carbohydrates and health has been fuelled by concerns about the potential relationship between carbohydrate intake (especially sugars intake; see later for definitions) and energy balance in light of the increasing prevalence of obesity around the world. It has also been driven by developments in understanding of the relationships between carbohydrates and cardio-metabolic disease; in particular, cardiovascular disease (CVD) and type 2 diabetes mellitus. Some of the cardio-

metabolic effects may be mediated through metabolism in the large bowel, and so this chapter makes brief reference to the effects of carbohydrates on gut health.

In the UK, the prevalence of obesity increased sharply during the 1990s and early 2000s. For example, in England, the proportion of adults who were categorised as obese – body mass index (BMI) $\geq 30\,kg/m^2$ – was less than 10% in the 1980s and increased from 13.2% of men in 1993 to 24.7% in 2011–2013 and from 16.4% of women in 1993 to 24.9% in 2011–2013; 6 in 10 men and 5 in 10 women are overweight or obese (BMI $>25\,kg/m^2$).

Public Health Nutrition, Second Edition. Edited by Judith L Buttriss, Ailsa A Welch, John M Kearney and Susan A Lanham-New.
© 2018 by The Nutrition Society. Published 2018 by John Wiley & Sons, Ltd.
Companion website: www.wiley.com/go/buttriss/publichealth

In addition, in England, 9.7% of boys and 8.8% of girls (all children 9.3%) aged 4–5 years and 20.4% of boys and 17.4% of girls (all children 18.9%) aged 10–11 years are classified as obese. In both age groups, a doubling in the prevalence of obesity was observed in children living in the most deprived areas compared with those in the least deprived (www.noo.org.uk/slide_sets; Lifestyle Statistics Team, Health and Social Care Information Centre, 2014).

Obesity is a risk factor for CVD (an umbrella term for diseases of the heart and circulation, including coronary heart disease (CHD) and stroke) and type 2 diabetes mellitus, both of which are major causes of morbidity and premature mortality around the world. CVD is responsible for more than a quarter (27%) of all deaths in the UK, 25% of which occur in people under the age of 75 years (British Heart Foundation, 2016). The annual number of deaths from CVD has fallen by more than half since the early 1960s. Over this period, death rates have fallen more quickly (by more than three-quarters) because people in the UK are now living longer lives. But 7 million people (9.3% of the population; 50% men and 50% women) in the UK are living with diseases of the cardiovascular system, with annual associated health costs estimated at up to £11 billion. CHD is the UK's biggest killer and is also the leading cause of death worldwide. In the UK, more than one in seven men and nearly one in ten women die from CHD. CHD death rates are highest in Scotland and the north of England and lowest in the South East. Stroke causes nearly 40 000 deaths in the UK each year; and around 1.2 million people in the UK have survived a stroke, almost half of whom are under the age of 75 years (British Heart Foundation, 2016). Many of these people live with disability resulting from the stroke.

In 2013, 6% of the adult population had diagnosed diabetes, with an estimated 90% being type 2 diabetes mellitus (PHE, 2014), and it is estimated that a further half a million are living with undiagnosed diabetes. Obesity accounts for 80–85% of the overall risk of diabetes and underlies the current global spread and trends. Type 2 diabetes mellitus is six times more common in people of South Asian descent and three times more common in people of African or African-Caribbean origin, and the disease tends to develop around 10 years earlier (PHE, 2014). If uncontrolled, the disease can cause poor circulation, resulting in foot and lower limb amputation, retinopathy and blindness, and kidney damage. Furthermore, many with diabetes go on to develop CVD. Thus, the disease carries a considerable economic burden, estimated to be a cost to the National Health Service of £10 billion per year in the UK.

Prevention of CVD and type 2 diabetes mellitus is therefore of considerable importance. The main public health approach in the prevention of type 2 diabetes mellitus is weight management through diet and regular activity. For CVD, a range of approaches apply; in particular, not smoking, control of blood pressure and body weight, blood cholesterol reduction, dietary salt reduction and moderation if alcohol is consumed. Diet has a role to play in the majority of these strategies; this chapter focuses specifically on dietary carbohydrates.

In recent years, there have been several major reviews about carbohydrate and health (WHO, 2015; SACN, 2015). This chapter summarises the findings and implications of the UK's SACN (2015) report, which was informed by systematic reviews of the literature undertaken to identify the best quality evidence. The Scientific Advisory Committee on Nutrition (SACN) restricted its review to evidence from randomised controlled trials (which have the potential to demonstrate a causal relationship, e.g. between an aspect of diet and a risk factor for disease) and prospective cohort studies (which reveal associations, e.g. between an aspect of diet and a disease risk factor or endpoint) as these are considered to be the most robust study designs for diet and health research. Strict inclusion and exclusion criteria for individual studies were applied to ensure the evidence considered was of sufficient quality to enable sound conclusions to be reached. For example, the duration of the study was a criterion. Generally, there needed to be three or more randomised controlled trials to determine whether or not there was evidence of an effect. Where an effect appeared to be present, the evidence was graded by SACN as adequate, moderate or limited.

The evidence that emerged from a series of systematic reviews was assessed and graded by SACN. The evaluation considered whether intakes of specific carbohydrates are a factor in the risk for CVD (heart disease and stroke), obesity and type 2 diabetes mellitus. Gastrointestinal health – in particular colorectal (bowel) cancers (see Chapter 19 for more information on diet on cancer) and oral health (Chapter 21 covers dental health in more detail) – were also considered but are not discussed in detail in this chapter. SACN's recommendations are based on only those relationships where the evidence met the required standards. Where they existed, dose–response relationships between carbohydrate intakes and health outcomes were considered and used to inform the dietary recommendations.

A feature of the SACN report that achieved the greatest media attention was sugar, but the report looks at all types of carbohydrate, in particular dietary fibre.

17.2 Carbohydrate definitions

Figure 17.1 summarises the different members of the carbohydrate family (PHE, 2015).

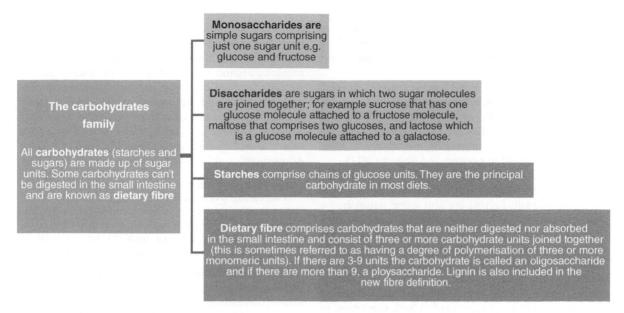

Figure 17.1 The carbohydrates family. *Source:* PHE (2015). Reproduced under Open Government Licence v3.0.

Starches

These comprise chains of glucose units, examples being amylose, amylopectin and modified starches used in food production. Starches are the principal carbohydrate in most diets, consumed as potatoes, bread, breakfast cereals, rice, other cereals and pasta.

Dietary fibre

Until 2016, recommendations in the UK were described in terms of non-starch polysaccharides (NSPs), the main components of which are mentioned shortly. Analytically, an NSP is defined using the Englyst method. This NSP definition does not include resistant starches, non-digestible oligosaccharides or lignin.

SACN has recently extended the definition of dietary fibre to include not only NSP and lignin but also non-digestible oligosaccharides, resistant starch and polydextrose, as there is now evidence to demonstrate similar beneficial physiological effects (e.g. stool bulking, decreasing intestinal transit time and constipation, or lowering total and low-density lipoprotein cholesterol) to those demonstrated for naturally integrated dietary fibre components of food (SACN, 2015). So the new definition for fibre (colloquially known as AOAC fibre, as this is the methodology used for its determination) includes all carbohydrates that are neither digested nor absorbed in the small intestine and have a degree of polymerisation of three or more monomeric units, plus lignin. SACN

also recommended that, for extracted natural carbohydrate components or synthetic carbohydrate products to be defined as dietary fibre, beneficial physiological effects similar to those demonstrated for the naturally integrated fibre component of foods must be demonstrated by accepted scientific evidence. Adopting this approach to defining fibre allows definitions to be aligned with the research bases and enables UK intakes to be compared more easily with those in other countries.

NSPs, which are plant cell wall constituents, comprise a diverse group of carbohydrates, the most widely distributed of which is cellulose. Also in this group are hemicelluloses such as arabinoxylan, pectins (common to all cell walls), beta-glucans, plant gums and storage polysaccharides; for example, gum Arabic, karaya, guar gum, plant mucilages such as psyllium and algal polysaccharides such as agar and carrageenans (Cummings and Stephen, 2007).

Oligosaccharides include maltodextrins, which principally occur from the hydrolysis of starch and are digested and absorbed in the small intestine (and so are not classed as dietary fibre). Oligosaccharides that are not digested and pass through to the large intestine include raffinose, stachyose and verbascose. These are found in a variety of plant seeds, such as peas, beans and lentils. Also in this group are inulin and fructo-oligosaccharides, which are the storage carbohydrates in artichokes and chicory. Human milk contains more than 100 different oligosaccharides, which are mainly galactose-containing, and it is thought that these may serve as substrates for colonic fermentation – see SACN (2015). Other sources of oligosaccharides, present in small amounts, are wheat, rye, asparagus and members of the leek, onion and garlic family (Cummings and Stephen, 2007).

Resistant starch is starch that is not absorbed in the small intestine. Some types are naturally present but inaccessible in foods, others form in cooked foods such as potatoes and pasta, especially when they are subsequently cooled, and yet other types are commercially manufactured. More details can be found in Lockyer and Nugent (2017).

Polyols are hydrogenated carbohydrates, otherwise known as sugar alcohols, such as sorbitol, xylitol, mannitol and isomalt. Polyols are also found naturally; for example, sorbitol in some fruits and also made commercially. Their digestibility varies considerably, reflected in their caloric values, with some being almost completely absorbed (e.g. erythritol), some partially (e.g. sorbitol) and others not at all (e.g. lactitol). With the exception of xylitol, polyols are less sweet than sugar and, because of their lower caloric value, are used as 'bulk sweeteners' to replace sugar, sometimes in combination with high-intensity sweeteners, which have little or no caloric value. There are some legislative restrictions to their use. For example, polyols are not permitted in all categories of foods, and use of a combination of sucrose and polyols is restricted. Also, if present at a concentration >10% (on a weight basis) a laxative warning needs to be made on the pack. For more details, see Burgos *et al.* (2016).

Even if a carbohydrate is not digested and absorbed in the small intestine, it can still provide energy because fermentation in the colon results in the formation of short-chain fatty acids. Energy value is dependent on carbohydrate sub-class, ranging up to 2.4 kcal/g (10 kJ/g) (SACN, 2015).

Sugars

SACN uses a new term to describe the types of sugars that need to be reduced in the diets of most of us, namely 'free sugars' (SACN, 2015). This term has also recently been adopted by the World Health Organization (WHO, 2015). 'Free sugars' replaces the term non-milk extrinsic sugars, which has been in use in the UK for almost 25 years (Committee on Medical Aspects of Food Policy, 1991). Although the definitions capture similar components, there are some subtle differences. 'Free sugars' includes all monosaccharides and disaccharides added to foods and beverages by the manufacturer, cook or consumer, plus sugars naturally present in honey, syrups, fruit juices and fruit juice concentrates. Under this definition, lactose (milk sugar), when naturally present in milk and milk products, and sugars contained within the cellular structure of foods (particularly fruits and

vegetables) are excluded. Detailed principles of how the definition is applied in practice are expected to be published shortly by Public Health England.

Different definitions for sugars are used in different countries around the world. The term 'total sugars' is typically required by law in nutrition labelling on pre-packaged foods and captures all of the sugars present; that is, free sugars as well as those present in intact fruit and in milk. In the USA, labels will in future show added sugars as well as total sugars. The US Food and Drug Administration defines added sugars thus (FDA, 2016):

> sugars that are either added during the processing of foods, or are packaged as such, and include sugars (free, mono- and disaccharides), sugars from syrups and honey, and sugars from concentrated fruit or vegetable juices that are in excess of what would be expected from the same volume of 100 percent fruit or vegetable juice of the same type.

So an obvious difference between the US definition of added sugars and the new UK and World Health Organization definitions of free sugars is that pure fruit juice is not included in the US added sugars definition (but is in the free sugars definitions). More information about the different sugar definitions and their application can be found in Buttriss (2016a).

Digestion and absorption

Only glucose and galactose are actively absorbed in humans, via sodium-dependent transporters. Fructose is not actively absorbed but is taken up by a specific transport pathway (SACN, 2015). Other dietary carbohydrates have to be hydrolysed to component monosaccharides. Carbohydrates with glycosidic linkages within their structure are resistant to cleavage in the small intestine, making them non-digestible. They travel through the gut into the large intestine, where they are fermented to varying degrees by the resident bacteria that have enzymes capable of hydrolysing the glycosidic linkages.

17.3 Recommendations on total carbohydrate

Concern has been raised by some that high intakes of total carbohydrate may be deleterious to health, but SACN concludes that total carbohydrate intakes, at levels generally recommended in the UK diet, are not associated with the cardio-metabolic health outcomes examined (or colorectal cancer or oral health). Specifically in relation to cardio-metabolic health, total carbohydrate intake shows no association with the incidence of CVD endpoints, type 2 diabetes mellitus or glycaemia. In children and adolescents, limited evidence indicates that there is no association between total carbohydrate intake and BMI or body fatness.

Overall, SACN concluded that there is no evidence to warrant a change to the total carbohydrate dietary reference value previously set by the Committee on Medical Aspects of Food Policy (1991) of 50% dietary energy from carbohydrate.

Summary of the evidence presented by the Scientific Advisory Committee on Nutrition

Total dietary carbohydrate

Prospective cohort studies indicate no association between total carbohydrate intake and the incidence of CVD endpoints, type 2 diabetes mellitus, glycaemia (or colorectal cancer). Cohort studies and trials conducted in children and adolescents provide limited evidence to show no association between total carbohydrate intake and BMI or body fatness.

Randomised controlled trials have assessed the effect of varying total carbohydrate intake by reciprocally varying fat type and quantity, and/or protein intake. These provide evidence that an energy-restricted higher carbohydrate, lower fat diet, as compared with a lower carbohydrate and average fat diet, may be effective in reducing BMI, but the evidence is based on only four trials and there is high heterogeneity between them. The hypothesis that diets higher in carbohydrate cause weight gain is not supported by the evidence from randomised controlled trials. Trials also showed no effect of varying total carbohydrate intake on vascular function, inflammation markers or risk of type 2 diabetes mellitus.

Overall, the evidence from both prospective cohort studies and randomised controlled trials indicates that total carbohydrate intake is neither detrimental nor beneficial to cardio-metabolic health (or colorectal health). Randomised controlled trials do suggest some effects on cardiovascular risk factors, but it is not possible to exclude confounding by a concomitant reduction in saturated fatty acid or total fat intake and/or differences in weight loss.

Starch and starch-rich foods

Cereals, rich in starch, are the dominant dietary source of carbohydrate worldwide, and starch is the major source of dietary carbohydrate. Overall, the available evidence in relation to cardio-metabolic outcomes indicates no association with dietary starch intake when consumed in the amounts typical of the UK diet.

In its comprehensive review, SACN found that prospective cohort studies suggest there is no association between total starch intake and incidence of coronary events or type 2 diabetes mellitus or between the intake of refined grains and risk of type 2 diabetes mellitus. There is insufficient evidence to draw a conclusion on the association between starch intake and weight gain. Consumption of brown rice is associated with a reduction in risk of type 2 diabetes, but the evidence is limited to a small number of studies. Prospective cohort studies indicate an association between greater consumption of white rice and increased risk of type 2 diabetes mellitus in Asian populations (in Japan and China) consuming amounts of white rice that are not generally achieved in the UK, for example. It is therefore uncertain whether the detrimental association is relevant to other populations. There was also evidence, limited to a small number of studies, of associations with other starch-rich foods, but again it is not possible to exclude confounding by other dietary variables (e.g. cooking methods such as frying).

Glycaemic index and glycaemic load

Glycaemic index (GI) and glycaemic load (GL) are measures of the glycaemic characteristics of foods; in other words, the blood sugar response to consumption of the food. GI is a relative measure of the capillary blood glucose response to a specific ingredient, food or portion of a meal, compared with the response to a reference food having the same amount of available carbohydrate (usually 50 g), and is used to rank carbohydrate according to its effect on postprandial glycaemia. The reference food can be either pure glucose or a carbohydrate-rich food such as white bread. A food's GL is the product of its GI and its available carbohydrate content, so takes account of both the amount present and the types and structures of carbohydrate present in the food. Influences on a food's GI are the amounts of protein, fat and fibre present, and so adding fat to a carbohydrate-containing food changes its GI. GI is also influenced by milling of grain, cooking, cooling and storage conditions – see Brouns et al. (2005). Variation in GI among foods reflects differences in rates of carbohydrate digestion and absorption, as well as effects on variation in rates of glucose production and disposal from the circulation into tissues. It is sometimes assumed that a low-GI diet will automatically be high in fibre or based on wholegrains, and vice versa, but this is not the case as many factors coalesce to determine predicted GI values. Seale (2016) has published a review on steps to define wholegrains, and GI values can be found in the Foster-Powell tables (http://ajcn.nutrition.org/cgi/content-nw/full/76/1/5/T1).

Overall, limited evidence from cohort studies and randomised controlled trials (summarised later) suggests there may also be some adverse health effects. However, higher and lower GI/GL diets will, in most cases, differ in many ways other than the carbohydrate component, and therefore study results are difficult to interpret. SACN concluded it was not possible to exclude confounding by other dietary variables and cautioned that the associations described in the meta-analysis cannot be specifically attributed to GI. A subsequent updated meta-analysis of three prospective cohorts confirmed this (Bhupathiraju *et al.*, 2014) and also indicated that participants who consumed diets low in cereal fibre but with a high GI/GL have an elevated risk of type 2 diabetes mellitus.

So, prospective cohort studies indicate that a diet with a higher GI or GL is associated with a greater risk of type 2 diabetes mellitus, but SACN found no evidence from prospective cohort studies to suggest an association between GI and CVD or CHD. GL is associated with a greater risk of CVD, but the evidence is limited to a small number of studies. SACN suggested that the relationships seen may be a result of other associated factors, such as dietary fibre, protein or fat content of the diet, as well as cooking method or extent of food processing or characteristics of storage.

Randomised controlled trials (mainly weight loss trials) have assessed the effect of varying the GI primarily by changing the source of dietary carbohydrate. Trials assessing the effect of varying GL have reduced carbohydrate intake, reciprocally varied fat (type and quantity) and/or protein intake, as well as changed the quality of dietary carbohydrate. These trials indicate no effect of varying GI or GL on vascular function, inflammatory markers or risk factors for type 2 diabetes mellitus and obesity. The trials indicate a higher GI diet may affect fasting blood lipid concentrations, but it is not possible to exclude confounding due to differential weight changes between the groups. A higher GL diet has been shown to reduce diastolic blood pressure and fasting blood triacylglycerol concentration to a lesser degree than the lower GL diet, but it is not possible to exclude confounding by other dietary variables and the evidence is limited due to the small number of trials. Consequently, a cause-and-effect relationship cannot be established from these trials exploring GI and GL in relation to cardio-metabolic risk factors (SACN, 2015).

Meeting carbohydrate recommendations

Current intakes of total carbohydrate for different age groups can be found in Table 17.1, which reveals that average intakes in adults fall slightly short of the recommendation made by SACN, which states that about 50% of dietary energy should be derived from carbohydrate. Currently, the top contributors to total dietary carbohydrate intakes among UK adults are white bread (11.8%), fruit (5.9%), soft drinks (5.7%), chips and fried/roast potatoes (5.2%), vegetables and vegetable-based dishes (4.9%), boiled/mashed/baked potatoes (4.4%), and rice and rice-based dishes (4.1%). The main dietary sources of starch among adults are bread, potatoes and breakfast cereals (SACN, 2015).

17.4 Recommendations on dietary fibre

Based on the quality of the evidence now available, SACN has recommended an increase in the UK population's

Table 17.1 Comparison of recommendations for intakes of total carbohydrate, free sugars (as a percentage of dietary energy) and dietary fibre with current intakes for children, teenagers and adults.

	Recommendation		Current intakes			
	Old	New	Children	Teenagers	Adults	
			4–10 years	11–18 years	19–64 years	≥65 years
Total carbohydrate (% total dietary energy)[a]	~50	~50	52.1	50.6	45.7	45.8
Dietary fibre[b] (g/day)						
Adults	~23–24	30	—	—	~18	~18
Children						
2–5 years	—	15	~14.5	—	—	—
5–11 years		20				
Teenagers						
11–16 years	—	25	—	~15	—	—
16–18 years		30				
Free sugars (% total dietary energy)[a]	≤10[c]	≤5	14.7	15.4	11.5	11.2

Sources: Committee on Medical Aspects of Food Policy (1991), SACN (2015) and Bates *et al.* (2014).

[a] Including energy from alcohol.
[b] Expressed as AOAC fibre.
[c] Expressed as non-milk extrinsic sugars.

fibre intake to an average of 30 g AOAC fibre per day for adults. This is a substantial increase from the previous recommendation, which was equivalent to 23–24 g/day AOAC fibre. No age group in the UK is achieving this currently; average intakes in adults are around 18 g AOAC fibre (Table 17.1). Socio-economic disparities exist, with lower intakes in the lowest income quintile compared with the highest, in all age groups and in both sexes. Similar trends are evident in fruit and vegetable intakes, which may partly explain these findings. For children, the recommended intakes are 15 g/day for ages 2–5 years, 20 g/day for ages 5–11 years, 25 g/day for ages 11–16 years and 30 g/day for ages 16–18 years. These recommendations have been rounded to the nearest 5 g, are proportional to the adult values and are informed by the UK's National Diet and Nutrition Survey (NDNS).

The new UK recommendation of 30 g/day for those over the age of 16 years is higher than that set by the European Food Safety Authority (EFSA) and in Ireland, but is comparable with recommended intakes in other nations (Table 17.2).

Most of the evidence for the range of health benefits linked to fibre, summarised shortly, comes from studies where the exposure reflects dietary fibre intakes achieved through a variety of foods where the fibre is present as a naturally integrated component of the food. However, there is also growing interest in particular carbohydrate fractions, such as resistant starch (for a review, see Lockyer and Nugent (2017)), and beta-glucans. There is also emerging evidence to show that particular extracted and isolated fibres have positive effects on blood lipids and bowel function but, owing to the smaller evidence base, it is not yet known whether these components confer the full range of health benefits associated with the

consumption of a mix of dietary fibre-rich foods. Therefore, SACN's recommendation is that fibre intakes should be achieved through a variety of food sources.

The Scientific Advisory Committee on Nutrition's findings on fibre

SACN reported that, since the UK dietary reference value for fibre was last considered in 1991, the quality of evidence has strengthened considerably for CVD, type 2 diabetes mellitus (and also colorectal cancer). There is a lack of randomised controlled trials with hard endpoints, but there is strong evidence from prospective cohort studies that increased intakes of total dietary fibre, and particularly cereal fibre and wholegrains, are associated with a lower risk of cardio-metabolic disease (CVDs, coronary events, stroke and type 2 diabetes mellitus – and of colorectal cancer). See Table 17.3. The evidence for wholegrains is based on a smaller number of studies than for dietary fibre, and the evidence is more limited for individual dietary fibre constituents due to the smaller number of studies available. SACN found no association of fibre intake with change in body weight in adults or body fatness in children.

Based on prospective studies ($n = 10$), SACN reported a biologically relevant 9% reduction in risk of CVD with every 7 g of additional fibre consumed (Table 17.3). For coronary events the reduction was also 9%, and for stroke it was 7%. The effect sizes were greater still for insoluble fibre specifically; a reduction of 18% in risk for each 7 g/day increase for CVD and coronary events, for example. This suggests a greater protective effect in comparison with other dietary components often promoted for cardiovascular health. For example, the prospective US Women's Health Study ($n = 39\,876$) reported a 17% reduction in CVD risk with each 10 g increment in daily intake of

Table 17.2 Recommendations for daily fibre intake in adults.

Nation/ region	Recommendation	Issuing body
UK	30 g	SACN
Europe	25 g	EFSA
Ireland	25 g	Food Safety Authority of Ireland
Nordic countries	25–35 g (3 g/MJ)	The Nordic Council
USA	28 g (women), 33.6 g (men) (14 g/1000 kcal)	US Department of Agriculture (USDA)
Australia and New Zealand	25 g (women), 30 g (men)	National Health and Medical Research Council of the Australian Government

Sources: EFSA Panel on Dietetic Products, Nutrition and Allergies (2010), USDA (2015), Food Safety Authority of Ireland (2011), Fagt *et al.* (2012) and NHMRC (2006).

Table 17.3 Relative risk of disease with every 7 g/day increase in fibre consumption using data from prospective studies (derived from SACN (2015)).

CVD	RR: 0.91; 95% CI: 0.88, 0.94; $p < 0.001$; 10 studies
Coronary events	RR: 0.91; 95% CI: 0.87, 0.94; $p < 0.001$; 13 studies
Stroke	RR: 0.93; 95% CI: 0.88, 0.98; $p = 0.002$; 7 studies
Type 2 diabetes	RR: 0.94; 95% CI: 0.90, 0.97; $p = 0.001$; 13 studies
Colorectal cancer	RR: 0.92; 95% CI: 0.87, 0.97; $p = 0.002$; 13 studies

RR: relative risk; CI: confidence interval.

dietary fibre (RR: 0.83; 95% CI: 0.69, 1.01) (Liu *et al.*, 2002) compared with a reduction in risk of 6% (RR: 0.94; 95% CI: 0.85, 1.02) with each additional daily serving of fruits and vegetables (Liu *et al.*, 2000).

Randomised controlled trials indicate that total dietary fibre, wheat fibre and other cereal fibres increase faecal mass and decrease intestinal transit times (this is mentioned here as some cardio-metabolic effects may be mediated at least in part through gut-related mechanisms such as short-chain fatty acid production in the colon, as mentioned later; Wolever *et al.*, 1996). Randomised trials indicate that dietary fibre intake has no effect on body weight or energy intake. Although there is limited evidence from trials that a higher intake of wholegrains (definitions vary between studies) may decrease total energy intake, more evidence is required before firm conclusions can be drawn.

Randomised controlled trials also indicate that higher intake of oat bran and isolated beta-glucans have beneficial effects on fasting blood lipid concentrations and blood pressure. SACN found no prospective cohort studies that had examined the relationship between non-digestible oligosaccharides or resistant starch and the health/disease outcomes SACN considered. But randomised controlled trials in adults, in which diets were supplemented with non-digestible oligosaccharides (arabinoxylan-oligosaccharide, fructo-oligosaccharide and galacto-oligosaccharide) demonstrated improvement in blood lipid concentrations, and increase in faecal mass and faecal bacterial content. SACN noted that the level of supplementation exceeded current estimated intakes of these carbohydrates in the UK. Resistant starch supplementation increases faecal mass and short-chain fatty acid content, and polydextrose and polyol supplementation increase faecal mass. The health significance of the effects on faecal parameters, however, is unclear. Trials also indicate that non-digestible oligosaccharides or inulin supplementation increases net calcium absorption in children, but the physiological relevance of this is unclear.

It has been suggested for some time that the physiological effects of different non-digested carbohydrate fractions overlap but also vary, as summarised in Table 17.4. In its analysis, SACN also considered high-fibre and wholegrain foods. One of the challenges with the latter is that there is currently no agreed definition of the term 'wholegrain'; this is discussed in a recent review by Seale (2016). From cohort studies there was limited evidence that a serving each day of high-fibre breakfast cereals (comprising 25% or more wholegrains or bran content by weight) is associated with reduced incidence of coronary events and type 2 diabetes mellitus, and that a serving per day of wholemeal bread is associated with reduced incidence of type 2 diabetes mellitus. Evidence from cohort studies also supported a benefit of wholegrain consumption (one

serving a day) in relation to incidence of CVD, type 2 diabetes mellitus, stroke and hypertension, and possibly energy intake.

Implications of the new UK fibre recommendation

Fibre intakes in adults are currently about 18 g AOAC fibre per day (~13.7 g NSP: 14.7 g in men and 12.8 g in women) and so fall well short of the 30 g/day now recommended in the UK – for more discussion, see Lockyer *et al.* (2016). The sources of fibre are predominantly plant-derived foods, and Figure 17.2 shows the main contributors of fibre in the UK diet for different age groups. Current average intakes in adults are about 12 g below the new recommendation, at 18 g, meaning that intakes need to increase substantially to meet the 30 g level. Table 17.1 shows current intakes in the UK compared with the new recommendations for different age groups.

To aid public understanding and implementation of the new recommendations, the British Nutrition Foundation developed a 7-day menu plan that illustrates, in practice, what a diet that provides 30 g of AOAC fibre and meets all other dietary recommendations looks like for adults (Hooper *et al.*, 2015). See later for more details. However, the required dietary pattern is not reflective of typical diets in the UK at present, and encouraging sufficient behaviour change to meet the new recommendation will be challenging. Some of the barriers and challenges are discussed in Lockyer *et al.* (2016).

17.5 Recommendations on sugars

UK recommendations on sugars have in the past been based on the association between intake and oral health, in particular the observation that dental caries was rare in populations whose intakes of sugar were estimated to be below 10% of total energy consumed. In 1991, the dietary reference value for non-milk extrinsic sugars was set at 10% of total energy (Committee on Medical Aspects of Food Policy, 1991). In 2015, the basis for setting the reference value and the value itself changed. As discussed in more detail shortly, a meta-analysis of randomised controlled trials resulted in a new recommendation: free sugars intake should be restricted to no more than 5% of energy intake (SACN, 2015). The recommendation, subsequently adopted by the UK Government, applies to age groups from 2 years upwards.

Summary of the Scientific Advisory Committee on Nutrition's findings on sugars

The majority of the evidence on sugars and sugar-sweetened foods and beverages is derived from cohort

Table 17.4 Summary of evidence presented in the SACN report describing biological effects of fibre consumption on cardio-metabolic and gut-related markers.

Fibre type	Findings	
	Randomised controlled trials[a]	Prospective cohort studies[b]
Total dietary fibre	• Increase faecal mass • Decrease intestinal transit times • No effect on body weight or energy intake	• Biologically relevant decreases in incidence of CVD, coronary events, haemorrhagic and ischaemic stroke, type 2 diabetes mellitus, colorectal cancer • No association with body weight change or energy intake, fasting blood lipids, blood glucose, fasting insulin • Increases faecal weight and decreases intestinal transit time
Wheat fibre	• Increase faecal mass • Decrease intestinal transit times	• No studies reported/met the criteria
Non-wheat cereal fibre	• Increase faecal mass • Decrease intestinal transit times	• No studies reported/met the criteria
Cereal fibre	• Reduces constipation	• Biologically relevant association with reduced coronary events, type 2 diabetes mellitus and colorectal cancer
Legume fibre/legumes	• Increase faecal weight	• No association with CVD events
Oat bran and beta-glucans	• Improve lipid profile • Lower blood pressure	• No studies reported/met the criteria
Fruit and vegetable fibre (evidence available for carrots, potatoes, prunes and citrus fruits)	• Increase faecal mass • Decrease intestinal transit times	• Biologically relevant association between increased intake of vegetable fibre and CVD incidence and coronary events
Non-digestible oligosaccharides	• Improve lipid profile • Increase faecal mass and bacterial content	• No studies reported/met the criteria
Resistant starch	• Increase faecal mass and short-chain fatty acid content	• No studies reported/met the criteria
Polydextrose and polyols	• Increase faecal mass	• No studies reported/met the criteria

Source: derived from SACN (2015).

[a] A study in which subjects are assigned to different experimental intervention groups by chance (randomly) and outcomes are compared after sufficient follow-up time. These intervention studies are designed to test a hypothetical cause-and-effect relationship by modifying a supposed causal factor in a population. Randomisation is important to minimise the differences between groups.

[b] A type of observational study in which the subjects are identified, baseline measurements taken (e.g. diet) and then subjects are followed forward in time, without any particular intervention. Observational studies such as these are prone to sources of bias and confounding by other dietary and lifestyle factors, whereby factors other than the specific ones being studied influence the associations found in the study. Therefore, any associations must be interpreted with caution.

studies. Very few studies on the effects of individual sugars, such as glucose, fructose or sucrose, met the inclusion criteria. There was also insufficient evidence of appropriate quality to draw conclusions on the impact of sugars intake on the majority of cardio-metabolic outcomes in adults, including body weight.

Relationship between dietary sugars intake and energy intake

SACN reported that randomised controlled trials conducted in adults indicate that increasing or decreasing the percentage of total dietary energy consumed as sugars, when eating an unrestricted diet, leads to a corresponding increase or decrease in energy intake. Change in the percentage of dietary energy provided as sugars was achieved in these trials either through

adjustment of other macronutrient (energy-providing) components or by replacing sugars with non-caloric sweeteners. Meta-analyses were undertaken using the randomised controlled trials identified, and used to inform the new free sugars recommendation. Details can be found in Annex 9 of the SACN report (SACN 2015) and are summarised herein.

Sugars-sweetened drinks and weight gain in children and adolescents

Randomised controlled trials conducted in children and adolescents indicate that consumption of sugars-sweetened drinks, compared with non-calorically sweetened drinks, results in greater weight gain and increases in BMI (SACN, 2015). The findings, which are limited to a small number of studies and not supported by the limited

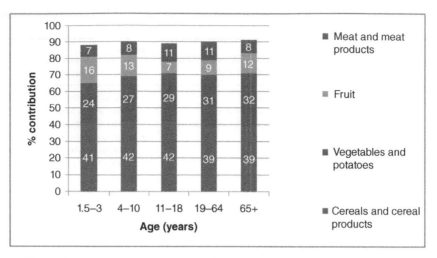

Figure 17.2 Sources of fibre in the UK diet. *Source:* Bates *et al.* (2014).

evidence from prospective studies, suggest that there is inadequate energy compensation for energy delivered as sugars. In other words, the degree of voluntary reduction in intake of other foods or drinks is insufficient.

Cardio-metabolic outcomes

Randomised controlled trials examining cardiovascular risk factors, body weight, inflammatory markers and risk factors for type 2 diabetes mellitus demonstrate no effects of increasing sugars intake. SACN also concluded that there is insufficient evidence to assess the link between individual sugars and sugars-sweetened foods and drinks and cardio-metabolic outcomes.

Cardiovascular disease, colorectal cancer and type 2 diabetes

Most of the evidence was from prospective studies, which indicated that there is insufficient evidence to enable conclusions to be drawn in relation to CVD risk factors or endpoints (events) and sugars; there is no association between the incidence of type 2 diabetes mellitus and total or individual sugars intake, but a greater risk of type 2 diabetes mellitus is associated with a higher intake of sugars-sweetened beverages. This finding was not supported by the limited evidence from randomised trials, which showed no effect of diets differing in sugars content on blood sugar and insulin levels or on insulin resistance (SACN, 2015). SACN comments that the reason for this discrepancy with type 2 diabetes mellitus, between the results of prospective studies and randomised controlled trials, is not clear. In a meta-analysis of prospective cohort studies, incidence of type 2 diabetes mellitus increased by 23% for each additional 330 mL/day of sugars-sweetened drinks consumed (Greenwood

et al., 2014). Although the majority of the cohort studies took place in North America, the association has also been found in Europe in the EPIC study (InterAct Consortium, 2013).

SACN concluded that free sugars intake is a dietary factor that increases energy intake in situations where food intake is unrestricted. No association was found between the incidence of type 2 diabetes mellitus and total or individual sugars intake. But prospective cohort studies associate greater consumption of sugars-sweetened drinks with increased risk of type 2 diabetes mellitus. Based on this, SACN advised that the consumption of sugars-sweetened drinks should be minimised in children and adults.

Fructose

Fructose is metabolised differently to other monosaccharides, and some commentators suggest it promotes lipid production and insulin resistance. Despite the interest in fructose in the popular press, where parallels have been drawn between use of high-fructose corn syrup in North America and increases in obesity prevalence (high-fructose corn syrup use has been much less common in Europe), very few trials on fructose met the inclusion criteria for the SACN report because many were either not randomised or they were of insufficient duration. No studies specifically investigating the effects of high-fructose corn syrup were identified that met the inclusion criteria. However, as concern has been expressed around fructose consumption and its implications for cardio-metabolic health, evidence from trials that did not meet the inclusion criteria for SACN's report were considered. It was concluded that, on balance, there was insufficient evidence to demonstrate that fructose intake, at levels consumed in the normal UK diet, leads to adverse health outcomes independently of any effects related to fructose's presence as a component of total and free sugars. Details are provided in Annex 3 of the SACN report (SACN 2015).

A subsequent systematic review and meta-analysis of 59 controlled feeding trials with fructose reported that there was no significant effect of fructose on blood lipid parameters in *isocaloric* comparisons with other carbohydrates but that there was evidence of a significant increase in triacylglycerol and apo B in *hypercaloric* comparisons, in which fructose supplemented diets with excess calorie content. In the absence of an effect in *isocaloric* comparisons, the authors suggest the effect of fructose appears more attributable to the excess energy rather than the fructose per se (Chiavaroli *et al.*, 2015).

Why 5% as the new reference value?

SACN arrived at this recommendation after considering the results of 11 randomised controlled trials that presented evidence on diets differing in the proportion of sugars in relation to energy intake. In five of the trials, the sugars content of participants' diets was manipulated by adjusting other sources of energy (starches, protein and fat). In six of the trials, the amount of sugars participants consumed was altered predominantly by replacing sugars with non-caloric sweeteners, particularly in drinks.

Data from the 11 trials were analysed together, using a technique known as meta-analysis, which is a statistical analysis applied to separate but similar experiments/studies that combines the individual results into a single piece of evidence. This statistical analysis indicated that in these studies there was an association between sugars consumption and energy intake. It demonstrated that relative changes (increases and decreases) in sugars intake resulted in corresponding relative changes in energy intake and that there was approximately a 19 kcal (78 kJ) change in energy intake for each one unit change in percentage energy consumed as sugars. With the exception of one study, the same direction of effect was observed in each of the trials. SACN's interpretation of this finding is that participants in these studies made inadequate energy compensation for energy derived from sugars; in other words, the extent of voluntary reduction in their consumption of other foods and drinks was insufficient. To test the conclusion, SACN conducted a second meta-analysis using slightly different data from the 11 randomised controlled trials. This showed the same relationship between sugars and energy intake as in the first analysis but gave a slightly larger quantitative effect. SACN used the more conservative result, from the first meta-analysis, as the basis for deriving its new recommendation for the population's free sugars intake. Details of the 11 randomised controlled trials and SACN's meta-analyses can be found in Annex 9 of the SACN report (SACN 2015).

To quantify the dietary recommendation, SACN considered advice from the Calorie Reduction Expert Group, which had estimated that a 100 kcal per person per day (418 kJ per person per day) reduction in energy intake, averaged across the population, would address energy imbalance and lead to a moderate degree of weight loss in the majority of individuals (Calorie Reduction Expert Group, 2011). SACN calculated that free sugars intake would need to be reduced by approximately 5% of total dietary energy in order to achieve an average reduction in population energy intake from free sugars of 100 kcal per person per day (418 kJ per person per day). Details of SACN's calculations can be found in Annex 9 of its report (SACN 2015). Using this 5% figure and the then current recommendation for non-milk extrinsic sugars of 10% of total energy intake, SACN arrived at its dietary recommendation that the population average intake of free sugars should not exceed 5% of total dietary energy.

Implications of the sugars recommendations

Data from the NDNS indicate that only 13% (one in eight) of adults and just 4% of young people already achieve this 5% dietary energy from free sugars recommendation – see PHE (2015). Average intakes of free sugars (measured in the NDNS as non-milk extrinsic sugars – the previously used definition referred to earlier) across all age groups range from 49 to 64 g/day in females and 63 to 84 g/day in males. Highest intakes are in children aged 4–10 years (14.7% of dietary energy intake) and 11- to 18-year-olds (15.4% of dietary energy, on average). See Figure 17.3.

Current average intakes in all age groups are at least twice the new sugars recommendation and three times higher in 11- to 18-year-olds. The main sources are sugars-sweetened drinks (including carbonated drinks, juice drinks, energy drinks, squashes and cordials), cereal-based products (biscuits, cakes, pastries and sweetened breakfast cereals), table sugar and confectionery, and fruit juice. Figure 17.4 shows the main sources in the diets of teenagers. The main sources are consistent across age groups but the proportions vary. For example, sugars-sweetened drinks provide 29% of non-milk extrinsic sugars intake in the 11–18 years age group and 16% in younger children and adults. Fruit juice provides a further 10% of energy in the 11–18 years age group and 13% in younger children. Cereals and cereal products provide about a quarter (22–29%) of non-milk extrinsic sugars intake in children, mainly from sugars added to biscuits, buns, cakes, pastries and breakfast cereals. Older adults (≥65 years) had

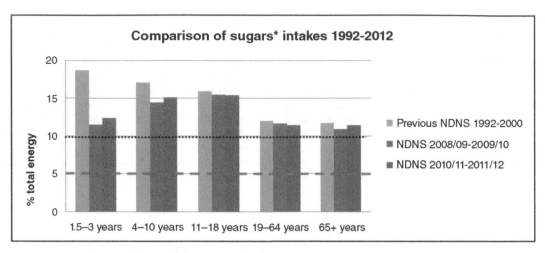

Figure 17.3 Comparison of sugars intakes (measured as non-milk extrinsic sugars) over the period 1992–2012. Dashed line is the new recommendation. Dotted line is the previous (10% of total dietary energy) recommendation. *Source:* Bates *et al.* (2014).

the lowest average free sugars intake (11.2% of total dietary energy). In this age group, the contribution from cereals and cereal products was higher and that from drinks was lower than in other age groups.

Public Health England has calculated that the 5% dietary energy recommendation means no more than 19 g/day of free sugars for children aged 4–6 years, no more than 24 g/day for 7- to 10-year-olds and no more than 30 g/day for children from age 11 years and adults. Table 17.5 compares the quantities with current intakes.

Free sugars are not the same as 'total sugars', as illustrated in Table 17.6. There is the potential for confusion as food labelling legislation requires the declaration of total sugars, not free sugars. For example, a plain yogurt contains 9.9 g total sugars but none of these are 'free sugars' as they are all derived from milk. The same applies to an individual portion of fresh fruit salad that might contain around 20 g of sugars, depending on the fruits selected, all of which are naturally present within the cellular structure of the fruit (rather than 'free'). The practical challenges of communicating the free sugars content of foods is discussed by Buttriss (2016a,b).

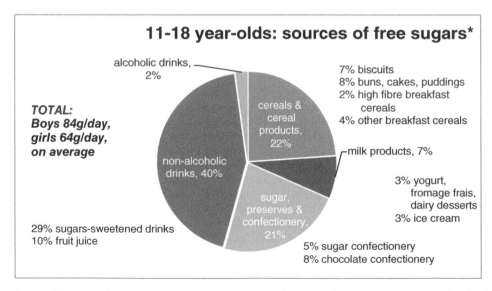

Figure 17.4 Sources of free sugars (measured as non-milk extrinsic sugars in the NDNS *Rolling Programme 2008–2012*) in the diets of 11- to 18-year-olds in the UK. *Source:* Bates *et al.* (2014).

Table 17.5 A comparison of current intakes with the new recommendations for free sugars.

Age	Recommended maximum free sugars intake[b] (g/day)	Current intakes of free sugars[a] (g/day)	
		Males	Females
4–6 years	≤19	63 (4–10 years)	58.5 (4–10 years)
7–10 years	≤24		
From 11 years, including adults	≤30	84 (11–18 years) 68.4 (19–64 years) 58.5 (≥65 years)	63.9 (11–18 years) 49.2 (19–64 years) 46.2 (≥65 years)

Source: data from Bates *et al.* (2014).

[a] Expressed as non-milk extrinsic sugars.
[b] Also see Table 17.1.

17.6 The carbohydrate recommendations in context

The new free sugars recommendations have been adopted by UK Department of Health and are part of a broader set of recommendations for carbohydrate intake, in which total digestible carbohydrate (comprising all sugars and all starches) should provide around half the energy we consume in total and that dietary fibre intake should increase to 30 g/day; an additional 12 g on top of the current estimated average intake of about 18 g/day (expressed as AOAC fibre). These carbohydrate recommendations sit within a set of reference values for other sources of energy (e.g. fat and protein), vitamins and minerals, which together describe a healthy and varied diet that is important for growth, health and well-being.

Table 17.6 Comparison of the total and free sugars content of foods.

	Portion size	Total sugars (per portion)	Free sugars (per portion)	Comment
Regular cola	330 mL	36.0 g	36.0 g	All of the sugars are present as free sugars
Calorie-free cola	330 mL	0	0	No sugars present
Lemonade	330 mL	27.4 g	27.4 g	All of the sugars are present as free sugars
Calorie-free lemonade	330 mL	0	0	No sugars present
Semi-skimmed milk	200 mL	9.4 g	0	None of the sugars are free sugars; all of the sugar is lactose from milk, which is excluded from the definition of free sugars
Flavoured milk	200 mL	28.0 g	16.2 g	The sugars are a mix of added 'free sugars' and lactose (from milk). Flavoured milk is permitted within the School Food Standards if it does not contain more than 5% added sugars
Plain yogurt (low fat)	125 g	9.9 g	0	None of the sugars are free sugars; all of the sugar is lactose from milk, which is excluded from the definition of free sugars
Fruit yogurt	125 g	15.9 g	11.25 g	The sugars present are a mix of free sugars, sugars from the fruit pieces (not 'free') and lactose from the milk (also excluded from the free sugars definition). Levels of free sugars vary and can be low when non-caloric sweeteners are used, but typically are 8–10 g/100 g; 9 g/100 g has been used here
Diet fruit yogurt (low fat, no added sugar)	125 g	7.8 g	0	None of the sugars are free sugars. The sugars present are from milk (lactose) and fruit pieces, which are both excluded from the definition of fruit sugars
Portion of fresh fruit salad	140 g	19.6 g	0	None of the sugars are free sugars. The sugars present are within the fruit structure (a mixture of fructose, glucose and sucrose)
Banana	100 g	18.1 g	0	None of the sugars are free sugars
Orange	160 g	13.6 g	0	None of the sugars are free sugars
Orange juice (150 mL)	150 mL	12.9 g	12.9 g	All the sugars are classed as free sugars, released from the fruit during juicing
Honey (5 g)	5 g	3.8 g	3.8 g	All the sugars are classed as free sugars

Source: compositional data derived from Finglas *et al.* (2015).

The new carbohydrate recommendations mean that most people need to reduce the amount of free sugars they consume and increase the amount of fibre. The new dietary recommendation for sugars is designed to minimise the risks associated with high free sugars intakes and to result in improved management of energy intake, by reducing energy (calorie) intake across the population by an estimated 100 kcal/day (418 kJ/day). For people who are maintaining a healthy body weight, SACN advises that the reduction in free sugars (to achieve the 5% energy level) should be replaced by starches (especially higher fibre starchy foods such as wholegrain cereals, wholemeal bread and pasta, brown rice, jacket potatoes and pulses), by sugars contained within the cellular structure of fruits and vegetables and by lactose naturally present in milk and milk products (such as plain yogurt and cheeses). For overweight individuals, SACN advises that reducing the amount of energy consumed as free sugars, without increasing energy intake from other sources, could contribute to a reduction in total energy intake and result in weight loss.

In light of the new fibre and free sugars recommendations, Public Health England recently reviewed and launched a revised healthy eating guide for the UK population, *The Eatwell Guide* (PHE, 2016). This depicts increased segment sizes for the starchy carbohydrates and fruit and vegetables groups compared with the previous version, the *eatwell plate*. Selection of beans, pulses and other sustainable plant proteins is also encouraged – see Buttriss (2016b).

A feature of dietary recommendations to increase fibre intake is a focus on wholegrains and wholemeal-based starchy carbohydrates (e.g. wholemeal bread, brown pasta and high-fibre breakfast cereals). However, there is no specific definition of 'wholegrain' and there are no specific recommendations on the amount of wholegrains that should be consumed each day in the UK (Seale, 2016). This is in contrast to recommendations in other countries. In Denmark, for example, adults are recommended to consume at least 75 g of wholegrain per day (Mejborn *et al.*, 2008) and US guidelines specify 48 g/day (USDHHS/USDA, 2010). A recent analysis of NDNS data suggested that median wholegrain intake in the UK is 20 g/day for adults and 13 g/day for children/teenagers (Mann *et al.*, 2015), with 18% of adults defined as non-consumers. In the UK (Mann *et al.*, 2015) and elsewhere (Bellisle *et al.*, 2014), there are socio-economic differences in wholegrain consumption, with higher intakes reported in those with higher education and income.

Is 5% achievable?

Average intakes of free sugars currently exceed the 5% level by a substantial margin in all age groups; two to three times higher than 5% total energy. In terms of carbohydrate, SACN's findings endorse a dietary pattern that is based on wholegrains, pulses, potatoes, vegetables and fruits, but limiting the amounts of free sugars consumed in the form of table sugar, preserves and sweet spreads, fruit juice, confectionery, biscuits, cakes and desserts.

Dietary modelling with everyday foods shows that a diet that provides 5% or less of energy as free sugars, the new target for fibre of 30 g/day (in itself a challenging target given current intake levels) and also meets other dietary reference values for nutrients is possible, although it will inevitably result in a dietary pattern that is dissimilar to the diets consumed by many in the UK currently. Example menus can be found at: https://www.nutrition.org.uk/attachments/article/881/SACN%20guidelines%20meal%20planner.pdf. Specific points to note are that the menus feature high-fibre varieties of starchy foods and more than five portions of fruit and vegetables daily (on average over eight) to achieve 30 g fibre, with fruit juice limited to one 150 mL glass a day. But current fruit and vegetable intakes are only 4.1 portions per day on average, in adults aged 19–64 years, with only 30% of both men and women achieving five a day (Bates *et al.*, 2014). Mean consumption of fruit and vegetables for children aged 11–18 years was 3.0 portions per day for boys and 2.7 portions per day for girls, with only 9% of this age group meeting the five a day recommendation (Bates *et al.*, 2014) (see Chapter 8 for more on dietary pattens). The majority of drinks in the diet plan are water, low-calorie drinks and unsweetened tea and coffee with milk. Some snacks and desserts with added sugars are included, but most snacks are fibre-rich ones. The type of diet that emerges in the dietary modelling is not representative of the average diet eaten in the UK and will require a substantial change in dietary habits for most people and considerable support and practical advice from multiple stakeholders. Innovative food solutions from manufactures and retailers may also be needed to help consumers achieve the recommendations (see Chapter 24 on the effects of the wider environment on consumption).

References

Bates, B., Lennox, A., Prentice, A. *et al.* (eds) (2014) *National Diet and Nutrition Survey. Results from Years 1, 2, 3 and 4 (Combined) of the Rolling Programme (2008/2009–2011/2012)*. Public Health England, London.

Bellisle, F., Hébel, P., Colin, J. *et al.* (2014) Consumption of whole grains in French children, adolescents and adults. *The British Journal of Nutrition*, **112**, 1674–1684.

Bhupathiraju, S., Tobias, D.K., Malik, V.S. *et al.* (2014) Glycemic index, glycemic load, and risk of type 2 diabetes: results from 3 large US cohorts and an updated meta-analysis. *The American Journal of Clinical Nutrition*, **100** (1), 218–232.

British Heart Foundation (2016) *CVD Statistics – BHF UK Factsheet*. https://www.bhf.org.uk/-/media/files/research/heart-statistics/bhf-cvd-statistics---uk-factsheet.pdf?la=en (accessed 10 December 2016).

Brouns, F., Bjorck, I., Frayn, K.N. *et al.* (2005) Glycaemic index methodology. *Nutrition Research Reviews*, **18**, 145–171.

Burgos, K., Subramaniam, P. and Arthur, J. (2016) *Reformulation Guide: Spotlight on Sugars*. Report, Leatherhead Food Research. https://www.fdf.org.uk/corporate_pubs/Reformulation-Guide-Sugars-Aug2016.pdf (accessed 11 December 2016).

Buttriss, J.L. (2016a) Nutrition labels to change in the US. *Nutrition Bulletin*, **41** (3), 197–201.

Buttriss, J. (2016b) The Eatwell Guide refreshed. *Nutrition Bulletin*, **41** (2), 135–141.

Calorie Reduction Expert Group (2011) *Statement of the Calorie Reduction Expert Group*. https://www.gov.uk/government/uploads/system/uploads/attachment_data/file/215561/dh_127554.pdf (accessed 11 December 2016).

Chiavaroli, L., de Souza, R.J., Ha, V. *et al.* (2015) Effect of fructose on established lipid targets: a systematic review and meta-analysis of controlled feeding trials. *Journal of the American Heart Association*, **4** (9), e001700.

Committee on Medical Aspects of Food Policy (1991) *Dietary Reference Values for Food Energy and Nutrients for the United Kingdom. Report On Health and Social Subjects*. HMSO, London.

Cummings, J. and Stephen, A. (2007) Carbohydrate terminology and classification. *European Journal of Clinical Nutrition*, **61** (Suppl 1), S5–S18.

EFSA Panel on Dietetic Products, Nutrition and Allergies (2010) Scientific Opinion on dietary reference values for carbohydrates and dietary fibre. *EFSA Journal* **8**: 1462.

Fagt, S., Gunnarsdottir, I., Hallas-Møller, T. *et al.* (2012) *Nordic Dietary Surveys. Study Designs, Methods, Results and Use in Food-based Risk Assessments*. Nordic Council of Ministers, Copenhagen. http://norden.diva-portal.org/smash/get/diva2:701738/FULLTEXT01.pdf (accessed 11 December 2016).

FDA (2016) *Changes to the Nutrition Facts Label*. http://www.fda.gov/food/guidanceregulation/guidancedocumentsregulatoryinformation/labelingnutrition/ucm385663.htm (accessed 11 December 2016).

Finglas, P.M., Roe, M.A., Pinchen, H.M. *et al.* (2015) *McCance and Widdowson's The Composition of Foods*, 7th summary edn. Royal Society of Chemistry, Cambridge.

Food Safety Authority of Ireland (2011) *Scientific Recommendations for Healthy Eating Guidelines in Ireland*. Food Safety Authority of Ireland, Dublin. https://www.fsai.ie/science_and_health/healthy_eating.html (accessed 11 December 2016).

Greenwood, D., Threapleton, D.E., Evans, C.E. *et al.* (2014) Association between sugar-sweetened and artificially sweetened soft drinks and type 2 diabetes: systematic review and dose–response meta-analysis of prospective studies. *British Journal of Nutrition*, **112** (5), 725–734.

Hooper, B., Spiro, A. and Stanner, S. (2015) 30 g of fibre a day: an achievable recommendation? *Nutrition Bulletin*, **40**, 118–129.

InterAct Consortium (2013) Consumption of sweet beverages and type 2 diabetes incidence in European adults: results from EPIC-InterAct. *Diabetologia*, **56** (7), 1520–1530.

Lifestyle Statistics Team, Health and Social Care Information Centre (2014). *National Child Measurement Programme:*

England, 2013/14 School Year. http://content.digital.nhs.uk/catalogue/PUB16070/nati-chil-meas-prog-eng-2013-2014-rep.pdf (accessed 10 December 2016).

Liu, S., Manson, J.E., Lee, I.-M. *et al.* (2000) Fruit and vegetable intake and risk of cardiovascular disease: the Women's Health Study. *The American Journal of Clinical Nutrition*, **72**, 922–928.

Liu, S., Buring, J.E., Sesso, H.D. *et al.* (2002) A prospective study of dietary fiber intake and risk of cardiovascular disease among women. *Journal of the American College of Cardiology*, **39**, 49–56.

Lockyer, S. and Nugent, A.P. (2017) Health effects of resistant starch. *Nutrition Bulletin*, **42**, 10–41. doi:10.1111/nbu.12244

Lockyer, S., Spiro, A. and Stanner, S. (2016) Dietary fibre and the prevention of chronic disease – should health professionals be doing more to raise awareness? *Nutrition Bulletin*, **41** (3), 214–231.

Mann, K.D., Pearce, M.S., McKevith, B. *et al.* (2015) Low whole grain intake in the UK: results from the National Diet and Nutrition Survey rolling programme 2008–11. *British Journal of Nutrition*, **113**, 1643–1651.

Mejborn, H., Biltoft-Jensen, A., Trolle, E. and Tetens, I.F. (2008) *Wholegrain – definition and scientific background for recommendations of wholegrain intake in Denmark*. Fødevareinstituttet, Danmarks Tekniske Universitet, Søborg (in Danish).

NHMRC (2006) *Nutrient Reference Values for Australia and New Zealand: Including Recommended Dietary Intakes*. National Health and Medical Research Council, Canberra. https://www.nhmrc.gov.au/_files_nhmrc/publications/attachments/n35.pdf (accessed 11 December 2016).

PHE (2014) *Adult Obesity and Type 2 Diabetes*. Public Health England, London. https://www.gov.uk/government/uploads/system/uploads/attachment_data/file/338934/Adult_obesity_and_type_2_diabetes_.pdf (accessed 10 December 2016).

PHE (2015) *Why 5%? An Explanation of the Scientific Advisory Committee on Nutrition's Recommendations about Sugars and Health, in the Context of Current Intakes of Free Sugars, Other Dietary Recommendations and the Changes in Dietary Habits Needed to Reduce Consumption of Free Sugars to 5% of Dietary Energy*. Public Health England, London. https://www.gov.uk/government/uploads/system/uploads/attachment_data/file/489906/Why_5__-_The_Science_Behind_SACN.pdf (accessed 11 December 2016).

PHE (2016) *The Eatwell Guide. Helping You Eat a Healthy, Balanced Diet*. www.gov.uk/government/uploads/system/uploads/attachment_data/file/510366/UPDATED_Eatwell-23MAR2016_England.pdf (accessed 11 December 2016).

SACN (2015) *Carbohydrates and Health*. The Stationery Office, London.

Seale, C. (2016) Whole grains and CVD risk. *Proceedings of the Nutrition Society*, **65** (1), 24–34.

USDA (2015) *2015-2020 Dietary Guidelines for Americans*, 8th edition. US Department of Agriculture, Washington, DC. http://health.gov/dietaryguidelines/2015/guidelines/(accessed 11 December 2016).

USDHHS/USDA (2010) *Dietary Guidelines for Americans 2010*. Government Printing Office, Washington, DC.

WHO (2015) *Guideline: Sugars Intake for Adults and Children*. World Health Organization, Geneva.

Wolever, T.M., Fernandes, J. and Rao, A.V. (1996) Serum acetate: propionate ratio is related to serum cholesterol in men but not women. *Journal of Nutrition*, **126** (11), 2790–2797.

18
Cardiovascular Disease: Dietary Fat Quality

Tom Sanders

Key messages

- Cardiovascular disease (CVD) is the leading cause of death world-wide. Besides the key role of blood pressure, the development of type 2 diabetes and CVD are associated with changes in lipid metabolism that cause atherosclerosis.
- Atherosclerosis develops over several decades, but the pathological processes leading to clinical events (heart attack, stroke) are usually the consequence of thrombosis resulting from the acute rupture of an atherosclerotic plaque or arterial aneurisms.
- Apolipoprotein-B-containing lipoproteins (low-density lipoprotein (LDL), very low density lipoprotein, intermediate-density lipoprotein) are causally involved in the generation of atherosclerotic plaques.
- Replacing C12–C16 saturated fatty acids with carbohydrates, monounsaturated or polyunsaturated fatty acids lowers LDL-cholesterol.
- Replacing fat with carbohydrate in the diet lowers high-density lipoprotein cholesterol and raises fasting plasma triacylglycerol concentrations. High intakes of dietary fat contribute to post-prandial lipaemia and have adverse effects on endothelial function, fibrinolytic activity and pro-coagulant activity.
- Excess accumulation of body fat accelerates the progression of atherosclerosis
- Prospective cohort studies show an association between reduced CVD mortality when: (a) trans fatty acids are replaced with saturated, monounsaturated or polyunsaturated fatty acids; (b) saturated fatty acids are replaced with linoleic acid; (c) the intake long-chain n-3 polyunsaturated fatty acids provided by oily fish is >0.2 g/day.
- Intervention trials show: (a) replacement of saturated fatty acids with polyunsaturated fatty acids lowers ischaemic heart disease incidence; (b) an intake of ~1 g long-chain n-3 polyunsaturated fatty acids decrease ischaemic heart disease mortality by 9%; (c) a Mediterranean dietary pattern, where monounsaturated fatty acids partially replace saturated fatty acids, reduces CVD mortality and events by 30%.

18.1 Introduction

Cardiovascular disease (CVD) is the leading cause of death worldwide, and in most developed economies ischaemic heart disease (IHD) is more prevalent than cerebrovascular disease (stroke). However, stroke is more prevalent than IHD in many emerging economies in Africa and in the Far East. CVD mortality rates have declined in many western countries but are rising in emerging economies and remain high in eastern Europe. In the UK, there have been changes in major risk factors over the past 20–30 years, with notably fewer people smoking and falls in blood pressure and serum cholesterol concentrations. In the UK, CVD mortality fell from 141/100 000 under 75 years in 1995–1997 to 85/100 000 between 2009 and 2011, which is a fall of about 55%.

Most of the reduction in mortality can be explained by better treatment and reductions in smoking habit, blood pressure and serum cholesterol, but about 14% of the fall remains unexplained.

Atherosclerosis is the underlying pathology leading to IHD and the more common form of stroke (cerebral infarction). The relationship between fat intake and atherosclerosis was recognised in the late 19th century and instigated an enormous body of work developing experimental models of atherosclerosis in animals which involved manipulating the level and type of fat as well as cholesterol in the diet. The major impact of this work was to establish the pathological pathways resulting in atherosclerosis, particularly the role of plasma lipids in the process of foam cell formation and progression to complex atherosclerotic plaques.

Public Health Nutrition, Second Edition. Edited by Judith L Buttriss, Ailsa A Welch, John M Kearney and Susan A Lanham-New.
© 2018 by The Nutrition Society. Published 2018 by John Wiley & Sons, Ltd.
Companion website: www.wiley.com/go/buttriss/publichealth

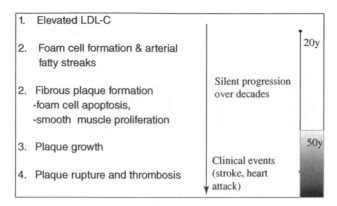

Figure 18.1 Relationship between elevated LDL-cholesterol (LDL-C) and the development of atherosclerosis and its consequences.

Human atherosclerosis is a chronic inflammatory process that develops over several decades, with clinical events becoming evident in the fifth decade of life and beyond. It begins with the accumulation of fatty streaks in large/medium arteries, which progress to form fibrous plaques over time. These fatty streaks consist of collections of foam cells, which are derived from tissue macrophages (a type of white blood cell) that have taken up low-density lipoprotein (LDL), which is rich in lipids, especially cholesteryl esters. The current view is that LDL needs to be modified (glycated) or oxidised before being taken up by macrophages. Fatty streaks can disappear with time or can progress to form fibrous atherosclerotic plaques. Plaques grow over many years and can develop large lipid-rich necrotic cores, making them unstable. Large plaques protrude into the lumen of the artery, impede the delivery of oxygenated blood to the tissues and cause turbulence in blood flow, which in turn increases the likelihood of blood clotting. The rupture of an atherosclerotic plaque causes a blood clot (thrombosis) to block the artery and is usually the event that precipitates a heart attack of stroke (Figure 18.1). Inflammation, which activates white blood cells, contributes to the erosion of the cap of atherosclerotic plaques, making them less stable as well as increasing the risk of thrombosis by increasing plasma fibrinogen concentrations. This partly explain why inflammation (i.e. smoking) or acute infections (i.e. influenza) can precipitate cardiovascular events. As shall be discussed, dietary fat intake can influence both the atherosclerotic and thrombotic pathways that influence risk of CVD.

18.2 Relationship between diet and plasma lipid concentrations

Elevated total cholesterol (TC) concentration, or specifically LDL-C concentration, is well established in the

promotion of atherosclerosis. The Seven Countries Study first showed that a population's median serum cholesterol concentration is a major predictor of its risk of IHD, and later prospective studies showed LDL-C to be a stronger predictor of risk. LDL-C-lowering therapies (by blood-cholesterol-lowering drugs such as statins, plasma apherisis and diet) slow the progression of atherosclerosis and decrease the incidence of IHD. Plasma LDL-C concentrations are determined by the rate of cholesterol synthesis in the liver and the activity of the LDL receptor, which is regulated by dietary, hormonal and genetic factors. The predominant role of fat is to promote cholesterol synthesis in the liver. Insulin also stimulates 3-hydroxy-3-methyl-glutaryl–coenzyme A reductase (the rate-limiting enzyme in cholesterol synthesis), very low density lipoprotein (VLDL) synthesis and secretion and lipoprotein lipase activity. Receptor-mediated clearance of LDL is promoted by oestradiol and thyroxine, whereas stress hormones, such as corticosteroids and glucagon, have the opposite effect. Plasma LDL-C concentrations are low in infancy and remain so until after puberty, after which they rise; they reach a plateau around the age of 40 years in men but continue to rise in women. Some of the age-related increase in LDL-C can be attributed to the decline in thyroid hormone levels, and in women after the menopause the decline in oestrogen secretion. Some of the age-related increase in LDL-C can be avoided by maintaining a body mass index (BMI) within healthy limits (18.5–25 kg/m²). LDL-C concentrations rise linearly with increasing BMI up to about 30 kg/m².

Cholesterol, trans and dietary saturated fatty acids (C12–C16) raise LDL-C. Over the range of normal intake up to 400 mg/day, each 100 mg dietary cholesterol raises LDL-C by 0.05 mmol/L and each 1% energy raises it by 0.04 mmol/L. Lauric (14:0), myristic (16:0) and palmitic (16:0) acids raise LDL-C by 0.052 mmol/L, 0.048 mmol/L and 0.039 mmol/L respectively for each 1% energy they

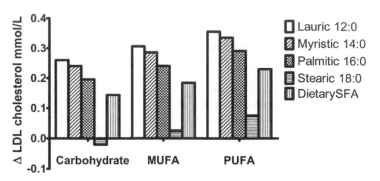

Figure 18.2 Effect of exchanging 5% energy lauric (12:0), myristic (14:0), palmitic (16:0), stearic (18:0) or a mixture typical of dietary saturated fatty acids on LDL-C compared with an equivalent proportion of energy from carbohydrate, MUFAs and PUFAs. *Source:* data based on Mensink *et al.* (2003) taken from Sanders (2013).

replace carbohydrates, or by 0.061 mmol/L, 0.057 mmol/L and 0.048 mmol/L respectively when they replace monounsaturated fatty acids (MUFAs) or by 0.071 mmol/L, 0.067 mmol/L and 0.058 mmol/L respectively when they replace polyunsaturated fatty acids (PUFAs) (mainly linoleic acid). However, short- and medium-chain fatty acids (<C12) and stearic acid (18:0) have no effect on LDL-C (Figure 18.2). Replacing C12–C16 saturated fatty acids with PUFAs, mainly linoleic acid, has a slightly greater LDL-C lowering effect than replacement with MUFAs In mixed diets, about 65% of saturated fatty acids are cholesterol raising, and exchanging each 1% energy (about 2 g/day) saturated fatty acids with carbohydrate, MUFAs and PUFAs lowers LDL-C by about 2%. However, long-chain *n*-3 PUFAs, particularly docosahexaenoic acid, raise LDL-C by about 10% when supplied as dietary supplements.

Palmitic, stearic and myristic acids are the major saturated fatty acids in animal fats. However, milk fat from cows, sheep and goats also contains significant amounts of short- and medium-chain fatty acids. Tropical oils (palm, coconut and cocoa butter) are high in saturated fatty acids: coconut oil contains about 90% saturated fatty acids (about 58% of which are medium-chain fatty acids), crude palm oil contains about 48% saturated fatty acids (mainly palmitic acid) and cocoa butter contains a similar proportion (mainly stearic and palmitic acids).

Vegetable seed oils are generally low in saturated fatty acids but contain corresponding higher proportions of oleic acid or PUFAs and tend to be liquid at room temperature. Consequently, exchanging solid fats for liquid oils in the diet reduces the intake of saturated fatty acids. However, in the UK, most of the saturated fatty acid intake comes from meat and milk fat.

Among communities living under conditions of primitive agriculture, where intakes of fat are very low (around 15% energy), there is limited accumulation of body fat and serum cholesterol levels are low. However, when energy intake exceeds expenditure and the proportion of fat in the diet is higher, body fat accumulates, mainly as palmitic and oleic acids, and LDL-C concentrations rise. In most economically developed countries, the majority of the middle-aged and older population have raised LDL-C concentrations (>3.0 mmol/L). Carriage of the apolipoprotein ε4 allele for apolipoprotein E, which is a common polymorphism affecting up to 30% of the population, results in higher LDL-C than those who are homozygous for the more common ε3 allele. However, groups such as vegans, who have low intakes of saturated fatty acids (~6% energy) and a low prevalence of obesity, tend to have much lower LDL-C concentrations (about 1 mmol/L lower) compared with meat-eaters.

18.3 Atherogenic lipoprotein phenotype

In addition to raised LDL-C there are other lipoprotein phenotypes associated with atherosclerosis. The second most common is the atherogenic lipoprotein phenotype (ALP), characterised by predominance of small, dense LDL particles and elevated plasma triacylglycerol (TAG) and low high-density lipoprotein (HDL) cholesterol (HDL-C) concentration. It occurs at a lower prevalence rate in middle-aged and older subjects than elevated LDL-C, but it may affect 10–15% of the population. It is commonly observed in people with type 2 diabetes. The ALP is characterised by persistently high concentrations of TAG-rich lipoproteins, which, as shall be explained, generate small, dense LDL particles. The main source of these TAG-rich lipoproteins is from VLDLs secreted from the liver to export TAG. TAG synthesis in the liver is mainly determined by the input of non-esterified fatty acids (NEFAs) derived from adipose tissue rather than *de novo* synthesis of fatty acids from carbohydrate in the liver, which is low (typically <10 g/day) in humans (although VLDL secretion is enhanced on a high carbohydrate intake, especially by sucrose and fructose).

High plasma insulin concentrations promote fat storage, particularly in the visceral depots, and the ALP is strongly linked to the amount of visceral body fat. The reasons why visceral adiposity causes the ALP is uncertain, but it may be more sensitive to stress-induced lipolysis, which would elevate plasma NEFAs, and in turn stimulate TAG synthesis and VLDL secretion. When plasma VLDL TAG concentrations are high, the exchange of TAG for cholesteryl esters between VLDL and cholesteryl-ester-rich lipoproteins occurs by the action of cholesterol ester transfer protein. VLDLs exchange TAG for cholesterol esters from LDL and HDL. The resulting HDL particles and LDL particles are enriched with TAG, but because they are much smaller than VLDLs they can pass into hepatic sinusoids where they react with hepatic lipase, which hydrolyses the TAG, causing the HDL and LDL particles to shrink. The small HDL particles are more rapidly removed from the circulation, but small LDL particles remain in circulation for longer. Thus, elevated VLDL TAG secretion induced by high insulin concentrations reduces HDL concentrations and promotes the formation of harmful small, dense LDL particles. Inflammation, which results in the production of cytokines such as such as interleukin-6, also has a similar effect because it stimulates the release of NEFAs from adipose tissue and thus increases VLDL TAG secretion.

The ALP is one of the features of the metabolic syndrome that describes the constellation of clinical features associated with increased risk of CVD: central obesity, insulin resistance or glucose intolerance, raised blood pressure, low HDL (usually ≤0.8 mmol/L) and high TAG (>1.7 mmol/L), gout and microalbuminuria (an indicator of microvascular disease and renal dysfunction), increased procoagulant activity, measured as raised fibrinogen and factor VII coagulant activity, and decreased fibrinolytic activity, and impaired endothelial function. These latter factors cause a hypercoaguable state and a reduced capacity to break down blood clots and are associated with increased risk of coronary events. The underlying disorder that results in metabolic syndrome is probably insulin resistance, which results in elevated plasma insulin concentrations. Eventually, the capacity to synthesise sufficient amounts of insulin to maintain normal glucose concentrations fails and type 2 diabetes is diagnosed based on elevated plasma glucose. However, there may be a long period prior to the diagnosis of type 2 diabetes where elevated levels of plasma insulin are causing vascular damage.

The International Diabetes Federation proposed a pragmatic definition for identifying individuals likely to have metabolic syndrome (waist circumference ≥94 cm for men and ≥80 cm for women or BMI >30 kg/m^2 plus at least two of the following: raised TAG (≥1.7 mmol/L), low HDL (<1.09 mmol/L in men and <1.29 in women), raised BP >130/85 mmHg or fasting glucose >5.6 mmol/L. The prevalence of the International Diabetes Federation metabolic syndrome is somewhere in the region of 25–30% of the middle-aged and older population in the UK. However, typically only 15% of individuals meeting this definition of metabolic syndrome have the ALP, and raised LDL-C is more common.

The ALP can be corrected by weight loss and exercise, but not by replacing saturated with MUFAs or PUFAs. The ALP is, however, improved by energy-restricted very low carbohydrate diets (10–25% energy) in conjunction with increased physical activity, probably because these diets reduce insulin secretion.

Replacing saturated fatty acids, especially lauric, myristic and palmitic acids, with carbohydrates lowers HDL-C. As low HDL-C is associated with a greater risk of CVD this might be thought to offset the benefit resulting from increased LDL-C. However, trials with drugs that raise HDL-C have failed to show any benefit in terms of decreasing CVD, and genetic variations associated with slightly higher HDL-C levels are not associated with a lower risk. The significance of changes in HDL-C brought about by changes in dietary fat intake, therefore, is uncertain. Nevertheless, the TC : HDL-C ratio is twice as informative of CVD than LDL-C or HDL-C alone. This may be because the ratio captures the common phenotype of raised LDL-C as well as the ALP. Trans fatty acids acid have an adverse effect on the ratio (Figure 18.3), but there is little difference between myristic and palmitic acids and carbohydrate. Lauric acid, on the other hand, appears to have a favourable effect comparable to MUFAs and PUFAs. A difference in the TC : HDL-C ratio of 1.33 is equivalent to a 30% difference in risk of CVD. In practice, replacing 10% saturated fatty acids with MUFAs results in a reduction in the ratio of about 0.12, which might be predicted to reduce risk of CVD death by 3%. However, these risk predictions are based on a single surrogate risk marker, not on evidence from trials.

18.4 Postprandial lipids

Measurements of plasma lipids are usually made in the fasting state, which does not reflect what happens for most of the day when humans are in the fed state.

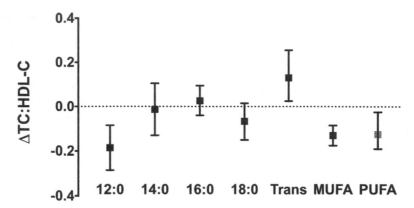

Figure 18.3 The effect of exchanging lauric (12:0), myristic (14:0), palmitic (16:0), stearic (18:0), trans, saturated fatty acids, MUFAs and PUFAs on the TC:HDL-C ratio compared with a similar proportion of energy from carbohydrate. *Source:* data based on Mensink *et al.* (2003) taken from Sanders (2013). Data are mean values with 95% confidence intervals.

Meals high in fat (>30 g per meal) elevated plasma TAG 3–4 h following a meal. In healthy individuals the increases in plasma TAG after a fatty meal are modest even following meals containing 50 g fat, and values return to normal 5–6 h following the meal. However, in older adults, and particularly in people with type 2 diabetes, meals high in fat often result in prolonged elevations in plasma TAG. Prolonged postprandial lipaemia has been shown to be associated with increased risk of CVD and affects several pathological process associated with arterial damage and thrombosis (Figure 18.4). For example, postprandial lipaemia causes elevations in factor VII coagulant activity, impairs fibrinolysis and endothelial function and has an inflammatory effect.

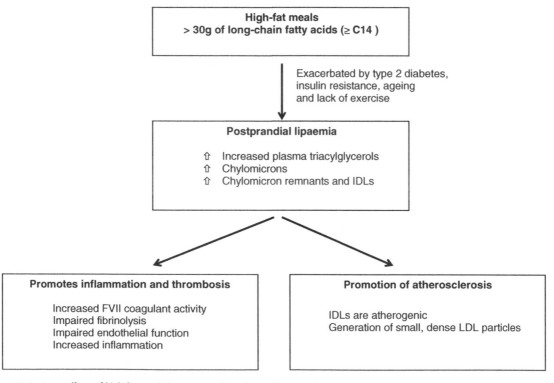

Figure 18.4 Acute effects of high-fat meals (IDL: intermediate-density lipoprotein).

The accumulation of TAG-rich lipoproteins, especially IDL, also contributes to causing atherosclerosis, particularly of the peripheral circulation affecting the limbs. Limb amputation as a consequence of atherosclerosis obliterans is a common complication of type 2 diabetes mellitus. The dietary management of raised IDL involves restricting the dietary intake of long-chain fatty acids. There is little difference between long-chain saturated, monounsaturated and linoleic acid with regard to their effects on postprandial lipaemia. However, long-chain n-3 PUFAs do reduce postprandial lipaemia indirectly by reducing VLDL TAG secretion. Short- and medium-chain saturated fatty acids, which are absorbed via the portal vein, however, do not result in postprandial lipaemia. Brisk walking 30 min/day also helps reduce postprandial lipaemia.

18.5 Increased adiposity and cardiovascular disease risk factors

The accumulation of excess amounts of adipose tissue in the body, most of which is derived from dietary fat intake, is associated with a number of physiological changes that increase risk of CVD. Increased adiposity is associated with raised TAG concentrations, lower HDL-C and higher fibrinogen concentrations and impaired fibrinolytic activity. While there is no convincing evidence to show that varying proportion of energy derived from fat influences the risk of obesity on isocaloric diets, the addition of fat does increase the energy density of food. Consequently, selecting reduced-fat alternatives (which have a reduced energy content) rather than high-fat products can be helpful in maintaining a healthy weight.

18.6 Evidence from cohort studies and trials with clinical endpoints

Prospective cohort studies are able to assess risk of the usual diet on subsequent risk of CVD. Most cohort studies have relied upon a single measurement of intake at baseline: either a 24 h dietary recall or more frequently a food frequency questionnaire. The ability to capture information about the level of quality of fat consumed may be limited by the detail provided. A further limitation is the assumption that fat intake has not changed in the follow-up period. There have been marked changes over the past 40 years in many countries owing to increased use of vegetable oils in place of animal fats, and the decline in the consumption of butter and full-fat milk. In the UK, total fat intakes have been reduced from ~42 to ~35% energy and saturated fatty acid intakes increased from ~10% to 12% energy. The intake of

PUFAs has risen from 4% energy to 6% energy. Intakes of trans fatty acids from partially hydrogenated fats have markedly declined from around 2% energy to well below 1% energy. Over the same time period, average serum cholesterol concentrations have fallen in the UK and many other western countries. These changes are thus likely to confound the interpretation of prospective cohort studies.

Chowdhury *et al.* (2014) conducted a systematic review of prospective studies and confirmed the adverse effect of trans fatty acid intake on CVD risk but surprisingly were unable to find any significant association between reported saturated fatty acid intake and risk of CVD mortality. They concluded that the evidence did not support recommendations to replace saturated fatty acid with PUFAs. However, a second meta-analysis by Farvid *et al.* (2014) that included new data from large cohort studies shows that the replacement of 5% energy as saturated fatty acids with linoleic acid (18:2n-6) was associated with 9% and 11% lower risks of CVD incidence and mortality respectively.

In the 1960s and 1970s, several randomised controlled trials evaluated the impact of replacing saturated fatty acids with PUFAs. They showed these lowered TC and had a favourable effect on IHD incidence but not mortality. However, because these were relatively small studies they did not have sufficient statistical power to detect an effect on CVD mortality. It is unlikely that any further trials will be conducted in the future because of the enormous resources required and the complexity of maintaining dietary change over many years, especially when there are more effective means of lowering LDL-C (e.g. statins).

High intakes of long-chain n-3 polyunsaturated fatty acids (3–14 g/day) plausibly explained the low incidence of acute myocardial infarction in Inuit groups on their traditional diets because of their pharmacological effects on eicosanoid synthesis. However, more recent studies have not found CVD prevalence to be lower among Inuit people, possibly because their traditional lifestyle has changed. Nevertheless, there is a large body of evidence demonstrating that high intakes (>3 g/day) of eicosapentaenoic acid (20:5n-3) and docosahexaenoic acid (22:6n-3) have blood-pressure-lowering, TAG-lowering, anti-thrombotic and anti-inflammatory effects. However, low intakes of fish providing well below 1 g long-chain n-3 PUFAs per day have been associated with a lower risk of CVD, with as little as one serving a week showing a 16% reduction in risk of death from IHD. However, it is hard to gauge the specific contribution to risk reduction made by long-chain n-3 PUFAs from other nutrients/compounds present in fish. There is some more limited data to suggest that alpha-linolenic acid (18:3n-3) may also be associated with a 14% lower risk of fatal CVD, as with long-chain n-3 PUFAs, and

Table 18.1 Recommended intakes expressed as percentage energy intake for fat and fatty acids for prevention of CVD.

	Recommended energy intake (%)						Recommended intake (g)
	Total fat	Trans	Saturated	PUFA	Linoleic acid	Linolenic acid	n-3 LCP
UK DoH 1994	≤35	<2	<11	6	No DRV	No DRV	0.45
WHO/FAO 2010	25–35	<1	≤10	6–11.5	2.5–9.0	0.5–2.0	0.25–2
EFSA 2010	≤35	<1	<10	No DRV	4.0 (AI)	0.5 (AI)	0.25 (AI)
Dietary Guidelines for Americans 2015	25–35	<1	≤10	No DRV	5–9	0.6—1.2	No DRV

AI: acceptable intake; DRV: dietary reference value; LCP: long-chain PUFA.

there appears to be a threshold effect where the increase in risk is seen only with an intake of 1 g/day. There have been several large placebo-controlled randomised trials of long-chain n-3 PUFA supplementation in patients who already have CVD; overall, these show a trend for a 9% lower risk of cardiac death but no effect on incident CVD. However, the more recent trials have failed to show any benefit, but these were in patients whose blood lipids, blood pressure and diabetes were well controlled by medication. It seems likely that any effect of n-3 fatty acids is likely to be mediated via pathways other than lipoprotein metabolism. Most likely are those affecting the acute processes of thrombosis and heart rhythm.

18.7 Current dietary guidelines

Most guidelines recommend consuming no more than 10% energy from saturated fatty acids and minimising the intake of trans fatty acids (<1% energy) (see Table 18.1). With regard to total, an acceptable macronutrient intake range of between 25 and 35% from fat has been recommended. The upper limit of 35% energy is because a higher proportion of fat may promote obesity. UK and European recommendations suggest consuming at least one portion of oily fish per week, and this has been translated into the equivalent of between 0.25 and 0.45 g long-chain PUFAs per day. There is less agreement regarding specifying intakes for other PUFAs. The USA and World Health Organization give a range of intakes for linoleic acid with an upper limit of 9% energy, whereas the European Food Safety Authority specifies an acceptable intake as being 4% energy. There are no specific recommendations for MUFAs.

It would appear that there has been a shift in current dietary thinking away from dietary advice focused on fat reduction and modification towards food-based guidelines that focus on changing the overall dietary pattern; for example, the DASH diet. This type of dietary pattern is typical of that recommended and it is not unlike a Mediterranean dietary pattern. A Mediterranean dietary pattern was first shown in the Seven Countries study to be associated with a lower risk of CVD. The Mediterranean diet contains between 35 and 42% energy as fat but is low in saturated fatty acids (~10% energy). The slightly lower carbohydrate content also has favourable effects on cardiovascular risk factors for people with type 2 diabetes. The Lyon Diet Heart Study was the first trial to show that a Mediterranean diet is more effective in patients with IHD than advice focusing on reducing total fat intake to 30% energy and saturated fatty acid intake to 10%; in that study, the fat was provided by rapeseed oil not olive oil. More recently, a large primary prevention trial (PREDIMED) found CVD mortality (mainly from stroke) was reduced by 30% when they adopted a Mediterranean diet compared with advice just focus on reducing total and saturated fat. They were encouraged to consume virgin olive oil as the main dietary fat as well as consume plenty of fruit and vegetables, nuts, legumes, fish and poultry and less red meat and processed foods, such as cakes and biscuits.

Despite the major reductions in CVD worldwide, there are now more people living with CVD. The obesity epidemic is resulting in more people developing type 2 diabetes, which in turn will increase CVD morbidity and mortality. The role of diet, including fat intake, in the prevention of CVD is likely to continue to be of importance.

References

Chowdhury, R., Warnakula, S., Kunutsor, S. et al. (2014) Association of dietary, circulating, and supplement fatty acids with coronary risk: a systematic review and meta-analysis. *Annals of Internal Medicine*, **160** (6), 398–406.

Farvid, M.S., Ding, M., Pan, A. et al. (2014) Dietary linoleic acid and risk of coronary heart disease: a systematic review and meta-analysis of prospective cohort studies. *Circulation*, **130** (18), 1568–1578.

Mensink, R.P., Zock, P.L., Kester, A.D. and Katan, M.B. (2003) Effects of dietary fatty acids and carbohydrates on the ratio of serum total to HDL cholesterol and on serum lipids and apolipoproteins: a meta-analysis of 60 controlled trials. *The American Journal of Clinical Nutrition*, **77**, 1146–1155.

Sanders, T.A. (2013) Reappraisal of SFA and cardiovascular risk. *Proceedings of the Nutrition Society*, **72** (4), 390–398.

19
Diet and Cancer

Farah Naja and Lara Nasreddine[1]

Key messages

- A third of the most common cancers in the world could be prevented by a healthy diet, being physically active and maintaining a healthy body weight.
- Epigenetic changes (including DNA methylation, histone modification and micro RNA) are postulated to modulate the protective effect of selected dietary compounds on cancer.
- Gut microbiota may have a role in modulating the cancer-promoting or cancer-inhibiting behaviour of dietary constituents, namely carbohydrates, proteins, fats, alcohol and phytoestrogens.
- Common to all guidelines of cancer prevention are to keep the weight within the healthy range, be physically active, limit alcohol consumption, limit intake of processed and red meat, and increase intake of fruits and vegetables.
- It has been estimated that 14% of all cancer deaths in men and 20% of all cancer deaths in women are attributable to overweight and obesity and that the relationship between body fatness and cancer is continuous across the range of body mass index.
- Even though the exact type, dose and timing of physical activity in cancer prevention remain unclear, there is ample evidence to recommend physical activity as a means for primary prevention of cancer.

- Alcohol drinking is associated with increased risk of several types of cancer, whereby ethanol metabolism, nutritional deficiencies, impaired gene expression and defective immune surveillance seem to be the major mechanisms involved in alcohol-related carcinogenesis.
- Available evidence has implicated high red and processed meat intake in promoting carcinogenesis, whereby a role for proteins, haem iron, N-nitroso compounds, heterocyclic aromatic amines and polycyclic aromatic hydrocarbons may be implicated.
- Fruits and vegetables contain a wide array of potentially cancer-preventive compounds, including phytochemicals (such as polyphenols, organosulphur compounds, terpenoids), antioxidant nutrients (such as carotenoids and vitamin C), as well as dietary fibre.
- There is convincing evidence that foods containing dietary fibre reduce colorectal cancer risk, but future studies on the types of fibre and fibre components are still needed to provide a better understanding of how and why dietary fibre may decrease the risk of cancer.

19.1 Global burden of cancer

Cancer is a global term for a variety of diseases that share some similar characteristics, such as uncontrolled cellular growth, enhanced angiogenesis and/or reduced programmed cell death. The site of origin is used to define general categories of disease (e.g. breast cancer, skin cancer). It is increasingly apparent that, despite the variation across cancer types, the majority of cancers proceed from the first initiated tumour cell (e.g. mutated DNA) to mild, moderate, and severe dysplasia, invasive

carcinoma (invasion of cells through the basement membrane) and metastatic disease. Over the last couple of decades, cancer has become one of the most important, burdensome, expensive non-communicable diseases facing populations and health-care systems globally. In high-income countries, cancer became the major cause of premature deaths among non-communicable diseases, surpassing cardiovascular diseases and chronic obstructive pulmonary disease (IARC, 2014).

Worldwide, the incidence of cancer is increasing from year to year (WHO, 2015). While epidemiological data

---

[1] Both authors contributed equally to this chapter.

Public Health Nutrition, Second Edition. Edited by Judith L Buttriss, Ailsa A Welch, John M Kearney and Susan A Lanham-New.
© 2018 by The Nutrition Society. Published 2018 by John Wiley & Sons, Ltd.
Companion website: www.wiley.com/go/buttriss/publichealth

on incidence of cancer and deaths caused by cancer vary enormously in coverage and quality between countries and regions, GLOBOCAN 2012 is considered the most updated appraisal of cancer worldwide (Ferlay *et al.*, 2013; IARC, 2014). In 2012, there were an estimated 14.1 million new cases of cancer diagnosed worldwide (excluding melanoma skin cancer), 32.6 million with a diagnosis of cancer in the previous 5 years and 8.2 million estimated deaths from cancer. There were slightly more incident cases (53%) and deaths (57%) among men than among women. Among men, the five most common cancer sites were the lung (16.7%), prostate (15.0%), colorectum (10.0%), stomach (8.5%) and liver (7.5%). The same sites were the most common causes of cancer deaths among men. Among women, the five most common incident sites of cancer were the breast (25.2%), colorectum (9.2%), lung (8.7%), cervix (7.9%) and stomach (4.8%). These sites also represented the most common causes of cancer deaths among women (Ferlay *et al.*, 2013).

In general, and with some exceptions, the highest incidence rates are observed in North America and western Europe. Intermediate rates are seen in Central and South America, eastern Europe and much of South East Asia. Such a gradient in cancer incidence has been linked to human development. The United Nations development programme (UNDP) in 1990 proposed the Human Development Index (HDI), as a multi-dimensional measure of human development which included a long and healthy life, education and decent standard of living. The UNDP report using the GLOBOCAN estimates from WCRF/AICR (2007) showed that countries with higher HDI suffer higher rates of cancer overall and of specific types. For instance, cancers of the lung, breast, prostate and colorectum are more common in countries with a high HDI, while cancers with infectious aetiology, such as stomach, liver and cervix, are seen more in less developed countries (UNDP, 2013). As for cancer mortality, less contrast exists between various parts of the world, probably due to better clinical care in high-income countries, leading to lower mortality and better survival, and to the fact that cancers of the industrialised countries have a relatively better prognosis than other cancers more common in low- and middle-income countries (Edwards *et al.*, 2005). By year 2025, the global population will reach 8.3 billion increasing by 1.3 billion from year 2012. This population growth will be accompanied by a predicted 20 million new cancer cases compared with 14.1 million new cases in 2012. Countries with medium and low HDI will experience the greatest proportion of population growth and consequently the greatest increase in cancer burden. These countries are undergoing rapid societal, economic and lifestyle transition and will most likely face a double burden of the cancer – that is, cancer associated with infectious agents combined with that associated with an increasingly westernised lifestyle.

This rising burden of cancer and its disproportionate increase in low- and middle-income countries has gained a considerable political momentum leading to the United Nations Resolution in 2011, whereby governments have approved a global monitoring framework and an updated Global Action Plan 2013–2020 for the prevention and control of non-communicable diseases, including cancer. One strong arguement in favour of cancer prevention is that the cause could be removed or greatly reduced in the long term (Vineis and Wild, 2014). Examples in support of this argument are the decrease in male lung cancer with the fall in tobacco smoking and the reduction in bladder cancer among dye workers after the elimination of aromatic amines exposure. Furthermore, prevention is an important means to improve public health, and it is by far the most cost-effective and sustainable intervention for reducing the burden of cancer globally. At least one-third of cancer cases that occur annually throughout the world could be prevented (Danaei *et al.*, 2005). A World Health Organization (WHO) study found that at least 1.3 million cancer deaths annually could be prevented through healthy working and living environments (Prüss-Üstün and Corvalán, 2006). Paramount to prevention in general and to cancer prevention in particular, is a better understanding of the aetiology of the disease as well as the identification of the modifiable risk factors associated with its development.

19.2 Aetiology

The aetiology of cancer is complex and multifactorial. Cancer results from multiple genetic alterations that ultimately affect the coding of oncogenes for growth factors, growth factor receptors or tumour suppressor genes, which, when inactivated, fail to control the normal processes of cell death and turnover. Exhaustive study of the factors that contribute to the onset of cancer has determined that inherited germ-line mutations account only for 5% of tumours, while 95% is due to environmental factors (Anand *et al.*, 2008).

Early evidence for the role of environmental factors was derived from immigrant studies to the USA and Australia. These studies showed that the incidence in common cancers changes to the level of the new host country in one or two generations. Women who immigrate to the USA from Asian countries, where the rates are four to seven times lower, experience an 80% increase in risk after living in the USAs a decade or more (Ziegler *et al.*, 1993). A generation later, the risk for their daughters approaches that of women born in the USA. Hispanic women born in the USA have a significantly higher rate of breast cancer than do immigrant Hispanic women, but the longer the period of time immigrant Hispanic women spend in the USA, the greater their risk for breast cancer. This is especially true for women who immigrate before the age of 20 years (John *et al.*, 2005). Another example is the increase in colon cancer among Japanese who immigrated to the USA (Tomatis, 1990). These findings were fundamental to the understanding of the environmental aetiology of human cancer. Another argument in the favour of environmental factors as key players in the aetiology of cancer is related to the substantial change in age-adjusted rates of cancer over a relatively short period of time within confined populations. For instance, the sharp increase in colon cancer rates in economically developed countries within a relatively short duration cannot be explained by genetic factors alone and hence verifies the role of environmental factors.

These environmental factors include, in addition to external stimuli (radiation, pollution, infections, etc.), lifestyle factors (tobacco, alcohol, physical activity) and diet (WCRF/AICR, 2007; Anand *et al.*, 2008). The latest figures from the World Cancer Research Fund (WCRF) and the American Institute for Cancer Research (AICR) show that a third of the most common cancers in the world could be prevented by a healthy diet, being physically active and maintaining a healthy body weight (WCRF/AICR, 2007). The cancers most preventable by appropriate food, nutrition, physical activity and body fatness include those of the oesophagus, mouth, pharynx, and larynx, of colon and rectum, and of the breast. Therefore, diet and lifestyle factors are second only to the abstinence of tobacco smoking to reduce the risk of cancer (Friedenreich, 2001; WCRF/AICR, 2007; Steindorf *et al.*, 2013).

The role of diet in cancer aetiology depends on how it impacts fundamental cellular processes and influences the balance between cell proliferation, death and differentiation. Food, nutrition, body fatness and physical activity may have an impact on one or more of fundamental cellular processes, including cell signalling, gene expression, epigenetic regulation, cellular differentiation and DNA repair, as well as the regulation of the normal cell cycle, which ensures correct DNA replication. The capability of a cell to perform efficient cancer prevention or repair depends on its extracellular microenvironment, including the availability of energy and the presence of appropriate macro- and micronutrients (WCRF/AICR, 2007).

Understanding the links between diet and cancer is complex. Traditionally, epidemiologists have dealt with risk factors such as smoking, which could be easily quantified. In contrast, diet represents thousands of dietary components that are ingested each day, with each food item composed of a very different combination and concentration of these dietary components (WCRF/AICR, 2007). The diet–cancer association is further complicated by the fact that a single bioactive food constituent can alter multiple steps in the cancer process and that many of these processes can be affected by several food components (WCRF/AICR, 2007).

The WCRF/AICR (2007) report on the association between food, nutrition, physical activity and the prevention of cancer is considered one of the most rigorous reports and will be referred to in most of the diet–cancer associations discussed in this section. A brief description of the WCRF/AICR (2007) terminology in classifying evidence for a causal relationship with varying levels of confidence follows.

1. **Convincing.** For evidence strong enough to support a judgement of a convincing causal relationship, which justifies goals, and recommendations designed to reduce the incidence of cancer. A convincing relationship should be robust enough to be highly unlikely to be modified in the foreseeable future as new evidence accumulates.
2. **Probable.** For evidence strong enough to support a judgment of a probable causal relationship, which would generally justify goals and recommendations designed to reduce the incidence of cancer.
3. **Limited–suggestive.** Evidence that is too limited to permit a probable or convincing causal judgment, but where there is evidence suggestive of a direction of effect. The evidence may have methodological flaws, or be limited in amount, but shows a generally consistent direction of effect. This almost always does not justify recommendations designed to reduce the incidence of cancer. Any exceptions to this require special explicit justification.
4. **Limited–non-conclusion.** Evidence is so limited that no firm conclusion can be made. This category represents an entry level, and is intended to allow any exposure for which there are sufficient data to warrant panel consideration, but where insufficient evidence exists to permit a more definitive grading.

The association between food, nutrition, physical activity and cancer has been updated since the WCRF/AICR (2007) report for specific cancer sites as part of the Continuous Update Project. So far, update reports have been published for breast cancer (WCRF/AICR, 2010), colorectal cancer (WCRF/AICR, 2011), pancreatic cancer (WCRF/AICR, 2012), endometrium cancer (WCRF/AICR, 2013) and ovarian cancer (WCRF/AICR, 2014) and are available on the WCRF/AICR web site (http://wcrf.org/int/research-we-fund/continuous-update-project-cup).

Energy balance and physical activity

Weight gain and body fatness

Weight gain and increased body fatness often result from a state of chronic positive energy balance that may be due to excessive energy intake and/or decreased energy expenditure (Hursting, 2014). Numerous anthropometry-based measures are used as markers of body fatness, the most common being the body mass index (BMI), which is calculated as weight in kilograms divided by height in metres squared (WHO, 2006). The WCRF/AICR (2007) panel highlights that the risk of cancer is modified not only by obesity (BMI > 30 kg/m²), but by overweight as well (25.0 ≤ BMI ≤ 29.9 kg/m²), and that the relationship between body fatness and cancer is continuous across the range of BMI. It is important to note that the WHO has modified the range of BMI cut-off values for specific racial/ethnic groups based on differences in body composition patterns. For example, in subjects with Asian ancestry, a BMI greater than 23.0 kg/m² is considered as the cut-off value for overweight (Alberti and Zimmet, 1998). In addition to BMI, the level of abdominal fatness and visceral fat was also highlighted as an important modulator of cancer risk (WCRF/AICR, 2007; Kushi et al., 2012).

The strongest evidence, which corresponds to judgements of 'convincing' and 'probable' by the WCRF/AICR, indicates that higher levels of body fatness cause cancers of the oesophagus (adenocarcinomas), pancreas, colorectum, breast (postmenopausal women), endometrium, kidney and (probably) the gallbladder and ovaries (WCRF/AICR, 2007; http://wcrf.org/int/research-we-fund/continuous-update-project-cup). Overall, it has been estimated that 14% of all cancer deaths in men and 20% of all cancer deaths in women are attributable to overweight and obesity (Calle et al., 2003; Hursting, 2014). In a large prospective study examining the role of excess adiposity in increasing cancer-related deaths, it was shown that increased body weight was associated with increased death rates for all cancers combined and for cancers at multiple specific sites (Calle et al., 2003; Vucenik and Stains, 2012). Other studies also showed that obesity was associated with increased mortality from cancer of the prostate and stomach in men; breast (postmenopausal), endometrium, cervix, uterus, and ovaries in women; and kidney (renal cell), colon, oesophagus (adenocarcinoma), pancreas, gallbladder and liver in both genders (Calle et al., 2003; Hursting, 2014). The Metabolic Syndrome and Cancer Project, a European cohort study of approximately 580 000 adults, documented associations between obesity in metabolic syndrome and risks of colorectal, thyroid and cervical cancer (Stocks et al., 2010).

There are several plausible mechanisms through which body fatness could modulate the risk of cancer. For instance, increases in body fatness and abdominal fatness may affect the levels of certain hormones and growth factors, influence insulin sensitivity, raise the levels of circulating oestrogens and heighten the body's inflammatory response, thus affecting cancer cell promotion and progression (WCRF/AICR, 2007; Vucenik and Stains, 2012). Obesity is associated with increases in the levels of a number of hormones and growth factors which can promote the growth of cancer cells, including insulin-like growth factor-1 (IGF-1), insulin and leptin (Hursting et al., 2003; WCRF/AICR, 2007: 39). IGF-1 may act as a mitogen, increasing cell proliferation and decreasing cell apoptosis (Kruk and Czerniak, 2013). Furthermore, obesity and particularly abdominal fatness increase insulin resistance, which triggers the pancreas to compensate by increasing insulin production. The resultant hyperinsulinaemia is associated with increased risk of cancers of the colon and endometrium, and possibly of the pancreas and kidney (Calle and Kaaks, 2004). Leptin has also been extensively investigated as a potential mediator of obesity-related cancer, with higher circulating leptin levels being associated with increased risk of colorectal (Stattin et al., 2004) and prostate cancers (Chang et al., 2001; Vucenik and Stains, 2012). Adiponectin, a hormone that is inversely associated with adiposity levels, was suggested to exert anticancer effects by decreasing insulin/IGF-1 signalling, and by exerting anti-inflammatory actions (Vucenik and Stains, 2012).

Sex steroid hormones, including oestrogens, androgens and progesterone, could also play a role in linking obesity to cancer. Adipose tissue is the major site of oestrogen production in postmenopausal women, and men, via aromatase-catalysed conversion of gonadal and adrenal androgens to oestrogen (Kaaks et al., 2002). Similarly, obesity-associated increases in the levels of insulin and IGF-1 lead to increased oestradiol levels in both men and women (Calle and Kaaks, 2004) and may also lead to higher testosterone levels in women (WCRF/AICR, 2007). Higher levels of sex steroids are strongly associated with increased risk of endometrial and postmenopausal breast cancers (Kaaks et al., 2002; Key et al., 2002) and were suggested to be associated with colon and other cancers (WCRF/AICR, 2007). Interestingly, it was indicated that body fatness probably plays a protective role against premenopausal breast cancer (WCRF/AICR, 2007, 2010), possibly because obese women tend to have anovulatory menstrual cycles, which result in reduced levels of oestrogen (WCRF/AICR, 2007).

Obesity is associated with a low-grade chronic state of inflammation, characterised by increased circulating free fatty acids and chemoattraction of immune cells, such as macrophages, which also produce inflammatory mediators (Hursting and Dunlap, 2012). The adipocyte produces pro-inflammatory cytokines such as tumour necrosis factor-alpha, interleukin-6, and monocyte chemoattractant protein-1 (Rexrode et al., 2003; Hursting and Dunlap, 2012; Vucenik and Stains, 2012), as well as leptin, which also functions as an inflammatory cytokine (Loffreda et al., 1998; WCRF/AICR, 2007). The presence of chronic inflammation promotes cancer development, thus providing one additional link between excess body fat and the risk of cancer (WCRF/AICR, 2007; Hardman, 2014). Finally, adipocytes communicate with endothelial cells by producing a variety of vascular permeability-enhancing factors, including plasminogen activator inhibitor-1 (PAI-1) and vascular endothelial growth factor (VEGF) (Hursting and Dunlap, 2012). Increased circulating levels of PAI-1 and VEGF, as frequently found in obese individuals, may contribute to obesity-associated enhancement of tumour angiogenesis and may increase the risk of several cancers (Carter and Church, 2009; Hursting and Dunlap, 2012; Iwaki et al., 2012).

Available evidence therefore suggests that several hormones, growth factors, cytokines and other obesity-associated mediators enable crosstalk between adipocytes, endothelial cells, macrophages and epithelial cells and contribute to cancer-related processes (including growth signalling, inflammation and vascular alterations) (Ford et al., 2013). Components of these interrelated pathways are promising mechanism-based targets for disrupting the link between obesity and tumour development.

Physical activity

In contrast to the evidence linking overweight and obesity to increased cancer risk, several studies have suggested that physical activity and regular exercise can exert protective effects against cancer. Physical activity, which can be classified as occupational, household related, transport related or recreational, increases energy expenditure and is thus one of the main factors modulating energy balance. Physical activity may protect against weight gain and obesity, and may play a protective role against certain types of cancer, particularly cancers associated with body fatness. In addition, available evidence on physical activity and the risk of cancer indicates that regular, sustained physical activity protects against colon cancer and female hormone-related cancers, with this protective effect being independent of other factors such as body fatness (WCRF/AICR, 2007).

Large epidemiological studies showed that physical inactivity is associated with increases in overall cancer incidence and mortality (Paffenbarger et al., 1987; Albanes et al., 1989; Blair et al., 1989), and animal studies have provided support to these findings (Cohen et al.,

1992). Available literature suggests that the relationship between physical activity and health is continuous, implying that the more physically active people are the better, while excluding extreme levels of activity (Vainio and Bianchini, 2002; WHO, 2003; WCRF/AICR, 2007). According to the judgment of the WCRF/AICR panel, there is convincing evidence that physical activity protects against colorectal cancer (WCRF/AICR, 2011). In fact, epidemiological studies have consistently reported an inverse association between physical activity and the risk of colorectal cancer, with risk reductions ranging from 20 to 70%, comparing the most- versus the least-active individuals (Wolin et al., 2009; Clague and Bernstein, 2012; Kruk and Czerniak, 2013; Steindorf et al., 2013). In addition, it has been indicated that physical activity of all types probably protects against postmenopausal breast cancer and cancer of the endometrium (WCRF/AICR, 2007, 2010, 2013; Kruk and Czerniak, 2013). Comparing the most- with the least-active female study participants, the magnitude of risk reduction in postmenopausal breast cancer was estimated at 25% and the magnitude of risk reduction in endometrial cancer at 30–35%, with available evidence pointing towards a dose–response effect for both types of cancer (Clague and Bernstein, 2012; Steindorf et al., 2013). Unlike the protective associations just described, there is little evidence for an association between physical activity and the risk of developing premenopausal breast cancer and cancers of the lung and stomach (WCRF/AICR, 2007, 2010; O'Rorke et al., 2010; Steindorf et al., 2013; also see http://wcrf.org/int/research-we-fund/continuous-update-project-cup).

Aside from reduction in body weight, several other mechanisms were proposed to explain the protective effects of physical activity against certain types of cancer (McTiernan, 2008; Rundle, 2011; Kruk and Czerniak, 2013). These mechanisms include increased metabolic efficiency and capacity, decreases in abdominal fat depots, enhanced antioxidant defence mechanisms, decreased levels of reproductive hormones, reductions in insulin resistance, altered growth factor hormones (e.g. IGF-1), reduction in chronic inflammation, decreases in gut transit time and changes in bile acid metabolism (Kavazis and Powers, 2013). It has also been postulated that higher physical activity levels are associated with greater nutrient adequacy and higher intakes of nutrients with cancer preventive potential, including folate, calcium and vitamin D (Csizmadi et al., 2014). It is important, however, to note that some concerns were raised regarding exhaustive exercise and its potential association with increased risk of tumour growth (Ulrich et al., 2013). Exhaustive and extreme levels of physical activity were suggested to cause sufficient increases in oxidative stress to increase inflammation, impair immune function and increase the risk of cancer development (Ulrich *et al.*, 2013). The molecular pathways explaining the cancer-preventive or cancer-promoting effects of exercise are not fully understood. One of the potential factors implicated in this controversy may be the levels of exercise-induced reactive oxygen species (ROS) and reactive nitrogen species (RNS) (Kavazis and Powers, 2013). High levels of ROS/RNS can damage cellular constituents and stimulate several inflammatory signal transduction pathways, while physiological levels of ROS/RNS play an important role in the normal functioning of cells, including the regulation of cell signalling pathways and the control of gene expression (Kavazis and Powers, 2013). Available evidence suggests that moderate exercise generates low, physiological levels of ROS/RNS that have the potential to induce antioxidant gene expression and increase tolerance to oxidative stress induced by carcinogenic insults (Kavazis and Powers, 2013). However, exhaustive types of exercise may be associated with high levels of ROS/RNS that increase oxidative stress and DNA damage, impair immune function and result in increased cancer risk (Kavazis and Powers, 2013). Accordingly, it has been suggested that physical activity may have different influences on carcinogenesis depending on energy supply, intensity and frequency of exercise, with moderate-intensity exercise being associated with cancer preventive effects, while single exhaustive bouts of exercise potentially increase the risk of cancer development (Kavazis and Powers, 2013).

The accumulating evidence on the benefits of moderate physical activity in preventing certain types of cancer can be equally interpreted as showing that sedentary lifestyles may increase the risk of these cancers. This is of concern given the recent evidence showing that sedentariness levels are increasing worldwide, with more reliance on mechanisation and industrialisation and with most people in urbanised settings leading sedentary ways of life. Occupational, household and transport related activities have become more sedentary with dependence on machines, cars and buses, while active recreation has been replaced by watching television, playing electronic games or engaging in other sedentary pursuits (WCRF/AICR, 2007).

To conclude, an overall strong and consistent body of evidence from both epidemiological and mechanistic studies shows that, compared with lower levels of physical activity, higher levels may protect against cancers of certain sites. Even though the exact type, dose and timing of physical activity in cancer prevention remain unclear, there is ample evidence to recommend physical activity as a means for primary prevention of cancer (Steindorf *et al.*, 2013). Further research and studies should help elucidate the optimal physical activity load (type,

frequency, intensity) for optimal risk reduction in cancer risk. Several mechanisms may explain the cancer-protective effects of physical activity, including improvement in antioxidant defence, decreases in insulin and reproductive hormone levels, reduction in chronic inflammation and decreases in body weight and body fatness. Evidence-based cancer prevention guidelines recommend engaging in regular physical activity, avoiding obesity and maintaining a healthy body weight as means for the primary prevention of cancer (WCRF/AICR, 2007).

The rest of this section will be dedicated for the discussion of the role of diet in the aetiology of cancer, covering selected macronutrients, micronutrients, food groups, alcohol and dietary patterns. The selection of the specific macronutrients, micronutrients and food groups was based on the availability of scientific evidence for their association with the disease.

Macronutrients

Dietary fats

Early reports suggested that dietary fat intake may modulate the risk of cancer and that, building on data stemming from rodent studies, altering the fat composition of the diet may affect the rate and number of tumours that may develop (Freedman *et al.*, 1990; Welsch, 1992; Kushi and Giovannucci, 2002). In addition, ecological studies have indicated that international differences in cancer rates were strongly associated with differences in per capita dietary fat intake (Prentice *et al.*, 1989; Kushi and Giovannucci, 2002). Based on these studies and observations, the National Academy of Sciences highlighted dietary fat reduction as one of the principal guidelines for the prevention of cancer in its 1982 report on diet, nutrition and cancer (National Research Council (US) Committee on Diet and Health, 1989). The associations between cancer and dietary fat intake appeared the strongest for breast, large bowel and prostate cancers, while being only suggestive for cancers at other sites (National Research Council (US) Committee on Diet and Health 1989; Kushi and Giovannucci, 2002). Since then, numerous studies have been conducted to examine the association of dietary fat with cancer, including several prospective studies. Data generated by these studies have highlighted the substantial discrepancy of their findings with those from earlier ecologic comparisons or animal studies and have provided little support for an important influence of dietary fat intake on cancer risk (WCRF/AICR, 2007; Kushi and Giovannucci, 2002).

Much controversy has surrounded the relation between breast cancer and dietary fat intake (WCRF/AICR, 2007;

Chajès and Romieu, 2014), with most prospective studies reporting no associations (Kushi and Giovannucci, 2002; WCRF/AICR, 2007; Khodarahmi and Azadbakht, 2014). The narrow ranges in dietary fat intake may be one of the possible factors explaining the lack of associations observed in these prospective studies (Khodarahmi and Azadbakht, 2014). Alternatively, errors and biases in dietary assessment could partially explain the discrepancies in the findings of epidemiological studies. For example, a pooled analysis of cohort studies reported a non-significant increase in the risk of breast cancer when dietary fat intake was assessed by a food frequency questionnaire, while a stronger significant increase was documented when fat intake was measured by food records (Bingham et al., 2003). There is also interest in examining the varying roles that different types of fatty acids might have on breast cancer risk (WCRF/AICR, 2007). Available studies suggest that saturated fats and trans fatty acids (TFAs) may be associated with an increased risk of breast cancer, while ω-3 fatty acids may be associated with a decreased risk (Zheng et al., 2013; Chajès and Romieu, 2014; Khodarahmi and Azadbakht, 2014). However, this evidence may be limited by the difficulties in obtaining exact estimates of intakes for the various types of fat and by the high correlation in the intakes of specific types of fat which co-exist in the same food sources. Another factor that may limit the interpretation of studies' findings is that dietary fat could have differential effects on different subtypes of breast cancer, as defined by oestrogen receptor (ER), progesterone receptor (PR) and human epidermal growth factor 2 receptor. Sieri et al. (2014) showed that high saturated fat intake increases the risk of receptor-positive disease, suggesting a potential role of saturated fat in the aetiology of a subtype of breast cancer. Several mechanisms have been proposed for the link between dietary fat and breast cancer risk, including their role on membrane fluidity and functions, stimulation of growth factors, regulation of immune function, modulation of gene expression and stimulation of the production of oestrogen and other endogenous hormones (Toniolo et al., 1989). Higher levels of endogenous oestrogen after menopause have been shown to cause breast cancer (Kaaks et al., 2002, Key et al., 2002) and there is strong evidence showing that dietary fat increases the production of endogenous oestrogen (Wu et al., 1999; Khodarahmi and Azadbakht, 2014). Another mechanism through which dietary fat could affect steroid hormone levels is that increased serum-free-fatty-acids could displace oestradiol from serum albumin, thus increasing the concentrations of free oestradiol (Bruning and Bonfrèr, 1986; WCRF/AICR, 2007; Parry et al., 2011). Some studies also suggest that saturated fat intake may increase breast cancer risk by increasing insulin resistance and consequently insulin levels (Khodarahmi and Azadbakht, 2014). The association between increased plasma concentrations of insulin and IGF-1 and increased risk of breast cancer has been indicated by several studies (Kaaks, 2005; Khodarahmi and Azadbakht, 2014). Similarly, fats are the most energy-dense constituents of foods and diets, and their role in weight gain, overweight and obesity may provide a further link with increased risk of breast cancer (WCRF/AICR, 2007). For instance, the levels of sex-hormone-binding globulin tend to decrease with increasing BMI and insulin resistance, and the serum concentration of sex-hormone-binding globulin is one of the important factors that determine the proportion of oestradiol that can enter the breast epithelial cell (WCRF/AICR, 2007). It is important to note that the majority of studies that have examined the association of fat intake and breast cancer risk have focused on dietary fat intake in adulthood, either in the recent past, such as in most case–control studies, or within a few years of follow-up, such as in most prospective studies (Kushi and Giovannucci, 2002). Recent interest, however, is shifting towards the possible role that dietary fat intake as well as the intake of other nutrients earlier in life may have on breast carcinogenesis (Kushi and Giovannucci, 2002) (refer to Section 19.4).

The association of fat intake with colorectal cancer risk has also received much attention in the literature. Experimental evidence supports the hypothesis that ω-3 fatty acids (i.e. α-linolenic acid, eicosapentaenoic acid, docosahexaenoic acid, and docosapentaenoic acid) may protect against colorectal cancer, while ω-6 polyunsaturated fatty acids (i.e. linoleic acid and arachidonic acid) may promote the development of this type of cancer (Larsson et al., 2004; Cockbain et al., 2012). The proposed biological mechanisms include modulation of inflammation, influence on cellular oxidative stress and cellular signalling, alteration of membrane dynamics and cell surface receptor function, and impact on insulin sensitivity (Larsson et al., 2004; Cockbain et al., 2012; Shen et al., 2012; Song et al., 2014b). However, in contrast to experimental evidence, recent epidemiological studies have provided mixed results and failed to document an association between fat intake and colorectal cancer risk (Kushi and Giovannucci, 2002; WCRF/AICR, 2007, 2011). Some reports have suggested that the association between dietary fat and colorectal cancer risk may be specific to fat from animal sources or may be attributed to meat intake, rather than fat per se (Potter, 1996; WCRF/AICR, 2007) (for a discussion of meat and cancer risk, refer to Section 19.2: 'Meat and processed meat'). When looking at the effects of polyunsaturated fats, Song *et al.* (2014b) showed that, based on a prospective study of 123 529 US adults who were followed for 24–26 years, no overall association was observed between ω-3 or ω-6 polyunsaturated fatty acid intake and colorectal cancer risk. The study by Song *et al.* has, however, suggested that the effects of marine ω-3 fatty acids may vary by subsite, with ω-3 fatty acids appearing to be positively associated with the risk of distal colon cancer and inversely associated with the risk of rectal cancer. A recent meta-analysis of seven prospective studies (489 465 participants) reported insufficient evidence of an overall protective effect of ω-3 fatty acids on colorectal cancer risk, while pointing towards a potential risk reduction amongst men (Shen *et al.*, 2012). Apart from gender, the duration of follow-up may also impact the observed associations in prospective studies (Song *et al.*, 2014b). Stronger association between baseline ω-3 fatty acids and reduced colorectal cancer risk have in fact been observed in studies with longer duration of follow-up, implying an early-acting role of ω-3 fatty acids against colorectal carcinogenesis (Larsson *et al.*, 2004; Cockbain *et al.*, 2012; Song *et al.*, 2014b). A role of ω-3 fatty acids in reducing the risk of lung cancer (Song *et al.*, 2014a) and skin cancer (Noel *et al.*, 2014) has also been proposed in the literature, but more well-designed studies are needed to verify the effects of these polyunsaturated fatty acids on cancer risk.

In conclusion, the role of dietary fat in modulating cancer risk remains inconclusive. There is, however, some evidence for plausible biological mechanisms, at least for certain types, such as breast cancer and colorectal cancer (WCRF/AICR, 2007; Khodarahmi and Azadbakht, 2014; Song *et al.*, 2014b). The associations of dietary fat with other cancers, such as prostate, lung or skin, are also unclear (Kushi and Giovannucci, 2002; WCRF/AICR, 2007; Mandair *et al.*, 2014). Of note is the growing interest in the associations of specific types of fat with the risk of cancer at different sites or even subsites, with some studies pointing towards a potential protective effect of ω-3 fatty acids against certain types of cancer (Azrad *et al.*, 2013; Jing *et al.*, 2013). More recently, TFA intake and its potential impact on cancer risk has gained more attention, particularly that TFAs may exert an influence on systemic inflammation, insulin resistance and adiposity (Laake *et al.*, 2013; Chajès and Romieu, 2014). However, the associations between TFA intake and cancer risk has not been sufficiently studied to date (Laake *et al.*, 2013). Overall, and according to the judgement of the WCRF/AICR panel, there is only 'limited evidence' suggesting that dietary fats may modulate cancer risk (WCRF/AICR, 2007; http://wcrf.org/int/research-we-fund/continuous-update-project-cup). Carefully designed studies are needed to account for the heterogeneity of the population and the numerous factors that may confound the association between dietary fats and the risk of cancer.

Carbohydrates, glycaemic index and glycaemic load

Several studies have suggested a potential role of glucose and insulin in promoting tumour growth (McKeown-Eyssen, 1994; Giovannucci, 1995; Hu *et al.*, 2013). It has therefore been proposed that the quantity and quality of carbohydrates (CHOs) consumed may play a role in carcinogenesis, due to their potential impact on insulin and glucose plasma levels as well as insulin resistance (Augustin *et al.*, 2002; Michels *et al.*, 2007; Hu *et al.*, 2013; Chajès and Romieu, 2014).

There has been a lot of debate in the literature on the optimal amount of dietary CHO for optimal reduction in disease risk, including cancer (Liebman, 2013). On the one hand, low-CHO diets are more likely to lead to decreased intakes of phytochemicals and non-digestible CHOs, which have been suggested to play a protective role against cancer (for a discussion on phytochemicals and fibre in relation to cancer risk, please refer to Section 19.2 'Micronutrients' and 'Fibre' respectively). On the other hand, high intakes of dietary CHOs were implicated in increasing cancer risk, but the evidence has so far been conflicting, with null, increased or decreased risk being reported (Johnson *et al.*, 2005; Aune *et al.*, 2012a,b; Coleman *et al.*, 2014). For instance, higher intake of sugar was suggested to increase the risk of developing certain types of cancer, such as pancreatic (Meinhold *et al.*, 2010) and colorectal cancer (Tuyns *et al.*, 1988; Franceschi and Favero, 1999; WCRF/AICR, 2011), while no associations were reported in others (Roberts-Thomson *et al.*, 1996; Terry *et al.*, 2001; Nöthlings *et al.*, 2007; Galeone *et al.*, 2012). The interpretation of findings stemming from studies examining the association of sugar with cancer risk is often complicated by the inconsistencies in the definition of 'sugar'. In fact, in some studies, sugar is equated with sucrose, while in others, sugar may refer to 'total sugars', to 'sugars added at the table', to 'sugary foods and/or drinks' or to 'added sugars' generally; and they may or may not include those sugars naturally present in foods. This inconsistency in the classification of 'sugar' makes it difficult to measure and assess the overall effect of sugar as a modifier of disease risk, including cancer (WCRF/AICR, 2007).

Some studies have suggested that high fructose intake may be associated with increased risk of insulin resistance and adiposity and may therefore play a role in carcinogenesis (Dekker *et al.*, 2010; Aune *et al.*, 2012a). A recent meta-analysis has reported a positive association between fructose intake and increased risk of pancreatic cancer (Aune *et al.*, 2012a), but further investigations are needed to confirm this association (WCRF/AICR, 2012).

Some of the mechanisms linking fructose intake to increased cancer risk remain speculative. The metabolism of fructose differs from that of other CHOs, such as glucose (Aune *et al.*, 2012a), and it has been recently shown that the contribution of fructose to nucleic acid synthesis through the pentose phosphate pathway is greater than that of glucose (Liu *et al.*, 2010). Synthesis of nucleic acids and nucleotides is necessary for the proliferation of tissues, and particularly cancer cells (Aune *et al.*, 2012a).

A plethora of studies have examined the association between glycaemic index (GI), glycaemic load (GL) and cancer risk (Aune *et al.*, 2012a,b; Choi *et al.*, 2012; Fedirko *et al.*, 2013; Hu *et al.*, 2013). The GI is a measure of the degree to which a food raises blood glucose compared with a reference food (usually glucose or white bread) under standard conditions (Liu *et al.*, 2000; Romieu *et al.*, 2012). The GI is therefore a measure of CHO quality (Romieu *et al.*, 2012). A related measure, the GL of a specific food is calculated as the product of the GI and the amount of dietary CHOs (grams) per serving. The GL reflects both the quality and quantity of dietary CHO (Foster-Powell *et al.*, 2002). It has been proposed that, compared with diets of high GI or high GL, low GI/GL diets may improve glycaemic control, decrease insulin output and inflammatory responses and lower the risk of several chronic diseases, including cancer (Brand-Miller *et al.*, 2003; Barclay *et al.*, 2008). The WCRF/AICR panel recently judged GL as probably increasing the risk of endometrial cancer (WCRF/AICR, 2013). In a meta-analysis of prospective studies, Dong and Qin (2011) reported a direct relationship between dietary GI and breast cancer risk, but this was not shown by Mulholland *et al.* (2008a). Similarly, other meta-analyses of several cancer sites reported no association of either GI or GL with colorectal or pancreatic cancer risk (Mulholland *et al.*, 2009; Hu *et al.*, 2013), but showed a positive association of GL with endometrial cancer risk (Mulholland *et al.*, 2008b; Hu *et al.*, 2013). A recent meta-analysis of prospective studies investigating the association between GI, GL and diabetes-related cancers (including bladder, breast, colon-rectum, endometrium, liver and pancreas) showed that GL was significantly positively associated with the risk of endometrial cancer, and GI positively significantly associated with breast and colorectal cancer, while stating that these associations were modest to weak (Choi *et al.*, 2012). Two other comprehensive meta-analyses of all major cancer sites reported direct associations of GI with colorectal and endometrial cancers (Gnagnarella *et al.*, 2008) and with breast cancer (Barclay *et al.*, 2008). Romieu *et al.* (2012) have argued that some of the inconsistencies between the studies' findings on breast cancer and CHO intake may be related to the differences in breast cancer phenotypes.

In fact, most studies did not classify breast cancer by hormone receptor status (ER and PR), which have been previously shown to influence the clinical, pathologic and molecular features of tumours and may, therefore, correspond to aetiologically distinct diseases with different risk factor profiles (Althuis *et al.*, 2004; Colditz *et al.*, 2004). Romieu *et al.* (2012) showed, based on data stemming from the European Prospective Investigation into Cancer and Nutrition (EPIC), that a diet with a high GL is positively associated with an increased risk of developing ER$^-$ and ER$^-$/PR$^-$ breast cancer among postmenopausal women, but not among premenopausal women and other types of breast cancer.

The overall evidence points towards conflicting data on the association between dietary CHO and cancer risk (WCRF/AICR, 2007; Coleman *et al.*, 2014), although experimental studies provide biologically plausible mechanisms. Apart from the potential association of dietary CHOs with weight gain and obesity (Ludwig *et al.*, 2001; Nooyens *et al.*, 2005), the mechanisms that may link CHOs to cancer risk include insulin resistance, hyperinsulinaemia and increased levels of IGF-1, all of which have been implicated as key mediators in the underlying pathways relating dietary and lifestyle factors to carcinogenesis (Giovannucci *et al.*, 2010; Choi *et al.*, 2012; Emond *et al.*, 2014). It is important to note that the majority of studies conducted on the link between CHO and cancer risk have been conducted in western countries, which may limit the generalisability of the findings to other geographical locations and populations, especially in Asian countries where the average diet typically consists of a greater proportion of CHO (Choi *et al.*, 2012). Further studies are needed to provide information on potential differences based on geographical locations or ethnic differences in the link between dietary CHO and cancer risk (Choi *et al.*, 2012).

Fibre

Findings from epidemiological and clinical studies document an inverse association between the consumption of dietary fibre (DF) and the risk of cancer (Park *et al.*, 2009; Lattimer and Haub, 2010). Naturally occurring DF is only obtained from plant foods (WCRF/AICR, 2007). Pulses, whole grains and minimally processed cereals are particularly concentrated sources of DF, but vegetables and fruits also contribute significant amounts (WCRF/AICR, 2007). Several definitions of DF have been proposed. It was traditionally defined as the edible parts of plants that are resistant to digestion by human digestive enzymes, thus including polysaccharides and lignin (Jones *et al.*, 2006; Ötles and Ozgoz, 2014). More recently, and based on nutrition physiology, the definition of DF has been expanded to include oligosaccharides, such as inulin, and resistant starches (Jones *et al.*, 2006; Ötles and Ozgoz, 2014). DFs have been further classified as soluble, such as viscous or fermentable fibres (e.g. pectin) that are fermented in the colon, and insoluble fibres, such as wheat bran, that have bulking action but may only be fermented to a limited extent in the colon (Anderson *et al.*, 2009; Ötles and Ozgoz, 2014).

Recent studies point towards an inverse association between DF and the development of several types of cancers, including colorectal, small intestine, oral, larynx and breast (Nomura *et al.*, 2007; Schatzkin *et al.*, 2008; Park *et al.*, 2009; Lattimer and Haub, 2010; Ötles and Ozgoz, 2014; Zeng *et al.*, 2014). Several modes of actions have been suggested to explain the anticancer effects of DF (Lattimer and Haub, 2010). First, since DF increases faecal bulking and viscosity, it helps to decrease the contact time between potential carcinogens and mucosal cells in the gastrointestinal tract and it reduces the time for proteolytic fermentation that results in harmful substances, (Lattimer and Haub, 2010; Zeng *et al.*, 2014). Second, DF fosters the binding between bile acids and carcinogens (Lattimer and Haub, 2010). Third, higher intakes of DF are usually associated with higher dietary nutritional quality and higher intakes of antioxidants (Lattimer and Haub, 2010). Fourth, DF may contribute to an increase in oestrogen faecal excretion by decreasing and inhibiting oestrogen absorption in the intestine (Adlercreutz *et al.*, 1987). Fifth, a high DF intake may decrease dietary energy density, caloric intake and metabolisable energy, thus contributing to the maintenance of a healthy body weight (Lattimer and Haub, 2010; Ötles and Ozgoz, 2014). Sixth, the fermentation of DF in the large intestine leads to the production of short-chain fatty acids (SCFAs), which have anti-carcinogenic properties, including the promotion of cancer cell cycle arrest, apoptosis, the inhibition of chronic inflammatory process and cancer cell migration/invasion (Young *et al.*, 2005; Lattimer and Haub, 2010; Zeng *et al.*, 2014). Seventh, DF modulates the microbial composition of the gut lumen, a factor that may also have an impact on the risk of cancer (this aspect is further discussed in Section 19.5).

A plethora of studies have highlighted a protective role of DF against certain types of cancer. In 2011, the WCRF/AICR updated its evidence on colorectal cancer and indicated that there is convincing evidence that foods containing DF reduce colorectal cancer risk (WCRF/AICR, 2011). However, not all types of fibre have the same properties, and the characteristics and components of specific DFs (e.g. arabinoxylan, β-glucan) may determine their specific modes of action against cancer cells (Zeng *et al.*, 2014). Future studies on types of fibre and fibre components may provide a better understanding of

how and why DF may decrease the risk of cancer (Zeng *et al.*, 2014). Future studies are also needed to clarify the microbiota changes that correlate with the beneficial effects of fibre, although it is possible that such changes may be dose, time and strain dependent (Zeng *et al.*, 2014).

Micronutrients

Vitamins and minerals

Several studies have suggested a role for specific vitamins and minerals in protecting against cancer (Ames and Wakimoto, 2002). Foods containing carotenoids were judged by the WCRF/AICR (2007) to probably protect against lung cancer and cancers of the mouth, pharynx and larynx. A recent study reported that higher levels of certain carotenoids in the blood may also decrease the risk of breast cancer, supporting a recommendation to consume deeply coloured plant foods, which tend to be rich sources of carotenoids, for breast cancer prevention (Kabat *et al.*, 2009; Brennan *et al.*, 2010; Kushi *et al.*, 2012). When looking at specific carotenoids, it was reported that foods containing beta-carotene probably protect against oesophageal cancer, and that foods containing lycopene probably protect against prostate cancer (WCRF/AICR, 2007). A recent meta-analysis has also suggested an inverse association between dietary intake of beta-carotene and colorectal adenoma (Xu *et al.*, 2013). Carotenoids exert antioxidant properties, which can protect against lipid oxidation and related oxidative stress (Kaulmann and Bohn, 2014). It is known that oxidative stress induced by free radicals can cause DNA damage (WCRF/AICR, 2007). If this initial damage is left unrepaired, base mutation, single- and double-strand breaks, DNA cross-linking, and chromosomal breakage can all occur (Block *et al.*, 1992; WCRF/AICR, 2007). In addition, several carotenoids, including beta-carotene, are also retinoid (vitamin A) precursors. These pro-vitamin A carotenoids may get converted to retinol and will thus play a role in cellular differentiation, immune enhancement and activation of carcinogen-metabolising enzymes (van Poppel and Goldbohm, 1995; Abnet *et al.*, 2003; WCRF/AICR, 2007; Kushi *et al.*, 2012). In addition to being the most potent carotenoid antioxidant, lycopene has antiproliferative effects and can improve immune function and reduce inflammation, thus potentially playing a role in cancer prevention (WCRF/AICR, 2007; Kelkel *et al.*, 2011). Evidence that the consumption of carotenoid-rich foods and particularly vegetable and fruit consumption reduces cancer risk has led to attempts to isolate specific carotenoids from these foods and investigate their effects as supplements, sometimes in very high doses (Kushi *et al.*, 2012). However, many of these chemoprevention studies and randomised controlled trials have shown that supplement use is unsuccessful in preventing cancer or its precursor lesions, and some studies have even illustrated adverse and harmful effects (Kushi *et al.*, 2012). Prototypical examples of such chemopreventive studies are the four randomised trials of beta-carotene for the prevention of lung cancer, which were initiated based on the observational epidemiologic evidence indicating a lower risk of lung cancer in subjects consuming foods high in beta-carotene (Albanes, 1999). Two of these trials have shown that individuals at high risk of lung cancer (such as heavy smokers, former heavy smokers and those with occupational exposure to asbestos) taking high doses of beta-carotene supplements developed lung cancer at higher rates than those taking a placebo (Heinonen and Albanes, 1994; Omenn *et al.*, 1996b). It has been suggested that micronutrients used in supplementation trials are isolated synthetic forms of nutrients which may have been different isomers from those naturally occurring and may consequently have differential health implications (WCRF/AICR, 2007). In observational studies that document a cancer-protective effect of beta-carotene-rich foods, beta-carotene may be serving as a proxy for other single nutrients or combinations of nutrients found in whole foods, or for other associated lifestyle exposures. These findings also suggest that taking a single nutrient in large amounts can be associated with harmful health effects, at least for some subgroups of the population (Kushi *et al.*, 2012).

Other antioxidant micronutrients were also proposed to exert cancer protective effects (Khuda-Bukhsh *et al.*, 2014). Several studies have proposed a link between the consumption of vitamin-C-rich foods and reduced risk of cancer, particularly oesophageal cancer (WCRF/AICR, 2007; Kushi *et al.*, 2012; Khuda-Bukhsh *et al.*, 2014). Vitamin C can trap free radicals and reactive oxygen molecules, protecting against oxidative damage and stimulating immune function (Terry *et al.*, 2000; Padayatty *et al.*, 2003; WCRF/AICR, 2007; Gonzalez and Miranda-Massari, 2014). Vitamin C can also recycle and regenerate other antioxidant vitamins, such as vitamin E (Padayatty *et al.*, 2003). In addition, it is reported to play a role in inhibiting the formation of carcinogens and in protecting DNA from mutagenic attack (Fountoulakis *et al.*, 2004). However, the studies in which vitamin C has been given as a supplement have not documented a reduction in the risk of cancer (Gaziano *et al.*, 2009; Kushi *et al.*, 2012).

Several anticancer properties have been attributed to vitamin E, an antioxidant that has been reported to enhance DNA repair, to protect against DNA damage and lipid peroxidation and to prevent the activation of carcinogens such as nitrosamines (WCRF/AICR, 2007; Aiub *et al.*, 2009; Niki, 2014). Vitamin E also protects other antioxidants in the body, such as vitamin A and selenium (WCRF/AICR, 2007). In addition to its ability to act as a free-radical scavenger, vitamin E improves the body's immune response, which may play a role in enhancing defences against cancer (Willis and Wians, 2003). Foods containing vitamin E were suggested to protect against oesophageal and prostate cancers (WCRF/AICR, 2007). A decrease in prostate cancer incidence was reported among men randomly assigned to receive alpha-tocopherol in the Alpha-Tocopherol, Beta-Carotene Cancer Prevention (ATBC) trial, a study that included only male smokers (Heinonen and Albanes, 1994; Kushi *et al.*, 2012). Selenium is another antioxidant that has been suggested to play a role in cancer prevention (Duffield-Lillico *et al.*, 2003; Dennert *et al.*, 2011; Hurst *et al.*, 2012). Foods containing selenium were judged by the WCRF/AICR to probably protect against prostate cancer, while there is limited evidence suggesting that it may protect against stomach cancer (WCRF/AICR, 2007; http://wcrf.org/int/research-we-fund/continuous-update-project-cup). Several mechanisms may explain this association. Dietary selenium deficiency results in decreased selenoprotein expression, and a number of these selenoproteins have important anti-inflammatory and antioxidant properties (Ganther, 1999). Four selenoproteins are glutathione peroxidases, which protect against oxidative damage to lipids, lipoproteins and DNA (WCRF/AICR, 2007; Davis *et al.*, 2012). In selenium deprivation or deficiency, these enzymes are rapidly degraded. Three selenoproteins are thioredoxin reductases which play a role in the regeneration of oxidised ascorbic acid back to its active antioxidant form, among other functions (WCRF/AICR, 2007; Davis *et al.*, 2012). The promising preliminary evidence that vitamin E and selenium may play a role in cancer prevention, and particularly prostate cancer, has led to the initiation of the Selenium and Vitamin E Cancer Prevention Trial (SELECT) (Kushi *et al.*, 2012). The results of the SELECT trial were disappointing, however, and failed to confirm any beneficial effects of these supplements in prostate cancer prevention (Lippman *et al.*, 2009). More recent analyses of the trial's data have even suggested that high doses of vitamin E supplements may promote a small increase in the risk of prostate cancer (Klein *et al.*, 2011; Kristal *et al.*, 2014). Similarly, the Heart Outcomes Prevention Evaluation trial showed no difference in cancer rates between the vitamin E supplement and placebo groups (Lonn *et al.*, 2005).

Foods containing folate were suggested to modulate cancer risk, with several mechanisms being proposed for this association (WCRF/AICR, 2007; Nazki *et al.*, 2014). Folate plays an important role in nucleic acid synthesis, methionine regeneration, shuttling and redox reactions of one-carbon units required for normal metabolism and regulation (Nazki *et al.*, 2014). It plays a pivotal role in the synthesis of *S*-adenosyl methionine (SAM) which serves as the methyl group donor in several methylation reactions, including DNA, RNA and protein methylation, and it is well known that abnormal DNA methylation leading to aberrant gene expression is one of the hallmarks of several types of cancer (WCRF/AICR, 2007; Nazki *et al.*, 2014). Folate deficiency may lead to misincorporation of uracil instead of thymine into DNA (WCRF/AICR, 2007; Jennings and Willis, 2014). It is suggested that the effects of folate deficiency and supplementation on DNA methylation are gene and site specific, and may depend on cell type, target organ, stage of transformation, and degree and duration of folate depletion (WCRF/AICR, 2007). The results of animal studies have indicated that the dose and timing of folate intervention are critical in determining its effect. For instance, it was shown that interventions with exceptionally high folate doses after the formation of microscopic neoplastic foci may promote rather than suppress colorectal carcinogenesis, at least in the studies animal models (Kim, 2003). In agreement with these experimental findings, some randomised controlled trials suggest that folic acid supplements may increase the risk of prostate cancer, colorectal adenomas (Cole *et al.*, 2007; Figueiredo *et al.*, 2009) and possibly breast cancer (Stolzenberg-Solomon *et al.*, 2006). A recent meta-analysis reported a significantly increased risk of prostate cancer with high blood folate levels (Tio *et al.*, 2014a), while another showed that blood folate levels are not associated with breast cancer risk (Tio *et al.*, 2014b). Given these potential harmful effects of folic acid supplements, it is recommended that folate be best obtained through the consumption of vegetables, fruits and whole-grain products (Kushi *et al.*, 2012). The 2011 and 2012 Continuous Update Project reports of WCRF/AICR concluded that the available evidence on folate and its association with cancer are too inconsistent to allow meaningful conclusions to be drawn (WCRF/AICR, 2011, 2012).

There is increasing evidence suggesting that vitamin D deficiency raises the risk of developing cancer and particularly colorectal cancer (WCRF/AICR, 2007, 2011; Chung *et al.*, 2009; USDA and HHS, 2010; Feldman *et al.*, 2014). Observational studies are also increasingly suggesting that vitamin D deficiency increases the risk of breast cancer development and its progression (Narvaez *et al.*, 2014). Several mechanisms have been suggested to explain the postulated protective effects of vitamin D against cancer. Vitamin D is the precursor of the potent steroid hormone calcitriol, which regulates gene expression and multiple signalling pathways involved in proliferation, apoptosis, differentiation, inflammation, invasion, angiogenesis and metastasis (Feldman *et al.*,

2014). Recent findings also indicate that calcitriol regulates microRNA (miRNA) expression and may exert an effect on cancer stem cell biology (Feldman *et al.*, 2014). Evidence stemming from cell culture and animal models of cancer suggest a role for dietary vitamin D and calcitriol in delaying cancer development and progression. However, data from human clinical trials have thus far been inconsistent (Feldman *et al.*, 2014), and epidemiological studies have provided conflicting findings on the association between vitamin D and incidence of cancer (Feldman *et al.*, 2014). Recent studies have even suggested that very high levels of circulating vitamin D may be associated with an increased risk of pancreatic cancer (Stolzenberg-Solomon *et al.*, 2010; Kushi *et al.*, 2012). Given the rising interest in the association between vitamin D and cancer risk, further research is needed, especially randomised controlled trials, to confirm in humans whether individuals with low levels of circulating vitamin D are at increased risk of developing cancer and whether calcitriol or vitamin D supplements can reduce cancer risk and progression (Feldman *et al.*, 2014). It is important to note that the effects of vitamin D may be strongly interrelated with those of calcium. In fact, an adequate vitamin D status is required for proper calcium absorption, and calcium-mediated effects are strongly dependent on vitamin D levels (Kushi *et al.*, 2012). In addition, both vitamin D and calcium exert growth-restraining effects and induce differentiation and apoptosis in intestinal cells (WCRF/AICR, 2007). In agreement with the evidence on vitamin D, calcium intake was reported to be associated with a lower risk of colorectal cancer (Cho *et al.*, 2004; Chung *et al.*, 2009; Aune *et al.*, 2012d). However, a potential increase in the risk of prostate cancer was suggested to be associated with a high calcium intake (Giovannucci *et al.*, 2006; WCRF/AICR, 2007). Accordingly, the American Cancer Society (ACS) guidelines do not recommend the use of calcium supplements or increasing calcium or dairy food intake for overall cancer prevention, although it may be helpful in decreasing the risk of developing colorectal cancer (Kushi *et al.*, 2012).

Based on the overall evidence on specific vitamins and minerals, it may be possible to conclude that foods and nutrients have additive or synergistic effects on cancer prevention and interact in complex ways that are difficult to capture in single nutrient interventions (Kushi *et al.*, 2012). The roles of individual nutrients and dietary factors are best to be considered and understood within the broader context of the total diet.

Polyphenolic compounds

Polyphenols, an important group of phytochemicals, are plant secondary metabolites which are characterised by the presence of one or more hydroxyl groups attached to a benzene ring in their chemical structure (Fraga *et al.*, 2010). More than 8000 different polyphenols from plant foods are present in the human diet, and several polyphenols showed the capacity to block the initiation of carcinogenesis and to suppress the promotion and progression of cancer (Pandey and Rizvi, 2009; González-Vallinas *et al.*, 2013). More recently, polyphenols were suggested to indirectly modulate the epigenome by miRNAs which target specific epigenetic modifier enzymes (Parasramka *et al.*, 2012; Vanden Berghe, 2012). Flavonoids, phenolic acids, stilbenes and curcuminoids are the most important polyphenols in relation to cancer (González-Vallinas *et al.*, 2013; Martin *et al.*, 2013).

- *Flavonoids* represent 60% of dietary polyphenols with more than 4000 varieties, classified into seven main groups: flavones, flavonols, flavanones, isoflavones, catechins, anthocyanins and chalcones (Murakami *et al.*, 2008; Ramos, 2008). Cocoa and its main flavonoids (epicatechin, catechin and procyanidins B2 and B1, among others) have been shown to possess a free radical scavenging ability and to regulate signal transduction pathways, thereby stimulating apoptosis and inhibiting inflammation, cellular proliferation and metastasis (Martin *et al.*, 2013). Epigallocatechin-3-gallate (EGCG), the major catechin found in green tea, was suggested to exert antitumour effects in multiple cancer types, including colorectal cancer (Khan *et al.*, 2006; Shimizu *et al.*, 2008; González-Vallinas *et al.*, 2013). However, the chemopreventive activity required, in most cases, a concentration of EGCG that is greater than that achieved in plasma after two or three cups of tea (0.1–0.3 μM), thus suggesting that alternative methods of administration may be needed in order to increase its bioavailability (Cao and Cao, 1999; González-Vallinas *et al.*, 2013). The anticancer properties of EGCG are related to its ability to modulate cancer cell proliferation, apoptosis, immune evasion, invasion, metastasis and angiogenesis (González-Vallinas *et al.*, 2013).

Luteolin is one of the most effective antitumour flavones and is found in many vegetables, such as parsley, celery and pepper (González-Vallinas *et al.*, 2013). At the molecular level, luteolin was shown to inhibit several tumour-related signalling pathways and to exert anti-inflammatory and antioxidant effects (Lin *et al.*, 2008). Diets rich in flavones, including luteolin, were associated with a lower risk of breast cancer, and luteolin intake was shown to significantly decrease the incidence of ovarian cancer (Seelinger *et al.*, 2008; González-Vallinas *et al.*, 2013).

Quercetin is a flavonol found in apple, onion and broccoli, among other plants, representing the most abundant flavonoid in fruits and vegetables (González-Vallinas *et al.*, 2013). It was shown to have a free radical scavenging effect and to protect against multiple age-related diseases, including cancer (Jan *et al.*, 2010; González-Vallinas *et al.*, 2013). Several anticancer properties have been attributed to quercetin, including antimutagenic, antioxidant and antiproliferative effects, as well as regulation of several cell-signalling pathways, cell cycle and apoptosis (Murakami *et al.*, 2008; González-Vallinas *et al.*, 2013). Based on case–control and cohort studies, the WCRF/AICR (2007) panel concluded that there is limited evidence suggesting that foods containing quercetin protect against lung cancer. Experimental studies based on *in vitro* assays and animal models have also suggested an inhibitory effect of quercetin on other cancer types (González-Vallinas *et al.*, 2013). The combination of quercetin with EGCG was found to produce a synergistic effect on the inhibition of prostate cancer stem cells (Tang *et al.*, 2010), thus illustrating the potentiating effects that some polyphenols may exert on others.

Isoflavones have also been suggested to play a protective role against carcinogenesis. Genistein is one of the most commonly encountered isoflavones and is the predominant isoflavone of soybean. The relatively lower incidence of prostate and breast cancers in Asian compared with western countries, was partially attributed to the consumption of soy (Banerjee *et al.*, 2008). Because genistein is endowed with a weak oestrogenic activity, it is commonly included in the group of phytoestrogens. Accordingly, most studies have focused on genistein and its relationship with hormone-related cancers, such as prostate and breast cancer, but inhibitory effects on other cancer types have also been suggested (González-Vallinas *et al.*, 2013). The antitumour activities of genistein include effects on prevention and progression (Banerjee *et al.*, 2008) and particularly effects on antioxidant/detoxification enzymes, apoptosis, cell cycle, hormone signalling and cytokine signalling (González-Vallinas *et al.*, 2013). *In vitro* and *in vivo* studies have shown that a concentration near 50 μM of genistein is needed to significantly inhibit the proliferation of most tumour cell types (González-Vallinas *et al.*, 2013). Taking into account that, in Japanese men, normal average plasma concentrations of genistein are of 0.28 μM (Hedlund *et al.*, 2003), the intake of supplements, or alterative administration routes, would be necessary to achieve the doses that are associated with chemopreventive effects. In vitro studies have documented genistein's synergistic effects with other phytochemicals, such as indole-3-carbinol (Nakamura *et al.*, 2009). Even though most of the epidemiological and experimental evidence showed that genistein inhibits carcinogenesis (Sarkar and Li, 2004), other studies have suggested an increased risk of cancer with increased genistein intake. For instance, genistein was reported to increase the growth of breast cancer cells in a postmenopausal animal model (Ju *et al.*, 2006) and its use in breast cancer is sometimes questioned because of genistein's oestrogen-like effects (Rimando and Suh, 2008).

- *Phenolic acids*, which contain in their structure a phenol ring and a carboxylic acid functional group, represent 30% of dietary polyphenols (Ramos, 2008). Ellagic acid, the main polyphenol in pomegranate, is one of the most studied phenolic acids in relation to cancer. More than 50% of the antioxidant activity of pomegranate juice is attributed to ellagic acid (González-Vallinas *et al.*, 2013). It has mainly been shown to exert antiproliferative activity in prostate cancer (Bell and Hawthorne, 2008), but it was also suggested to induce cell cycle arrest and apoptosis and exert antiproliferative effects in several other cancer types (González-Vallinas *et al.*, 2013). These effects were observed at physiological concentrations that are within or below those found in plasma after oral intake (Strati *et al.*, 2009).

- *Stilbenes* are reported to possess several pharmacological activities, such as increasing insulin sensitivity, preventing cancer and extending lifespan (Rimando and Suh, 2008). Resveratrol is the most important stilbene in relation to cancer and is mainly found in red wine and grapes (González-Vallinas *et al.*, 2013). Experimental evidence suggests that resveratrol plays a role in controlling proliferation, apoptosis, cell cycle progression, inflammation, angiogenesis, invasion and metastasis in multiple cancer cell types (González-Vallinas *et al.*, 2013). Clinical studies provided support to these findings and showed that resveratrol consumption from grapes resulted in decreased breast cancer incidence (Levi *et al.*, 2005), although studies on resveratrol from wine failed to document such protective effects (Levi *et al.*, 2005). Interestingly, resveratrol was shown to be more potent in inhibiting already established lung cancer than in its prevention, while the opposite was reported for skin and breast cancers (Bishayee, 2009; González-Vallinas *et al.*, 2013). A role for resveratrol in colon cancer prevention has also been suggested (Nguyen *et al.*, 2009). Available evidence suggests that resveratrol effects may be influenced by environmental and genetic factors. For instance, resveratrol was found to down regulate the *ErbB2* gene (a member of a family of genes that dictates the production of growth factor receptors, therefore stimulating cell growth and division) in oestrogen-free medium, and to upregulate it in the presence of oestrogens (Choi *et al.*, 2006), thus suggesting that resveratrol may differentially affect pre- and post-menopausal women (González-Vallinas *et al.*, 2013).

- *Curcuminoids* are obtained from turmeric as a yellow crystalline powder and are usually used to give flavour and/or colour to spice blends, such as curry (Shehzad *et al.*, 2010; González-Vallinas *et al.*, 2013). The main curcuminoids found in turmeric include curcumin, demethoxycurcumin, bisdemethoxycurcumin and cyclocurcumin (Shehzad *et al.*, 2010). Most of these curcuminoids were shown to exert anticancer effects, with curcumin being the most widely studied (González-Vallinas *et al.*, 2013). Curcumin has the ability to inhibit cell growth in a wide range of cancers and to possess anti-inflammatory, antioxidant and antitumour effects (González-Vallinas *et al.*, 2013). The multiplicity of curcumin's molecular targets renders it capable of inhibiting most of the stages of carcinogenesis (González-Vallinas *et al.*, 2013). Clinical trials showed that it may play protective effects against pancreatic and colon cancers (Shehzad *et al.*, 2010), while further studies are needed to confirm its antitumour effects in other types of cancer (González-Vallinas *et al.*, 2013). It is important to note that curcumin was found to have a tumour-promoting effect in damaged lung epithelium, thus underlining the need to exclude smokers and ex-smokers in future clinical studies (Omenn *et al.*, 1996a).

In conclusion, several polyphenols have been shown to exert antitumor effects through multiple pathways and mechanisms (González-Vallinas *et al.*, 2013). However, more studies are needed to identify the most important molecular targets for these polyphenols in order to perform tailored clinical studies, generate more consistent findings and potentially recommend the use of polyphenol supplements in the target population and patients (González-Vallinas *et al.*, 2013). Health benefits of dietary polyphenols as epigenetic modulators, particularly when used as nutraceutical agents, will depend on our further understanding of their epigenetic effects in early life, ageing and carcinogenesis (Vanden Berghe, 2012).

Food groups

Meat and processed meat

Available evidence has implicated high red and processed meat intake in promoting carcinogenesis. Among all cancers, colorectal cancer appears to have the strongest association with meat intake, with a clear dose–response relationship being documented in cohort studies (WCRF/AICR, 2007, 2011; Kim *et al.*, 2013). Based on a meta-analysis of cohort studies, it was estimated that the risk of colorectal cancer increases by 29% for every

100 g/day increase in red meat and by 21% for every 50 g/day increase in processed meat consumption (WCRF/AICR, 2007; Kim *et al.*, 2013). In a longitudinal study over the period of 5 years, the EPIC, which included 478,040 men and women from 10 European countries, showed that, compared with a low intake of red and processed meat (<20 g/day), the high intake group (>160 g/day) had 1.35-fold higher risk to develop colorectal cancer (Norat *et al.*, 2005). Based on this, as well as several other studies, the association with colorectal cancer was reported to be stronger for processed than for unprocessed red meat (Norat *et al.*, 2005; Ferguson, 2010). It is important to note that, although there is no generally agreed definition of 'processed meat' and although this term is inconsistently used in epidemiological studies, it usually refers to meats preserved by smoking, curing or salting, or by the addition of preservatives (WCRF/AICR, 2007). Ham, bacon, pastrami, salami, sausages, bratwursts, frankfurters and 'hot dogs' are examples of processed meats.

Based on the overall accumulating evidence, the WCRF/AICR panel concluded that there is convincing evidence that red meat and processed meat are causes of colorectal cancer (WCRF/AICR, 2007, 2011). As for other types of cancer, there is limited evidence suggesting that high red and processed meat consumption may cause cancers of the oesophagus, lung and pancreas (WCRF/AICR, 2007, 2012); processed meat may further cause cancers of the stomach and prostate; and foods containing iron may cause colorectal cancer (WCRF/AICR, 2007, 2011). There is also limited evidence that the consumption of grilled, barbecued (charbroiled) or smoked animal foods may cause stomach cancer (WCRF/AICR, 2007).

Several plausible mechanisms may explain the association between meat, and particularly red or processed meat, with increased cancer risk. These mechanisms underline a role for proteins, haem iron, *N*-nitroso compounds (NOCs), heterocyclic aromatic amines and polycyclic aromatic hydrocarbons (PAHs; WCRF/AICR, 2007; Kim *et al.*, 2013). Meat is high in protein, and a role of high-protein diets in promoting colorectal cancer was suggested (McIntosh and Le Leu, 2001; Toden *et al.*, 2006; Kim *et al.*, 2013). This suggested association may be partially explained by protein-induced genetic damage in colonocytes (Kim *et al.*, 2013). Toden *et al.* (2005, 2006) showed that animal-derived proteins may enhance colonocyte DNA damage and induce a thinning of the mucus barrier in rats. The metabolism of the protein fraction that reaches the colon, its relationship with the gut microbiota and its potential association with cancer risk is further discussed in Section 19.5: 'Protein'.

Other potential mechanisms linking red meat consumption to increased cancer risk include the higher exposure to carcinogenic NOCs (nitrosamines or nitrosamides). NOCs are formed by the reaction of nitrite and nitrogen oxides with secondary amines and *N*-alkylamides (Ferguson, 2010). Nitrite is used to preserve processed meats against bacterial contamination and gives cured meats their typical colour and flavour (WCRF/AICR, 2007). Nitrite can react with the degradation products of amino acids to produce NOCs (WCRF/AICR, 2007). These NOCs may be formed in meat during the curing process itself or endogenously in the body, and particularly in the stomach, from dietary nitrite (or nitrate). Several NOCs are categorised as human or animal carcinogens (IARC, 2010), and there is concern that nitrites and preformed nitrosamines (e.g. from processed meats) may be involved in carcinogenesis, particularly in the stomach (WCRF/AICR, 2007).

The rate of NOC formation is influenced by other dietary factors, including haem iron, which may catalyse the production of NOCs from natural precursors in the gut (Santarelli *et al.*, 2008). In addition to this potential effect of haem iron, there is evidence that haem iron may increase cell proliferation in the mucosa through lipoperoxidation and/or cytotoxicity (Ferguson, 2010). Some studies have also reported a strong association between iron overload and increased cancer risk in humans (Huang, 2003). Iron overload can activate oxidative responsive transcription factors, pro-inflammatory cytokines and iron-induced hypoxia signalling (Huang, 2003; WCRF/AICR, 2007).

Red meats are sometimes cooked at high temperatures, leading to the production of heterocyclic amines and PAHs. Several of the heterocyclic amines produced have so far been identified as risk factors for cancer (Kim *et al.*, 2013). Temperature is the most crucial factor in the formation of these compounds, with frying, grilling and barbecuing (charbroiling) producing the largest amounts (WCRF/AICR, 2007). PAHs are formed when organic substances like meat are incompletely burnt. Grilling and barbecuing (charbroiling) animal foods with intense heat over a direct flame result in fat dropping on the hot fire, thus leading to the production of PAHs that stick to the surface of the food. Similarly, during traditional smoking processes, the PAHs are transferred into a range of meats (Ferguson, 2010). Available data support a role for PAHs in increasing cancer risk (Santarelli *et al.*, 2008).

Based on the above-relayed evidence, the WCRF/AICR (2007) recommended an upper limit of 500 g/week of cooked red meat intake, while avoiding the consumption of processed meats. This same conclusion was reinforced by the more recent publication of the policy document (WCRF/AICR, 2009; Ferguson, 2010). It should be stated that the relationship between meat consumption and cancer risk is still the subject of scientific debate, with some reviews indicating that the association between meat intake and cancer risk, if detected, is rather weak (Alexander *et al.*, 2010; Alexander and Cushing, 2011). However, it may be possible that the overall association between meat intake and cancer risk is modified or confounded by other dietary or lifestyle factors (e.g. high intake of sugars and alcohol, low intake of fruits and vegetables, low physical activity, smoking) (Kim *et al.*, 2013). It is also possible that the association between cancer risk and meat consumption observed in some studies is reflecting an overall dietary pattern rather than revealing the effects of meat consumption per se (Ferguson, 2010). For instance, De Stefani *et al.* (2008) showed that a western dietary pattern, characterised by high levels of red meat, fried eggs, potatoes and red wine, was associated with a significantly increased risk of bladder cancer. Future epidemiological and experimental research is needed to improve our understanding of cancer and its association with meat intake.

Fruits and vegetables

Fruits and non-starchy vegetables may exert protective effects against several types of cancer (WCRF/AICR, 2007; Aune *et al.*, 2011, 2012c; Wu *et al.*, 2013a,b; Shimazu *et al.*, 2014). A large systematic review on fruit and vegetable intake in relation to cancer risk concluded that the overall evidence provided by case–control studies is in support of the hypothesis that fruit and vegetable consumption is associated with a lower risk of cancers of the oesophagus, lung, stomach and colorectum (Riboli and Norat, 2003; Norat *et al.*, 2014). Breast cancer risk was reported to be inversely associated with the intake of vegetables but not with fruits, while bladder cancer was inversely associated with fruit but not with vegetable intake (Riboli and Norat, 2003; Norat *et al.*, 2014). The evidence provided by cohort studies, although suggestive of a potential protective effect of both fruits and vegetables against cancer, was not as convincing as that from case–control studies (Riboli and Norat, 2003; Norat *et al.*, 2014). In fact, based on cohort studies, the only significant protective associations were reported for fruit intake in relation to lung and bladder cancer (Riboli and Norat, 2003; Norat *et al.*, 2014). The discrepancy in the findings between case–control and cohort studies may be partially due to recall and selection biases (Norat *et al.*, 2014). Alternatively, it may be possible that some diet–disease associations may get underestimated in prospective cohort studies as a result of limited variability in dietary intakes within each cohort and/or diet measurement error (Day *et al.*, 2004; Norat *et al.*, 2014). In fact, multiple epidemiological studies have reported stronger associations between diet and disease endpoints when using biomarkers of

dietary intakes compared with the associations stemming from the use of dietary assessment questionnaire (Jenab *et al.*, 2006; Bingham *et al.*, 2008; Harding *et al.*, 2008).

The 2007 WCRF/AICR report and updated reports concluded that the evidence that fruit and vegetables intake modifies the risk of cancer is not 'convincing' (WCRF/AICR, 2007; Norat *et al.*, 2014; see also http://wcrf.org/int/research-we-fund/continuous-update-project-cup). Accordingly, it was judged that non-starchy vegetables and fruits probably protect against cancers of the mouth, larynx, pharynx, oesophagus and stomach, and that fruits probably protect against lung cancer (WCRF/AICR, 2007). The evidence also indicated that allium vegetables, and particularly garlic, probably protect against stomach cancer and against colorectal cancer (WCRF/AICR, 2007, 2011).

Fruits and vegetables contain a wide array of potentially cancer-preventive compounds, including phytochemicals (such as polyphenols, organosulphur compounds, terpenoids), antioxidant nutrients (such as carotenoids and vitamin C), as well as DF – for discussion of DF in relation to cancer risk, refer to Section 19.2: 'Fibre' – (WCRF/AICR, 2007; González-Vallinas *et al.*, 2013; Grosso *et al.*, 2013).

Phytochemicals are able to exert cancer protective effects by acting at different stages of the carcinogenic process, from tumour initiation to cell proliferation, apoptosis, invasion and metastasis (Kroemer and Pouyssegur, 2008; Hanahan and Weinberg, 2011; González-Vallinas *et al.*, 2013). Phytochemicals may protect against the tumorigenic action of carcinogens, blocking their mutagenic activity and suppressing cell proliferation (Surh, 2003). In addition, phytochemicals exert antioxidant properties and may modulate immune and inflammatory responses (Ho *et al.*, 2002; Issa *et al.*, 2006; Ferguson and Philpott, 2007). Several fruits and vegetables contain high levels of polyphenols (such as quercetin in apples, naringenin in citrus and luteolin in parsley) that, in addition to their antioxidant effects, can inhibit carcinogen-activating enzymes and alter the metabolism of other dietary agents. For instance, it was reported that the consumption of apples in physiological quantities inhibits carcinogen-induced mammary cancer in rodents in a dose–response manner (Liu *et al.*, 2005). Similarly, laboratory studies showed that citrus can inhibit the growth of several tumours, including breast and colorectal cancer (Kocic *et al.*, 2010; Vitale *et al.*, 2013) through the inhibition of several cancer-related biological pathways, such as carcinogen bioactivation, cell signalling, cell cycle regulation, angiogenesis and inflammation (Galvano *et al.*, 2009; Masella *et al.*, 2012). Citrus flavonoids have also been hypothesised to exert pro-apoptotic activity (Park *et al.*, 2008; Leonardi *et al.*, 2010; Ghorbani *et al.*, 2012; Sivagami *et al.*, 2012) (the role of polyphenols in cancer prevention is discussed further in Section 19.2: 'Polyphenolic compounds').

High consumption of organosulphur compounds, and particularly glucosinolate from cruciferous vegetables, such as Brussels sprouts (*Brassica oleraceae*), has been associated with a decreased cancer risk (Latté *et al.*, 2011; Grosso *et al.*, 2013; Wu *et al.*, 2013a,b). Experimental studies have shown that indoles and isothiocyanates, two main groups of glucosinolate breakdown products, were found to reduce the carcinogenic effects of PAHs and nitrosamines (Steinkellner *et al.*, 2001; Grosso *et al.*, 2013). In addition, indole-3-carbinol was found to prevent the progression of different cancers, particularly breast cancer, and to exert antitumoural effects (Nguyen *et al.*, 2008; Grosso *et al.*, 2013). The anticancer properties of garlic were attributed to its content of diallyl disulphide and other organosulphur compounds. Case–control and cohort studies have consistently shown an inverse relationship between garlic intake and colorectal cancer risk (Ngo *et al.*, 2007), and experimental evidence stemming from in vitro and in vivo studies documented antiproliferative effects of diallyl disulphide and inhibition of colon and gastric cancers (González-Vallinas *et al.*, 2013). A study evaluating the inhibitory effects of extracts isolated from 34 different vegetables on the proliferation of eight different tumour cell lines showed that the extracts from cruciferous vegetables as well as from vegetables of the genus *Allium* inhibited the proliferation of all cancer cell lines tested, whereas extracts from vegetables most commonly consumed in western countries were much less effective (Boivin *et al.*, 2009). The antiproliferative effect of these vegetables was found to be specific to cells of cancerous origin and to be largely independent of their antioxidant properties (Boivin *et al.*, 2009).

Fruits and vegetables are good sources of terpenoids (such as carotenoids) and several micronutrients that may also exert cancer-preventive effects. For instance, non-starchy vegetables and fruits are a good source of folate, which is known to play a crucial role in synthesis and methylation of DNA (WCRF/AICR, 2007; Nazki *et al.*, 2014). Abnormal DNA methylation has been related to aberrant gene expression and to cancers at several sites (WCRF/AICR, 2007). Beta-carotene and other carotenoids are found in carrots, tomatoes (lycopene) and several fruits. The cancer protective effects of carotenoids may be mediated by their antioxidant properties and by ligand-dependent signalling through retinoid receptors (WCRF/AICR, 2007; Kushi *et al.*, 2012; Kaulmann and Bohn, 2014). Lycopene, which is the red pigment present in several red fruits and vegetables and the major carotenoid in tomatoes, is a very efficient singlet oxygen quencher (Stahl *et al.*, 2006). It was found to lower biomarkers of oxidative stress (Basu and

Imrhan, 2006), to protect against tissue damage and to decrease the risk of many chronic diseases, including several types of cancer (Jamshidzadeh *et al.*, 2008; Talvas *et al.*, 2010). Tomatoes and fruits, in particular citrus fruits, are good sources of vitamin C, which is able to trap free radicals and reactive oxygen molecules, thus protecting against oxidative damage (WCRF/AICR, 2007; Gonzalez and Miranda-Massari, 2014). Vitamin C can also regenerate other antioxidant vitamins, such as vitamin E (Padayatty *et al.*, 2003), inhibit the formation of carcinogens and protect DNA from mutagenic attack (Fountoulakis *et al.*, 2004) (for more discussion of micronutrients in relation to cancer risk, refer to section 19.2: 'Micronutrients').

It is important to note that there is a complex mixture of phytochemicals and nutrients in fruits and vegetables and these may have additive and synergistic effects in reducing cancer risk (WCRF/AICR, 2007). It is therefore difficult to decipher the relative importance of each compound alone, and it is likely that the protective effects of fruits and vegetables may result from a combination of effects on several pathways involved in carcinogenesis (WCRF/AICR, 2007). It is likely that additional bioactive phytochemicals have yet to be identified and that those that are already known may have additional anticancer properties that are yet to be understood (WCRF/AICR, 2007).

Alcohol

A wealth of evidence has shown that alcohol drinking is associated with increased risk of several types of cancer (Cuomo *et al.*, 2014, Pelucchi *et al.*, 2011, WCRF/AICR, 2007, WCRF/AICR, 2014). This association is supported by epidemiological studies as well as animal experiments that have identified ethanol, or its metabolites, as promoting factors of human carcinogenesis (Pelucchi *et al.*, 2011; Cuomo *et al.*, 2014). It has recently been estimated that 3.6% of all cases of cancer are attributable to alcohol drinking (5.2% in men and 1.7% in women) worldwide (Boffetta and Hashibe, 2006; Cuomo *et al.*, 2014). The evidence does not only implicate high or excessive alcohol intakes as risk factors for cancer development but also shows that moderate or even light intakes of alcohol may increase the risk of certain cancers (WCRF/AICR, 2007; Pelucchi *et al.*, 2011; Bagnardi *et al.*, 2013; Brooks and Zakhari, 2013). A recent meta-analysis showed that light alcohol drinking increases the risk of cancer of the oral cavity and pharynx, oesophagus and breast. This meta-analysis estimated that approximately 5000 deaths from oropharyngeal cancer, 24 000 from oesophageal cancer and 5000 from breast cancer were attributed to light alcohol drinking in 2004 worldwide (Bagnardi *et al.*, 2013). These findings support the hypothesis that alcohol acts as a cumulative carcinogen (Brooks and Zakhari, 2013). The WCRF/AICR panel states that alcoholic drinks are a cause of cancers of a number of sites, with the evidence being rated as 'convincing' for the association between alcohol and cancers of the mouth, pharynx, larynx, oesophagus, colorectum (men) and breast (WCRF/AICR, 2007, 2010, 2011). In addition, alcohol drinking was described as a 'probable' cause of colorectal cancer in women and of liver cancer (WCRF/AICR, 2007, 2011). Available evidence suggests that there is no 'safe limit' of alcohol intake and that the carcinogenic effects are from ethanol, irrespective of the type of drink (WCRF/AICR, 2007). Accordingly, ethanol has been classified as a human carcinogen by the WCRF/AICR (2007). It is important to note, however, that the interpretation of some of the epidemiological findings may be complicated by the fact that, at high levels of consumption, the effects of alcohol are considerably confounded by other high-risk behaviours, such as tobacco smoking (WCRF/AICR, 2007).

The mechanisms underlying the carcinogenic effects of alcohol are not fully understood and may differ by target organs (Cuomo et al., 2014). Strong evidence suggests that alcohol may act as a solvent, thus enhancing the penetration of carcinogens into cells (WCRF/AICR, 2007; Cuomo et al., 2014). In fact, acute administration of ethanol was shown to increase the permeability of biological membranes and to facilitate the entry of carcinogenic molecules into epithelial cells (Wight and Ogden, 1998; Cuomo et al., 2014). These local effects of ethanol could help explain the frequently described synergistic effects of alcohol and smoking in the carcinogenesis of head and neck (Cuomo et al., 2014).

Apart from the aforementioned local effects of alcohol, ethanol metabolism is also known to play an important role in alcohol-related carcinogenesis. Acetaldehyde is the main metabolite of ethanol, and numerous studies have documented its direct mutagenic and carcinogenic effects (Fang and Vaca, 1997; Cuomo et al., 2014): acetaldehyde has the capacity to bind to DNA and to make stable adducts by which it could elicit replication errors and mutations in oncogenes or oncosuppressors (Fang and Vaca, 1997; Cuomo et al., 2014). Acetaldehyde production depends on the activity of the enzymes alcohol dehydrogenase and aldehyde dehydrogenase, which are encoded by multiple genes (Cuomo et al., 2014). Since these genes exist in several variants, some polymorphisms may cause high acetaldehyde levels and thus increase the risk of alcohol-related cancers (Cuomo et al., 2014). An increasing body of evidence highlights an interaction between genetic susceptibility and alcohol drinking on cancer risk in human beings (Druesne-Pecollo et al., 2009; Cuomo et al., 2014).

Ethanol metabolism is also known to increase oxidative stress and the production of ROS, thus inducing lipid peroxidation (Cuomo et al., 2014). Products of lipid peroxidation are known to interact with DNA, forming exocyclic DNA adducts. This mechanism may be of particular relevance to liver carcinogenesis (Hoek and Pastorino, 2002; Molina et al., 2003). Similarly, chronic consumption of alcohol is suggested to interact with the metabolism of pro-carcinogens such as nitrosamines and aflatoxins. In fact, alcohol consumption induces cytochrome P450 2E1 (CYP2E1), which is normally involved in the metabolism of various xenobiotics and pro-carcinogenic compounds (Pöschl and Seitz, 2004). The interaction between ethanol and pro-carcinogen metabolism is complex and depends on several factors, including the degree of CYP2E1 induction, the chemical structure of the pro-carcinogen and the presence or absence of ethanol in the body during pro-carcinogen metabolism (Seitz and Meier, 2007; Cuomo et al., 2014).

Ethanol metabolism may also have implications on gene expression, particularly through its effects on DNA methylation. It is known that DNA methylation hampers gene expression, whereas reduced DNA methylation enhances it (Varela-Rey et al., 2013) (DNA methylation is further discussed in Section 19.3: 'DNA methylation'). There is evidence showing that chronic alcohol use induces important changes in the degree of DNA methylation (Choi et al., 1999; Varela-Rey et al., 2013; Cuomo et al., 2014). For instance, it has been hypothesised that decreased methylation of tumour promoter genes provides a mechanism linking alcohol consumption to cancer development (Cuomo et al., 2014). There are several ways through which alcohol ingestion may impact DNA methylation, including reduction in the activity of methionine synthetase (the enzyme that remethylates homocysteine to methionine), inhibition of DNA methylase (which transfers methyl groups to DNA) (Pöschl and Seitz, 2004) and reduction of SAM (the methyl donor for DNA methylation reactions). SAM deficiency results in DNA hypomethylation and increased DNA instability, which is associated with increased risk for cancer (Morgan et al., 2004; Cuomo et al., 2014).

Another link between alcohol, DNA methylation and increased cancer risk may be mediated by nutritional deficiencies that often accompany chronic alcohol consumption. Heavy alcohol drinking may affect folate metabolism, given that the intake of this vitamin is typically low in chronic alcohol drinkers and given its destruction by acetaldehyde (Varela-Rey et al., 2013; Cuomo et al., 2014). Folate deficiency, through affecting the inhibition of transmethylation, may impact gene expression and thus play a potential role in carcinogenesis (Stickel and Seitz, 2004) (folate and its link with cancer is further discussed in Section 19.2: 'Vitamins and minerals'). Similarly, impaired intake and metabolism of vitamin B_{12} and vitamin B_6, commonly encountered in chronic alcoholics, may also contribute to impaired DNA methylation (Boffetta and Hashibe, 2006). Several studies have also highlighted a role for vitamin A and beta-carotene deficiency in alcohol carcinogenesis (Wang, 2003). Available evidence suggests that chronic use of alcohol is associated with a low intake of retinoids and carotenoids, and with a breakdown of retinol through ROS production (Leo and Lieber, 1999). Therefore, through its impact on retinoid status, alcohol drinking may adversely alter cellular growth, cellular differentiation and apoptosis (WCRF/AICR, 2007). Finally, chronic alcohol intake is associated with an immunodeficient state, and a reduction of both innate and specific immune responses, which facilitate cancer cell growth (Cook, 1998).

In conclusion, ethanol metabolism, nutritional deficiencies, impaired gene expression and defective immune surveillance seem to be the major mechanisms involved in alcohol-related carcinogenesis (Cuomo et al., 2014). For all these mechanisms, genetic polymorphisms might modulate the risk (Dumitrescu and Shields, 2005; WCRF/AICR, 2007). The variants in genes for alcohol metabolism have prompted interest in examining the interaction between individual susceptibility and the cellular toxic effects mediated by exposure to ethanol (Druesne-Pecollo et al., 2009; Cuomo et al., 2014).

Dietary patterns in relation to cancer risk

Traditional nutrition epidemiology investigating the association between diet and cancer has focused on a single or few nutrients and foods. Nutrition epidemiologists have proposed studying dietary patterns as an alternative approach to evaluate diet–disease associations (Hu et al., 1999, 2000; Jacques and Tucker, 2001). This alternate approach looks beyond the single nutrient or food and attempts to capture the broader picture of diet that is hypothesised to discriminate between health and disease (Slattery, 2008). This section offers an overview of the methodological and public health advantages of using the dietary patterns approach, a brief description of dietary patterns derivation, as well as the association between dietary patterns and cancer risk.

Limitations and challenges of the single nutrient approach
Until recently, nutrition research has largely focused on the reductionist approach, with investigations into the relationship between diet and cancer addressing single nutrients or food groups and specific biological effects or markers (Hoffmann, 2003). While this type of research

has greatly advanced the understanding of the dietary risk factors for cancer, this approach has several conceptual and methodological limitations for implementing changes. In the real world, foods are consumed in various characteristic combinations that deliver a variety of nutrients which can have either synergistic or interactive metabolic actions. For example, diets high in fibre tend to be high in vitamin C, folate, carotenoids, magnesium and potassium. The traditional approach, based on single nutrient or food, resorts to multiple linear and logistic regression models to account for the interaction and synergistic effects of nutrients and foods. However, with many correlated exogenous variables, these models may be unstable and could result in large confidence intervals for the regression parameters (Hoffmann et al., 2002). Furthermore, when a large number of variables are entered in a regression model, it is possible to obtain significant association simply by chance (Hu, 2002).

As a result of these limitations, the single nutrient approach resulted in some inconsistent relationships between diet and cancer. Studies at the nutrient levels have sometimes reported null associations or findings inconsistent with established knowledge with regard to the role of specific foods or nutrients in the aetiology of cancer, such as the association between beta-carotene intake and the risk of lung cancer. Epidemiological studies have provided evidence for a positive association between high beta-carotene uptake, or a high beta-carotene plasma concentration, and reduced risks for cancer, especially lung cancer. In addition, animal studies have demonstrated anti-carcinogenic activity for beta-carotene. Unexpectedly in three large clinical intervention trials, beta-carotene supplementation either showed no effect (Physician Health Study), or was associated with an increased incidence of lung cancer (ATBC; Beta-Carotene and Retinol Efficacy Trial) (Goralczyk, 2009). Another example is the association between dietary intake of fatty acids and the risk of breast cancer, despite the strong biological plausibility, this association remains controversial as population-based studies have been inconsistent (Chajès and Romieu, 2014).

Advantages of the dietary pattern approach
Consequently, there has been a growing appreciation that the overall dietary pattern, rather than any single nutrient, should be considered in relation to studying the association between diet and disease. Cancer, in particular, has complex aetiology and it is unlikely that its development will be mediated by a single nutrient or food (Hu, 2002; Newby and Tucker, 2004; Moeller et al., 2007; Jones-McLean et al., 2010; Kant, 2010). So, conceptually, the evaluation of the overall dietary patterns appears closer to real world as people 'do not eat nutrients they eat food' (Hu, 2002). The use of the dietary

pattern approach to study diet–disease association might help capture the complexity of diet that is often lost in nutrient-based analyses. Furthermore, this approach accounts for the collinearity or intercorrelations between nutrients or foods (Tucker, 2010). It is important to note that recent dietary intervention studies have indicated that interventions focused on the dietary patterns, compared with a single nutrient approach, led to more consistent findings in relation to other chronic diseases, such as cardiovascular diseases. These interventions resulted in a decreased blood pressure and reduction of cardiovascular complications (Appel et al., 1997; de Lorgeril et al., 1999; Reidlinger et al., 2015).

Lastly, studying dietary patterns could have important public health implications because the overall patterns of dietary intake might be easy to interpret or translate into diets by the public as well as by health-care professionals (National Research Council (US) Committee on Diet and Health, 1989). Furthermore, given the fact that recommendations stemming from the dietary pattern approach are culturally sensitive, their integration and adoption by the general public are more likely. In fact, the prevailing dietary guidelines emphasise dietary patterns in the prevention of cancer (WCRF/AICR, 2007). Studying dietary patterns in relation to disease outcomes thus provides a practical way to evaluate the health effects of adherence to dietary guidelines by individuals (Huijbregts et al., 1997).

Derivation of dietary patterns

The derivation and analysis of dietary patterns have been done either empirically using data-driven methods or theoretically using hypothesis-driven methods (Hu, 2002; Newby and Tucker, 2004; Moeller et al., 2007; Kant, 2010; Tucker, 2010). Cluster analysis and factor analysis are broadly categorised as 'empirically driven' approaches that derive a posteriori patterns, while index analysis is a 'hypothesis-driven' approach that creates patterns based on a priori decisions (Reedy et al., 2010). Whether derived theoretically or empirically, dietary patterns analysis has been consistently shown in the literature to be a valid and reproducible approach of investigating diet–disease associations. Recently, a few studies examined the reproducibility and validity of dietary patterns over periods of time varying from 1 to 7 years. In these studies, confirmatory factor analysis and discriminant analysis, as well as correlation analysis between pattern scores at baseline and pattern scores at different points of time, showed good reproducibility and stability of the derived patterns (Hu et al., 1999; Quatromoni et al., 2002; Khani et al., 2004; Togo et al., 2004; Newby et al., 2006; Weismayer et al., 2006; Okubo et al., 2010; Nanri et al., 2012).

Dietary patterns and cancer risk: western, prudent and traditional patterns

Regardless of what method was used to derive dietary patterns, most of the studies depicted two main patterns: the 'prudent' pattern, generally characterised by vegetables, fruit, legumes, fish, poultry and whole grains, and the 'western', an energy-dense pattern rich in red meat, processed meat, refined grains, French fries and sweets/desserts. Though no final judgment could be made by WCRF/AICR (2007) regarding the association between dietary patterns and cancer risk, recent meta-analyses (after 2007) have consistently conferred a protective effect of the prudent/healthy diet for most cancer sites.

A recent review of 26 studies examining the association between dietary patterns and breast cancer concluded that prudent dietary patterns or diets composed largely of vegetables, fruit, fish and soy were associated with a decreased risk of breast cancer (Albuquerque et al., 2014). In fact, a meta-analysis of cohort and case–control studies showed a decreased risk of breast cancer in the highest compared with the lowest categories of prudent/healthy dietary patterns (odds ratio (OR): 0.89; 95% confidence interval (CI): 0.82–0.99; $p = 0.02$) (Brennan et al., 2010). Similar results were reported for gastric cancer, where a meta-analysis showed a favourable role for the 'prudent/healthy', with an OR of 0.75 (95% CI: 0.63–0.90), for the highest versus the lowest category. On the other hand, a western-type diet was associated with an increased risk of this cancer (OR: 1.5; 95% CI: 1.21–1.89) (Bertuccio et al., 2013). For colorectal cancer, a review of all studies between the years 2000 and 2011, examining the effect of various dietary patterns, concluded that diets high in fruits and vegetables and low in fat were most likely to be protective against colorectal cancer, while diets high in pork, processed meat, potatoes and refined grain were associated with an increased risk of the disease (Yusof et al., 2012). These associations were confirmed by the results of a pooled analysis of eight cohort and eight case–control studies, whereby the risk of colon cancer for highest versus lowest levels of exposure of prudent and western dietary patters were 0.80 (95% CI: 0.70–0.90) and 1.29 (95% CI: 1.13–1.48) respectively (Magalhaes et al., 2012). In line with these associations between dietary patterns and cancer risk, the results of the Shanghai Women's and Men's Health Studies conferred a protective effect of a vegetable-based dietary pattern against liver cancer (H: 0.58; 95% CI: 0.40–0.84) for highest versus lowest quartiles of intake (Zhang et al., 2013). As dietary patterns analysis has moved beyond North America and Europe, many studies have identified ethnic- or country-specific 'traditional' patterns in addition to the western and the prudent patterns (Tucker, 2010). The association between 'traditional' patterns and the risk of cancer depends to a large extent on the population studied (Bhupathiraju and Tucker, 2011).

The aforementioned associations between dietary patterns and cancer risk are of particular public health concern in countries undergoing nutrition transition, whereby a shift in dietary intake is taking place mainly from a healthy- to a western-type diet. This shift is tied to factors such as rapid urbanisation, economic growth and technological advances (Mehio Sibai *et al.*, 2010). Latin America, the Middle East and North Africa, as well as a few countries of the Far East (i.e. Thailand) were reported to witness some forms of nutrition transition. Alarmingly, the shift from a healthy to a western pattern in these countries is mainly affecting the younger populations (Naja *et al.*, 2013). As will be discussed later in this chapter, it is during early life that exposures to various dietary components are shown to most influence cancer risk.

Mediterranean dietary pattern and the risk of cancer

In addition to the empirically derived patterns described in Section 19.2: 'Dietary patterns and cancer risk: western, prudent, and traditional patterns', *a posteriori* dietary patterns, such as the Mediterranean diet (MD), have also been studied in association with cancer risk. The MD has been widely used to describe the dietary pattern that dominated in olive-tree-growing areas of the Mediterranean coastline (Willett *et al.*, 1995; Bach *et al.*, 2006). Recently, this pattern was recognised by UNESCO as an 'Intangible Cultural Heritage of Humanity' (Turmo, 2012: 115). While many definitions of the MD exist, this pattern has been mainly described as (i) daily consumption of unrefined cereals and cereal products, vegetables (two to three servings), fruit (four to six servings), olive oil, dairy products (one or two servings), and red or white wine (one to two wine glasses); (ii) weekly consumption of potatoes (four to five servings), fish (four to five servings), olives, pulses and nuts (more than four servings), and eggs and sweets (one to three servings); (iii) monthly consumption of red meat and meat products (four to five servings) (Dontas *et al.*, 2007). Since 1975, when Ancel Keys first used the term Mediterranean pattern (Keys, 1975), a plethora of studies have investigated the health effects of this dietary pattern. These studies conferred substantial evidence for a protective effect of the MD against the incidence of several non-communicable diseases, including neoplastic diseases (Bhupathiraju and Tucker, 2011). Historically, populations living in the area of the Mediterranean Sea had a lower cancer incidence compared with those living in the regions of northern Europe and the USA (Keys *et al.*, 1986). This singular condition has been attributed to the traditional dietary pattern of populations living in this area, which has also been recognised to protect from cardiovascular diseases (Pauwels, 2011).

Epidemiological studies strongly support the hypothesis that the MD plays a role in preventing several types of cancers, especially those of the digestive tract, whereas contradictory results were reported for hormone-related cancers, such as breast cancer. The most recent meta-analysis, aiming at evaluating the effects of adherence to MD on overall cancer risk as well as on different cancer types, covered 21 cohort studies including 1 368 736 subjects and 12 case–control studies with 62 725 subjects. Results of this meta-analysis have shown that the highest adherence to the MD category resulted in a significant reduction in the risk of overall cancer mortality (10%) and the incidence of colorectal cancer (14%), prostate cancer (4%) and aerodigestive cancer (56%) (Schwingshackl and Hoffmann, 2014). This protective effect of the MD could be due to the constituents of this diet being mainly fruits and vegetables, fish, whole grains, olive oil and red wine (Grosso *et al.*, 2013). Consumed together, these food components resulted in a significant and consistent reduction in cancer risk. The biological and physiological mechanisms by which these elements exert their effect have been discussed earlier in this chapter.

In conclusion, findings from dietary pattern research provide invaluable evidence which can be used to develop recommendations to reverse the trend in nutrition transition. Such recommendations are particularly beneficial in the primary prevention of distinct types of cancer by dietary measures. The usefulness of the dietary patterns approach was reported by James (2009), who stated: 'Examining dietary patterns rather than specific nutrients may better allow public health professionals to translate dietary goals into practical dietary recommendations that are culturally relevant'.

19.3 Diet, epigenetics and cancer

As described throughout this chapter, diet has been shown to affect cancer risk. Recent evidence suggests that dietary factors, as well as other environment and lifestyle stressors, could induce heritable changes in gene expression without affecting DNA sequence. These changes are known as epigenetic changes and seem to play an important role in modulating the effect of diet on cancer risk (Lee and Herceg, 2014). Distinctive features of these epigenetic changes, in comparison with genetic mutations, relate to their reversible and gradual nature, making them an attractive target for cancer prevention. The three main mechanisms that have been described in modulating epigenetic changes are DNA methylation, histone modifications and RNA interference.

DNA methylation

DNA methylation is an epigenetic mechanism that allows for the regulation of transcription via the addition of methyl groups from S-adenosyl-L-methionine to the 5-carbon (C5) of the nucleotide cytosine. In general, DNA methylation in specific gene promoter regions results in transcriptional silencing of tumour suppressor genes, causing their inactivation, potentially resulting in malignant transformation and cancer (Rassoulzadegan et al., 2007). This epigenetic silencing of tumour suppressor genes is a common feature of the cancer epigenome and represents an alternative to mutations as a cause of gene function loss. Furthermore, general DNA hypomethylation in the highly repeated DNA sequences is associated with triggering chromosomal instability and expression of normally silent genes, including oncogenes (Ehrlich, 2009). Such epigenetic alteration can occur early in the neoplastic process and disrupt key cell signalling pathways favouring clonal expansion (Baylin and Ohm, 2006).

Several dietary factors have been studied in relation to their potential effect on DNA methylation, including folate, polyphenols, selenium, retinoids, fatty acids, isothiocyanates and allyl compounds (Ross, 2003; Davis and Uthus, 2004; Dashwood et al., 2006; Myzak and Dashwood, 2006; Chen and Xu, 2010; Link et al., 2010). The chemopreventive effect of folic acid supplementation has been demonstrated in a few cancer models, including the liver, cervix and breast. In rats fed a folic-acid-enriched diet followed by the chemical initiation of liver cancer, cell growth and the number of preneoplastic lesions as well as c-myc oncogene expression were diminished compared with a control group (Chagas et al., 2011). Furthermore, folic acid supplementation has been found to reverse cervical dysplasia in patients using oral contraceptives and prevent cervical cancer (Whitehead et al., 1973; Butterworth et al., 1982). Recent prospective and epidemiological studies indicated that high folate intake reduces breast cancer risk in premenopausal women (Shrubsole et al., 2011), particularly in ER-negative cancer (Maruti et al., 2009). Recent studies advocated the use of certain polyphenols as complementary to existing cancer therapies (Dorai and Aggarwal, 2004). These polyphenols include catechins (catechin, epicatechin, EGCG), coffee polyphenols (caffeic acid, chlorogenic acid), curcumin (from curry) and resveratrol (from grapes and berries). Using in vitro and in vivo models, these dietary botanicals were shown to exert an inhibitory effect on DNA methylation and gene silencing and restore expression in various tumour-suppressing genes (Link et al., 2010). Though the epidemiological evidence for a protective role for selenium has been inconsistent, in vitro studies showed that selenium supplementation induced global hypomethylation and promoter methylation of the p53 gene (Davis et al., 2000). Similar to selenium, retinoids may exert their cancer-preventive activity through epigenetic modulation. Animal studies showed that retinoids may alter the DNA methylation processes by enhancing the 1-carbon metabolism, thus optimising methyl group supply (Rowling et al., 2002; Johanning and Piyathilake, 2003). Such an effect was observed with various cancer sites, including hepatic carcinoma, leukaemia, and colorectal and breast cancer (Di Croce et al., 2002; Esteller et al., 2002; Moreno et al., 2002; Fazi et al., 2005; Stefanska et al., 2010).

Histone modifications

Histones have an active function in the regulation of chromatin structure and gene expression. Histone modifications typically occur as post-translational modifications at the N-terminal of histones. These modifications include acetylation, methylation, phosphorylation, biotinylation and ubiquitination and are essential during development (Feinberg et al., 2006; Hassan and Zempleni, 2006; Doi et al., 2009). Disruption of histone modifications has been implicated in carcinogenesis by its ability to induce aberrant gene expression, encourage loss of genomic instability, impair DNA repair and diminish cell cycle checkpoint stability (Füllgrabe et al., 2011). Specifically, histone acetylation is an essential step for a relaxed chromatin structure that is more readily accessible to transcriptional factors for subsequent DNA transcription/gene expression (Tollefsbol, 2009). Suboptimal histone acetylation has been association with cancer pathology (Mahlknecht and Hoelzer, 2000).

A few food compounds were found to inhibit histone deacetylation, namely isothiocyanate from cruciferous vegetables and broccoli, allyl compounds found in garlic, and butyrate. In vitro and in vivo studies have shown that sulphoraphane, an isothiocyanate, inhibited histone deacetylase (HDAC) in human colon, prostate and breast cancer cells (Myzak and Dashwood, 2006; Dashwood and Ho, 2007; Nian et al., 2009). Other isothiocyanates, such a phenylhexyl isothiocyanate and phenethyl isothiocyanate, have also shown significant reduction of HDAC activity and histone markers (Ma et al., 2006; Wang et al., 2008). Allyl compounds, namely diallyl sulphide, were associated with increased histone acetylation and growth arrest in colon cancer and leukaemia cells (Druesne-Pecollo et al., 2006; Zhao et al., 2006). Butyrate, a three-carbon chain attached to a carboxylic acid group, represents one of the first anticancer agents to be identified with histone acetylation properties. It is the smallest-identified HDAC inhibitor, and its effect has been reported in several cell lines (Myzak and Dashwood, 2006). Butyrate has been considered for combinatorial anticancer interventions with diverse agents such as retinoids (de Conti *et al.*, 2012). Similar effects were observed with polyphenols, tea catechins, resveratrol, as well as curcumin, making them potential cancer chemopreventive agents (Ong *et al.*, 2011).

MicroRNA

The human genome contains only 20 000 protein-coding genes, representing less than 2% of the total genome, whereas a substantial fraction of the human genome can be transcribed, yielding many short RNAs with limited protein-coding capacity (Krutovskikh and Herceg, 2010). Among them, the most extensively studied are miRNAs (20–22 nucleotides), which play a role in post-transcriptional regulation (Shivdasani, 2006; Negrini *et al.*, 2007). miRNA acts either by the complete complementary base pairing, which results in messenger RNA degradation, or by a partial base pairing, which leads to translational inhibition of the targeted messenger RNA (Shivdasani, 2006; Negrini *et al.*, 2007). Numerous miRNA expression profiling and functional studies have associated miRNA with cancer progression, diagnosis, prognosis and treatment (Calin *et al.*, 2004). Downregulation of subsets of miRNAs in cancers suggests that some of them may act as putative tumour-suppressor genes, while upregulation suggests that many miRNAs may act as oncogenes, depending on their targets (Shivdasani, 2006; Negrini *et al.*, 2007). A few diet-derived compounds were shown to decrease the risk of cancer through downregulation of a few miRNAs associated with an elevated risk of cancer. Such an effect was observed with folate, EGCG, genistein, curcumin and selenium (Supic *et al.*, 2013).

The accumulating evidence for the protective effect of selected dietary compounds on cancer through modulating epigenetic changes suggests their use in conjunction with other cancer prevention and chemotherapeutic strategies (Hardy and Tollefsbol, 2011; Tollefsbol, 2014). Despite the promising future for therapeutic applications of natural dietary components, many unresolved questions ought to be considered for dietary recommendations in cancer prevention: Are the protective effects, observed with intracellular concentrations of these compounds, attainable with dietary intake of the food items rich in these compounds? What are the critical times for exposure: during fetal development, throughout a lifespan, or during ageing? Which cancer site and at which stage do such compounds deliver their postulated protective effects? What is a safe upper limit of intake?

19.4 Early life diet and cancer

Recently, clear evidence has emerged showing that exposure of developing tissues or organs to an adverse stimulus or insult during crucial periods of development can increase the risk of many diseases. This evidence is in line with the developmental origins of health and disease (DOHAD) hypothesis stating that an adverse developmental environment early in life can reprogramme cellular and tissue responses to normal physiological signals in a manner that increases disease susceptibility (Swanson *et al.*, 2009). A growing body of literature identifies early childhood and adolescence as stages of the life cycle where energy balance, diet composition and other exposures are of significance in determining adult risk of many diseases, including cancer (WCRF/AICR, 2007; Fuemmeler *et al.*, 2009; Potischman and Linet, 2013; Lillycrop and Burdge, 2014). Furthermore, even nutrition in the prenatal stage has been implicated in the mediation of one's risk of cancer.

Diet and cancer: childhood and adolescence

Among other dietary factors, energy restriction during early life is speculated to modulate the risk of various cancers in adulthood. During the Dutch famine in World War II, severe energy restriction in childhood and adolescence was associated with a decreased risk of colorectal and pancreatic cancer, an increased risk of breast cancer and had no effect on prostate cancer risk (Dirx *et al.*, 2001; Hughes *et al.*, 2010; Heinen *et al.*, 2011). The famine-related energy restriction in childhood and adolescence resulted in persistent epigenetic changes, which were shown to be highly correlated to the observed reduction in colorectal cancer risk (Hughes *et al.*, 2009; Simons *et al.*, 2014). On the other hand, elevated body mass in childhood and adolescence is associated with an increased risk of colon, renal, colorectal, endometrial, ovarian and pancreatic cancers as well as glioma and lymphoma in adulthood (Maskarinec *et al.*, 2008; Fuemmeler *et al.*, 2009; Moore *et al.*, 2009; Thomas *et al.*, 2009; Kanda *et al.*, 2010). Some studies show an even stronger association of adolescent overweight to future cancer risk than overweight in adulthood (Maskarinec *et al.*, 2008; Fuemmeler *et al.*, 2009). Interestingly, a reduced risk of breast and prostate cancer has been associated with higher body mass in adolescence independent of weight status in adulthood (Giovannucci *et al.*, 1997; Li *et al.*, 2010).

In addition to energy balance, various studies investigated the association between intake of specific food groups/foods in early life and cancer risk. These studies suggest that diets high in fruits and vegetables are associated with a lower risk of cancer (Potischman and Linet, 2013). For instance, girls with higher intake of fruits and vegetables at the age of 12–13 years have a lower risk of breast cancer later in life (Potischman *et al.*, 1998). Furthermore, based on results from the National Institutes of Health–AARP Diet and Health Study cohort, a reduced colon cancer risk was observed for individuals with a higher intake of vegetables and vitamin A in adolescence but not in adulthood (Ruder *et al.*, 2011). A high intake of vegetable protein has also been associated with a delayed onset of puberty in girls (de Ridder *et al.*, 1991; Berkey *et al.*, 2000; Günther *et al.*, 2010) and boys (Günther *et al.*, 2010). Such a delay is implicated in reducing the risk of hormone-related cancers such as breast, ovarian, prostate and testicular cancers (Forman *et al.*, 1994; Berkey *et al.*, 1999; Giles *et al.*, 2003; Garner *et al.*, 2005; Velie *et al.*, 2006; Barker *et al.*, 2008; Ruder *et al.*, 2008).

In addition to fruits and vegetables, among plant-based foods, soy intake in childhood and adolescence has received attention for its benefits in reducing breast cancer risk (Wu *et al.*, 2002; Thanos *et al.*, 2006; Korde *et al.*, 2009; Lee *et al.*, 2009) and colorectal cancer risk (Cotterchio *et al.*, 2006). Soy intake was shown to be most protective against breast cancer when consumed in childhood (Korde *et al.*, 2009). Not only is soy a rich source of plant protein, it also contains high concentrations of phytoestrogen isoflavones. A prospective study in Germany showed that the highest tertile ($\geq$423 mg/day) of isoflavone intake in girls delayed peak height development and the Tanner stage 2 of breast development by 7–8 months compared with girls with the lowest tertile ($\leq$22 mg/day). This delay in pubertal onset was estimated to reduce breast cancer risk by around 6%. Such an association between soy intake and age at puberty was not found among boys (Cheng *et al.*, 2010).

As opposed to diets rich in fruits and vegetables, a high consumption of animal based foods in early life is associated with an increased risk of some cancers in adulthood (Potischman and Linet, 2013). The Nurses' Health Study II found a positive association between increased consumption of red meat and fat during adolescence and adult premenopausal breast cancer risk (Linos *et al.*, 2008, 2010). In a case–control study of early-onset breast cancer, premenopausal breast cancer risk has also been linked to adolescent chicken and fish intake (Potischman *et al.*, 1998). Furthermore, an increased risk of pancreatic cancer in men was associated with a high intake of nitrate and nitrite from processed meats in adolescence (Aschebrook-Kilfoy *et al.*, 2011). In the 65-year follow-up of the Boyd Orr cohort, a high dairy intake during childhood was associated with an increased risk of colorectal cancer, but not with stomach and breast cancer (van der Pols *et al.*, 2007). Animal protein, particularly dairy protein, can indirectly affect cancer risk by affecting growth and development in early life. High intake of animal protein, especially from cows' milk and dairy products, in children is associated with an increased circulation of IGF-1 (Hoppe *et al.*, 2004a,b). Serum IGF-1 concentrations in childhood and adolescence are positively associated with height (Hoppe *et al.*, 2004b) and are suspected to reduce the age of pubertal onset (Günther *et al.*, 2010; Cheng *et al.*, 2012). Adult attained height is positively associated with overall cancer risk (Kabat *et al.*, 2013), particularly colorectal, breast, ovarian and pancreatic cancers (WCRF/AICR, 2010, 2011, 2012, 2014). Moreover, early puberty increases the risk of hormone-related cancers (Forman *et al.*, 1994; Berkey *et al.*, 1999; Giles *et al.*, 2003; Garner *et al.*, 2005; Velie *et al.*, 2006; Barker *et al.*, 2008; Ruder *et al.*, 2008). Furthermore, a positive association between dairy protein intake and body weight has been found (Michaelsen and Greer, 2014). A high intake of dairy protein at the age of 12 months was associated with excess body weight at the age of 7 years, demonstrating its potential effect on long-term weight status (Günther *et al.*, 2010).

Diet and cancer: prenatal environment

In the context of the DOHAD hypothesis, the prenatal environment is an additional crucial phase of the life cycle where diet is postulated to influence disease risk later in life, possibly through the reprogramming of the epigenome. During the early stages of organogenesis and even embryogenesis, DNA methylation and histone modifications occur at a high rate and in a dynamic fashion. It is thought that this plasticity affords opportunities for modifying epigenetic programming in response to environmental cues, including energy balance and dietary exposures, and thus can modulate the effect of diet on cancer later in life.

Prenatal exposure to severe energy restriction seems to influence cancer risk, although evidence is inconclusive. For instance, while women born during the Dutch famine in World War II had a higher risk of breast cancer, those exposed to the famine in Norway had a lower risk of the disease. However, the two famine conditions are, in a way, different as the Dutch famine was more severe and ended more abruptly than the Norwegian famine, which may have had an influence on future cancer risk (Lillycrop and Burdge, 2014). Birth weight, an indirect measure of the prenatal nutritional environment of the individual, was also investigated in relation to cancer risk. High birth weight was found to be associated with an increased *in utero* concentration of growth factors and hormones, including oestrogens, insulin, IGF-I, leptin and adiponectin (Delvaux *et al.*,

2003; Sivan *et al.*, 2003; Troisi *et al.*, 2003; Vatten *et al.*, 2005). Such an environment seems to predispose the individual to various cancers, including premenopausal breast cancer in women (Michels and Xue, 2006; Xu *et al.*, 2009; WCRF/AICR, 2010). On the other hand, low birth weight was associated with maternal under-nutrition, which is hypothesised to reprogramme the epigenome to adapt to an environment with little nourishment. When in a nutrient-rich environment later in life, accelerated growth may take place (Walker and Ho, 2012). This catch-up growth pattern is associated with higher levels of hormones and growth factors similar to those observed in high birth weight children (Park, 2005), predisposing the individual to obesity, diabetes and various cancers in adulthood (Walker and Ho, 2012).

In addition to energy balance, intake of specific foods by the mother may cause epigenetic alterations in the offspring, hence affecting cancer risk later in life. For instance, phytoestrogens, such as the soy isoflavone genistein, are suspected to increase the risk of hor-mone-related cancer in woman. Animal studies have shown that prenatal exposure of genistein in female mice fetuses (gestational age of 1–5 days) resulted in hypomethylation of the *Nsbp1* gene promoter region. After reaching puberty, where high concentrations of circulating oestrogen levels activate the *Nsbp1* gene, mice exposed prenatally to phytoestrogens were hyperrespon-sive to circulating hormone levels. This increased their risk of uterine tumours relative to the control mice (Tang *et al.*, 2008). This effect of phytoestrogen is reversed should exposure take place during the postnatal period (as discussed earlier in this section).

In summary, prenatal, childhood and adolescent energy balance and diet are increasingly implicated in the risk of cancer, particularly hormone-related cancers, later in life. Their effect seems to be mediated via metabolic and epigenetic adjustments to nutritionally unfavourable conditions. The contribution of develop-mental reprogramming to the risk of cancers that are not hormonally regulated is currently mostly unknown.

19.5 Gut microbiota as a modulator of the effect of diet on cancer risk

The gut microbiota, also called the 'forgotten organ' (O'Hara and Shanahan, 2006), outnumber human cells tenfold (Khan *et al.*, 2012) and are most abundant in the colon (He *et al.*, 2013). Gut microbiota play many key roles in maintaining the health of the colon and the rest of the body – including harvesting nutrients and energy that would otherwise be inaccessible – and inhibiting the growth of pathogens in the colon (Matsuki and Tanaka,

2014). Recently, new evidence shows that the gut micro-biota may have a role in modulating the cancer-promot-ing or cancer-inhibiting behaviour of dietary constituents, namely CHOs, proteins, fats, alcohol and phytoestrogens.

Carbohydrates

DFs are the main form of CHOs reaching the colon and include resistant starches, non-starch polysaccharides and oligosaccharides (Scott *et al.*, 2013). DF constitutes the main energy source for gut microbiota and has the largest impact on the profile and metabolic activity of the gut microbiota. A diet high in DF increases the growth of healthy gut microbiota (Zeng *et al.*, 2014) and therefore limits the growth of pathogens by increasing demand on colonic attachment sites and nutrients, including dietary amino acids, needed for cellular growth (Hullar *et al.*, 2014).

The fermentation of DFs results in the production of biomass, lower colonic pH and the production of SCFAs (Gibson and Macfarlane, 1995; Zeng *et al.*, 2014). The production of biomass increases the faecal bulk and viscosity, resulting in a decreased colonic transit time, which in turn dilutes and reduces the exposure time of carcinogens in the colon (Lattimer and Haub, 2010; Macfarlane and Macfarlane, 2012). The lower colonic pH from fibre fermentation inhibits several carcinogenic metabolic processes (Section 19.5: 'Protein' and 'Fat') and inhibits the growth of patho-gens (Nicholson *et al.*, 2012). SCFAs, consisting of butyrate, propionate and acetate (Gibson and Macfar-lane, 1995; Zeng *et al.*, 2014), are the preferred energy source for colonocytes and play an important role in gut microbiota and colonic health. SCFAs were shown to have strong anticancer properties, including the inhibition of chronic inflammation, inhibition of can-cer cell migration and invasion, and the enhancement of cancer cell cycle arrest and apoptosis (Macfarlane and Macfarlane, 2011; Zeng *et al.*, 2014).

With respect to specific cancers, the evidence for the anticancer effect of DF is most convincing for colorectal cancers (WCRF/AICR, 2007, 2011). Recent studies suggest a preventive effect of the DF for breast cancer risk. DF reduces the level of free oestrogens in the circulation by directly binding to oestrogens and also indirectly by promoting the growth of bifidobacteria, which convert oestrogens to phytoestrogens (Adler-creutz, 2007; Wang *et al.*, 2010). Based on epidemio-logic studies (Milder *et al.*, 2007; Ward and Kuhnle, 2010), high serum concentrations of phytoestrogens are negatively associated with breast cancer risk. Further-more, DFs are rich sources of cancer-preventive vita-mins, minerals and phytochemicals (Section 19.2:

'Fibre' and 'Micronutrients') which are made accessible to humans by the gut microbiota (Liu, 2003; Stevenson *et al.*, 2012; Zeng *et al.*, 2014).

Protein

Around 10% of ingested protein reaches the colon, where it undergoes bacterial fermentation and decomposition (Walker *et al.*, 2005), resulting in branched-chain fatty acids, phenols, indoles, ammonia, amines and sulphides (Hamer *et al.*, 2012), in addition to similar products as CHO fermentation (SCFAs, biomass, gas). The ammonia, amines and sulphides produced by protein fermentation have been investigated for their potential role in cancer risk, as will be discussed shortly.

Most ammonia produced in the colon is rapidly absorbed and metabolised into urea by the liver (Scott *et al.*, 2013). However, some of this ammonia remains in the colon and may act as a tumour promoter by altering the morphology of the intestinal tissues (Scott *et al.*, 2013). Among amines, polyamine produced from the fermentation of amino acid ornithine can be oxidised to form ROS, which are pro-inflammatory. Gut microbiota plays an essential role in *N*-nitrosation, where amines, amides, nitrates and nitrites are metabolised to carcinogenic NOCs (Catsburg *et al.*, 2014b). NOCs induce mutations by forming DNA adducts (Hullar *et al.*, 2014). Some dietary factors can promote or inhibit *N*-nitrosation. For instance, red and especially processed meats tend to result in a higher faecal NOC concentration than other source of dietary proteins. Haem iron, which is rich in red meat and many processed meats, is suspected to act as a catalyst in *N*-nitration. Furthermore, nitrate and nitrite, often used as salts for processing meat, are substrates in *N*-nitration. On the other hand, consumption of soy has shown to have a strong inhibitory effect on NOC production. While many plant-based foods are also rich sources of nitrate and nitrite, vitamins C and E and some polyphenols in the plant counteract this effect (to a certain extent) by inhibiting *N*-nitration (Hughes *et al.*, 2002). Sulphated amino acids and inorganic sulphur from water and processed food reaching the colon are metabolised by the sulphur-reducing bacteria to yield the highly cytotoxic and genotoxic hydrogen sulphide. Hydrogen sulphide inhibits respiration by the mitochondria in the colon cells, thus reducing energy harvest. This undermines the colonic cell roles of mucus production, ion absorption and cellular detoxification (Hullar *et al.*, 2014). Furthermore, hydrogen sulphide damages DNA directly (Attene-Ramos *et al.*, 2006), alters cell proliferation (Deplancke and Gaskins, 2003), stimulates the production of ROS and promotes chronic inflammation in the colon (Fiorucci *et al.*, 2006).

DF has multiple effects on reducing protein fermentation, and hence the production of its associated carcinogens. First, protein fermentation is reduced by the lower pH, resulting from fibre fermentation, possibly by inhibiting the bacterial growth and/or metabolic functions involved in protein fermentation. Second, the increased bacterial growth associated with DF results in greater demand on amino acids for biosynthesis. Third, decreased transit time results in some dietary proteins being excreted before their full fermentation.

Fat

The majority of dietary fat ingested is absorbed in the small intestine and undergoes enterohepatic circulation in the presence of bile fluids which act as emulsifiers (Yokota *et al.*, 2012). While most of the bile fluids (around 95%) are recycled in the ileum, 5% escape into the large intestine and are then converted by anaerobic bacteria to secondary bile acids (SBAs), including deoxycholic acid (DCA) (Reddy, 1981; Hullar *et al.*, 2014). SBAs promote tumour formation and are associated with increased colon cancer risk (McGarr *et al.*, 2005). DCA has been shown to alter the epigenetic mechanisms responsible for tumour suppression and regulation of cell growth in the colon (Hague *et al.*, 1995; Hullar *et al.*, 2014). Furthermore, DCA has strong antibacterial properties, which reduce the biodiversity and cell density of the gut microbiota. Bacteria in the gut microbiota have different levels of tolerance to DCA, resulting in selective pressure on the gut microbial community. For instance, *Escherichia coli*, a carcinogenic pathogen, is resistant to the antimicrobial effects of DCA, giving it advantage over healthy gut microbiota, which are inhibited by DCA. The associations between the gut microbiota and DCA concentration in the colon were confirmed in animal studies where rats were administered cholic acid (cholic acid is converted to DCA in the gut) (Islam *et al.*, 2011).

Overall, lower consumption of dietary fat is recommended to reduce the concentration of SBAs in the colon in order to maintain healthy gut microbiota and reduce the risk of colon cancer. The production of SBAs can also be reduced by an increased consumption of DF, which lowers the colonic pH. Bile fluids are less soluble at low pH, resulting in less conversion of bile fluids to SBAs (Windey *et al.*, 2012; Wong *et al.*, 2006).

Phytochemicals

The literature supports a cancer protective role for many of the identified phytochemicals, as discussed in Section

19.2: 'Micronutrients'. Gut microbiota release many of these phytochemicals from plant material (mostly fibre) and often metabolise them to forms which can be absorbed and used by the host (Bosscher *et al.*, 2009; Crozier *et al.*, 2010). The metabolism of phytochemicals to more bioactive forms has been well documented in the conversion of isoflavone daidzein (found in soy) to equol and of glucosinolates (found in cruciferous vegetables) to isothiocyanates, both of which have more potent anticancer properties than their precursors (Navarro *et al.*, 2011; Hullar *et al.*, 2014). Equol has strong antioxidant and oestrogenic properties and is associated with reducing breast and prostate cancer risk (Hullar *et al.*, 2014). Isothiocyanates' anticancer properties include inducing apoptosis, causing cell cycle arrest and inhibiting angiogenesis (Molina-Vargas, 2013; Hullar *et al.*, 2014). Phytochemicals can also play a role in modulating the gut microbial profile through antimicrobial effects observed in many polyphenols in vitro (Puupponen-Pimiä *et al.*, 2001, 2005; Vaquero *et al.*, 2007; Selma *et al.*, 2009; Duda-Chodak, 2012). In vivo, however, the effects of dietary polyphenols and other phytochemicals on the gut microbiota are difficult to isolate from the effect of fibre, which also comes in high concentrations in foods with phytochemicals (He *et al.*, 2013).

Alcohol

While moderate alcohol consumption has not been shown to affect the gut microbiota in healthy individuals, studies have shown that excess alcohol consumption leads to abnormal gut microbiota and bacterial overgrowth (Yan *et al.*, 2011). This can initiate or worsen the impaired gut barrier function ('leaky gut') that is characteristic of excess alcohol consumption (Hartmann *et al.*, 2012). Chronic alcohol consumption alters the metabolism of the gut microbiota, producing endotoxins and pro-inflammatory factors (Mutlu *et al.*, 2012). Furthermore, chronic alcohol consumption increases faecal pH (Bull-Otterson *et al.*, 2013), which in turn could alter the gut microbiota profile and promote some carcinogenic processes which are pH dependent (Section 19.5: 'Protein' and 'Fat').

19.6 Dietary recommendations

Though many of the associations between dietary intake and the risk of the disease are still controversial, a few scientific and public health associations have released guidelines to advise health-care professionals, policy makers, and the general public about dietary and other lifestyle practices that reduce cancer risk. This section

presents an overview for the guidelines of the ACS, the WCRF/AICR, the European Code Against Cancer (ECAC) and the WHO (WHO, 2002; Boyle *et al.*, 2003; WCRF/AICR, 2007; Kushi *et al.*, 2012) summarised in Table 19.1.

Common to all four guidelines are recommendations regarding weight, physical activity, alcohol consumption, animal- and plant-based food consumption. With different wordings, it was advised to keep the weight within the healthy range, be physically active, limit alcohol consumption, limit intake of processed and red meat, and increase intake of fruits and vegetables ($\geq$400 g/day vegetables and fruits). In line with maintaining a healthy weight, the WCRF/AICR (2007) added a specific recommendation to limit the intake of energy-dense foods and to avoid sugary drinks. The ACS (Kushi *et al.*, 2012) and WCRF/AICR (2007) both encouraged the consumption of unprocessed and whole grains. Furthermore, both the WCRF/AICR (2007) and WHO (2002) guidelines included limiting sodium intake to moderate level. Recommendations regarding dietary supplements and breastfeeding were exclusive to the WCRF/AICR (2007) guidelines. Consumption of dietary supplements was not recommended for cancer prevention, and efforts should be made to meet nutritional needs through dietary intake. Exclusive breastfeeding for a period of 6 months was encouraged for its benefits for both mothers and children.

Rigorous evidence supports the association between adherence to dietary cancer prevention guidelines and reduced cancer risk and mortality (Cerhan *et al.*, 2004; Catsburg *et al.*, 2014a; Hastert *et al.*, 2014); however, the prevalence of adherence to these guidelines remains of major public health concern. In fact, a study on compliance with dietary and lifestyle guidelines for cancer prevention in population samples of Europeans and Mesoamericans showed that overall compliance with the WCRF/AICR was low in all samples, with 28%, 63%, 77% and 81% of subjects adhering to at least half of the selected recommendation components in the Netherlands, Scotland, Mexico and Guatemala respectively (Vossenaar *et al.*, 2011). Similarly low adherence rates to the WCRF/AICR (2007) cancer prevention guidelines were observed across 18 countries in Africa, with particularly low adherence to the nutrition, physical activity and weight status recommendations (Akinyemiju *et al.*, 2014). Future research is needed to further investigate adherence to guidelines and its determinants in other populations, mainly populations with increasing trend in cancer prevalence. The observed poor adherence to cancer prevention guidelines raises important concerns that ought to be addressed at the levels of the individual, the practitioner, the community and policy makers.

Table 19.1 A summary of four main cancer prevention guidelines.

Category	ACS[a]	WCRF/AICR[b]	ECAC[c]	WHO[d]
Weight (BMI)	'Achieve and maintain a healthy weight throughout life' (BMI: 18.5 to <25.0 kg/m²)	'Be as lean as possible within the normal range of body weight' (BMI: 18.5 to <25.0 kg/m²)	'Avoid obesity'	'Maintain BMI in range of 18.5 to 25 kg/m², and avoid weight gain' (BMI: 18.5 to <25.0 kg/m²)
Physical activity	'Adopt a physically active lifestyle' (≥150 min/week moderate or ≥75 min/week vigorous-intensity physical activity)	'Be physically active as part of everyday life' (≥30 min/day moderate intensity physical activity)	'Undertake some brisk, physical activity every day'	'Engage in regular physical activity'
Alcohol	'If you drink alcoholic beverages, limit consumption' (≤1 drink/day)[e]	'Limit alcoholic drinks' (≤1 drink/day for women, ≤2 drinks/day for men)[e]	'If you drink alcohol, . . . moderate your consumption . . . ' (≤1 drink/day for women, ≤2 drinks/day for men)[e]	'Consumption of alcoholic beverages is not recommended' (≤2 drinks/day)[e]
Animal foods	'Limit consumption of processed meat and red meat'	'Limit intake of red meat and avoid processed meat.' (<500 g/week red meat)	'Limit your intake of foods containing fats from animal sources'	'Those who are not vegetarian are advised to moderate consumption of preserved meat and red meat'
Vegetable and fruit	'Eat at least 2.5 cups of vegetables and fruits each day' (≥400 g/day vegetables and fruits)	'Eat mostly foods of plant origin. Eat . . . a variety of non-starchy vegetables and of fruits every day' (≥400 g/day vegetables and fruits)	'Increase your daily intake and variety of vegetables and fruits' (≥400 g/day vegetables and fruits)	'Have a diet which includes at least 400 g/day of fruit and vegetables' (≥400 g/day vegetables and fruits)
Whole grain	'Choose whole grains instead of refined grain products'	'Eat relatively unprocessed cereals (grains) and/or pulses (legumes) with every meal. Limit refined starchy foods' (≥25 g non-starch polysaccharides)	N/A	N/A
Sodium intake	N/A	'Limit consumption of salt' (<6 g salt/day, <2.4 g sodium/day)	N/A	'Overall consumption of salt-preserved foods and salt should be moderate'
Dietary supplements	N/A	'Aim to meet nutritional needs through diet alone. Dietary supplements are not recommended for cancer prevention'	N/A	N/A
Breastfeeding	N/A	'Mothers to breastfeed; children to be breastfed' (age 0–6 months: exclusive breastfeeding)	N/A	N/A
Energy density	N/A	'Limit consumption of energy-dense foods. Avoid sugary drinks'	N/A	N/A

[a] Kushi et al. (2012).
[b] WCRF/AICR (2007).
[c] Boyle et al. (2003).
[d] WHO (2002).
[e] Drink is equivalent to 10 g ethanol.

19.7 Future research directions

The last couple of decades have witnessed major advances in understanding diet–cancer association, with evidence from epidemiological and clinical studies suggesting that diet may be associated with both increases and reductions of cancer risk. However, such associations are not conclusively resolved. Major impediments to diet and cancer research include the complex nature of dietary exposures and the scarcity of objective measures of dietary intake (biomarkers). Furthermore, the mechanisms of action of certain dietary components, the dosages of intake and the period in the life cycle that affect cancer risk remain to be elucidated. The following contains a brief description of the main research challenges and directions proposed in the field of diet and cancer.

Dietary intake assessment constitutes a considerable challenge for nutrition research in the 21st century. Many methods are proposed to assess dietary intake, including food frequency questionnaires, diet records and multiple 24-h dietary recalls. However, these methods are limited by their subjectivity, reliance on memory and lack of accuracy, in addition to being subject to unknown degrees of reporting bias. New studies are required to improve the existing dietary intake assessment tools and the methods for defining dietary intake, whether in terms of nutrients, foods, food groups or dietary patterns. With such limitations in dietary assessment, the identification of objective biomarkers of dietary intake becomes crucial for the advancement of the field, especially biomarkers for foods and nutrients that are postulated to affect cancer risk, such as fruits and vegetables. Biomarkers are needed not only to better assess exposure but also to indicate outcome (cancer), as the time required for tumour development presents another challenge in this field. Major cancers take years to develop, and prevention approaches are difficult to follow for longer periods. Maintaining strict dietary regimens for long periods is also difficult. A proper prevention trial can be lengthy and very expensive. Furthermore, for randomised clinical trials, a large number of participants is needed to reach statistically significant findings (the percentage of cases who develop cancer from a pool of undiagnosed participants). Studying high-risk populations is not optimal for prevention trials because of the possibility that some participants may already have developed cancer. Therefore, the identification of cancer biomarkers or precursor lesions that express early during cancer development is important for nutritional epidemiologic studies to develop intervention studies and to control cancer by evaluating biomarker profiles (Verma, 2013). In addition, there is a need for well-designed cohort studies linking with the identified

biomarkers to cancer risk as well as for controlled nutrition intervention trials to compare change in biomarker concentrations from baseline with the several follow-up time points in exposed individuals versus the control group. These studies can give answers for many basic questions, like what are the optimal dosages that may lead to cancer prevention, whether impact of a certain dietary component depends on cancer subtype, and at what age consumption is most impactful. The latter issue regarding critical times for exposure, whether during fetal development, throughout a lifespan or during ageing, has topped cancer research agendas specifically, with increasing evidence pointing to exposures in the first 1000 days of life, including *in utero*, as a significant determinant in disease risk.

An important aspect of diet and cancer research is the generation of mechanistic evidence to support associations. This aspect is paramount to establishing causality and ultimately to develop strategies for cancer prevention. Examples of associations lacking clear and definite mechanistic validation were discussed in earlier sections of this chapter, mainly related to the observed effect of obesity, physical activity, various fatty acids, alcohol, phytochemicals (cocoa), and so on. It is important to note, however, that the recent advances in the field of epigenetics constitute a quantum leap in the understanding of mechanistic pathways of diet–cancer associations, thus creating a promising research terrain for the exploration of these associations. Future studies addressing the effects of dietary compounds in animal models of human disease as well as in humans are warranted. Important factors that should be determined include the optimal dose and timing of exposure to attain cancer-preventive epigenetic effects. The duration and specificity of epigenetic modulation by these dietary agents are also important topics in nutritional epigenomics and cancer research. In addition to epigenetics, the gut microbiome is another promising mediator of the effect of diet on cancer risk. Future research is needed to elucidate more clearly the exact impact of the selection of different diets on qualitative changes in the gut microbiota. In addition, it is important to characterise the metabolic activity of the gut microbiota and its effects on the host immune function and metabolism.

Recently, there has been an increasing inclination towards international collaborations to study diet–cancer association. This approach is advantageous as it encompasses countries from different 'diet/lifestyle zones' of the world and with varying cancer disease profiles. Hence, differences and similarities in dietary practices and lifestyle behaviours can be explored across cultures, and the effects of societal beliefs and practices can be examined. For instance, EPIC is an international collaboration between 23 centres from 10 European countries. It is a multicentre prospective study aimed at investigating the relationships between diet, lifestyle, genetic and environmental factors and the incidence of cancer. Another example illustrating the trend in global strategies to address diet cancer associations is the International Breast Cancer and Nutrition (IBCN) initiative. The latter gathers scientists and clinicians from different backgrounds and world regions. It represents a global endeavour that will not only bring the diversity necessary to pinpoint important diet–gene relationships, but will also provide momentum to develop the models, detection and assessment tools, and funding and public policy framework necessary to advance primary prevention research for the benefit of all populations affected by breast cancer. The IBCN paradigm can be adapted to understanding diet–gene relationships for other cancers as well as other chronic diseases. The results of the international endeavours are anticipated to make significant contributions to the already accumulated evidence, and in combination with data from other prospective studies as well as from studies using biomarkers, they will provide the scientific knowledge for appropriate public health policies and strategies aimed at reducing the global burden of cancer.

Acknowledgements

We would like to thank Bayan Rafii for her assistance in the literature review and referencing of this chapter.

References

Abnet, C.C., Qiao, Y.-L., Dawsey, S.M. et al. (2003) Prospective study of serum retinol, β-carotene, β-cryptoxanthin, and lutein/zeaxanthin and esophageal and gastric cancers in China. Cancer Causes & Control, 14, 645–655.

Adlercreutz, H. (2007) Lignans and human health. Critical Reviews in Clinical Laboratory Sciences, 44, 483–525.

Adlercreutz, H., Hämäläinen, E., Gorbach, S. et al. (1987) Association of diet and sex hormones in relation to breast cancer. European Journal of Cancer and Clinical Oncology, 23, 1725–1726.

Aiub, C.A.F., Pinto, L.F.R. and Felzenszwalb, I. (2009) DNA-repair genes and vitamin E in the prevention of N-nitrosodiethylamine mutagenicity. Cell Biology and Toxicology, 25, 393–402.

Akinyemiju, T.F., McDonald, J.A., Tsui, J. and Greenlee, H. (2014) Adherence to cancer prevention guidelines in 18 African countries. PloS One, 9 (8), e105209.

Albanes, D. (1999) β-Carotene and lung cancer: a case study. The American Journal of Clinical Nutrition, 69, 1345s–1350s.

Albanes, D., Blair, A. and Taylor, P.R. (1989) Physical activity and risk of cancer in the NHANES I population. American Journal of Public Health, 79, 744–750.

Alberti, K.G.M.M. and Zimmet, P. (1998) Definition, diagnosis and classification of diabetes mellitus and its complications. Part 1: diagnosis and classification of diabetes mellitus. Provisional report of a WHO consultation. Diabetic Medicine, 15, 539–553.

Albuquerque, R.C., Baltar, V.T. and Marchioni, D.M. (2014) Breast cancer and dietary patterns: a systematic review. Nutrition Reviews, 72, 1–17.

Alexander, D. and Cushing, C. (2011) Red meat and colorectal cancer: a critical summary of prospective epidemiologic studies. Obesity Reviews, 12, e472–e493.

Alexander, D.D., Miller, A.J., Cushing, C.A. and Lowe, K.A. (2010) Processed meat and colorectal cancer: a quantitative review of prospective epidemiologic studies. European Journal of Cancer Prevention, 19, 328–341.

Althuis, M.D., Fergenbaum, J.H., Garcia-Closas, M. et al. (2004) Etiology of hormone receptor-defined breast cancer: a systematic review of the literature. Cancer Epidemiology, Biomarkers & Prevention, 13, 1558–1568.

Ames, B.N. and Wakimoto, P. (2002) Are vitamin and mineral deficiencies a major cancer risk? Nature Reviews: Cancer, 2, 694–704.

Anand, P., Kunnumakara, A.B., Sundaram, C. et al. (2008) Cancer is a preventable disease that requires major lifestyle changes. Pharmaceutical Research, 25, 2097–2116.

Anderson, J.W., Baird, P., Davis Jr, R.H. et al. (2009) Health benefits of dietary fiber. Nutrition Reviews, 67, 188–205.

Appel, L.J., Moore, T.J., Obarzanek, E. et al. (1997) A clinical trial of the effects of dietary patterns on blood pressure. The New England Journal of Medicine, 336, 1117–1124.

Aschebrook-Kilfoy, B., Cross, A.J., Stolzenberg-Solomon, R.Z. et al. (2011) Pancreatic cancer and exposure to dietary nitrate and nitrite in the NIH–AARP Diet and Health Study. American Journal of Epidemiology, 174 (3), 305–315.

Attene-Ramos, M.S., Wagner, E.D., Plewa, M.J. and Gaskins, H.R. (2006) Evidence that hydrogen sulfide is a genotoxic agent. Molecular Cancer Research: MCR, 4, 9–14.

Augustin, L., Franceschi, S., Jenkins, D. et al. (2002) Glycemic index in chronic disease: a review. European Journal of Clinical Nutrition, 56, 1049–1071.

Aune, D., Lau, R., Chan, D.S.M. et al. (2011) Nonlinear reduction in risk for colorectal cancer by fruit and vegetable intake based on meta-analysis of prospective studies. Gastroenterology, 141, 106–118.

Aune, D., Chan, D.S., Vieira, A.R. et al. (2012a) Dietary fructose, carbohydrates, glycemic indices and pancreatic cancer risk: a systematic review and meta-analysis of cohort studies. Annals of Oncology, 23, 2536–2546.

Aune, D., Chan, D.S.M., Lau, R. et al. (2012b) Carbohydrates, glycemic index, glycemic load, and colorectal cancer risk: a systematic review and meta-analysis of cohort studies. Cancer Causes & Control, 23, 521–535.

Aune, D., Chan, D.S.M., Vieira, A.R. et al. (2012c) Fruits, vegetables and breast cancer risk: a systematic review and meta-analysis of prospective studies. Breast Cancer Research and Treatment, 134, 479–493.

Aune, D., Lau, R., Chan, D. et al. (2012d) Dairy products and colorectal cancer risk: a systematic review and meta-analysis of cohort studies. Annals of Oncology, 23, 37–45.

Azrad, M., Turgeon, C. and Demark-Wahnefried, W. (2013) Current evidence linking polyunsaturated fatty acids with cancer risk and progression. Frontiers in Oncology, 3, 224.

Bach, A., Serra-Majem, L., Carrasco, J.L. et al. (2006) The use of indexes evaluating the adherence to the Mediterranean diet in epidemiological studies: a review. Public Health Nutrition, 9, 132–146.

Bagnardi, V., Rota, M., Botteri, E. et al. (2013) Light alcohol drinking and cancer: a meta-analysis. Annals of Oncology, 24, 301–308.

Banerjee, S., Li, Y., Wang, Z. and Sarkar, F.H. (2008) Multi-targeted therapy of cancer by genistein. Cancer Letters, 269, 226–242.

Barclay, A.W., Petocz, P., McMillan-Price, J. *et al.* (2008) Glycemic index, glycemic load, and chronic disease risk – a meta-analysis of observational studies. *The American Journal of Clinical Nutrition*, **87**, 627–637.

Barker, D.J., Osmond, C., Thornburg, K.L. *et al.* (2008) A possible link between the pubertal growth of girls and ovarian cancer in their daughters. *American Journal of Human Biology*, **20**, 659–662.

Basu, A. and Imrhan, V. (2006) Tomatoes versus lycopene in oxidative stress and carcinogenesis: conclusions from clinical trials. *European Journal of Clinical Nutrition*, **61**, 295–303.

Baylin, S.B. and Ohm, J.E. (2006) Epigenetic gene silencing in cancer – a mechanism for early oncogenic pathway addiction? *Nature Reviews: Cancer*, **6**, 107–116.

Bell, C. and Hawthorne, S. (2008) Ellagic acid, pomegranate and prostate cancer – a mini review. *The Journal of Pharmacy and Pharmacology*, **60**, 139–144.

Berkey, C.S., Frazier, A.L., Gardner, J.D. and Colditz, G.A. (1999) Adolescence and breast carcinoma risk. *Cancer*, **85**, 2400–2409.

Berkey, C.S., Gardner, J.D., Frazier, A.L. and Colditz, G.A. (2000) Relation of childhood diet and body size to menarche and adolescent growth in girls. *American Journal of Epidemiology*, **152**, 446–452.

Bertuccio, P., Rosato, V., Andreano, A. *et al.* (2013) Dietary patterns and gastric cancer risk: a systematic review and meta-analysis. *Annals of Oncology*, **24**, 1450–1458.

Bhupathiraju, S.N. and Tucker, K.L. (2011) Coronary heart disease prevention: nutrients, foods, and dietary patterns. *Clinica Chimica Acta*, **412**, 1493–1514.

Bingham, S., Luben, R., Welch, A. *et al.* (2008) Associations between dietary methods and biomarkers, and between fruits and vegetables and risk of ischaemic heart disease, in the EPIC Norfolk Cohort Study. *International Journal of Cancer*, **37**, 978–987.

Bingham, S.A., Luben, R., Welch, A. *et al.* (2003) Are imprecise methods obscuring a relation between fat and breast cancer? *The Lancet*, **362**, 212–214.

Bishayee, A. (2009) Cancer prevention and treatment with resveratrol: from rodent studies to clinical trials. *Cancer Prevention Research*, **2**, 409–418.

Blair, S.N., Kohl, H.W., Paffenbarger, R.S. *et al.* (1989) Physical fitness and all-cause mortality: a prospective study of healthy men and women. *JAMA*, **262**, 2395–2401.

Block, G., Patterson, B. and Subar, A. (1992) Fruit, vegetables, and cancer prevention: a review of the epidemiological evidence. *Nutrition and Cancer*, **18**, 1–29.

Boffetta, P. and Hashibe, M. (2006) Alcohol and cancer. *The Lancet Oncology*, **7**, 149–156.

Boivin, D., Lamy, S., Lord-Dufour, S. *et al.* (2009) Antiproliferative and antioxidant activities of common vegetables: a comparative study. *Food Chemistry*, **112**, 374–380.

Bosscher, D., Breynaert, A., Pieters, L. and Hermans, N. (2009) Food-based strategies to modulate the composition of the intestinal microbiota and their associated health effects. *Journal of Physiology and Pharmacology*, **60**, 5–11.

Boyle, P., Autier, P., Bartelink, H. *et al.* (2003) European Code Against Cancer and scientific justification: third version (2003). *Annals of Oncology*, **14**, 973–1005.

Brand-Miller, J., Hayne, S., Petocz, P. and Colagiuri, S. (2003) Low-glycemic index diets in the management of diabetes: a meta-analysis of randomized controlled trials. *Diabetes Care*, **26**, 2261–2267.

Brennan, S.F., Cantwell, M.M., Cardwell, C.R. *et al.* (2010) Dietary patterns and breast cancer risk: a systematic review and meta-analysis. *The American Journal of Clinical Nutrition*, **91**, 1294–1302.

Brooks, P.J. and Zakhari, S. (2013) Moderate alcohol consumption and breast cancer in women: from epidemiology to mechanisms and interventions. *Alcoholism, Clinical and Experimental Research*, **37**, 23–30.

Bruning, P.F. and Bonfrèr, J.M. (1986) Free fatty acid concentrations correlated with the available fraction of estradiol in human plasma. *Cancer Research*, **46**, 2606–2609.

Bull-Otterson, L., Feng, W., Kirpich, I. *et al.* (2013) Metagenomic analyses of alcohol induced pathogenic alterations in the intestinal microbiome and the effect of *Lactobacillus rhamnosus* GG treatment. *PloS One*, **8** (1), e53028.

Butterworth, C., Hatch, K.D., Gore, H. *et al.* (1982) Improvement in cervical dysplasia associated with folic acid therapy in users of oral contraceptives. *The American Journal of Clinical Nutrition*, **35**, 73–82.

Calin, G.A., Sevignani, C., Dumitru, C.D. *et al.* (2004) Human micro-RNA genes are frequently located at fragile sites and genomic regions involved in cancers. *Proceedings of the National Academy of Sciences of the United States of America*, **101**, 2999–3004.

Calle, E.E. and Kaaks, R. (2004) Overweight, obesity and cancer: epidemiological evidence and proposed mechanisms. *Nature Reviews: Cancer*, **4**, 579–591.

Calle, E.E., Rodriguez, C., Walker-Thurmond, K. and Thun, M.J. (2003) Overweight, obesity, and mortality from cancer in a prospectively studied cohort of US adults. *The New England Journal of Medicine*, **348**, 1625–1638.

Cao, Y. and Cao, R. (1999) Angiogenesis inhibited by drinking tea. *Nature*, **398**, 381.

Carter, J.C. and Church, F.C. (2009) Obesity and breast cancer: the roles of peroxisome proliferator-activated receptor-γ and plasminogen activator inhibitor-1. *PPAR Research*, **2009**, 345320.

Catsburg, C., Miller, A.B. and Rohan, T.E. (2014a) Adherence to cancer prevention guidelines and risk of breast cancer. *International Journal of Cancer*, **135**, 2444–2452.

Catsburg, C.E., Gago-Dominguez, M., Yuan, J.M. *et al.* (2014b) Dietary sources of *N*-nitroso compounds and bladder cancer risk: findings from the Los Angeles Bladder Cancer Study. *International Journal of Cancer*, **134**, 125–135.

Cerhan, J.R., Potter, J.D., Gilmore, J.M. *et al.* (2004) Adherence to the AICR cancer prevention recommendations and subsequent morbidity and mortality in the Iowa Women's Health Study cohort. *Cancer Epidemiology, Biomarkers & Prevention*, **13**, 1114–1120.

Chagas, C.E.A., Bassoli, B.K., De Souza, C.A.S. *et al.* (2011) Folic acid supplementation during early hepatocarcinogenesis: cellular and molecular effects. *International Journal of Cancer*, **129**, 2073–2082.

Chajès, V. and Romieu, I. (2014) Nutrition and breast cancer. *Maturitas*, **77**, 7–11.

Chang, S., Hursting, S.D., Contois, J.H. *et al.* (2001) Leptin and prostate cancer. *Prostate*, **46**, 62–67.

Chen, J. and Xu, X. (2010) Diet, epigenetic, and cancer prevention. *Advances in Genetics*, **71**, 237–255.

Cheng, G., Remer, T., Prinz-Langenohl, R. *et al.* (2010) Relation of isoflavones and fiber intake in childhood to the timing of puberty. *The American Journal of Clinical Nutrition*, **92**, 556–564.

Cheng, G., Buyken, A.E., Shi, L. *et al.* (2012) Beyond overweight: nutrition as an important lifestyle factor influencing timing of puberty. *Nutrition Reviews*, **70**, 133–152.

Cho, E., Smith-Warner, S.A., Spiegelman, D. *et al.* (2004) Dairy foods, calcium, and colorectal cancer: a pooled analysis of 10 cohort studies. *Journal of the National Cancer Institute*, **96**, 1015–1022.

Choi, H.K., Yang, J.W. and Kang, K.W. (2006) Bifunctional effect of resveratrol on the expression of *ErbB2* in human breast cancer cell. *Cancer Letters*, **242**, 198–206.

Choi, S.-W., Stickel, F., Baik, H.W. *et al.* (1999) Chronic alcohol consumption induces genomic but not p53-specific DNA hypomethylation in rat colon. *The Journal of Nutrition*, **129**, 1945–1950.

Choi, Y., Giovannucci, E. and Lee, J.E. (2012) Glycaemic index and glycaemic load in relation to risk of diabetes-related cancers: a meta-analysis. *British Journal of Nutrition*, **108**, 1934–1947.

Chung, M., Balk, E.M., Brendel, M. *et al.* (2009) *Vitamin D and Calcium: A Systematic Review of Health Outcomes.* Evidence Report/Technology Assessment, no. 183. Agency for Healthcare Research and Quality, Rockville, MD. http://www.ahrq.gov/downloads/pub/evidence/pdf/vitadcal/vitadcal.pdf (accessed 13 December 2016).

Clague, J. and Bernstein, L. (2012) Physical activity and cancer. *Current Oncology Reports*, **14**, 550–558.

Cockbain, A., Toogood, G. and Hull, M. (2012) Omega-3 poly-unsaturated fatty acids for the treatment and prevention of colorectal cancer. *Gut*, **61**, 135–149.

Cohen, L.A., Boylan, E., Epstein, M. and Zang, E. (1992) Voluntary exercise and experimental mammary cancer. In M.M. Jacobs (ed.), *Exercise, Calories, Fat and Cancer.* Plenum Press, New York; pp. 41–59.

Colditz, G.A., Rosner, B.A., Chen, W.Y. *et al.* (2004) Risk factors for breast cancer according to estrogen and progesterone receptor status. *Journal of the National Cancer Institute*, **96**, 218–228.

Cole, B.F., Baron, J.A., Sandler, R.S. *et al.* (2007) Folic acid for the prevention of colorectal adenomas: a randomized clinical trial. *JAMA*, **297**, 2351–2359.

Coleman, H.G., Kitahara, C.M., Murray, L.J. *et al.* (2014) Dietary carbohydrate intake, glycemic index, and glycemic load and endometrial cancer risk: a prospective cohort study. *American Journal of Epidemiology*, **179**, 75–84.

Cook, R.T. (1998) Alcohol abuse, alcoholism, and damage to the immune system – a review. *Alcoholism, Clinical and Experimental Research*, **22**, 1927–1942.

Cotterchio, M., Boucher, B.A., Manno, M. *et al.* (2006) Dietary phytoestrogen intake is associated with reduced colorectal cancer risk. *The Journal of Nutrition*, **136**, 3046–3053.

Crozier, A., Del Rio, D. and Clifford, M.N. (2010) Bioavailability of dietary flavonoids and phenolic compounds. *Molecular Aspects of Medicine*, **31**, 446–467.

Csizmadi, I., Kelemen, L.E., Speidel, T. *et al.* (2014) Are physical activity levels linked to nutrient adequacy? *Implications for cancer risk. Nutrition and Cancer*, **66**, 214–224.

Cuomo, R., Andreozzi, P. and Zito, F.P. (2014) Alcoholic beverages and carbonated soft drinks: consumption and gastrointestinal cancer risks. In V. Zappia, S. Panico, G. L. Russo *et al.* (eds), *Advances in Nutrition and Cancer.* Cancer Treatment and Research 159. New York: Springer; pp. 97–120.

Danaei, G., Vander Hoorn, S., Lopez, A.D. *et al.* (2005) Causes of cancer in the world: comparative risk assessment of nine behavioural and environmental risk factors. *The Lancet*, **366**, 1784–1793.

Dashwood, R.H. and Ho, E. (2007) Dietary histone deacetylase inhibitors: from cells to mice to man. *Seminars in Cancer Biology*, **17** (5), 363–369.

Dashwood, R.H., Myzak, M.C. and Ho, E. (2006) Dietary HDAC inhibitors: time to rethink weak ligands in cancer chemoprevention? *Carcinogenesis*, **27**, 344–349.

Davis, C.D. and Uthus, E.O. (2004) DNA methylation, cancer susceptibility, and nutrient interactions. *Experimental Biology and Medicine*, **229**, 988–995.

Davis, C.D., Uthus, E.O. and Finley, J.W. (2000) Dietary selenium and arsenic affect DNA methylation in vitro in Caco-2 cells and in vivo in rat liver and colon. *The Journal of Nutrition*, **130**, 2903–2909.

Davis, C.D., Tsuji, P.A. and Milner, J.A. (2012) Selenoproteins and cancer prevention. *Annual Review of Nutrition*, **32**, 73–95.

Day, N., Wong, M., Bingham, S. *et al.* (2004) Correlated measurement error – implications for nutritional epidemiology. *International Journal of Epidemiology*, **33**, 1373–1381.

De Conti, A., Kuroiwa-Trzmielina, J., Horst, M.A. *et al.* (2012) Chemopreventive effects of the dietary histone deacetylase inhibitor tributyrin alone or in combination with vitamin A during the promotion phase of rat hepatocarcinogenesis. *Journal of Nutritional Biochemistry*, **23**, 860–866.

De Lorgeril, M., Salen, P., Martin, J.-L. *et al.* (1999) Mediterranean diet, traditional risk factors, and the rate of cardiovascular complications after myocardial infarction: final report of the Lyon Diet Heart Study. *Circulation*, **99**, 779–785.

De Ridder, C.M., Thijssen, J., van't Veer, P. *et al.* (1991) Dietary habits, sexual maturation, and plasma hormones in pubertal girls: a longitudinal study. *The American Journal of Clinical Nutrition*, **54**, 805–813.

De Stefani, E., Boffetta, P., Ronco, A.L. *et al.* (2008) Dietary patterns and risk of bladder cancer: a factor analysis in Uruguay. *Cancer Causes & Control*, **19**, 1243–1249.

Dekker, M.J., Su, Q., Baker, C. *et al.* (2010) Fructose: a highly lipogenic nutrient implicated in insulin resistance, hepatic steatosis, and the metabolic syndrome. *American Journal of Physiology. Endocrinology and Metabolism*, **299**, E685–E694.

Delvaux, T., Buekens, P., Thoumsin, H. *et al.* (2003) Cord C-peptide and insulin-like growth factor-I, birth weight, and placenta weight among North African and Belgian neonates. *American Journal of Obstetrics and Gynecology*, **189**, 1779–1784.

Dennert, G., Zwahlen, M., Brinkman, M. *et al.* (2011) Selenium for preventing cancer. *The Cochrane Database of Systematic Reviews*, (5) CD005195.

Deplancke, B. and Gaskins, H.R. (2003) Hydrogen sulfide induces serum-independent cell cycle entry in nontransformed rat intestinal epithelial cells. *FASEB Journal*, **17**, 1310–1312.

Di Croce, L., Raker, V.A., Corsaro, M. *et al.* (2002) Methyltransferase recruitment and DNA hypermethylation of target promoters by an oncogenic transcription factor. *Science*, **295**, 1079–1082.

Dirx, M.J., van den Brandt, P.A., Goldbohm, R.A. and Lumey, L. (2001) Energy restriction in childhood and adolescence and risk of prostate cancer: results from the Netherlands Cohort Study. *American Journal of Epidemiology*, **154**, 530–537.

Doi, A., Park, I.-H., Wen, B. *et al.* (2009) Differential methylation of tissue- and cancer-specific CpG island shores distinguishes human induced pluripotent stem cells, embryonic stem cells and fibroblasts. *Nature Genetics*, **41**, 1350–1353.

Dong, J.-Y. and Qin, L.-Q. (2011) Dietary glycemic index, glycemic load, and risk of breast cancer: meta-analysis of prospective cohort studies. *Breast Cancer Research and Treatment*, **126**, 287–294.

Dontas, A.S., Zerefos, N.S., Panagiotakos, D.B. and Valis, D.A. (2007) Mediterranean diet and prevention of coronary heart disease in the elderly. *Clinical Interventions in Aging*, **2**, 109–115.

Dorai, T. and Aggarwal, B.B. (2004) Role of chemopreventive agents in cancer therapy. *Cancer Letters*, **215**, 129–140.

Druesne-Pecollo, N., Pagniez, A., Thomas, M. *et al.* (2006) Diallyl disulfide increases CDKN1A promoter-associated histone acetylation in human colon tumor cell lines. *Journal of Agricultural and Food Chemistry*, **54**, 7503–7507.

Druesne-Pecollo, N., Tehard, B., Mallet, Y. *et al.* (2009) Alcohol and genetic polymorphisms: effect on risk of alcohol-related cancer. *The Lancet Oncology*, **10**, 173–180.

Duda-Chodak, A. (2012) The inhibitory effect of polyphenols on human gut microbiota. *Journal of Physiology and Pharmacology*, **63**, 497–503.

Duffield-Lillico, A., Dalkin, B., Reid, M. *et al.* (2003) Selenium supplementation, baseline plasma selenium status and incidence of prostate cancer: an analysis of the complete treatment period of the Nutritional Prevention of Cancer Trial. *BJU International*, **91**, 608–612.

Dumitrescu, R.G. and Shields, P.G. (2005) The etiology of alcohol-induced breast cancer. *Alcohol*, **35**, 213–225.

Edwards, B.K., Brown, M.L., Wingo, P.A. *et al.* (2005) Annual report to the nation on the status of cancer, 1975–2002, featuring population-based trends in cancer treatment. *Journal of the National Cancer Institute*, **97**, 1407–1427.

Ehrlich, M. (2009) DNA hypomethylation in cancer cells. *Epigenomics*, **1**, 239–259.

Emond, J.A., Pierce, J.P., Natarajan, L. *et al.* (2014) Risk of breast cancer recurrence associated with carbohydrate intake and tissue expression of IGF-1 receptor. *Cancer Epidemiology, Biomarkers & Prevention*, **23** (7), 1273–1279.

Esteller, M., Guo, M., Moreno, V. *et al.* (2002) Hypermethylation-associated inactivation of the cellular retinol-binding-protein 1 gene in human cancer. *Cancer Research*, **62**, 5902–5905.

Fang, J.-L. and Vaca, C.E. (1997) Detection of DNA adducts of acetaldehyde in peripheral white blood cells of alcohol abusers. *Carcinogenesis*, **18**, 627–632.

Fazi, F., Travaglini, L., Carotti, D. *et al.* (2005) Retinoic acid targets DNA-methyltransferases and histone deacetylases during APL blast differentiation in vitro and in vivo. *Oncogene*, **24**, 1820–1830.

Fedirko, V., Lukanova, A., Bamia, C. *et al.* (2013) Glycemic index, glycemic load, dietary carbohydrate, and dietary fiber intake and risk of liver and biliary tract cancers in western Europeans. *Annals of Oncology*, **24**, 543–553.

Feinberg, A.P., Ohlsson, R. and Henikoff, S. (2006) The epigenetic progenitor origin of human cancer. *Nature Reviews: Genetics*, **7**, 21–33.

Feldman, D., Krishnan, A.V., Swami, S. *et al.* (2014) The role of vitamin D in reducing cancer risk and progression. *Nature Reviews: Cancer*, **14**, 342–357.

Ferguson, L.R. (2010) Meat and cancer. *Meat Science*, **84**, 308–313.

Ferguson, L.R. and Philpott, M. (2007) Cancer prevention by dietary bioactive components that target the immune response. *Current Cancer Drug Targets*, **7**, 459–464.

Ferlay, J., Soerjomataram, I., Ervik, M. *et al.* (2013) *GLOBOCAN 2012 v1.0, Cancer Incidence and Mortality Worldwide: IARC CancerBase No. 11.* International Agency for Research on Cancer, Lyon. http://globocan.iarc.fr (accessed 12 July 2014).

Figueiredo, J.C., Grau, M.V., Haile, R.W. *et al.* (2009) Folic acid and risk of prostate cancer: results from a randomized clinical trial. *Journal of the National Cancer Institute*, **101**, 432–435.

Fiorucci, S., Distrutti, E., Cirino, G. and Wallace, J.L. (2006) The emerging roles of hydrogen sulfide in the gastrointestinal tract and liver. *Gastroenterology*, **131**, 259–271.

Ford, N.A., Lashinger, L.M., Allott, E.H. and Hursting, S.D. (2013) Mechanistic targets and phytochemical strategies for breaking the obesity-cancer link. *Frontiers in Oncology*, **3**, 209.

Forman, D., Pike, M., Davey, G. *et al.* (1994) Aetiology of testicular cancer: association with congenital abnormalities, age at puberty, infertility, and exercise. *BMJ*, **308**, 1393–1399.

Foster-Powell, K., Holt, S.H. and Brand-Miller, J.C. (2002) International table of glycemic index and glycemic load values: 2002. *The American Journal of Clinical Nutrition*, **76**, 5–56.

Fountoulakis, A., Martin, I., White, K. *et al.* (2004) Plasma and esophageal mucosal levels of vitamin C: role in the pathogenesis and neoplastic progression of Barrett's esophagus. *Digestive Diseases and Sciences*, **49**, 914–919.

Fraga, C.G., Galleano, M., Verstraeten, S.V. and Oteiza, P.I. (2010) Basic biochemical mechanisms behind the health benefits of polyphenols. *Molecular Aspects of Medicine*, **31**, 435–445.

Franceschi, S. and Favero, A. (1999) The role of energy and fat in cancers of the breast and colon–rectum in a southern European population. *Annals of Oncology*, **10**, S61–S63.

Freedman, L.S., Clifford, C. and Messina, M. (1990) Analysis of dietary fat, calories, body weight, and the development of mammary tumors in rats and mice: a review. *Cancer Research*, **50**, 5710–5719.

Friedenreich, C.M. (2001) Physical activity and cancer prevention from observational to intervention research. *Cancer Epidemiology, Biomarkers & Prevention*, **10**, 287–301.

Fuemmeler, B.F., Pendzich, M.K. and Tercyak, K.P. (2009) Weight, dietary behavior, and physical activity in childhood and adolescence: implications for adult cancer risk. *Obesity Facts*, **2**, 179–186.

Füllgrabe, J., kavanagh, E. and Joseph, B. (2011) Histone onco-modifications. *Oncogene*, **30**, 3391–3403.

Galeone, C., Pelucchi, C. and La Vecchia, C. (2012) Added sugar, glycemic index and load in colon cancer risk. *Current Opinion in Clinical Nutrition and Metabolic Care*, **15**, 368–373.

Galvano, F., Frigiola, A., Gazzolo, D. *et al.* (2009) Endothelial protective effects of anthocyanins: the underestimated role of their metabolites. *Annals of Nutrition and Metabolism*, **54**, 158–159.

Ganther, H.E. (1999) Selenium metabolism, selenoproteins and mechanisms of cancer prevention: complexities with thioredoxin reductase. *Carcinogenesis*, **20**, 1657–1666.

Garner, M.J., Turner, M.C., Ghadirian, P. and Krewski, D. (2005) Epidemiology of testicular cancer: an overview. *International Journal of Cancer*, **116**, 331–339.

Gaziano, J.M., Glynn, R.J., Christen, W.G. *et al.* (2009) Vitamins E and C in the prevention of prostate and total cancer in men: the Physicians' Health Study II randomized controlled trial. *JAMA*, **301**, 52–62.

Ghorbani, A., Nazari, M., Jeddi-Tehrani, M. and Zand, H. (2012) The citrus flavonoid hesperidin induces p53 and inhibits NF-κB activation in order to trigger apoptosis in NALM-6 cells: involvement of PPARγ-dependent mechanism. *European Journal of Nutrition*, **51**, 39–46.

Gibson, G.R. and Macfarlane, G.T. (1995) *Human Colonic Bacteria: Role in Nutrition, Physiology, and Pathology.* CRC Press, Boca Raton, FL.

Giles, G.G., Severi, G., English, D.R. *et al.* (2003) Early growth, adult body size and prostate cancer risk. *International Journal of Cancer*, **103**, 241–245.

Giovannucci, E. (1995) Insulin and colon cancer. *Cancer Causes & Control*, **6**, 164–179.

Giovannucci, E., Rimm, E.B., Stampfer, M.J. *et al.* (1997) Height, body weight, and risk of prostate cancer. *Cancer Epidemiology, Biomarkers & Prevention*, **6**, 557–563.

Giovannucci, E., Liu, Y., Stampfer, M.J. and Willett, W.C. (2006) A prospective study of calcium intake and incident and fatal prostate cancer. *Cancer Epidemiology, Biomarkers & Prevention*, **15**, 203–210.

Giovannucci, E., Harlan, D.M., Archer, M.C. *et al.* (2010) Diabetes and cancer: a consensus report. *CA: A Cancer Journal for Clinicians*, **60**, 207–221.

Gnagnarella, P., Gandini, S., La Vecchia, C. and Maisonneuve, P. (2008) Glycemic index, glycemic load, and cancer risk: a meta-analysis. *The American Journal of Clinical Nutrition*, **87**, 1793–1801.

Gonzalez, M.J. and Miranda-Massari, J.R. (2014) *New Insights on Vitamin C and Cancer.* Springer, New York.

González-Vallinas, M., González-Castejón, M., Rodríguez-Casado, A. and Ramírez de Molina, A. (2013) Dietary phytochemicals in cancer prevention and therapy: a complementary approach with promising perspectives. *Nutrition Reviews*, **71**, 585–599.

Goralczyk, R. (2009) β-Carotene and lung cancer in smokers: review of hypotheses and status of research. *Nutrition and Cancer*, **61**, 767–774.

Grosso, G., Buscemi, S., Galvano, F. *et al.* (2013) Mediterranean diet and cancer: epidemiological evidence and mechanism of selected aspects. *BMC Surgery*, **13** (Suppl 2), S14.

Günther, A.L., Karaolis-Danckert, N., Kroke, A. et al. (2010) Dietary protein intake throughout childhood is associated with the timing of puberty. *The Journal of Nutrition*, **140**, 565–571.

Hague, A., Elder, D.J., Hicks, D.J. and Paraskeva, C. (1995) Apoptosis in colorectal tumour cells: induction by the short chain fatty acids butyrate, propionate and acetate and by the bile salt deoxycholate. *International Journal of Cancer*, **60**, 400–406.

Hamer, H.M., de Preter, V., Windey, K. and Verbeke, K. (2012) Functional analysis of colonic bacterial metabolism: relevant to health? *American Journal of Physiology: Gastrointestinal and Liver Physiology*, **302**, G1–G9.

Hanahan, D. and Weinberg, R.A. (2011) Hallmarks of cancer: the next generation. *Cell*, **144**, 646–674.

Harding, A.-H., Wareham, N.J., Bingham, S.A. et al. (2008) Plasma vitamin C level, fruit and vegetable consumption, and the risk of new-onset type 2 diabetes mellitus: the European Prospective Investigation of Cancer–Norfolk prospective study. *Archives of Internal Medicine*, **168**, 1493–1499.

Hardman, W.E. (2014) Diet components can suppress inflammation and reduce cancer risk. *Nutrition Research and Practice*, **8**, 233–240.

Hardy, T.M. and Tollefsbol, T.O. (2011) Epigenetic diet: impact on the epigenome and cancer. *Epigenomics*, **3**, 503–518.

Hartmann, P., Chen, W.-C. and Schnabl, B. (2012) The intestinal microbiome and the leaky gut as therapeutic targets in alcoholic liver disease. *Frontiers in Physiology*, **3**, 402.

Hassan, Y.I. and Zempleni, J. (2006) Epigenetic regulation of chromatin structure and gene function by biotin. *The Journal of Nutrition*, **136**, 1763–1765.

Hastert, T.A., Beresford, S.A.A., Sheppard, L. and White, E. (2014) Adherence to the WCRF/AICR cancer prevention recommendations and cancer-specific mortality: results from the Vitamins and Lifestyle (VITAL) Study. *Cancer Causes & Control*, **25**, 541–552.

He, X., Marco, M.L. and Slupsky, C.M. (2013) Emerging aspects of food and nutrition on gut microbiota. *Journal of Agricultural and Food Chemistry*, **61**, 9559–9574.

Hedlund, T.E., Johannes, W.U. and Miller, G.J. (2003) Soy isoflavonoid equol modulates the growth of benign and malignant prostatic epithelial cells in vitro. *Prostate*, **54**, 68–78.

Heinen, M.M., Verhage, B.A., Goldbohm, R.A. et al. (2011) Physical activity, energy restriction, and the risk of pancreatic cancer: a prospective study in the Netherlands. *The American Journal of Clinical Nutrition*, **94**, 1314–1323.

Heinonen, O. and Albanes, D. (1994) The effect of vitamin E and beta carotene on the incidence of lung cancer and other cancers in male smokers. The Alpha-Tocopherol, Beta-Carotene Cancer Prevention Study Group. *The New England Journal of Medicine*, **330**, 1029–1035.

Ho, J.W., Leung, Y. and Chan, C. (2002) Herbal medicine in the treatment of cancer. *Current Medicinal Chemistry: Anti-Cancer Agents*, **2**, 209–214.

Hoek, J.B. and Pastorino, J.G. (2002) Ethanol, oxidative stress, and cytokine-induced liver cell injury. *Alcohol*, **27**, 63–68.

Hoffmann, I. (2003) Transcending reductionism in nutrition research. *The American Journal of Clinical Nutrition*, **78**, 514S–516S.

Hoffmann, K., Schulze, M., Boeing, H. and Altenburg, H. (2002) Dietary patterns: report of an international workshop. *Public Health Nutrition*, **5**, 89–90.

Hoppe, C., Mølgaard, C., Juul, A. and Michaelsen, K. (2004a) High intakes of skimmed milk, but not meat, increase serum IGF-I and IGFBP-3 in eight-year-old boys. *European Journal of Clinical Nutrition*, **58**, 1211–1216.

Hoppe, C., Udam, T.R., Lauritzen, L. et al. (2004b) Animal protein intake, serum insulin-like growth factor I, and growth in healthy 2.5-y-old Danish children. *The American Journal of Clinical Nutrition*, **80**, 447–452.

Hu, F.B. (2002) Dietary pattern analysis: a new direction in nutritional epidemiology. *Current Opinion in Lipidology*, **13**, 3–9.

Hu, F.B., Rimm, E., Smith-Warner, S.A. et al. (1999) Reproducibility and validity of dietary patterns assessed with a food-frequency questionnaire. *The American Journal of Clinical Nutrition*, **69**, 243–249.

Hu, F.B., Rimm, E.B., Stampfer, M.J. et al. (2000) Prospective study of major dietary patterns and risk of coronary heart disease in men. *The American Journal of Clinical Nutrition*, **72**, 912–921.

Hu, J., La Vecchia, C., Augustin, L.S. et al. (2013) Glycemic index, glycemic load and cancer risk. *Annals of Oncology*, **24**, 245–251.

Huang, X. (2003) Iron overload and its association with cancer risk in humans: evidence for iron as a carcinogenic metal. *Mutation Research: Fundamental and Molecular Mechanisms of Mutagenesis*, **533**, 153–171.

Hughes, L.A., van den Brandt, P.A., Goldbohm, R.A. et al. (2010) Childhood and adolescent energy restriction and subsequent colorectal cancer risk: results from the Netherlands Cohort Study. *International Journal of Epidemiology*, **39**, 1333–1344.

Hughes, L.A., van den Brandt, P.A., de Bruïne, A.P. et al. 2009. Early life exposure to famine and colorectal cancer risk: a role for epigenetic mechanisms. *PLoS One*, **4** (11), e7951.

Hughes, R., Pollock, J.R. and Bingham, S. (2002) Effect of vegetables, tea, and soy on endogenous N-nitrosation, fecal ammonia, and fecal water genotoxicity during a high red meat diet in humans. *Nutrition and Cancer*, **42**, 70–77.

Huijbregts, P., Feskens, E., Räsänen, L. et al. (1997) Dietary pattern and 20 year mortality in elderly men in Finland, Italy, and the Netherlands: longitudinal cohort study. *BMJ*, **315**, 13–17.

Hullar, M.A.J., Burnett-Hartman, A.N. and Lampe, J.W. (2014) Gut microbes, diet, and cancer. In V. Zappia, S. Panico, G. L. Russo et al. (eds), *Advances in Nutrition and Cancer*. Cancer Treatment and Research 159. New York: Springer; pp. 377–399.

Hurst, R., Hooper, L., Norat, T. et al. (2012) Selenium and prostate cancer: systematic review and meta-analysis. *The American Journal of Clinical Nutrition*, **96**, 111–122.

Hursting, S.D. (2014) Obesity, energy balance, and cancer: a mechanistic perspective. In V. Zappia, S. Panico, G. L. Russo et al. (eds), *Advances in Nutrition and Cancer*. Cancer Treatment and Research 159. Springer, New York; pp. 21–33.

Hursting, S.D. and Dunlap, S.M. (2012) Obesity, metabolic dysregulation, and cancer: a growing concern and an inflammatory (and microenvironmental) issue. *Annals of the New York Academy of Sciences*, **1271**, 82–87.

Hursting, S.D., Lavigne, J.A., Berrigan, D. et al. (2003) Calorie restriction, aging, and cancer prevention: mechanisms of action and applicability to humans. *Annual Review of Medicine*, **54**, 131–152.

IARC (2010) *Ingested Nitrate and Nitrite, and Cyanobacterial Peptide Toxins*. International Agency for Research on Cancer, Lyon.

IARC (2014) *World Cancer Report 2014*. International Agency for Research on Cancer, Lyon.

Islam, K.B.M., Fukiya, S., Hagio, M. et al. (2011) Bile acid is a host factor that regulates the composition of the cecal microbiota in rats. *Gastroenterology*, **141**, 1773–1781.

Issa, A.Y., Volate, S.R. and Wargovich, M.J. (2006) The role of phytochemicals in inhibition of cancer and inflammation: new directions and perspectives. *Journal of Food Composition and Analysis*, **19**, 405–419.

Iwaki, T., Urano, T. and Umemura, K. (2012) PAI-1, progress in understanding the clinical problem and its aetiology. *British Journal of Haematology*, **157**, 291–298.

Jacques, P.F. and Tucker, K.L. (2001) Are dietary patterns useful for understanding the role of diet in chronic disease? *The American Journal of Clinical Nutrition*, **73**, 1–2.

James, D. (2009) Cluster analysis defines distinct dietary patterns for African-American men and women. *Journal of the American Dietetic Association*, **109**, 255–262.

Jamshidzadeh, A., Baghban, M., Azarpira, N. *et al.* (2008) Effects of tomato extract on oxidative stress induced toxicity in different organs of rats. *Food and Chemical Toxicology*, **46**, 3612–3615.

Jan, A.T., Kamli, M.R., Murtaza, I. *et al.* (2010) Dietary flavonoid quercetin and associated health benefits – an overview. *Food Reviews International*, **26**, 302–317.

Jenab, M., Riboli, E., Ferrari, P. *et al.* (2006) Plasma and dietary carotenoid, retinol and tocopherol levels and the risk of gastric adenocarcinomas in the European Prospective Investigation into Cancer and Nutrition. *British Journal of Cancer*, **95**, 406–415.

Jennings, B.A. and Willis, G. (2014) How folate metabolism affects colorectal cancer development and treatment; a story of heterogeneity and pleiotropy. *Cancer Letters*, **356**, 224–230.

Jing, K., Wu, T. and Lim, K. (2013) Omega-3 polyunsaturated fatty acids and cancer. *Anti-Cancer Agents in Medicinal Chemistry*, **13**, 1162–1177.

Johanning, G.L. and Piyathilake, C.J. (2003) Retinoids and epigenetic silencing in cancer. *Nutrition Reviews*, **61**, 284–289.

John, E.M., Phipps, A.I., Davis, A. and Koo, J. (2005) Migration history, acculturation, and breast cancer risk in Hispanic women. *Cancer Epidemiology, Biomarkers & Prevention*, **14**, 2905–2913.

Johnson, K.J., Anderson, K.E., Harnack, L. *et al.* (2005) No association between dietary glycemic index or load and pancreatic cancer incidence in postmenopausal women. *Cancer Epidemiology, Biomarkers & Prevention*, **14**, 1574–1575.

Jones-McLean, E.M., Shatenstein, B. and Whiting, S.J. (2010) Dietary patterns research and its applications to nutrition policy for the prevention of chronic disease among diverse North American populations. *Applied Physiology, Nutrition, and Metabolism*, **35**, 195–198.

Jones, J.R., Lineback, D.M. and Levine, M.J. (2006) Dietary reference intakes: implications for fiber labeling and consumption: a summary of the International Life Sciences Institute North America Fiber Workshop, June 1–2 004, Washington, DC. *Nutrition Reviews*, **64**, 31–38.

Ju, Y.H., Allred, K.F., Allred, C.D. and Helferich, W.G. (2006) Genistein stimulates growth of human breast cancer cells in a novel, postmenopausal animal model, with low plasma estradiol concentrations. *Carcinogenesis*, **27**, 1292–1299.

Kaaks, R. (2005) Nutrition, insulin, IGF-1 metabolism and cancer risk: a summary of epidemiological evidence. Biology of IGF-1. *Novartis Foundation Symposium*, **262**, 247–264.

Kaaks, R., Lukanova, A. and Kurzer, M.S. (2002) Obesity, endogenous hormones, and endometrial cancer risk: a synthetic review. *Cancer Epidemiology, Biomarkers & Prevention*, **11**, 1531–1543.

Kabat, G.C., Kim, M., Adams-Campbell, L.L. *et al.* (2009) Longitudinal study of serum carotenoid, retinol, and tocopherol concentrations in relation to breast cancer risk among postmenopausal women. *The American Journal of Clinical Nutrition*, **90** (1), 162–169.

Kabat, G.C., Heo, M., Kamensky, V. *et al.* (2013) Adult height in relation to risk of cancer in a cohort of Canadian women. *International Journal of Cancer*, **132**, 1125–1132.

Kanda, J., Matsuo, K., Suzuki, T. *et al.* (2010) Association between obesity and the risk of malignant lymphoma in Japanese: a case–control study. *International Journal of Cancer*, **126**, 2416–2425.

Kant, A.K. (2010) Dietary patterns: biomarkers and chronic disease risk. *Applied Physiology, Nutrition, and Metabolism*, **35**, 199–206.

Kaulmann, A. and Bohn, T. (2014) Carotenoids, inflammation and oxidative stress – implications of cellular signaling pathways and relation to chronic disease prevention. *Nutrition Research*, **34**, 907–929.

Kavazis, A.N. and Powers, S.K. (2013) Impact of exercise, reactive oxygen and reactive nitrogen species on tumor growth. In C.M. Ulrich, K. Steindorf and N.A. Berger (eds), *Exercise, Energy Balance, and Cancer*. Springer, New York; pp. 7–20.

Kelkel, M., Schumacher, M., Dicato, M. and Diederich, M. (2011) Antioxidant and anti-proliferative properties of lycopene. *Free Radical Research*, **45**, 925–940.

Key, T., Appleby, P., Barnes, I. and Reeves, G. (2002) Endogenous sex hormones and breast cancer in postmenopausal women: reanalysis of nine prospective studies. *Journal of the National Cancer Institute*, **94**, 606–616.

Keys, A., Mienotti, A., Karvonen, M.J. *et al.* (1986) The diet and 15-year death rate in the seven countries study. *American Journal of Epidemiology*, **124**, 903–915.

Keys, A.K.M. (1975) *How to Eat Well and Stay Well the Mediterranean Way*. Doubleday, Garden City, NY.

Khan, A.A., Shrivastava, A. and Khurshid, M. (2012) Normal to cancer microbiome transformation and its implication in cancer diagnosis. *Biochimica et Biophysica Acta (BBA) – Reviews on Cancer*, **1826**, 331–337.

Khan, N., Afaq, F., Saleem, M. *et al.* (2006) Targeting multiple signaling pathways by green tea polyphenol (−)-epigallocatechin-3-gallate. *Cancer Research*, **66**, 2500–2505.

Khani, B.R., Ye, W., Terry, P. and Wolk, A. (2004) Reproducibility and validity of major dietary patterns among Swedish women assessed with a food-frequency questionnaire. *The Journal of Nutrition*, **134**, 1541–1545.

Khodarahmi, M. and Azadbakht, L. (2014) The association between different kinds of fat intake and breast cancer risk in women. *International Journal of Preventive Medicine*, **5**, 6–15.

Khuda-Bukhsh, A.R., Das, S. and Saha, S.K. (2014) Molecular approaches toward targeted cancer prevention with some food plants and their products: inflammatory and other signal pathways. *Nutrition and Cancer*, **66**, 194–205.

Kim, E., Coelho, D. and Blachier, F. (2013) Review of the association between meat consumption and risk of colorectal cancer. *Nutrition Research*, **33**, 983–994.

Kim, Y.-I. (2003) Role of folate in colon cancer development and progression. *The Journal of Nutrition*, **133** (11 Suppl 1), 3731S–3739S.

Klein, E.A., Thompson, I.M., Tangen, C.M. *et al.* (2011) Vitamin E and the risk of prostate cancer: the Selenium and Vitamin E Cancer Prevention Trial (SELECT). *JAMA*, **306**, 1549–1556.

Kocic, B., Filipovic, S., Nikolic, M. and Petrovic, B. (2010) Effects of anthocyanins and anthocyanin-rich extracts on the risk for cancers of the gastrointestinal tract. *Journal of BUON*, **16**, 602–608.

Korde, L.A., Wu, A.H., Fears, T. *et al.* (2009) Childhood soy intake and breast cancer risk in Asian American women. *Cancer Epidemiology, Biomarkers & Prevention*, **18**, 1050–1059.

Kristal, A.R., Darke, A.K., Morris, J.S. *et al.* (2014) Baseline selenium status and effects of selenium and vitamin E supplementation on prostate cancer risk. *Journal of the National Cancer Institute*, **106** (3), djt456.

Kroemer, G. and Pouyssegur, J. (2008) Tumor cell metabolism: cancer's Achilles' heel. *Cancer Cell*, **13**, 472–482.

Kruk, J. and Czerniak, U. (2013) Physical activity and its relation to cancer risk: updating the evidence. *Asian Pacific Journal of Cancer Prevention*, **14**, 3993–4003.

Krutovskikh, V.A. and Herceg, Z. (2010) Oncogenic microRNAs (OncomiRs) as a new class of cancer biomarkers. *Bioessays*, **32**, 894–904.

Kushi, L. and Giovannucci, E. (2002) Dietary fat and cancer. *American Journal of Medicine*, **113**, 63–70.

Kushi, L.H., Doyle, C., McCullough, M. *et al.* (2012) American Cancer Society guidelines on nutrition and physical activity for cancer prevention. *CA: A Cancer Journal for Clinicians*, **62**, 30–67.

Laake, I., Carlsen, M.H., Pedersen, J.I. et al. (2013) Intake of trans fatty acids from partially hydrogenated vegetable and fish oils and ruminant fat in relation to cancer risk. International Journal of Cancer, 132, 1389–1403.

Larsson, S.C., Kumlin, M., Ingelman-Sundberg, M. and Wolk, A. (2004) Dietary long-chain n-3 fatty acids for the prevention of cancer: a review of potential mechanisms. The American Journal of Clinical Nutrition, 79, 935–945.

Latté, K.P., Appel, K.-E. and Lampen, A. (2011) Health benefits and possible risks of broccoli – an overview. Food and Chemical Toxicology, 49, 3287–3309.

Lattimer, J.M. and Haub, M.D. (2010) Effects of dietary fiber and its components on metabolic health. Nutrients, 2, 1266–1289.

Lee, H.S. and Herceg, Z. (2014) The epigenome and cancer prevention: a complex story of dietary supplementation. Cancer Letters, 342, 275–284.

Lee, S.-A., Shu, X.-O., Li, H. et al. (2009) Adolescent and adult soy food intake and breast cancer risk: results from the Shanghai Women's Health Study. The American Journal of Clinical Nutrition, 89, 1920–1926.

Leo, M.A. and Lieber, C.S. (1999) Alcohol, vitamin A, and β-carotene: adverse interactions, including hepatotoxicity and carcinogenicity. The American Journal of Clinical Nutrition, 69, 1071–1085.

Leonardi, T., Vanamala, J., Taddeo, S.S. et al. (2010) Apigenin and naringenin suppress colon carcinogenesis through the aberrant crypt stage in azoxymethane-treated rats. Experimental Biology and Medicine, 235, 710–717.

Levi, F., Pasche, C., Lucchini, F. et al. (2005) Resveratrol and breast cancer risk. European Journal of Cancer Prevention, 14, 139–142.

Li, J., Humphreys, K., Eriksson, L. et al. (2010) Effects of childhood body size on breast cancer tumour characteristics. Breast Cancer Research: BCR, 12 (2), R23.

Liebman, M. (2013) When and why carbohydrate restriction can be a viable option. Nutrition, 30 (7–8), 748–754.

Lillycrop, K.A. and Burdge, G.C. (2014) Breast cancer and the importance of early life nutrition. In V. Zappia, S. Panico, G. L. Russo et al. (eds), Advances in Nutrition and Cancer. Cancer Treatment and Research 159. New York: Springer; pp. 269–285.

Lin, Y., Shi, R., Wang, X. and Shen, H.-M. (2008) Luteolin, a flavonoid with potentials for cancer prevention and therapy. Current Cancer Drug Targets, 8, 634–646.

Link, A., Balaguer, F. and Goel, A. (2010) Cancer chemoprevention by dietary polyphenols: promising role for epigenetics. Biochemical Pharmacology, 80, 1771–1792.

Linos, E., Willett, W.C., Cho, E. et al. (2008) Red meat consumption during adolescence among premenopausal women and risk of breast cancer. Cancer Epidemiology, Biomarkers & Prevention, 17, 2146–2151.

Linos, E., Willett, W.C., Cho, E. and Frazier, L. (2010) Adolescent diet in relation to breast cancer risk among premenopausal women. Cancer Epidemiology, Biomarkers & Prevention, 19 (3), 689–96.

Lippman, S.M., Klein, E.A., Goodman, P.J. et al. (2009) Effect of selenium and vitamin E on risk of prostate cancer and other cancers: the Selenium and Vitamin E Cancer Prevention Trial (SELECT). JAMA, 301, 39–51.

Liu, H., Huang, D., McArthur, D.L. et al. (2010) Fructose induces transketolase flux to promote pancreatic cancer growth. Cancer Research, 70, 6368–6376.

Liu, R.H. (2003) Health benefits of fruit and vegetables are from additive and synergistic combinations of phytochemicals. The American Journal of Clinical Nutrition, 78, 517S–520S.

Liu, R.H., Liu, J. and Chen, B. (2005) Apples prevent mammary tumors in rats. Journal of Agricultural and Food Chemistry, 53, 2341–2343.

Liu, S., Willett, W.C., Stampfer, M.J. et al. (2000) A prospective study of dietary glycemic load, carbohydrate intake, and risk of coronary heart disease in US women. The American Journal of Clinical Nutrition, 71, 1455–1461.

Loffreda, S., Yang, S., Lin, H. et al. (1998) Leptin regulates proinflammatory immune responses. FASEB Journal, 12, 57–65.

Lonn, E., Bosch, J., Yusuf, S. et al. (2005) Effects of long-term vitamin E supplementation on cardiovascular events and cancer: a randomized controlled trial. JAMA, 293, 1338–1347.

Ludwig, D.S., Peterson, K.E. and Gortmaker, S.L. (2001) Relation between consumption of sugar-sweetened drinks and childhood obesity: a prospective, observational analysis. The Lancet, 357, 505–508.

Ma, X., Fang, Y., Beklemisheva, A. et al. (2006) Phenylhexyl isothiocyanate inhibits histone deacetylases and remodels chromatins to induce growth arrest in human leukemia cells. International Journal of Oncology, 28, 1287–1293.

Macfarlane, G.T. and Macfarlane, S. (2011) Fermentation in the human large intestine: its physiological consequences and the potential contribution of prebiotics. Journal of Clinical Gastroenterology, 45 (Suppl), S120–S127.

Macfarlane, G.T. and Macfarlane, S. (2012) Bacteria, colonic fermentation, and gastrointestinal health. Journal of AOAC International, 95, 50–60.

Magalhaes, B., Peleteiro, B. and Lunet, N. (2012) Dietary patterns and colorectal cancer: systematic review and meta-analysis. European Journal of Cancer Prevention, 21, 15–23.

Mahlknecht, U. and Hoelzer, D. (2000) Histone acetylation modifiers in the pathogenesis of malignant disease. Molecular Medicine, 6, 623–644.

Mandair, D., Rossi, R.E., Pericleous, M., Whyand, T. and Caplin, M.E. (2014) Prostate cancer and the influence of dietary factors and supplements: a systematic review. Nutrition and Metabolism, 11, 30.

Martin, M.A., Goya, L. and Ramos, S. (2013) Potential for preventive effects of cocoa and cocoa polyphenols in cancer. Food and Chemical Toxicology, 56, 336–351.

Maruti, S.S., Ulrich, C.M. and White, E. (2009) Folate and one-carbon metabolism nutrients from supplements and diet in relation to breast cancer risk. The American Journal of Clinical Nutrition, 89, 624–633.

Masella, R., Santangelo, C., D'Archivio, M. et al. (2012) Protocatechuic acid and human disease prevention: biological activities and molecular mechanisms. Current Medicinal Chemistry, 19, 2901–2917.

Maskarinec, G., Erber, E., Gill, J. et al. (2008) Overweight and obesity at different times in life as risk factors for non-Hodgkin's lymphoma: the multiethnic cohort. Cancer Epidemiology, Biomarkers & Prevention, 17, 196–203.

Matsuki, T. and Tanaka, R. (2014) Function of the human gut microbiota. In J.R. Marchesi (ed.), The Human Microbiota and Microbiome. CABI, Wallingford; pp. 90–106.

McGarr, S.E., Ridlon, J.M. and Hylemon, P.B. (2005) Diet, anaerobic bacterial metabolism, and colon cancer: a review of the literature. Journal of Clinical Gastroenterology, 39, 98–109.

McIntosh, G.H. and Le Leu, R.K. (2001) The influence of dietary proteins on colon cancer risk. Nutrition Research, 21, 1053–1066.

McKeown-Eyssen, G. (1994) Epidemiology of colorectal cancer revisited: are serum triglycerides and/or plasma glucose associated with risk? Cancer Epidemiology, Biomarkers & Prevention, 3, 687–695.

McTiernan, A. (2008) Mechanisms linking physical activity with cancer. Nature Reviews: Cancer, 8, 205–211.

Mehio Sibai, A., Nasreddine, L., Mokdad, A.H. et al. (2010) Nutrition transition and cardiovascular disease risk factors in Middle East and North Africa countries: reviewing the evidence. Annals of Nutrition and Metabolism, 57, 193–203.

Meinhold, C.L., Dodd, K.W., Jiao, L. et al. (2010) Available carbohydrates, glycemic load, and pancreatic cancer: is there a link? American Journal of Epidemiology, 171, 1174–1182.

Michaelsen, K.F. and Greer, F.R. (2014) Protein needs early in life and long-term health. *The American Journal of Clinical Nutrition*, **99**, 718S–722S.

Michels, K.B. and Xue, F. (2006) Role of birthweight in the etiology of breast cancer. *International Journal of Cancer*, **119**, 2007–2025.

Michels, K.B., Mohllajee, A.P., Roset-Bahmanyar, E. *et al.* (2007) Diet and breast cancer: a review of the prospective observational studies. *Cancer*, **109**, 2712–2749.

Milder, I.E., Kuijsten, A., Arts, I.C. *et al.* (2007) Relation between plasma enterodiol and enterolactone and dietary intake of lignans in a Dutch endoscopy-based population. *The Journal of Nutrition*, **137**, 1266–1271.

Moeller, S.M., Reedy, J., Millen, A.E. *et al.* (2007) Dietary patterns: challenges and opportunities in dietary patterns research: an Experimental Biology workshop, April 1, 2006. *Journal of the American Dietetic Association*, **107**, 1233–1239.

Molina, P.E., Hoek, J.B., Nelson, S. *et al.* (2003) Mechanisms of alcohol-induced tissue injury. *Alcoholism, Clinical and Experimental Research*, **27**, 563–575.

Molina-Vargas, L.F. (2013) Mechanism of action of isothiocyanates. A review. *Agronomía Colombiana*, **31**, 68–75.

Moore, S.C., Rajaraman, P., Dubrow, R. *et al.* (2009) Height, body mass index, and physical activity in relation to glioma risk. *Cancer Research*, **69**, 8349–8355.

Moreno, F., S-Wu, T., Naves, M.M. *et al.* (2002) Inhibitory effects of beta-carotene and vitamin a during the progression phase of hepatocarcinogenesis involve inhibition of cell proliferation but not alterations in DNA methylation. *Nutrition and Cancer*, **44**, 80–88.

Morgan, T.R., Mandayam, S. and Jamal, M.M. (2004) Alcohol and hepatocellular carcinoma. *Gastroenterology*, **127** (5 Suppl 1), S87–S96.

Mulholland, H., Murray, L., Cardwell, C. and Cantwell, M. (2008a) Dietary glycaemic index, glycaemic load and breast cancer risk: a systematic review and meta-analysis. *British Journal of Cancer*, **99**, 1170–1175.

Mulholland, H., Murray, L., Cardwell, C. and Cantwell, M. (2008b) Dietary glycaemic index, glycaemic load and endometrial and ovarian cancer risk: a systematic review and meta-analysis. *British Journal of Cancer*, **99**, 434–441.

Mulholland, H.G., Murray, L.J., Cardwell, C.R. and Cantwell, M.M. (2009) Glycemic index, glycemic load, and risk of digestive tract neoplasms: a systematic review and meta-analysis. *The American Journal of Clinical Nutrition*, **89**, 568–576.

Murakami, A., Ashida, H. and Terao, J. (2008) Multitargeted cancer prevention by quercetin. *Cancer Letters*, **269**, 315–325.

Mutlu, E.A., Gillevet, P.M., Rangwala, H. *et al.* (2012) Colonic microbiome is altered in alcoholism. *American Journal of Physiology: Gastrointestinal and Liver Physiology*, **302**, G966–G978.

Myzak, M.C. and Dashwood, R.H. (2006) Histone deacetylases as targets for dietary cancer preventive agents: lessons learned with butyrate, diallyl disulfide, and sulforaphane. *Current Drug Targets*, **7**, 443–452.

Naja, F., Nasreddine, L., Itani, L. *et al.* (2013) Dietary patterns in cardiovascular diseases prevention and management: review of the evidence and recommendations for primary care physicians in Lebanon. *Le Journal Médical Libanais*, **62**, 92–99.

Nakamura, Y., Yogosawa, S., Izutani, Y. *et al.* (2009) A combination of indol-3-carbinol and genistein synergistically induces apoptosis in human colon cancer HT-29 cells by inhibiting Akt phosphorylation and progression of autophagy. *Molecular Cancer*, **8**, 1476–4598.

Nanri, A., Shimazu, T., Ishihara, J. *et al.* (2012) Reproducibility and validity of dietary patterns assessed by a food frequency questionnaire used in the 5-year follow-up survey of the Japan Public Health Center-Based Prospective Study. *Journal of Epidemiology*, **22**, 205.

Narvaez, C.J., Matthews, D., Laporta, E. *et al.* (2014) The impact of vitamin D in breast cancer: genomics, pathways, metabolism. *Frontiers in Physiology*, **5**, 213.

National Research Council (US) Committee on Diet and Health (1989) *Diet and Health: Implications for Reducing Chronic Disease Risk*. National Academies Press, Washington, DC.

Navarro, S.L., Li, F. and Lampe, J.W. (2011) Mechanisms of action of isothiocyanates in cancer chemoprevention: an update. *Food & Function*, **2**, 579–587.

Nazki, F.H., Sameer, A.S. and Ganaie, B.A. (2014) Folate: metabolism, genes, polymorphisms and the associated diseases. *Gene*, **533**, 11–20.

Negrini, M., Ferracin, M., Sabbioni, S. and Croce, C.M. (2007) MicroRNAs in human cancer: from research to therapy. *Journal of Cell Science*, **120**, 1833–1840.

Newby, P. and Tucker, K.L. (2004) Empirically derived eating patterns using factor or cluster analysis: a review. *Nutrition Reviews*, **62**, 177–203.

Newby, P., Weismayer, C., Åkesson, A. *et al.* (2006) Long-term stability of food patterns identified by use of factor analysis among Swedish women. *The Journal of Nutrition*, **136**, 626–633.

Ngo, S.N., Williams, D.B., Cobiac, L. and Head, R.J. (2007) Does garlic reduce risk of colorectal cancer? A systematic review. *The Journal of Nutrition*, **137**, 2264–2269.

Nguyen, A.V., Martinez, M., Stamos, M.J. *et al.* (2009) Results of a phase I pilot clinical trial examining the effect of plant-derived resveratrol and grape powder on Wnt pathway target gene expression in colonic mucosa and colon cancer. *Cancer Management and Research*, **1**, 25–37.

Nguyen, H.H., Aronchik, I., Brar, G.A. *et al.* (2008) The dietary phytochemical indole-3-carbinol is a natural elastase enzymatic inhibitor that disrupts cyclin E protein processing. *Proceedings of the National Academy of Sciences of the United States of America*, **105**, 19750–19755.

Nian, H., Delage, B., Ho, E. and Dashwood, R.H. (2009) Modulation of histone deacetylase activity by dietary isothiocyanates and allyl sulfides: studies with sulforaphane and garlic organosulfur compounds. *Environmental and Molecular Mutagenesis*, **50**, 213–221.

Nicholson, J.K., Holmes, E., Kinross, J. *et al.* (2012) Host–gut microbiota metabolic interactions. *Science*, **336**, 1262–1267.

Niki, E. (2014) Role of vitamin E as a lipid-soluble peroxyl radical scavenger: in vitro and in vivo evidence. *Free Radical Biology & Medicine*, **66**, 3–12.

Noel, S.E., Stoneham, A., Olsen, C.M. *et al.* (2014) Consumption of omega-3 fatty acids and the risk of skin cancers: a systematic review and meta-analysis. *International Journal of Cancer*, **135**, 149–156.

Nomura, A.M., Hankin, J.H., Henderson, B.E. *et al.* (2007) Dietary fiber and colorectal cancer risk: the multiethnic cohort study. *Cancer Causes & Control*, **18**, 753–764.

Nooyens, A.C., Visscher, T.L., Schuit, A.J. *et al.* (2005) Effects of retirement on lifestyle in relation to changes in weight and waist circumference in Dutch men: a prospective study. *Public Health Nutrition*, **8**, 1266–1274.

Norat, T., Bingham, S., Ferrari, P. *et al.* (2005) Meat, fish, and colorectal cancer risk: the European Prospective Investigation into cancer and nutrition. *Journal of the National Cancer Institute*, **97**, 906–916.

Norat, T., Aune, D., Chan, D. and Romaguera, D. (2014) Fruits and vegetables: updating the epidemiologic evidence for the WCRF/AICR lifestyle recommendations for cancer prevention. In V. Zappia, S. Panico, G. L. Russo *et al.* (eds), *Advances in Nutrition and Cancer*. Cancer Treatment and Research 159. Springer, New York; pp. 35–50.

Nöthlings, U., Murphy, S.P., Wilkens, L.R. *et al.* (2007) Dietary glycemic load, added sugars, and carbohydrates as risk factors for pancreatic cancer: the Multiethnic Cohort Study. *The American Journal of Clinical Nutrition*, **86**, 1495–1501.

O'Hara, A.M. and Shanahan, F. (2006) The gut flora as a forgotten organ. *EMBO Reports*, **7**, 688–693.

O'Rorke, M.A., Cantwell, M.M., Cardwell, C.R. *et al.* (2010) Can physical activity modulate pancreatic cancer risk? A systematic review and meta-analysis. *International Journal of Cancer*, **126**, 2957–2968.

Okubo, H., Murakami, K., Sasaki, S. *et al.* (2010) Relative validity of dietary patterns derived from a self-administered diet history questionnaire using factor analysis among Japanese adults. *Public Health Nutrition*, **13**, 1080–1089.

Omenn, G.S., Goodman, G.E., Thornquist, M.D. *et al.* (1996a) Risk factors for lung cancer and for intervention effects in CARET, the Beta-Carotene and Retinol Efficacy Trial. *Journal of the National Cancer Institute*, **88**, 1550–1559.

Omenn, G.S., Goodman, G.E., Thornquist, M.D. *et al.* (1996b) Effects of a combination of beta carotene and vitamin A on lung cancer and cardiovascular disease. *The New England Journal of Medicine*, **334**, 1150–1155.

Ong, T.P., Moreno, F.S. and Ross, S.A. (2011) Targeting the epigenome with bioactive food components for cancer prevention. *Journal of Nutrigenetics and Nutrigenomics*, **4**, 275–292.

Ötles, S. and Ozgoz, S. (2014) Health effects of dietary fiber. *Acta Scientiarum Polonorum. Technologia Alimentaria*, **13**, 191–202.

Padayatty, S.J., Katz, A., Wang, Y. *et al.* (2003) Vitamin C as an antioxidant: evaluation of its role in disease prevention. *Journal of the American College of Nutrition*, **22**, 18–35.

Paffenbarger, R.S., Hyde, R. and Wing, A. (1987) Physical activity and incidence of cancer in diverse populations: a preliminary report. *The American Journal of Clinical Nutrition*, **45**, 312–317.

Pandey, K.B. and Rizvi, S.I. (2009) Plant polyphenols as dietary antioxidants in human health and disease. *Oxidative Medicine and Cellular Longevity*, **2**, 270–278.

Parasramka, M.A., Ho, E., Williams, D.E. and Dashwood, R.H. (2012) MicroRNAs, diet, and cancer: new mechanistic insights on the epigenetic actions of phytochemicals. *Molecular Carcinogenesis*, **51**, 213–230.

Park, C.S. (2005) Role of compensatory mammary growth in epigenetic control of gene expression. *FASEB Journal*, **19**, 1586–1591.

Park, H., Kim, M.-J., Ha, E. and Chung, J.-H. (2008) Apoptotic effect of hesperidin through caspase3 activation in human colon cancer cells, SNU-C4. *Phytomedicine*, **15**, 147–151.

Park, Y., Brinton, L.A., Subar, A.F. *et al.* (2009) Dietary fiber intake and risk of breast cancer in postmenopausal women: the National Institutes of Health–AARP Diet and Health Study. *The American Journal of Clinical Nutrition*, **90** (3), 664–671.

Parry, B.M., Milne, J.M., Yadegarfar, G. and Rainsbury, R.M. (2011) Dramatic dietary fat reduction is feasible for breast cancer patients: results of the randomised study, WINS (UK) – stage 1. *European Journal of Surgical Oncology*, **37**, 848–855.

Pauwels, E.K. (2011) The protective effect of the Mediterranean diet: focus on cancer and cardiovascular risk. *Medical Principles and Practice*, **20**, 103–111.

Pelucchi, C., Tramacere, I., Boffetta, P. *et al.* (2011) Alcohol consumption and cancer risk. *Nutrition and Cancer*, **63**, 983–990.

Pöschl, G. and Seitz, H.K. (2004) Alcohol and cancer. *Alcohol and Alcoholism*, **39**, 155–165.

Potischman, N. and Linet, M.S. (2013) Invited commentary: are dietary intakes and other exposures in childhood and adolescence important for adult cancers? *American Journal of Epidemiology*, **178**, 184–189.

Potischman, N., Swanson, C.A., Hoover, R.N. *et al.* (1998) Diet during adolescence and risk of breast cancer among young women. *Journal of the National Cancer Institute*, **90**, 226–233.

Potter, J.D. (1996) Nutrition and colorectal cancer. *Cancer Causes & Control*, **7**, 127–146.

Prentice, R.L., Pepe, M. and Self, S.G. (1989) Dietary fat and breast cancer: a quantitative assessment of the epidemiological literature and a discussion of methodological issues. *Cancer Research*, **49**, 3147–3156.

Prüss-Üstün, A. and Corvalán, C. (2006) *Preventing Disease through Healthy Environments: Towards an Estimate of the Environmental Burden of Disease*. World Health Organization, Geneva.

Puupponen-Pimiä, R., Nohynek, L., Meier, C. *et al.* (2001) Antimicrobial properties of phenolic compounds from berries. *Journal of Applied Microbiology*, **90**, 494–507.

Puupponen-Pimiä, R., Nohynek, L., Hartmann-Schmidlin, S. *et al.* (2005) Berry phenolics selectively inhibit the growth of intestinal pathogens. *Journal of Applied Microbiology*, **98**, 991–1000.

Quatromoni, P., Copenhafer, D., Demissie, S. *et al.* (2002) The internal validity of a dietary pattern analysis. The Framingham Nutrition Studies. *Journal of Epidemiology & Community Health*, **56**, 381–388.

Ramos, S. (2008) Cancer chemoprevention and chemotherapy: dietary polyphenols and signalling pathways. *Molecular Nutrition & Food Research*, **52**, 507–526.

Rassoulzadegan, M., Grandjean, V., Gounon, P. and Cuzin, F. (2007) Inheritance of an epigenetic change in the mouse: a new role for RNA. *Biochemical Society Transactions*, **35**, 623–625.

Reddy, B.S. (1981) Diet and excretion of bile acids. *Cancer Research*, **41**, 3766–3768.

Reedy, J., Wirfält, E., Flood, A. *et al.* (2010) Comparing 3 dietary pattern methods – cluster analysis, factor analysis, and index analysis – with colorectal cancer risk: the NIH–AARP Diet and Health Study. *American Journal of Epidemiology*, **171**, 479–487.

Reidlinger, D.P., Darzi, J., Hall, W.L. *et al.* (2015) How effective are current dietary guidelines for cardiovascular disease prevention in healthy middle-aged and older men and women? A randomized controlled trial. *The American Journal of Clinical Nutrition*, **101**, 922–930.

Rexrode, K.M., Pradhan, A., Manson, J.E. *et al.* (2003) Relationship of total and abdominal adiposity with CRP and IL-6 in women. *Annals of Epidemiology*, **13**, 674–682.

Riboli, E. and Norat, T. (2003) Epidemiologic evidence of the protective effect of fruit and vegetables on cancer risk. *The American Journal of Clinical Nutrition*, **78**, 559S–569S.

Rimando, A.M. and Suh, N. (2008) Biological/chemopreventive activity of stilbenes and their effect on colon cancer. *Planta Medica*, **74**, 1635–1643.

Roberts-Thomson, I.C., Khoo, K., Hart, W. *et al.* (1996) Diet, acetylator phenotype, and risk of colorectal neoplasia. *The Lancet*, **347**, 1372–1374.

Romieu, I., Ferrari, P., Rinaldi, S. *et al.* (2012) Dietary glycemic index and glycemic load and breast cancer risk in the European Prospective Investigation into Cancer and Nutrition (EPIC). *The American Journal of Clinical Nutrition*, **96**, 345–355.

Ross, S.A. (2003) Diet and DNA methylation interactions in cancer prevention. *Annals of the New York Academy of Sciences*, **983**, 197–207.

Rowling, M.J., McMullen, M.H. and Schalinske, K.L. (2002) Vitamin A and its derivatives induce hepatic glycine *N*-methyltransferase and hypomethylation of DNA in rats. *The Journal of Nutrition*, **132**, 365–369.

Ruder, E.H., Dorgan, J.F., Kranz, S. *et al.* (2008) Examining breast cancer growth and lifestyle risk factors: early life, childhood, and adolescence. *Clinical Breast Cancer*, **8**, 334–342.

Ruder, E.H., Thiebaut, A.C., Thompson, F.E. *et al.* (2011) Adolescent and mid-life diet: risk of colorectal cancer in the NIH–AARP Diet and Health Study. *The American Journal of Clinical Nutrition*, **94**, 1607–1619.

Rundle, A. (2011) Mechanisms underlying the effects of physical activity on cancer. In A. McTiernan (ed.), *Physical Activity, Dietary Calorie Restriction, and Cancer*. Springer, New York; pp. 143–163.

Santarelli, R.L., Pierre, F. and Corpet, D.E. (2008) Processed meat and colorectal cancer: a review of epidemiologic and experimental evidence. *Nutrition and Cancer*, **60**, 131–144.

Sarkar, F.H. and Li, Y. (2004) The role of isoflavones in cancer chemoprevention. *Frontiers in Bioscience*, **9**, 2714–2724.

Schatzkin, A., Park, Y., Leitzmann, M.F. *et al.* (2008) Prospective study of dietary fiber, whole grain foods, and small intestinal cancer. *Gastroenterology*, **135**, 1163–1167.

Schwingshackl, L. and Hoffmann, G. (2014) Adherence to Mediterranean diet and risk of cancer: a systematic review and meta-analysis of observational studies. *International Journal of Cancer*, **135**, 1884–1897.

Scott, K.P., Gratz, S.W., Sheridan, P.O. *et al.* (2013) The influence of diet on the gut microbiota. *Pharmacological Research*, **69**, 52–60.

Seelinger, G., Merfort, I., Wölfle, U. and Schempp, C.M. (2008) Anti-carcinogenic effects of the flavonoid luteolin. *Molecules*, **13**, 2628–2651.

Seitz, H.K. and Meier, P. (2007) The role of acetaldehyde in upper digestive tract cancer in alcoholics. *Translational Research*, **149**, 293–297.

Selma, M.V., Espin, J.C. and Tomas-Barberan, F.A. (2009) Interaction between phenolics and gut microbiota: role in human health. *Journal of Agricultural and Food Chemistry*, **57**, 6485–6501.

Shehzad, A., Wahid, F. and Lee, Y.S. (2010) Curcumin in cancer chemoprevention: molecular targets, pharmacokinetics, bioavailability, and clinical trials. *Archiv der Pharmazie*, **343**, 489–499.

Shen, X.-J., Zhou, J.-D., Dong, J.-Y. *et al.* (2012) Dietary intake of *n*-3 fatty acids and colorectal cancer risk: a meta-analysis of data from 489 000 individuals. *British Journal of Nutrition*, **108**, 1550–1556.

Shimazu, T., Wakai, K., Tamakoshi, A. *et al.* (2014) Association of vegetable and fruit intake with gastric cancer risk among Japanese: a pooled analysis of four cohort studies. *Annals of Oncology*, **25**, 1228–1233.

Shimizu, M., Fukutomi, Y., Ninomiya, M. *et al.* (2008) Green tea extracts for the prevention of metachronous colorectal adenomas: a pilot study. *Cancer Epidemiology, Biomarkers & Prevention*, **17**, 3020–3025.

Shivdasani, R.A. (2006) MicroRNAs: regulators of gene expression and cell differentiation. *Blood*, **108**, 3646–3653.

Shrubsole, M.J., Shu, X.O., Li, H.-L. *et al.* (2011) Dietary B vitamin and methionine intakes and breast cancer risk among Chinese women. *American Journal of Epidemiology*, **173**, 1171–1182.

Sieri, S., Chiodini, P., Agnoli, C. *et al.* (2014) Dietary fat intake and development of specific breast cancer subtypes. *Journal of the National Cancer Institute*, **106** (5), dju068.

Simons, C.C.J.M., van den Brandt, P.A., Stehouwer, C. *et al.* (2014) Body size, physical activity, early-life energy restriction, and associations with methylated insulin-like growth factor binding protein genes in colorectal cancer. *Cancer Epidemiology, Biomarkers & Prevention*, **23** (9), 1852–1862.

Sivagami, G., Vinothkumar, R., Preethy, C.P. *et al.* (2012) Role of hesperetin (a natural flavonoid) and its analogue on apoptosis in HT-29 human colon adenocarcinoma cell line – a comparative study. *Food and Chemical Toxicology*, **50**, 660–671.

Sivan, E., Mazaki-Tovi, S., Pariente, C. *et al.* (2003) Adiponectin in human cord blood: relation to fetal birth weight and gender. *The Journal of Clinical Endocrinology and Metabolism*, **88**, 5656–5660.

Slattery, M.L. (2008) Defining dietary consumption: is the sum greater than its parts? *The American Journal of Clinical Nutrition*, **88**, 14–15.

Song, J., Su, H., Wang, B.-L. *et al.* (2014a) Fish consumption and lung cancer risk: systematic review and meta-analysis. *Nutrition and Cancer*, **66**, 539–549.

Song, M., Chan, A.T., Fuchs, C.S. *et al.* (2014b) Dietary intake of fish, omega-3 and omega-6 fatty acids and risk of colorectal cancer: a prospective study in US men and women. *International Journal of Cancer*, **135**, 2413–2423.

Stahl, W., Heinrich, U., Aust, O. *et al.* (2006) Lycopene-rich products and dietary photoprotection. *Photochemical & Photobiological Sciences*, **5**, 238–242.

Stattin, P., Lukanova, A., Biessy, C. *et al.* (2004) Obesity and colon cancer: does leptin provide a link? *International Journal of Cancer*, **109**, 149–152.

Stefanska, B., Rudnicka, K., Bednarek, A. and Fabianowska-Majewska, K. (2010) Hypomethylation and induction of retinoic acid receptor beta 2 by concurrent action of adenosine analogues and natural compounds in breast cancer cells. *European Journal of Pharmacology*, **638**, 47–53.

Steindorf, K., Leitzmann, M.F. and Friedenreich, C.M. (2013) Physical activity and primary cancer prevention. In C.M. Ulrich, K. Steindorf and N.A. Berger (eds), *Exercise, Energy Balance, and Cancer*. Springer, New York; pp. 86–106.

Steinkellner, H., Rabot, S., Freywald, C. *et al.* (2001) Effects of cruciferous vegetables and their constituents on drug metabolizing enzymes involved in the bioactivation of DNA-reactive dietary carcinogens. *Mutation Research: Fundamental and Molecular Mechanisms of Mutagenesis*, **480**, 285–297.

Stevenson, L., Phillips, F., O'Sullivan, K. and Walton, J. (2012) Wheat bran: its composition and benefits to health, a European perspective. *International Journal of Food Sciences and Nutrition*, **63**, 1001–1013.

Stickel, F. and Seitz, H.K. (2004) Ethanol and methyl transfer: its role in liver disease and hepatocarcinogenesis. In R.R. Watson and V.R. Preedy (eds), *Nutrition and Alcohol: Linking Nutrient Interactions and Dietary Intake*. CRC Press, Boca Raton, FL; pp. 57–72.

Stocks, T., Borena, W., Strohmaier, S. *et al.* (2010) Cohort profile: the metabolic syndrome and cancer project (Me-Can). *International Journal of Epidemiology*, **39**, 660–667.

Stolzenberg-Solomon, R.Z., Chang, S.-C., Leitzmann, M.F. *et al.* (2006) Folate intake, alcohol use, and postmenopausal breast cancer risk in the Prostate, Lung, Colorectal, and Ovarian Cancer Screening Trial. *The American Journal of Clinical Nutrition*, **83**, 895–904.

Stolzenberg-Solomon, R.Z., Jacobs, E.J., Arslan, A.A. *et al.* (2010) Circulating 25-hydroxyvitamin D and risk of pancreatic cancer: Cohort Consortium Vitamin D Pooling Project of Rarer Cancers. *American Journal of Epidemiology*, **172**, 81–93.

Strati, A., Papoutsi, Z., Lianidou, E. and Moutsatsou, P. (2009) Effect of ellagic acid on the expression of human telomerase reverse transcriptase (*hTERT*) α+ β+ transcript in estrogen receptor-positive MCF-7 breast cancer cells. *Clinical Biochemistry*, **42**, 1358–1362.

Supic, G., Jagodic, M. and Magic, Z. (2013) Epigenetics: a new link between nutrition and cancer. *Nutrition and Cancer*, **65**, 781–792.

Surh, Y.-J. (2003) Cancer chemoprevention with dietary phytochemicals. *Nature Reviews: Cancer*, **3**, 768–780.

Swanson, J.M., Entringer, S., Buss, C. and Wadhwa, P.D. (2009) Developmental origins of health and disease: environmental exposures. *Seminars in Reproductive Medicine*, **27** (5), 391–402.

Talvas, J., Caris-Veyrat, C., Guy, L. *et al.* (2010) Differential effects of lycopene consumed in tomato paste and lycopene in the form of a purified extract on target genes of cancer prostatic cells. *The American Journal of Clinical Nutrition*, **91**, 1716–1724.

Tang, S.-N., Singh, C., Nall, D. *et al.* (2010) The dietary bioflavonoid quercetin synergizes with epigallocathechin gallate (EGCG) to inhibit prostate cancer stem cell characteristics, invasion, migration and epithelial-mesenchymal transition. *Journal of Molecular Signaling*, 5, 14.

Tang, W.-Y., Newbold, R., Mardilovich, K. *et al.* (2008) Persistent hypomethylation in the promoter of nucleosomal binding protein 1 (*Nsbp1*) correlates with overexpression of *Nsbp1* in mouse uteri neonatally exposed to diethylstilbestrol or genistein. *Endocrinology*, 149, 5922–5931.

Terry, P., Lagergren, J., Ye, W. *et al.* (2000) Antioxidants and cancers of the esophagus and gastric cardia. *International Journal of Cancer*, 87, 750–754.

Terry, P., Giovannucci, E., Michels, K.B. *et al.* (2001) Fruit, vegetables, dietary fiber, and risk of colorectal cancer. *Journal of the National Cancer Institute*, 93, 525–533.

Thanos, J., Cotterchio, M., Boucher, B.A. *et al.* (2006) Adolescent dietary phytoestrogen intake and breast cancer risk (Canada). *Cancer Causes & Control*, 17, 1253–1261.

Thomas, C.C., Wingo, P.A., Dolan, M.S. *et al.* (2009) Endometrial cancer risk among younger, overweight women. *Obstetrics and Gynecology*, 114, 22–27.

Tio, M., Andrici, J., Cox, M.R. and Eslick, G.D. (2014a) Folate intake and the risk of prostate cancer: a systematic review and meta-analysis. *Prostate Cancer and Prostatic Diseases*, 17, 213–219.

Tio, M., Andrici, J. and Eslick, G.D. (2014b) Folate intake and the risk of breast cancer: a systematic review and meta-analysis. *Breast Cancer Research and Treatment*, 145, 513–524.

Toden, S., Bird, A.R., Topping, D.L. and Conlon, M.A. (2005) Resistant starch attenuates colonic DNA damage induced by higher dietary protein in rats. *Nutrition and Cancer*, 51, 45–51.

Toden, S., Bird, A.R., Topping, D.L. and Conlon, M.A. (2006) Resistant starch prevents colonic DNA damage induced by high dietary cooked red meat or casein in rats. *Cancer Biology & Therapy*, 5, 267–272.

Togo, P., Osler, M., Sørensen, T. and Heitmann, B. (2004) A longitudinal study of food intake patterns and obesity in adult Danish men and women. *International Journal of Obesity*, 28, 583–593.

Tollefsbol, T.O. (2009) *Cancer Epigenetics*. CRC Press, Boca Raton, FL.

Tollefsbol, T.O. (2014) Dietary epigenetics in cancer and aging. In V. Zappia, S. Panico, G. L. Russo *et al.* (eds), *Advances in Nutrition and Cancer*. Cancer Treatment and Research 159. New York: Springer; pp. 257–267.

Tomatis L. (ed.) (1990) *Cancer: Causes, Occurrence and Control.* IARC Scientific Publications, 100. International Agency for Research on Cancer, Lyon.

Toniolo, P., Riboli, E., Protta, F. *et al.* (1989) Calorie-providing nutrients and risk of breast cancer. *Journal of the National Cancer Institute*, 81, 278–286.

Troisi, R., Potischman, N., Roberts, J. *et al.* (2003) Associations of maternal and umbilical cord hormone concentrations with maternal, gestational and neonatal factors (United States). *Cancer Causes & Control*, 14, 347–355.

Tucker, K.L. (2010) Dietary patterns, approaches, and multicultural perspective. *Applied Physiology, Nutrition, and Metabolism*, 35, 211–218.

Turmo, I.G. (2012) The Mediterranean diet: consumption, cuisine and food habits. In *Mediterra: The Mediterranean Diet for Sustainable Regional Development*. Presses de Sciences Po, Paris; pp. 115–132.

Tuyns, A.J., Kaaks, R. and Haelterman, M. (1988) Colorectal cancer and the consumption of foods: a case–control study in Belgium. *Nutrition and Cancer*, 11, 189–204.

Ulrich, C.M., Steindorf, K. and Berger, N.A. (eds) (2013) *Exercise, Energy Balance and Cancer*. Springer, New York.

UNDP (2013) *Human Development Report 2012. The Rise of the South: Human Progress in a Diverse World*. United Nations Development Programme, New York.

USDA and HHS (2010) *Dietary Guidelines for Americans, 2010*. US Government Printing Office, Washington, DC.

Vainio, H. and Bianchini, F. (2002) *Weight Control and Physical Activity*. IARC Press, Lyon.

Van der Pols, J.C., Bain, C., Gunnell, D. *et al.* (2007) Childhood dairy intake and adult cancer risk: 65-y follow-up of the Boyd Orr cohort. *The American Journal of Clinical Nutrition*, 86, 1722–1729.

Van Poppel, G. and Goldbohm, R.A. (1995) Epidemiologic evidence for beta-carotene and cancer prevention. *The American Journal of Clinical Nutrition*, 62, 1393S–1402S.

Vanden Berghe, W. (2012) Epigenetic impact of dietary polyphenols in cancer chemoprevention: lifelong remodeling of our epigenomes. *Pharmacological Research*, 65, 565–576.

Vaquero, M., Alberto, M. and de Nadra, M. (2007) Antibacterial effect of phenolic compounds from different wines. *Food Control*, 18, 93–101.

Varela-Rey, M., Woodhoo, A., Martinez-Chantar, M.L. *et al.* (2013) Alcohol, DNA methylation, and cancer. *Alcohol Research*, 35, 25–35.

Vatten, L.J., Nilsen, T.I.L., Tretli, S. *et al.* (2005) Size at birth and risk of breast cancer: prospective population-based study. *International Journal of Cancer*, 114, 461–464.

Velie, E.M., Nechuta, S. and Osuch, J.R. (2006) Lifetime reproductive and anthropometric risk factors for breast cancer in postmenopausal women. *Breast Disease*, 24, 17–35.

Verma, M. (2013) Cancer control and prevention: nutrition and epigenetics. *Current Opinion in Clinical Nutrition and Metabolic Care*, 16, 376–384.

Vineis, P. and Wild, C.P. (2014) Global cancer patterns: causes and prevention. *The Lancet*, 383, 549–557.

Vitale, D.C., Piazza, C., Melilli, B. *et al.* (2013) Isoflavones: estrogenic activity, biological effect and bioavailability. *European Journal of Drug Metabolism and Pharmacokinetics*, 38, 15–25.

Vossenaar, M., Solomons, N.W., Valdés-Ramos, R. and Anderson, A.S. (2011) Agreement between dietary and lifestyle guidelines for cancer prevention in population samples of Europeans and Mesoamericans. *Nutrition*, 27, 1146–1155.

Vucenik, I. and Stains, J.P. (2012) Obesity and cancer risk: evidence, mechanisms, and recommendations. *Annals of the New York Academy of Sciences*, 1271, 37–43.

Walker, A.W., Duncan, S.H., Leitch, E.C.M. *et al.* (2005) pH and peptide supply can radically alter bacterial populations and short-chain fatty acid ratios within microbial communities from the human colon. *Applied and Environmental Microbiology*, 71, 3692–3700.

Walker, C.L. and Ho, S.-M. (2012) Developmental reprogramming of cancer susceptibility. *Nature Reviews: Cancer*, 12, 479–486.

Wang, C.-Z., Ma, X.-Q., Yang, D.-H. *et al.* (2010) Production of enterodiol from defatted flaxseeds through biotransformation by human intestinal bacteria. *BMC Microbiology*, 10, 115.

Wang, L., Liu, X., Fang, Y. *et al.* (2008) De-repression of the p21 promoter in prostate cancer cells by an isothiocyanate via inhibition of HDACs and c-Myc. *International Journal of Oncology*, 33, 375–380.

Wang, X.-D. (2003) Retinoids and alcohol-related carcinogenesis. *The Journal of Nutrition*, 133 (1), 287S–290S.

Ward, H.A. and Kuhnle, G.G. (2010) Phytoestrogen consumption and association with breast, prostate and colorectal cancer in EPIC Norfolk. *Archives of Biochemistry and Biophysics*, 501, 170–175.

WCRF/AICR (2007) *Food, Nutrition, Physical Activity, and the Prevention of Cancer: A Global Perspective*. American Institute for Cancer Research, Washington, DC.

WCRF/AICR (2009) *Policy and Action for Cancer Prevention. Food, Nutrition, and Physical Activity: A Global Perspective.* American Institute for Cancer Research, Washington, DC. http://www.wcrf.org/sites/default/files/Policy_Report.pdf (accessed 12 December 2016).

WCRF/AICR (2010) *Food, Nutrition, Physical Activity, and the Prevention of Breast Cancer.* American Institute for Cancer Research, Washington, DC. http://www.aicr.org/continuous-update-project/reports/Breast-Cancer-2010-Report.pdf (accessed 12 December 2016).

WCRF/AICR (2011) *Food, Nutrition, Physical Activity, and the Prevention of Colorectal Cancer.* Institute for Cancer Research, Washington, DC. http://www.aicr.org/continuous-update-project/reports/Colorectal-Cancer-2011-Report.pdf (accessed 12 December 2016).

WCRF/AICR (2012) *Food, Nutrition, Physical Activity, and the Prevention of Pancreatic Cancer.* Institute for Cancer Research, Washington, DC. http://www.aicr.org/continuous-update-project/reports/pancreatic-cancer-2012-report.pdf (accessed 12 December 2016).

WCRF/AICR (2013) *Food, Nutrition, Physical Activity, and the Prevention of Endometrial Cancer.* http://www.aicr.org/continuous-update-project/reports/Endometrial-Cancer-2013-Report.pdf (accessed 12 December 2016).

WCRF/AICR (2014) *Food, Nutrition, Physical Activity, and the Prevention of Ovarian Cancer.* Institute for Cancer Research, Washington, DC. http://www.aicr.org/continuous-update-project/reports/ovarian-cancer-2014-report.pdf (accessed 12 December 2016).

Weismayer, C., Anderson, J.G. and Wolk, A. (2006) Changes in the stability of dietary patterns in a study of middle-aged Swedish women. *The Journal of Nutrition,* **136,** 1582–1587.

Welsch, C.W. (1992) Relationship between dietary fat and experimental mammary tumorigenesis: a review and critique. *Cancer Research,* **52,** 2040s–2048s.

Whitehead, N., Reyner, F. and Lindenbaum, J. (1973) Megaloblastic changes in the cervical epithelium: association with oral contraceptive therapy and reversal with folic acid. *JAMA,* **226,** 1421–1424.

WHO (2002) *National Cancer Control Programmes: Policies and Managerial Guidelines.* World Health Organization, Geneva.

WHO (2003) *Diet, Nutrition and the Prevention of Chronic Diseases: Report of a Joint WHO/FAO Expert Consultation.* World Health Organization, Geneva.

WHO (2006) *BMI classification.* http://apps.who.int/bmi/index.jsp?introPage=intro_3.html (accessed 12 December 2016).

WHO (2015) *Cancer.* Fact sheet no. 297. http://www.who.int/mediacentre/factsheets/fs297/en/ (accessed 13 December 2016).

Wight, A. and Ogden, G. (1998) Possible mechanisms by which alcohol may influence the development of oral cancer – a review. *Oral Oncology,* **34,** 441–447.

Willett, W.C., Sacks, F., Trichopoulou, A. *et al.* (1995) Mediterranean diet pyramid: a cultural model for healthy eating. *The American Journal of Clinical Nutrition,* **61,** 1402S–1406S.

Willis, M.S. and Wians Jr, F.H. (2003) The role of nutrition in preventing prostate cancer: a review of the proposed mechanism of action of various dietary substances. *Clinica Chimica Acta,* **330,** 57–83.

Windey, K., de Preter, V. and Verbeke, K. (2012) Relevance of protein fermentation to gut health. *Molecular Nutrition & Food Research,* **56,** 184–196.

Wolin, K., Yan, Y., Colditz, G. and Lee, I. (2009) Physical activity and colon cancer prevention: a meta-analysis. *British Journal of Cancer,* **100,** 611–616.

Wong, J.M., de Souza, R., Kendall, C.W. *et al.* (2006) Colonic health: fermentation and short chain fatty acids. *Journal of Clinical Gastroenterology,* **40,** 235–243.

Wu, A.H., Pike, M.C. and Stram, D.O. (1999) Meta-analysis: dietary fat intake, serum estrogen levels, and the risk of breast cancer. *Journal of the National Cancer Institute,* **91,** 529–534.

Wu, A.H., Wan, P., Hankin, J. *et al.* (2002) Adolescent and adult soy intake and risk of breast cancer in Asian-Americans. *Carcinogenesis,* **23,** 1491–1496.

Wu, Q.J., Xie, L., Zheng, W. *et al.* (2013a) Cruciferous vegetables consumption and the risk of female lung cancer: a prospective study and a meta-analysis. *Annals of Oncology,* **24,** 1918–1924.

Wu, Q.J., Yang, Y., Wang, J. *et al.* (2013b) Cruciferous vegetable consumption and gastric cancer risk: a meta-analysis of epidemiological studies. *Cancer Science,* **104,** 1067–1073.

Xu, X., Dailey, A.B., Peoples-Sheps, M. *et al.* (2009) Birth weight as a risk factor for breast cancer: a meta-analysis of 18 epidemiological studies. *Journal of Women's Health,* **18,** 1169–1178.

Xu, X., Yu, E., Liu, L. *et al.* (2013) Dietary intake of vitamins A, C, and E and the risk of colorectal adenoma: a meta-analysis of observational studies. *European Journal of Cancer Prevention,* **22,** 529–539.

Yan, A.W., Fouts, D.E., Brandl, J. *et al.* (2011) Enteric dysbiosis associated with a mouse model of alcoholic liver disease. *Hepatology,* **53,** 96–105.

Yokota, A., Fukiya, S., Islam, K.B. *et al.* (2012) Is bile acid a determinant of the gut microbiota on a high-fat diet? *Gut Microbes,* **3,** 455–459.

Young, G.P., Hu, Y., Le Leu, R.K. and Nyskohus, L. (2005) Dietary fibre and colorectal cancer: a model for environment–gene interactions. *Molecular Nutrition & Food Research,* **49,** 571–584.

Yusof, A.S., Isa, Z.M. and Shah, S.A. (2012) Dietary patterns and risk of colorectal cancer: a systematic review of cohort studies (2000–2011). *Asian Pacific Journal of Cancer Prevention,* **13,** 4713–4717.

Zeng, H., Lazarova, D.L. and Bordonaro, M. (2014) Mechanisms linking dietary fiber, gut microbiota and colon cancer prevention. *World Journal of Gastrointestinal Oncology,* **6,** 41–51.

Zhang, W., Xiang, Y.B., Li, H.L. *et al.* (2013) Vegetable-based dietary pattern and liver cancer risk: results from the Shanghai Women's and Men's Health Studies. *Cancer Science,* **104,** 1353–1361.

Zhao, J., Huang, W.G., He, J. *et al.* (2006) Diallyl disulfide suppresses growth of HL-60 cell through increasing histone acetylation and $p21^{WAF1}$ expression in vivo and in vitro. *Acta Pharmacologica Sinica,* **27,** 1459–1466.

Zheng, J.S., Hu, X.J., Zhao, Y.M. *et al.* (2013) Intake of fish and marine n-3 polyunsaturated fatty acids and risk of breast cancer: meta-analysis of data from 21 independent prospective cohort studies. *BMJ,* **346,** f3706.

Ziegler, R.G., Hoover, R.N., Pike, M.C. *et al.* (1993) Migration patterns and breast cancer risk in Asian-American women. *Journal of the National Cancer Institute,* **85,** 1819–1827.

20
Bone Health

Louise R Wilson, Andrea L Darling, and Susan A Lanham-New

Key messages

- Achieving and maintaining optimum bone health throughout the life cycle is critical for the prevention of rickets, osteomalacia and osteoporosis. Rickets and osteomalacia are usually a result of calcium and vitamin D deficiency, causing softening of bones, and both conditions are treatable with calcium and vitamin D supplementation.
- Osteoporosis is much more complex to treat. It is characterised by both a low bone mass and micro-architectural deterioration of bone tissue, leading to an increase in bone fragility and susceptibility to fracture. It is not reversible and results in a huge financial burden to public health-care systems.
- Nutrition is one of many factors that influence bone mass and risk of bone disease, and developing nutritional approaches and policies is a feasible option for the prevention and treatment of osteoporosis via population-based strategies.
- The importance of adequate calcium and vitamin D in promoting bone health throughout the life cycle has a robust evidence base, and emphasis of their importance has been included in several important European, American and global health reports. Poor vitamin D status in populations groups of all ages is widespread across many countries (developed and developing). Urgent public health strategies are required to address this growing epidemic

given that vitamin D plays a critical role in health outcomes other than just skeletal integrity.
- Dietary protein may be beneficial for bone due to its effect of increasing insulin like growth-factor 1. It may also be detrimental as it can cause calcium loss from bone via its effect on increasing net endogenous acid production. However, this depends on the type and amount of protein consumed, as well as the overall composition of the diet.
- There is some evidence from observational studies and small-scale intervention trials that increased dietary protein intake is associated with higher bone mineral content, but there is little evidence to date that increased protein intake reduces the risk of bone fracture in the longer term.
- Other nutritional factors and nutrients (such as potassium, magnesium, vitamins A, C, E and K, and acid–base balance), as well as lifestyle factors (alcohol and caffeine consumption), are also likely to have important roles in bone health. However, at present, the evidence base is less well developed in terms of the relationship between these factors and bone health.

20.1 Introduction

This chapter first briefly defines the principal diseases of poor bone health, and the burden of this on the individual and health-care services. It also introduces the fundamentals of bone structure, how this changes throughout life and how bone health is assessed. It then focuses on the importance of certain nutritional factors that have benefits, or are detrimental, to bone health and concludes with areas for further research.

20.2 Definition of bone diseases and public health impact of poor bone health

Rickets, osteomalacia and osteoporosis

Achieving and maintaining optimal bone health throughout the life course is important in the prevention of rickets in childhood, osteomalacia in adulthood and osteoporosis in older age. Both rickets and osteomalacia are defined as a softening of the bones, causing bone pain

Public Health Nutrition, Second Edition. Edited by Judith L Buttriss, Ailsa A Welch, John M Kearney and Susan A Lanham-New.
© 2018 by The Nutrition Society. Published 2018 by John Wiley & Sons, Ltd.
Companion website: www.wiley.com/go/buttriss/publichealth

and muscle weakness. In addition, rickets leads to bone deformity due to abnormal bone growth. Osteoporosis is defined by the World Health Organization (WHO) as a 'systemic skeletal disease characterised by low bone mass and micro-architectural deterioration of bone tissue, with a consequent increase in bone fragility and susceptibility to fracture' (Peck *et al.*, 1993).

Public health impact of osteoporosis in the UK

Poor bone health constitutes a major public health problem. In the UK, osteoporosis leads to over 200 000 fractures each year, causing disability and pain to sufferers, as well as an annual cost of over £1.73 billion to the National Health Service (NHS) (National Osteoporosis Guideline Group, 2016). This value excludes the high cost of social care, and in the case of hip fractures the hospital cost is thought to only represent a half of the total care cost. It is estimated that one in three women and one in five men aged >50 years worldwide will suffer from osteoporosis in their lifetime (International Osteoporosis Foundation, 2015) and will subsequently suffer one or more osteoporotic fractures; hence, this a disease of high public health importance.

Public health impact of osteoporosis worldwide

Osteoporosis is a global problem. For example, in the USA, osteoporosis results in an estimated 2 million fractures each year (Burge *et al.*, 2007). The hospitalisation burden of osteoporotic fractures (and other related health-care costs) is greater than that of myocardial infarction, stroke or breast cancer (Singer *et al.*, 2015). Across Europe, more disability-adjusted life years (DALY) are lost due to osteoporosis than for many other non-communicable diseases, such as rheumatoid arthritis, Parkinson's disease, and prostate and breast cancer (National Osteoporosis Guideline Group, 2016).

20.3 Fundamentals of bone physiology

The skeleton serves a variety of functions. The primary function of bone tissue is to provide structural support and allow movement, but it also functions to maintain calcium homeostasis and serves as a storage site for calcium and other minerals. It is also the primary site of blood cell formation.

The skeleton is made up of two types of bone tissue: 80% cortical bone and 20% trabecular bone. Cortical bone (also known as compact bone) is found in the shafts of the long bones, whereas trabecular bone (also known as cancellous bone) is found in the flat bones (e.g. pelvis) and in the ends

of long bones (e.g. head and neck of the femur). Trabecular bone is formed by a honeycomb-type structure of bone tissue called trabeculae. It is more metabolically active than cortical bone, with an annual bone turnover rate of 25%, compared with 2–3% in cortical bone.

20.4 Bone changes throughout the life course

Bone is continuously being remodelled, principally through the actions of osteoblast and osteoclast cells. Osteoblasts are responsible for bone formation, whereas osteoclasts cause bone resorption. Therefore, bone mass changes throughout the life cycle, as shown in Figure 20.1. Bone mass in later life is predominantly determined by three factors; (1) peak bone mass attained during adolescence and early adulthood, (2) bone mass maintenance during adulthood and (3) the progressive rate of bone loss with age. The menopausal transition is of considerable concern for women, as due to oestrogen deficiency there can be a loss of 3% of bone density each year over a period of 5–10 years. That represents, for some women, over one-fifth of their bone density being lost and thus increases the risk of developing osteoporosis and subsequent fractures.

20.5 Diagnosis of osteoporosis and assessment of bone health

Although the most clinically relevant endpoint in assessing bone health is actual bone fracture, by this stage preventative interventions are too late except in the prevention of further fracture. Most studies use intermediate outcome measures to assess bone health and subsequent risk of fracture. These intermediate outcomes include bone strength and density, biochemical markers and other musculoskeletal outcomes.

Bone strength and density

Osteoporosis is characterised by a loss in bone strength, and although bone quality is also a contributing factor, measuring bone density provides an indirect estimation of bone strength and is used in the diagnosis of osteoporosis. The most common measurement of bone strength used in clinical settings to diagnose osteoporosis is areal bone mineral density (aBMD), with the most common technique used to measure aBMD being dual X-ray absorptiometry. Osteoporosis is diagnosed when a patient's bone mineral density (BMD) is equal to or more than 2.5 standard deviations below a reference measurement derived from bone density measurements in a population of healthy young adults, indicated by a *T*-score of −2.5 or

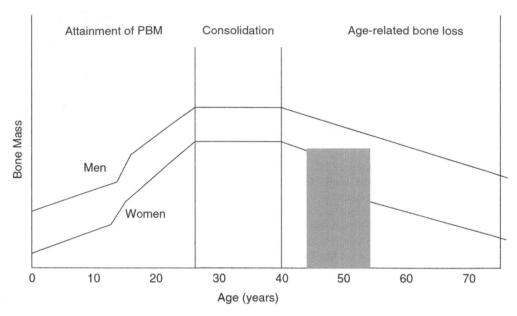

Figure 20.1 Changes in bone mass during the life course. The grey shaded area indicates the menopause.

lower (Kanis, 2002). However, measuring aBMD by dual X-ray absorptiometry has limitations in its assessment of bone strength as, although it accounts for 60–70% of the variation in bone strength, it does not take into account other factors that contribute to bone strength, such as bone size, shape, architecture and turnover (Ammann and Rizzoli, 2003). Moreover, aBMD underestimates bone density in persons with a small bone size.

Volumetric BMD is a more accurate estimate of bone density, and thus bone strength, as the measurement is three-dimensional and so takes account of bone size. This is measured using quantitative computed tomography and peripheral quantitative computed tomography, and can assess structural and geometric properties of the bone. However, as it only measures peripheral sites (e.g. radius, tibia) and not central sites (e.g. spine and hip), it is mainly used in scientific research rather than in clinical settings.

Biochemical markers

In addition to measuring 25-hydroxyvitamin D (25OHD) status, the active vitamin D hormone 1,25-di-hydroxyvitamin D (1,25(OH)$_2$D, calcitriol) and parathyroid hormone (PTH) levels are useful in the assessment of bone health (due to their role in regulating calcium and phosphorus homeostasis). Serum total calcium and albumin (to calculate albumin adjusted/corrected calcium) are often measured to detect conditions associated with hypercalcaemia (such as primary hyperparathyroidism) or hypocalcaemia and consequent secondary hyperparathyroidism, which may cause bone loss.

Bone markers

Bone turnover markers, which are measured in blood serum or urine, are by-products of the bone turnover process (e.g. enzymes, collagen breakdown products) and, therefore, can be used to assess bone turnover rate and to predict fracture risk (Vasikaran et al. 2011). Both bone formation markers, such as procollagen type 1 N-terminal propeptide, and bone resorption markers, such as C-terminal telopeptide of collagen type 1, can be measured (Johansson et al., 2014). Unfortunately, the use of these bone turnover markers gives limited information as it is not possible to determine the metabolic activity of different skeletal compartments (e.g. cortical versus trabecular) (Garnero, 2014) and they are costly to measure. They are mainly used in research settings, but in clinical medicine the particular value of bone resorption markers is to enable the measurement of osteoclastic activity in response to anti-resorptive therapy, such as bisphosphonates. However, there is a great deal of inter-individual variation, and hence this must be considered in the interpretation of such markers.

Musculoskeletal outcomes

Muscle strength and function has been shown to be an independent predictor of BMD, with decreased muscle strength being associated with lower BMD (Francis et al., 2015), and is therefore a musculoskeletal outcome that can be measured to assess bone strength and subsequent risk of fracture. Frailty (Ensrud et al., 2007), incidence of falls (Clark et al., 2011) and prior fractures (Gehlbach et al., 2012) are also determinants of fracture risk.

Risk assessment tools

The use of fracture risk assessment tools in the assessment of patients has been recommended in the UK by the National Institute of Clinical Excellence. The FRAX tool (https://www.shef.ac.uk/FRAX/tool.jsp) has been developed by the WHO Collaborating Centre for Metabolic Bone Disease at Sheffield using risk factors (including body mass index, history of prior fracture, parental history of fracture, smoking, glucocorticoids, alcohol and rheumatoid arthritis) to compute a 10-year probability of hip or major osteoporotic fracture. This has proved very useful in the clinical setting (McCloskey *et al.*, 2015), but further work is required, particularly to assess the validity of the tool in ethnic minority groups.

20.6 Regulation of calcium homeostasis

Body stores of calcium

Calcium is an important component of the skeleton, given that it is one of the predominant minerals found in bone tissue. Over 99% of the body's total calcium is found in the bone matrix (and teeth) as hydroxyapatite, and the remaining 1% of calcium circulates in the blood.

Phosphorus and magnesium also make up large percentages of the bone matrix, with over 88% and 60% respectively of the body's content of these minerals deposited in bone.

Calcium homeostasis

Circulating calcium is essential for a range of metabolic activities, such as blood coagulation, neuromuscular contraction, heart muscle function, cell adhesion, cell membrane stability and as a trigger for hormonal secretion. To perform these important physiological roles, the concentration of calcium within the blood is maintained within narrow limits of 2.2–2.5 nmol/L. This calcium balance, known as calcium homeostasis, is essential for adequate bone mineralisation, and is tightly regulated by the thyroid and parathyroid glands, which release calciotrophic hormones (PTH, calcitriol, calcitonin). This is shown schematically in Figure 20.2.

When low blood calcium levels are detected, the secretion of calcitonin (which stimulates osteoblast activity) is inhibited and PTH is secreted. PTH increases blood calcium levels through its effects on bone, the kidneys and the intestine. PTH causes an increase in bone resorption, resulting in a release of calcium from the skeleton into the blood. In the kidneys, PTH

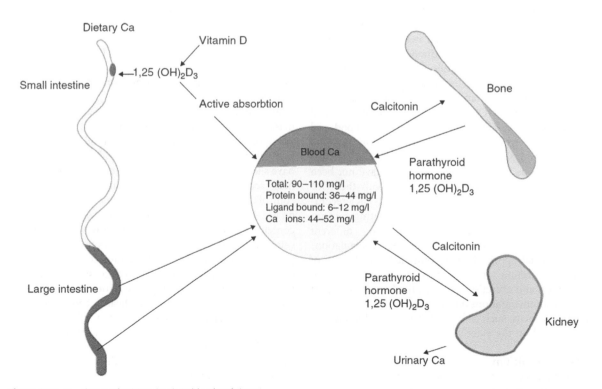

Figure 20.2 Regulation of calcium levels in blood and tissue.

enhances active reabsorption of calcium from the distal tubules and the thick ascending limb, and also stimulates the conversion of 25OHD to the active form of vitamin D (calcitriol, 1,25(OH)$_2$D). Calcitriol increases the absorption of dietary calcium in the intestine, but also stimulates the release of calcium from bone via increased bone resorption.

When blood calcium levels are high, the opposing effect is seen. Calcitonin is secreted by the thyroid gland and PTH secretion is suppressed, which leads to lower calcium levels through the inhibition of: calcium absorption in the intestine, osteoclast activity and renal tubular reabsorption of calcium, as well as by the stimulation of osteoblast activity by calcitonin.

20.7 Nutritional influences on bone health

Calcium

As calcium is one of the main bone-forming minerals, an adequate supply to the bones is essential at all stages of life: to support the attainment of optimal peak bone mass in childhood and adolescence, and to minimise bone losses to maintain bone mass during adulthood.

Calcium requirements: what are they based on?

Calcium requirements, therefore, vary throughout an individual's lifetime, with greater needs during the periods of rapid growth in childhood and adolescence, during pregnancy and lactation, and in later adult life. Recommendations on dietary calcium intake for adults are consistent across many leading organisations – Institute of Medicine (IOM), USA; National Health and Medical Research Council, Australia; WHO/Food and Agriculture Organization of the United Nations (FAO) – although the UK recommendations differ. The UK recommendations have been reviewed, but have not been updated since 1991. Table 20.1 shows both the IOM (USA) and Department of Health (DoH, UK) recommendations for dietary calcium. In estimating calcium requirements, committees have used different approaches; the UK DoH report based recommendations on a factorial approach that combined calculations of skeletal accretion and turnover rates with calcium absorption and excretion, whereas the USA IOM report based recommendations on varying outcomes relevant to the age of focus, such as bone density in childhood and fracture risk in the elderly.

Intakes of calcium

Inadequate calcium intake is a worldwide problem, having been reported in children, adolescents and adults

Table 20.1 Dietary calcium recommendations from the USA (IOM) and the UK (DoH).

Age	IOM RDA (mg) All	IOM RDA (mg) Female[a]	Age	DoH RNI (mg) All	DoH RNI (mg) Female[a]
0-6 months	1000[b]		0–12 months	525	
6–12 months	1500[b]				
1–3 years	700		1–3 years	350	
4–8 years	1000		4–6 years	450	
			7–10 years	550	
9–18 years	1300		11–18 years	1000	800
19–50 years	1000		19–50 years	700	
51–70 years	1000	1200	>50 years	700	
>70 years	1200				

RDA: recommended dietary allowance; RNI: reference nutrient intake.
[a] Where different from recommendation for males.
[b] Upper level intake.

across Europe, North America, Asia and Oceania (Peterlik *et al.*, 2009). In older adults, calcium intakes vary between countries (Peterlik *et al.*, 2009). In the UK, adolescents aged 11–18 years have been reported to have dietary calcium intakes below the relative UK DoH reference nutrient intake (RNI), whereas younger and older adults are meeting the UK RNI (Bates *et al.*, 2014). Although pre-school children are also meeting the UK RNI, a decline in calcium intake between the ages of 18 months and 3.5 years has been shown (Cribb *et al.*, 2015).

Calcium intakes and supplementation on bone health

Low calcium intakes during growth will affect peak bone mass attainment, and consequently have an effect on osteoporosis and fracture risk later in life. Clinical trials with calcium supplements in both children and teenagers have shown an overall positive effect of calcium on bone mass accrual, although a meta-analysis of randomised controlled trials (RCTs) found that calcium had no effect on BMD, and only a small positive effect on bone mineral content (Winzenberg *et al.*, 2006). However, the role of calcium supplementation in the prevention of osteoporosis and fracture has been the subject of considerable debate. Further research is required to establish the risk/benefit ratio of calcium supplementation with respect to the beneficial effects on bone health compared with suggested adverse effects on cardiovascular health; to date there has not been an RCT with the primary aim of determining the effect of calcium supplementation on cardiovascular health, and the evidence to date is not sufficient to warrant change to recommendations. The current consensus across professional bodies (National

Osteoporosis Society, UK; International Osteoporosis Foundation, USA) is that calcium supplements should only be used on an individual basis to bring total calcium intake to the recommended level in healthy adults.

Vitamin D

Sources and metabolism and of vitamin D

In the diet vitamin D is naturally present in two forms: vitamin D_2, which is found in plants and fungi, and vitamin D_3, which is found in fish, meat and eggs. However, there are limited natural dietary sources of either forms and vitamin D is a unique nutrient, with the main source not being diet but rather ultraviolet B-rays (UVB) from sunlight. Vitamin D_3 is formed as the result of direct skin exposure to UVB, which causes the conversion of 7-dehydrocholesterol to pre-vitamin D_3. This is then metabolised to vitamin D_3 by a temperature-dependent isomerisation. Both vitamin D_2 and D_3, irrespective of source, go through the same two-step hydroxylation process to become the biologically active form of vitamin D: $1,25(OH)_2D$ (calcitriol).

Once in the circulatory system both vitamins D_2 and D_3 bind to the vitamin-D-binding protein (VDBP) and are transported to the liver. At the liver, both vitamins D_2 and D_3 are converted to 25-hydoxyvitamin D (25OHD) via the action of 25-hydroxylase enzymes, such as those from the cyctochrome P450 (CYP) group (CYP2R1 and CYP27A1). 25OHD is the serum marker used to determine vitamin D status. Following hydroxylation in the liver, 25OHD then binds to VDBP in the circulation and is transported to the kidney. In the kidneys, 25OHD is converted to $1,25(OH)_2D$, the active form of vitamin D, by 25-hydroxyvitamin D-1-α-hydroxylases, such as CYP27B1 (DeLuca, 2004). This critical step is under the tight homeostatic regulation of circulating PTH concentrations (Deeb et al., 2007). The available $1,25(OH)_2D$ is then able to elicit the biologic functions of vitamin D, including the important role in calcium homeostasis discussed previously.

Vitamin D and musculoskeletal health

Vitamin D deficiency has been associated with skeletal conditions and other musculoskeletal health outcomes. In children, rickets is associated with low 25OHD levels of <12 nmol/L in the majority of cases (SACN, 2016). The IOM concluded that if calcium intake was adequate, the risk of rickets was increased at serum 25OHD concentration <30 nmol/L (IOM, 2011). In adults, osteomalacia is present when 25OHD levels are ≤20 nmol/L (SACN, 2016). Based on findings from a post-mortem analysis of bone biopsies the IOM concluded that all individuals were free of osteomalacia when serum 25OHD levels were >50 nmol/L and that a

significant increase in the number of people displaying osteomalacia was observed when serum 25OHD levels were <30 nmol/L (Priemel et al., 2010).

In addition, epidemiological studies and RCTs have reported associations between vitamin D levels and muscle strength and function (Ward et al., 2010; Tomlinson et al., 2014), fracture risk (Chapuy et al., 1992; Dawson-Hughes, 2008) and risk of falls (Stein et al., 1999), as well as stress fracture risk in military personnel (Dao et al., 2015). Specifically, supplementation with vitamin D has been shown to have a positive effect on BMD (Chapuy et al., 1992; Ooms et al., 1995; Dawson-Hughes et al., 1997), with a recent meta-analysis of 23 studies showing a small beneficial effect on femoral neck BMD (Reid et al., 2014).

Optimal vitamin D status for health

25OHD is the major circulating vitamin D metabolite measured to determine vitamin D status, being considered the gold standard (Seamans and Cashman, 2009). Nonetheless, internationally, there is a lack of consensus and definition on the suggested thresholds (cut-offs) used to define 25OHD levels, from deficiency to optimal levels, and the range of terminology and associated values used make comparisons of reported prevalence difficult.

The WHO and the UK's Scientific Advisory Committee on Nutrition (SACN) state that 25OHD levels <25 nmol/L (10 mg/mL) is the deficiency threshold (WHO Scientific Group on the Prevention and Management of Osteoporosis, 2003; SACN, 2007, 2016) with regard to the prevention of rickets and osteomalacia, and the WHO also define vitamin D insufficiency as 25OHD levels <50 nmol/L. However, the US IOM defines 25OHD levels <30 nmol/L as deficiency, 30–50 nmol/L as inadequacy and >50 nmol/L as sufficient (IOM, 2011).

The UK National Osteoporosis Society has recently agreed with the IOM thresholds and proposed that the UK practitioners should also adopt these (Francis et al., 2013). Commonly, vitamin D deficiency is defined by a 25OHD threshold of <25–30 nmol/L, with insufficiency defined by 25OHD levels in the range of 25–49 nmol/L (Spiro and Buttriss, 2014). Conversely, the Endocrine Society Task Force (USA/Canada) defines deficiency as 25OHD levels <50 nmol/L and advocates that 25OHD levels should exceed 75 nmol/L (Holick et al., 2011).

The differences in opinions of researchers in the field of vitamin D have previously been highlighted, specifically in relation to the optimal 25OHD levels for fracture prevention (Dawson-Hughes et al., 2005). Using this outcome measure, 'optimal' levels ranging from 50 to 80 nmol/L were reported. In a review of evidence from studies that evaluated thresholds for 25OHD levels in relation to BMD, lower-extremity function, dental health, and risk of falls, fractures and colorectal cancer it was found that the most advantageous 25OHD level for all health outcomes was at least 75 nmol/L, but 90–100 nmol/L was optimal (Bischoff-Ferrari et al., 2005). Despite one-off studies and individual researchers suggesting optimal 25OHD levels on the higher range of 70–100 nmol/L, many organisations and researchers consider a desirable level of 25OHD to be above 25 nmol/L, due to the limited number of RCTs investigating higher levels and a lack of long-term safety data for them (Lanham-New et al., 2011).

Dietary vitamin D recommendations internationally and in the UK

As there is no international consensus on the optimal 25OHD level for health among researchers, there is also variation in opinions across the world as to the dietary vitamin D intakes required to reach an optimal 25OHD status, with suggested daily doses ranging from 10 to 40 μg/day (Dawson-Hughes et al., 2005).

Most official vitamin D dietary recommendations worldwide, as shown in Table 20.2, are established based on ensuring adequate serum 25OHD levels to support skeletal health (Spiro and Buttriss, 2014; Buttriss, 2015).

Despite this same basis, there is still variation in recommendations from country to country. However, as illustrated in Table 20.2, the newly proposed UK recommendation of 10 μg/day (SACN, 2016) will bring the UK into alignment with other European and international recommendations.

The UK was previously the only country in Europe not to have any dietary recommendations for those aged 4–65 years, unless they were pregnant or breastfeeding, or considered specifically 'at risk' of vitamin D deficiency (e.g. individuals who get little sun exposure, such as older adults or those from ethnic groups). The recommendation had not been updated since 1991, as it had been assumed that free-living individuals attained adequate body stores of vitamin D from cutaneous synthesis during the summer to sustain 25OHD levels during the winter months (DoH, 1991). However, this is now known not to be the case for many individuals in the UK (Hyppönen and Power, 2007; Darling et al., 2013).

Vitamin D$_2$ versus vitamin D$_3$

Historically, it has been assumed that vitamin D$_2$ and vitamin D$_3$ were equally effective at raising vitamin D status (25OHD levels), but following recent controversy

Table 20.2 Dietary reference values for vitamin D (μg/day) in the UK, other European countries and internationally, at different life stages.

Reference		Children				Adults	Older adults	Pregnancy and lactation
		<1 year	1–3 years	4–10 years	11–18 years			
UK								
1991	DoH (1991)	8.5	7	–	–	–	10	10
2016[a]	SACN (2016)	8.5–10	10	10	10	10	10	10
European								
Austria/ Germany/ Switzerland[a]	DACH (2013)	10	20	20	20	20	20	20
Belgium	Hoge Gezondheidsraad (2009)	10	10	10	10–15	10–15	15	20
France	Afssa (2001)	20–25	10	5	5	5	5	10
Ireland	FSAI (1999)	7.0–8.5	10	0–10	0–15	0–10	10	10
Spain	Moreiras . (2013). (2013)	10	15	15	15	15	20	15
Netherlands	Health Council of the Netherlands (2012)	10	10	10	10	10	20	10
NNR	Nordic Council of Ministers (2014)	10	10	10	10	10	20	10
EC	SCF (1993)	7.0–8.5	10	0–10	0–15	0–10	10	10
Other								
OM	IOM (2011)	10	15	15	15	15	20	15
WHO/FAO	WHO Scientific Group on the Prevention and Management of Osteoporosis (2003)	5	5	5	5	5	10–15	5
NHMRC	NHMRC (2006)	5	5	5	5	5	10–15	5

Source: Modified from Spiro and Buttriss (2014).

NNR: Nordic Nutrition Recommendations; EC: European Commission; NHMRC, National Health and Medical Research (Australia).
[a] Specified without endogenous synthesis.

and several RCTs it is now clear that vitamin D_3 is almost twice as effective at raising status than vitamin D_2 is (Tripkovic et al., 2014). This increased efficacy is present when the vitamin D is delivered via both daily (Tripkovic et al., 2014) and bolus dosing (Tripkovic et al., 2012). Thus, it is speculated that they may not have equal effects on bone health. Previous studies that have shown differential responses in 25OHD levels to vitamin D_2 and D_3 have shown no difference in PTH concentrations between the groups (Logan et al., 2013) nor in 1,25 $(OH)_2D$ levels (Trang et al., 1998). However, very few of these studies have measured or published levels of all three key biochemical markers (25OHD, PTH and 1,25 $(OH)_2D$) together, which therefore has limited the ability to determine (i) the impact of and (ii) differences in impact of vitamin D_2 and D_3 on markers of bone health beyond the effect on 25OHD levels alone.

Current vitamin D status and dietary intakes

Low levels of vitamin D are highly prevalent in children, adolescents and adults throughout the world; making this a global concern (Mithal et al., 2009). Within the UK alone, one in five people are known to have low vitamin D levels (<25 nmol/L) (Bates et al., 2014), with a greater prevalence of deficiency found in those living at a higher latitude (Hyppönen and Power, 2007) and those of ethnic minority groups, such as South Asian women (Darling et al., 2013). The ability to synthesise vitamin D_3 from the sun's UVB rays has its limitations; latitude, season, weather and even air pollution limit the availability of UVB rays. Most notably, between the months of October and April the required UVB rays are not available in the UK for the synthesis of vitamin D_3. During these months, individuals are dependent on dietary sources of vitamin D to maintain 25OHD levels. However, these are also limited. The latest National Diet and Nutrition Survey data shows mean dietary intakes of vitamin D in British men and women to be 3.9 µg/day and 3.4 µg/day respectively (Bates et al., 2014), with approximately 0.8 µg of this, for both the men and women, coming from fortified foods such as meats and breakfast cereals. These intakes are well below the proposed UK recommendation of 10 µg/day and the SACN have recognised that it will be difficult for the UK population to achieve this proposed intake from natural dietary sources alone and recommend that consideration is given to strategies to help the UK population achieve the recommendation. As discussed in more detail in two recent reviews, the next steps will be to determine whether public health policies, such as mandatory fortification, need to be implemented to tackle the issue of low vitamin D status across the UK (Buttriss, 2015; Lanham-New and Wilson, 2016).

Acid–base balance and skeletal health

The human body is required to maintain physiological acidity at a pH of 7.35–7.45, which it achieves via three processes: kidney excretion of hydrogen ions, carbon dioxide expired from the lungs and the use of alkaline buffers such as bicarbonate. The skeleton acts as a reservoir of alkaline mineral, which is available for the body to use to reduce excess physiological acidity. During periods of higher physiological acidity, calcium is released from the bone to neutralise the acid and bring the body back to the correct pH. Hence, in the long term, excess physiological acidity could theoretically lead to reduced bone mass, through the continual loss of calcium from the bone that is not being replaced.

It is known that physiological acidity increases with ageing, due to poorer ability of the kidneys to remove acid ions from the body, which is likely to contribute to the process of osteoporosis with ageing. However, diet may also play a role in establishing physiological acid load in the body in persons of all ages. Some research has investigated whether diets producing high levels of physiological acidity – net endogenous acid production (NEAP) – are associated with poorer bone health. Some studies suggest an inverse relationship between NEAP and bone health (New et al., 2004; Wynn et al., 2008), but others suggest no relationship (McLean et al., 2011; Jia et al., 2015). Therefore, the evidence is still inconsistent, and further long-term intervention studies with good participant dietary compliance to a reduced NEAP diet are required.

Protein and bone health

Dietary protein and insulin-like growth factor-1
Historically, there has been much debate as to whether dietary protein is good or bad for bone health. Insulin-like growth factor-1 is a hormone that has an anabolic effect on bone, and is stimulated by dietary protein intake. In terms of epidemiology, many studies have found a positive association between dietary protein intake and bone health (Cooper et al., 1996; Hannan et al., 2000), but some have found no association (Zhu et al., 2011). In particular, there is conflicting evidence as to whether protein intake is associated with hip fracture risk, with a systematic review and meta-analysis finding a positive association between dietary protein intake and BMD, but not fracture risk (Darling et al., 2009). Therefore, dietary protein may have beneficial effects on bone density in the shorter term, but in the longer term this benefit may not necessarily translate into reduced risk of fracture.

Dietary protein and acid–base
High dietary protein intakes may theoretically cause increased physiological acid load in the body, leading

to calcium loss in the urine (calciuria) and loss of bone density. In a landmark study, Arnett and Dempster (1986) found that bone osteoclasts from rats increased in activity when placed in a more acidic environment, implying that bone resorption in humans would be increased with a higher physiological acid load. Moreover, some human studies have found poorer markers of bone health in persons with higher dietary protein intake (Kerstetter *et al.*, 1999; Zhang *et al.*, 2010), as well as increased calciuria with higher protein intakes (Ince *et al.*, 2004).

Conversely, it is probable that some of this increased calciuria is caused by dietary protein increasing calcium absorption from the gut (Kerstetter *et al.*, 1998), rather than calcium loss from bone. Also, the acid–base balance of the body is affected not only by dietary protein but also by other food components, such as phosphorus and potassium (Massey, 2003). In particular, a higher dietary calcium and fruit and vegetable intake may reduce the acid-increasing effect of high dietary protein intakes (Thorpe and Evans, 2011), with higher NEAP from high protein diets likely to detriment bone health most when calcium intakes are low (Mangano *et al.*, 2014).

Animal, vegetable and soy protein

There is also debate as to whether animal protein is more detrimental to bone health than vegetable protein, with studies finding animal protein is either detrimental (Feskanich *et al.*, 1996; Sellmeyer *et al.*, 2001) or better (Munger *et al.*, 1999) for bone health compared with vegetable protein intake. It is only protein sources that are high in sulphur amino acid content that have acid-raising potential, which includes all animal protein sources, and some vegetable protein sources (grains). Hence, vegetable-protein-based diets may have acid-raising potential if they contain a lot of grains, which may partly explain some of the conflicting results between studies. It also suggests that vegetarian diets may not necessarily be better for bone health, unless they contain a lot of alkaline-producing foods (e.g. fruit and vegetables).

The relationship between soy protein intake and bone health has also been of interest, due to the large consumption of soy-based foods in East Asia. Some studies have found a positive relationship between soy protein intake and bone health (Ho *et al.*, 2003; Spence *et al.*, 2005), whereas others have found no relationship (Vupadhyayula *et al.*, 2009). Soy protein contains other components (e.g. isoflavones) that may have beneficial effects on bone density via their ability to behave like oestrogen in the body. Therefore, it is difficult to interpret whether soy protein itself, when separate from the other components of soy foods, has an effect on bone

health or not. Further research examining supplements containing soy protein alone is required to establish the true effect of soy protein on bone.

Other micronutrients relevant to bone health

Vitamin K

Vitamin K comes in two main forms – K_1 (phylloquinone) and K_2 (menaquinones) – and is an essential cofactor enabling the addition of γ-carboxyglutamyl (Gla) residues to a variety of proteins in the body. Some of these proteins are important for bone health, including osteocalcin, protein S and matrix Gla protein. It is important, therefore, that the body has adequate vitamin K for bone health.

Systematic reviews and meta-analyses have shown a benefit of vitamin K_2 supplementation on reduced fracture risk in observational studies (Cockayne *et al.*, 2006) and improved BMD in RCTs (Huang *et al.*, 2015). On the other hand, the role of K_1, which is the form mostly found in western diets, is less clear, with less evidence of a benefit to bone health of increasing dietary K_1 intake compared with taking a vitamin K_2 supplement. This discrepancy between the two forms of vitamin K may be due to differences in biochemical structure as well as dose, which is higher in supplements than the usual western diet.

Magnesium

Adequate magnesium status is required for normal PTH secretion, and thus calcium homeostasis. Thus, a lack of magnesium can contribute to low serum calcium, a loss of calcium from the bones and poorer bone health. A recent systematic review and meta-analysis of observational studies showed a positive association between dietary magnesium intake and femoral neck BMD, but there was no relationship with lumbar spine BMD or fracture risk (Farsinejad-Marj *et al.*, 2016). Moreover, magnesium may help reduce the sarcopenia associated with ageing (Welch *et al.*, 2016), which could help prevent falls, and thus prevent fractures. Randomised, placebo-controlled trials of magnesium supplementation are now required to establish the supplemental dose or dietary intake of magnesium required for optimal bone health, in order to inform public health messages for reducing osteoporosis risk.

Phosphorus

The skeleton contains a large reservoir of phosphorus, which is important for a multitude of physiological processes (e.g. cell signalling, DNA structure, adenine triphosphate). Lack of phosphate can arise from inherited genetic conditions that cause pathological renal loss of phosphate; these conditions also cause severe bone disease due to the associated hypophosphataemia (e.g. hypophosphataemic rickets).

Hyperphosphataemia can occur in end-stage renal disease, or in the healthy population consuming western diets whereby there is an overconsumption of phosphorus compared with calcium (e.g. due to displacement of dairy products with soda drinks, high phosphorus content of food additives) (Calvo and Tucker, 2013). Of concern is that higher phosphorus intake is associated with increased PTH levels. Therefore, the high levels of phosphorus found in many processed foods may be contributing to increased osteoporosis risk (Calvo and Tucker, 2013) as phosphorus intake increases NEAP and thus increases bone resorption. Therefore, public health messages focusing on the reduction of processed food consumption to tackle obesity and cardiovascular disease may potentially also be extended to highlight the prevention of osteoporosis, subject to further evidence for a clear detrimental effect of high phosphorus intakes on bone health.

Potassium

Potassium in the diet is alkaline forming; thus, it will theoretically reduce NEAP and reduce the amount of calcium that is lost from bone to maintain acid–base homeostasis, helping to preserve bone health. A recent systematic review and meta-analysis of supplementation trials indicated that potassium bicarbonate or potassium citrate supplementation led to reduced urinary calcium excretion and lower bone resorption (Lambert et al., 2015). However, there is a lack of evidence as to whether potassium affects BMD and fracture risk in the long term. Also, it is unclear as to how effective increasing consumption of potassium-rich foods in the diet is for promoting bone health, although some recent research suggests higher dietary potassium intakes are beneficial for bone health (Hayhoe et al., 2015). Longer term trials assessing the effect of alkaline potassium supplements and dietary potassium on BMD and fracture risk are now required before increasing potassium intake can be recommended as a public health message for improvement of bone health in the general population.

Other nutrients

There is some evidence for a positive association between higher vitamin C levels and bone health, but supplementation trials are required to confirm that such associations are causal (Finck et al., 2014) before increased vitamin C can be recommended for improved bone health. There is conflicting evidence as to whether vitamin E is good or bad for bone, with research suggesting either that vitamin E may reduce bone mass, via its stimulatory effect on osteoclast cells (Fujita et al., 2012), or alternatively that it may increase bone mass (Kasai et al., 2015). Similarly, it has been suggested that vitamin

A may both stimulate and reduce osteoclast activity (Conaway et al., 2013), with a recent meta-analysis showing both high and low intakes of vitamin A are associated with increased fracture risk (Wu et al., 2014). Overall, a lot more research is now required into the actions of vitamins A, C and E on bone health.

Other lifestyle factors

Smoking

Smoking is associated with lower bone density (Eleftheriou et al., 2013) and increased risk of fracture (Kanis et al., 2005). Strong evidence of an association between increased smoking and reduced BMD comes from a meta-analysis which predicted that one in eight hip fractures may result from cigarette smoking (Law and Hackshaw, 1997). This study showed that current smokers lose bone at a faster rate than non-smokers, and by the age of 80 years this can translate into a 6% lower BMD, and greater fracture risk (Law and Hackshaw, 1997). Also, male smokers may be at even higher risk than women, with a recent study finding that male smokers had a small, but significantly greater risk of low bone density, and more vertebral fractures, than female smokers (Jaramillo et al., 2015).

Alcohol

High/excessive intakes of alcohol are known to have adverse effects on skeletal health, causing low BMD and an increased fracture risk (Malik et al., 2009), most likely due to the toxic effects of alcohol on osteoblasts (Rico et al., 1987). However, the effects of moderate consumption are less clear. At intakes above two units daily, alcohol intake has been associated with an increased risk of any fracture (Kanis et al., 2005). Conversely, beneficial associations between moderate drinking of alcohol and bone health have also been shown consistently across many studies (Williams et al., 2005), which may be due to the oestrogen-promoting effects of alcohol consumption (Maurel et al., 2012). Therefore, the role of alcohol in bone health is not clear, and further research is required to assess the level of alcohol intake that is safe for good bone health.

Caffeine

A high intake of caffeine may increase the amount of calcium excreted in urine, which could be detrimental to bone health, although studies in postmenopausal women have shown that adequate dietary calcium may counteract much of the negative effect of higher caffeine consumption. A recent meta-analysis found increased daily coffee consumption was associated with increased risk of fractures (Lee et al., 2014). The evidence is less clear for tea consumption, although one meta-analysis has found a reduced risk of fractures in people who drink one to four cups of tea daily (Sheng *et al.*, 2014).

Exercise

For a review of the effects of exercise on bone health, refer to Sanborn *et al.* (2011) in the Sports and Exercise Nutrition textbook within the Nutrition Society Textbook series.

20.8 Concluding remarks and areas for further research

Given that populations around the world are rapidly ageing, the burden of osteoporosis and subsequent fragility fractures is expected to increase dramatically across the world. This will impose an ever-increasing burden on already stretched health care services and be at an enormous cost to the world economy. As a modifiable factor affecting bone health, nutrition and lifestyle interventions play a key role in the promotion of optimal bone health and prevention of osteoporosis across the population.

The roles of calcium and vitamin D are well established in terms of their roles in bone health, but less is known about the effects of dietary protein, acid–base balance, micronutrients (such as magnesium, phosphorus and potassium), and vitamins A, C, E and K. Further research is required into the effects of these nutrients on bone tissue in order to establish their potential role as well as required intakes to promote bone health. More research is also required as to the effects of lifestyle choices on bone health (e.g. alcohol and caffeine consumption).

References

Afssa (Agence française de sécurité sanitaire des aliments) (2001) *Apports Nutritionnels Conseillés pour la Population Française.* Editions Tec&Doc, Paris.

Ammann, P. and Rizzoli, R. (2003) Bone strength and its determinants. *Osteoporosis International*, 14 (3), 13–18.

Arnett, T.R. and Dempster, D.W. Effect of pH on bone resorption by rat osteoclasts in vitro. *Endocrinology*, 119 (1), 119–124.

Bates, B., Lennox, A., Prentice, A. *et al.* (eds) (2014) National Diet and Nutrition Survey. Results from Years 1, 2, 3 and 4 (Combined) of the Rolling Programme (2008/2009-2011/2012). A Survey Carried Out on Behalf of Public Health England and the Food Standards Agency. Public Health England, London. https://www.gov.uk/government/uploads/system/uploads/attachment_data/file/310995/NDNS_Y1_to_4_UK_report.pdf (accessed 30 November 2016).

Bischoff-Ferrari, H.A., Willett, W.C., Wong, J.B. *et al.* (2005) *Fracture prevention with vitamin D supplementation: a meta-analysis of randomized controlled trials.* JAMA, 293 (18), 2257–2264.

Burge, R., Dawson-Hughes, B., Solomon, D.H. *et al.* (2007) Incidence and economic burden of osteoporosis related fractures in the United States, 2005–2025. *Journal of Bone and Mineral Research*, 22 (3), 465–475.

Buttriss, J.L. (2015) Vitamin D: sunshine vs. diet vs. pills. *Nutrition Bulletin*, 40, 279–285.

Calvo, M.S. and Tucker, K.L. (2013) Is phosphorus intake that exceeds dietary requirements a risk factor in bone health? *Annals of the New York Academy of Sciences*, 1301, 29–35.

Chapuy, M.C., Arlot, M.E., Duboeuf, F. *et al.* (1992) Vitamin D_3 and calcium to prevent hip fractures in elderly women. *The New England Journal of Medicine*, 327 (23), 1637–1642.

Clark, E.M., Gould, V.C., Morrison, L. *et al.* (2011) Determinants of fracture risk in a UK-population-based cohort of older women: a cross-sectional analysis of the Cohort for Skeletal Health in Bristol and Avon (COSHIBA). *Age and Ageing*, 41 (1), 46–52.

Cockayne, S., Adamson, J., Lanham-New, S. *et al.* (2006) Vitamin K and the prevention of fractures: systematic review and meta-analysis of randomized controlled trials. *Archives of Internal Medicine*, 166 (12), 1256–1261.

Conaway, H.H., Henning, P. and Lerner, U.H. (2013) Vitamin A metabolism, action, and role in skeletal homeostasis. *Endocrine Reviews*, 34 (6), 766–797.

Cooper, C., Atkinson, E.J., Hensrud, D.D. *et al.* (1996) Dietary protein intake and bone mass in women. *Calcified Tissue International*, 58 (5), 320–325.

Cribb, V.L., Northstone, K., Hopkins, D. and Emmett, P.M. (2015) Sources of vitamin D and calcium in the diets of preschool children in the UK and the theoretical effect of food fortification. *Journal of Human Nutrition and Dietetics*, 28 (6), 583–592.

DACH (Deutsche Gesellschaft für Ernährung – Österreichische Gesellschaft für Ernährung – Schweizerische Gesellschaft für Ernährungsforschung – Schweizerische Vereinigung für Ernährung) (2013) *Referenzwerte für die Nährstoffzufuhr.* Umschau Braus Verlag, Frankfurt am Main.

Dao, D., Sodhi, S., Tabasinejad, R. *et al.* (2015) Serum 25-hydroxyvitamin D levels and stress fractures in military personnel: a systematic review and meta-analysis. *The American Journal of Sports Medicine*, 43 (8), 2064–2072.

Darling, A.L., Millward, D.J., Torgerson, D.J. *et al.* (2009) Dietary protein and bone health: a systematic review and meta-analysis. *The American Journal of Clinical Nutrition*, 90 (6), 1674–1692.

Darling, A.L., Hart, K.H., Macdonald, H.M. *et al.* (2013) Vitamin D deficiency in UK South Asian women of childbearing age: a comparative longitudinal investigation with UK Caucasian women. *Osteoporosis International*, 24 (2), 477–488.

Dawson-Hughes, B. (2008) Serum 25-hydroxyvitamin D and functional outcomes in the elderly. *The American Journal of Clinical Nutrition*, 88 (2), 537S–540S.

Dawson-Hughes, B., Harris, S.S., Krall, E.A. and Dallal, G.E. (1997) Effect of calcium and vitamin D supplementation on bone density in men and women 65 years of age or older. *The New England Journal of Medicine*, 337 (10), 670–676.

Dawson-Hughes, B., Heaney, R.P., Holick, M.F. *et al.* (2005) Estimates of optimal vitamin D status. *Osteoporosis International*, 16 (7), 713–716.

Deeb, K.K., Trump, D.L. and Johnson, C.S. (2007) Vitamin D signalling pathways in cancer: potential for anticancer therapeutics. *Nature Reviews Cancer*, 7 (9), 684–700.

DeLuca, H.F. (2004) Overview of general physiologic features and functions of vitamin D. *The American Journal of Clinical Nutrition*, 80 (6), 1689S–1696S.

DoH (1991) *Dietary Reference Values for Food Energy and Nutrients for the United Kingdom. Report of the Panel on Dietary Reference Values of the Committee on Medical Aspects of Food Policy.* Report on Health and Social Subjects 41. HM Stationery Office, London.

Eleftheriou, K.I., Rawal, J.S., James, L.E. *et al.* (2013) Bone structure and geometry in young men: the influence of smoking, alcohol intake and physical activity. *Bone*, **52** (1), 17–26.

Ensrud, K.E., Ewing, S.K., Taylor, B.C. *et al.* (2007) Frailty and risk of falls, fracture, and mortality in older women: the study of osteoporotic fractures. *The Journals of Gerontology Series A: Biological Sciences and Medical Sciences*, **62** (7), 744–751.

Farsinejad-Marj, M., Saneei, P. and Esmaillzadeh, A. (2016) Dietary magnesium intake, bone mineral density and risk of fracture: a systematic review and meta-analysis. *Osteoporosis International*, **27** (4), 1389–1399.

Feskanich, D., Willett, W.C., Stampfer, M.J. and Colditz, G.A. (1996) Protein consumption and bone fractures in women. *American Journal of Epidemiology*, **143** (5), 472–479.

Finck, H., Hart, A.R., Jennings, A. and Welch, A.A. (2014) Is there a role for vitamin C in preventing osteoporosis and fractures? A review of the potential underlying mechanisms and current epidemiological evidence. *Nutrition Research Reviews*, **27** (2), 268–283.

Francis, R., Aspray, T., Fraser, W. *et al.* (2013) *Vitamin D and Bone Health: A Practical Clinical Guideline for Patient Management.* National Osteoporosis Society, Bath.

FSAI (1999) *Recommended Dietary Allowances for Ireland.* Food Safety Authority of Ireland, Dublin.

Fujita, K., Iwasaki, M., Ochi, H. *et al.* (2012) Vitamin E decreases bone mass by stimulating osteoclast fusion. *Nature Medicine*, **18** (4), 589–594.

Garnero, P. (2014) New developments in biological markers of bone metabolism in osteoporosis. *Bone*, **66**, 46–55.

Gehlbach, S., Saag, K.G., Adachi, J.D. *et al.* (2012) Previous fractures at multiple sites increase the risk for subsequent fractures: the Global Longitudinal Study of Osteoporosis in Women. *Journal of Bone and Mineral Research*, **27** (3), 645–653.

Hannan, M.T., Tucker, K.L., Dawson-Hughes B. *et al.* (2000) Effect of dietary protein on bone loss in elderly men and women: the Framingham Osteoporosis Study. *Journal of Bone and Mineral Research*, **15** (12), 2504–2512.

Hayhoe, R.P., Lentjes, M.A., Luben, R.N. *et al.* (2015) Dietary magnesium and potassium intakes and circulating magnesium are associated with heel bone ultrasound attenuation and osteoporotic fracture risk in the EPIC–Norfolk cohort study. *The American Journal of Clinical Nutrition*, **102** (2), 376–384.

Health Council of the Netherlands (2012) *Evaluation of Dietary Reference Values for Vitamin D.* Publication no. 2012/15E. Health Council of the Netherlands, The Hague. https://www.gezondheidsraad.nl/sites/default/files/201215EEvaluationDietaryReferenceVitaminD.pdf (accessed 10 January 2017).

Ho, S.C., Woo, J., Lam, S. *et al.* (2003) Soy protein consumption and bone mass in early postmenopausal Chinese women. *Osteoporosis International*, **14** (10), 835–842.

Holick, M.F., Binkley, N.C., Bischoff-Ferrari, H.A. *et al.* (2011) Evaluation, treatment, and prevention of vitamin D deficiency: an Endocrine Society clinical practice guideline. *The Journal of Clinical Endocrinology & Metabolism*, **96** (7), 1911–1930.

Huang, Z.B., Wan, S.L., Lu, Y.J. *et al.* (2015) Does vitamin K2 play a role in the prevention and treatment of osteoporosis for postmenopausal women: a meta-analysis of randomized controlled trials. *Osteoporosis International*, **26** (3), 1175–1186.

Hyppönen, E. and Power, C. (2007) Hypovitaminosis D in British adults at age 45 y: nationwide cohort study of dietary and lifestyle predictors. *The American Journal of Clinical Nutrition*, **85** (3), 860–868.

Ince, B.A., Anderson, E.J. and Neer, R.M. (2004) Lowering dietary protein to U.S. recommended dietary allowance levels reduces urinary calcium excretion and bone resorption in young women.

The Journal of Clinical Endocrinology and Metabolism, **89** (8), 3801–3807.

International Osteoporosis Foundation (2015) *Facts and Statistics.* http://www.iofbonehealth.org/facts-statistics#category-15 (accessed 16 December 2016).

IOM (2011) *Dietary Reference Intakes for Calcium and Vitamin D.* The National Academies Press, Washington, DC.

Jaramillo, J.D., Wilson, C., Stinson, D.S. *et al.* (2015) Reduced bone density and vertebral fractures in smokers. Men and COPD patients at increased risk. *Annals of the American Thoracic Society*, **12** (5), 648–656.

Jia, T., Byberg, L., Lindholm, B., *et al.* (2015) Dietary acid load, kidney function, osteoporosis, and risk of fractures in elderly men and women. *Osteoporosis International*, **26** (2), 563–570.

Johansson, H., Odén, A., Kanis, J.A. *et al.* (2014) A meta-analysis of reference markers of bone turnover for prediction of fracture. *Calcified Tissue International*, **94** (5), 560–567.

Kanis, J.A. (2002) Diagnosis of osteoporosis and assessment of fracture risk. *The Lancet*, **359** (9321), 1929–1936.

Kanis, J.A., Johnell, O., Oden, A. *et al.* (2005) Smoking and fracture risk: a meta-analysis. *Osteoporosis International*, **16** (2), 155–162.

Kasai, S., Ito, A., Shindo, K. *et al.* (2015) High-dose α-tocopherol supplementation does not induce bone loss in normal rats. *PloS One*, **10** (7), e0132059.

Kerstetter, J.E., O'Brien, K.O. and Insogna, K.L. (1998) Dietary protein affects intestinal calcium absorption. *The American Journal of Clinical Nutrition*, **68** (4), 859–865.

Kerstetter, J.E., Mitnick, M.E., Gundberg, C.M. *et al.* (1999) Changes in bone turnover in young women consuming different levels of dietary protein. *The Journal of Clinical Endocrinology and Metabolism*, **84** (3), 1052–1055.

Lambert, H., Frassetto, L., Moore, J.B. *et al.* (2015) The effect of supplementation with alkaline potassium salts on bone metabolism: a meta-analysis. *Osteoporosis International*, **26** (4), 1311–1318.

Lanham-New, S.A. and Wilson, L.R. (2016) Vitamin D – has the new dawn for dietary recommendations arrived? *Journal of Human Nutrition and Dietetics*, **29** (1), 3–6.

Lanham-New, S.A., Buttriss, J.L., Miles, L.M. *et al.* (2011) Proceedings of the rank forum on vitamin D. *British Journal of Nutrition*, **105** (1), 144–156.

Law, M.R. and Hackshaw, A.K. (1997) A meta-analysis of cigarette smoking, bone mineral density and risk of hip fracture: recognition of a major effect. *BMJ*, **315**, 841–846.

Lee, D.R., Lee, J., Rota, M. *et al.* (2014) Coffee consumption and risk of fractures: a systematic review and dose–response meta-analysis. *Bone*, **63**, 20–28.

Logan, V.F., Gray, A.R., Peddie, M.C. *et al.* (2013) Long-term vitamin D_3 supplementation is more effective than vitamin D_2 in maintaining serum 25-hydroxyvitamin D status over the winter months. *British Journal of Nutrition*, **109** (6), 1082–1088.

Malik, P., Gasser, R.W., Kemmler, G. *et al.* (2009) Low bone mineral density and impaired bone metabolism in young alcoholic patients without liver cirrhosis: a cross-sectional study. *Alcoholism, Clinical and Experimental Research*, **33**, 375–381.

Mangano, K.M., Walsh, S.J., Kenny, A.M. *et al.* (2014) Dietary acid load is associated with lower bone mineral density in men with low intake of dietary calcium. *Journal of Bone and Mineral Research*, **29** (2), 500–506.

Massey, L.K. (2003) Dietary animal and plant protein and human bone health: a whole foods approach. *The Journal of Nutrition*, **133** (3), 862S–865S.

Maurel, D.B., Boisseau, N., Benhamou, C.L. and Jaffre, C. (2012) Alcohol and bone: review of dose effects and mechanisms. *Osteoporosis International*, **23** (1), 1–16.

McCloskey, E.V., Odén, A., Harvey, N.C. *et al.* (2015) A meta-analysis of trabecular bone score in fracture risk prediction and its relationship to FRAX. *Journal of Bone and Mineral Research*, **31** (5), 940–948.

McLean, R.R., Qiao, N., Broe, K.E. *et al.* (2011) Dietary acid load is not associated with lower bone mineral density except in older men. *The Journal of Nutrition*, **141** (4), 588–594.

Mithal, A., Wahl, D.A., Bonjour, J.P. *et al.* (2009) Global vitamin D status and determinants of hypovitaminosis D. *Osteoporosis International*, **20** (11), 1807–1820.

Moreiras, O., Carbajal, A., Cabrera, L. and Cuadrado, C. (2013) *Tablas de Composición de Alimentos: Guía de Prácticas*, 16th edn. Ediciones Pirámide, Madrid.

Munger, R.G., Cerhan, J.R. and Chiu, B.C. (1999) Prospective study of dietary protein intake and risk of hip fracture in post-menopausal women. *The American Journal of Clinical Nutrition*, **69** (1), 147–152.

National Osteoporosis Guideline Group (2016) *Osteoporosis: Clinical Guideline for Prevention and Treatment, Executive Summary*. https://www.shef.ac.uk/NOGG/NOGG_Executive_Summary.pdf (accessed 16 December 2016).

New, S.A., MacDonald, H.M., Campbell, M.K. *et al.* (2004) Lower estimates of net endogenous non-carbonic acid production are positively associated with indexes of bone health in premenopausal and perimenopausal women. *The American Journal of Clinical Nutrition*, **79** (1), 131–138.

NHMRC (National Health and Medical Research Council) (2006) Nutrient Reference Values for Australia and New Zealand: Including Recommended Dietary Intakes. https://www.nhmrc.gov.au/_files_nhmrc/publications/attachments/n35.pdf (accessed 10 January 2016).

Nordic Council of Ministers (2014) *Nordic Nutrition Recommendations 2012. Integrating Nutrition and Physical Activity*, 5th edn. Norden, Copenhagen. https://www.norden.org/en/theme/nordic-nutrition-recommendation/nordic-nutrition-recommendations-2012 (accessed 10 January 2016).

Ooms, M.E., Roos, J.C., Bezemer, P.D. *et al.* (1995) Prevention of bone loss by vitamin D supplementation in elderly women: a randomized double-blind trial. *The Journal of Clinical Endocrinology & Metabolism*, **80** (4), 1052–1058.

Peck, W.A., Burckhardt, P., Christiansen, C. *et al.* (1993) Conference report: Consensus Development Conference: Diagnosis, Prophylaxis, and Treatment of Osteoporosis. *The American Journal of Medicine*, **94**, 646–650.

Peterlik, M., Boonen, S., Cross, H.S. and Lamberg-Allardt, C. (2009) Vitamin D and calcium insufficiency-related chronic diseases: an emerging world-wide public health problem. *International Journal of Environmental Research and Public Health, 2009*; **6** (10), 2585–2607.

Priemel, M., von Domarus, C., Klatte, T.O. *et al.* (2010) Bone mineralization defects and vitamin D deficiency: histomorphometric analysis of iliac crest bone biopsies and circulating 25-hydroxyvitamin D in 675 patients. *Journal of Bone and Mineral Research.*, **25** (2), 305–312.

Reid, I.R., Bolland, M.J. and Grey, A. (2014) Effects of vitamin D supplements on bone mineral density: a systematic review and meta-analysis. *The Lancet*, **383** (9912), 146–155.

Rico, H., Cabranes, J.A., Cabello, J. *et al.* (1987) Low serum osteocalcin in acute alcohol intoxication: a direct toxic effect of alcohol on osteoblasts. *Bone and Mineral*, **2** (3), 221–225.

SACN (2007) *Update on Vitamin D. Position Statement by the Scientific Advisory Committee on Nutrition*. The Stationary Office, London. https://www.gov.uk/government/uploads/system/uploads/attachment_data/file/339349/SACN_Update_on_Vitamin_D_2007.pdf (accessed 10 January 2017).

SACN (2016) Vitamin D and Health. https://www.gov.uk/government/uploads/system/uploads/attachment_data/file/537616/SACN_Vitamin_D_and_Health_report.pdf (accessed 29 November 2016).

Sanborn, C., Nichols, D.I. and DiMarco, N.M. (2011) Bone health. In S.A. Lanham-New, S.J. Stear, S.M. Shirreffs and A.L. Collins (eds), *Sport and Exercise Nutrition*. Wiley-Blackwell, Chichester; pp. 244–263.

SCF (Scientific Committee for Food) (1993) Vitamin D. In *Nutrient and Energy Intakes of the European Community*. Commission of the European Communities, Brussels/Luxembourg; pp. 132–139.

Seamans, K.M. and Cashman, K.D. (2009) Existing and potentially novel functional markers of vitamin D status: a systematic review. *The American Journal of Clinical Nutrition*, **89** (6), 1997S–2008S.

Sellmeyer, D.E., Stone, K.L., Sebastian, A. and Cummings, S.R. (2001) A high ratio of dietary animal to vegetable protein increases the rate of bone loss and the risk of fracture in postmenopausal women. Study of Osteoporotic Fractures Research Group. *The American Journal of Clinical Nutrition*, **73** (1), 118–122.

Sheng, J., Qu, X., Zhang, X. *et al.* (2014) Coffee, tea, and the risk of hip fracture: a meta-analysis. *Osteoporosis International*, **25** (1), 141–150.

Singer, A., Exuzides, A., Spangler, L. *et al.* (2015) Burden of illness for osteoporotic fractures compared with other serious diseases among postmenopausal women in the United States. *Mayo Clinic Proceedings*, **90** (1), 53–62.

Spence, L.A., Lipscomb, E.R., Cadogan, J. *et al.* (2005) The effect of soy protein and soy isoflavones on calcium metabolism in postmenopausal women: a randomized crossover study. *The American Journal of Clinical Nutrition*, **81** (4), 916–922.

Spiro, A. and Buttriss, J. (2014) Vitamin D: an overview of vitamin D status and intake in Europe. *Nutrition Bulletin*, **39** (4), 322–350.

Stein, M.S., Wark, J.D., Scherer, S.C. *et al.* (1999) Falls relate to vitamin D and parathyroid hormone in an Australian nursing home and hostel. *Journal of the American Geriatrics Society*, **47** (10), 1195–1201.

Tomlinson, P.B., Joseph, C. and Angioi, M. (2014) Effects of vitamin D supplementation on upper and lower body muscle strength levels in healthy individuals. A systematic review with meta-analysis. *Journal of Science and Medicine in Sport*, **18** (5), 575–580.

Trang, H.M., Cole, D.E., Rubin, L.A. *et al.* (1998) Evidence that vitamin D_3 increases serum 25-hydroxyvitamin D more efficiently than does vitamin D_2. *The American Journal of Clinical Nutrition*, **68** (4), 854–858.

Tripkovic, L., Lambert, H., Hart, K. *et al.* (2012) Comparison of vitamin D_2 and vitamin D_3 supplementation in raising serum 25-hydroxyvitamin D status: a systematic review and meta-analysis. *The American Journal of Clinical Nutrition*, **95** (6), 1357–1364.

Tripkovic, L., Wilson, L.R., Hart, K. *et al.* (2015) The D2-D3 Study: a randomised, double-blind, placebo-controlled food fortification trial in women, comparing the efficacy of 15ug/d vitamin D_2 vs vitamin D_3 in raising serum 25OHD levels. *Proceedings of the Nutrition Society*, **74** (OCE1), E16.

Thorpe, M.P. and Evans, E.M. (2011) Dietary protein and bone health: harmonizing conflicting theories. *Nutrition Reviews*, **69** (4), 215–230.

Vasikaran, S., Eastell, R., Bruyère, O. *et al.* (2011) Markers of bone turnover for the prediction of fracture risk and monitoring of osteoporosis treatment: a need for international reference standards. *Osteoporosis International*, **22** (2), 391–420.

Vupadhyayula, P.M., Gallagher, J.C., Templin, T. *et al.* (2009) Effects of soy protein isolate on bone mineral density and physical performance indices in postmenopausal women – a

2-year randomized, double-blind, placebo-controlled trial. *Menopause*, **16** (2), 320–328.

Ward, K.A., Das, G., Roberts, S.A. *et al.* (2010) A randomized, controlled trial of vitamin D supplementation upon musculoskeletal health in postmenarchal females. *The Journal of Clinical Endocrinology & Metabolism*, **95** (10), 4643–4651.

Welch, A.A., Kelaiditi, E., Jennings, A. *et al.* (2016) Dietary magnesium is positively associated with skeletal muscle power and indices of muscle mass and may attenuate the association between circulating C-reactive protein and muscle mass in women. *Journal of Bone and Mineral Research*, **31** (2), 317–325.

WHO Scientific Group on the Prevention and Management of Osteoporosis (2003) *Prevention and Management of Osteoporosis: Report of a WHO Scientific Group*. WHO Technical Report Series, No. 921. World Health Organization, Geneva.

Williams, F.M.K., Cherkas, L.F., Spector, T.D. and MacGregor, A.J. (2005) The effect of moderate alcohol consumption on bone mineral density: a study of female twins. *Annals of the Rheumatic Diseases*, **64**, 309–310.

Winzenberg, T., Shaw, K., Fryer, J. and Jones, G. (2006) Effects of calcium supplementation on bone density in healthy children: meta-analysis of randomised controlled trials. *BMJ*, **333**, 775.

Wu, A.M., Huang, C.Q., Lin, Z.K. *et al.* (2014) The relationship between vitamin A and risk of fracture: meta-analysis of prospective studies. *Journal of Bone and Mineral Research*, **29** (9), 2032–2039.

Wynn, E., Lanham-New, S.A., Krieg, M.A. *et al.* (2008) Low estimates of dietary acid load are positively associated with bone ultrasound in women older than 75 years of age with a lifetime fracture. *The Journal of Nutrition*, **138** (7), 1349–1354.

Zhang, Q., Ma, G., Greenfield, H. *et al.* The association between dietary protein intake and bone mass accretion in pubertal girls with low calcium intakes. *The British Journal of Nutrition*, **103** (5), 714–723.

Zhu, K., Meng, X., Kerr, D.A. *et al.* (2011) The effects of a two-year randomized, controlled trial of whey protein supplementation on bone structure, IGF-1, and urinary calcium excretion in older postmenopausal women. *Journal of Bone and Mineral Research*, **26** (9), 2298–2306.

21
Dental Health

Anja Heilmann and Richard G Watt

Key messages

- Oral diseases, in particular dental caries, are major public health problems that affect populations worldwide.
- Dental caries is caused by the consumption of free sugars.
- Current advice stipulates that intake of free sugars should not exceed 5% of total dietary energy for all age groups from 2 years upwards.

- Fluoride has a protective effect against dental caries. The mechanism of fluoride action is mainly topical (directly in the mouth). Exposure to fluoride does not, however, eliminate the caries risk posed by free sugars in the diet.
- Urgent public health action is needed to reduce free sugars consumption across the population to promote both oral and general health.

21.1 Introduction

Oral health is an essential and integral component of overall health and well-being. Oral health refers not just to the teeth, but the entire mouth, including the periodontal tissues (gums) and supporting hard and soft tissues. Oral diseases include dental caries (tooth decay), periodontal (gum) diseases, dental erosion (loss of surface enamel and dentine) and oral cancers. Despite being largely preventable, oral diseases and especially dental caries remain major public health problems in many parts of the world. There is an urgent need to adopt effective preventive measures, as treatment services will never eradicate this problem. Oral diseases, as is the case for other non-communicable chronic conditions, are caused by common risk factors including diet. The most important aetiological factor for dental caries is the consumption of dietary sugars. Official UK guidelines for the average population intake of sugars were updated in 2015, following a comprehensive review of the evidence on the role of sugars for both general and oral health. The current advice is that intake of free sugars (all added sugars plus those in fruit juice, honey and syrups) should not exceed 5% of total dietary energy, for all age groups from 2 years upwards. This represents a halving of the previous recommendation (SACN, 2015).

This chapter will highlight the public health significance of oral diseases and will present an overview of the evidence linking diet to the main oral conditions. Consensus policy and practice recommendations on the need to reduce free sugars consumption will be outlined. Finally, possible public health measures to improve diet to promote better oral health both at a clinical and population level will be presented.

21.2 Public health significance of oral diseases

At a United Nations summit in September 2011 on the prevention and control of non-communicable diseases, oral conditions were highlighted as one of the major global health priorities (United Nations, 2012). Dental caries and periodontal disease are both highly prevalent conditions affecting a significant proportion of the world's population. Dental caries is the most common chronic disease of humankind (Marcenes et al., 2013). In the USA, caries is estimated to be five times as common as asthma and seven times more common than allergic rhinitis (Benjamin, 2010).

With the exception of oral cancers, dental diseases are rarely life threatening but have a significant negative impact on quality of life. Untreated dental caries can cause severe pain, discomfort and infection (both acute and chronic), leading to eating and sleep disruption, which in children can adversely affect their ability to concentrate in school and ultimately affect their educational performance. Severe dental caries can also negatively impact on a child's growth and development. Amongst adults and older people, tooth loss caused by dental caries can severely restrict dietary intakes, particularly of fresh fruit and vegetables. The treatment of caries is costly and time consuming. In the UK, the multiple extraction of carious teeth is the main reason for administering general anaesthesia among young children, a very traumatic and unpleasant experience. In addition to the negative effect on the individual and their family, dental diseases also impose a major economic burden in terms of the costs to the health system of providing dental treatment. It is estimated that dental care accounts for about 5% of global health expenditure and that dental caries is the fourth most expensive disease to treat worldwide (WHO, 2003; Listl *et al.*, 2015). In addition to the direct costs of treatment, indirect costs are also very high. For example, in the USA it is estimated that 2.4 million days of work were lost due to oral disease (Beaglehole *et al.*, 2009).

Dental diseases are, however, largely preventable. Indeed, in recent decades there has been a dramatic overall improvement in levels of both caries and periodontal diseases in middle- and high-income countries (WHO, 2003). The major reason for the overall decline in caries has been the widespread use of fluoride toothpastes, whereas with periodontal diseases the key factors have been reductions in smoking and improvements in hygiene. Increasingly, dental diseases are a particular problem amongst socially disadvantaged and marginalised populations. Global epidemiological data show a consistent pattern of inequalities in oral diseases by socioeconomic status (Watt *et al.*, 2015). In low-income countries, dental caries is steadily increasing largely as a consequence of the nutrition transition and the subsequent rise in consumption of processed foods and drinks that are high in free sugars (WHO, 2003).

21.3 Diet and oral diseases: overview of the evidence

The oral disease that is inextricably linked to diet is dental caries, as the main cause of caries is the consumption of free sugars. Diet also plays a role in the development of dental erosion, oral cancer and, to a lesser extent, periodontal disease.

Dental caries

Dental caries is a chronic, cumulative lifelong disease that is caused by dietary sugars (Sheiham and James, 2015). The evidence for the link between consumption of free sugars and caries is strong and comes from a multitude of scientific studies, including observational and experimental research across different countries and populations (Moynihan and Kelly, 2014; PHE, 2014b; SACN, 2015; WHO, 2015).

The caries process
Dental caries is a dynamic process and the result of an imbalance between the demineralisation and remineralisation of dental hard tissue. The Keyes diagram shown in Figure 21.1 depicts the factors that are necessary for caries to occur and whose properties influence a person's susceptibility to the disease (Keyes and Jordan, 1963). Bacteria present in the dental plaque (mutans streptococci and other acidogenic and acid-tolerating species) metabolise free sugars from the diet and produce acids, causing the pH in the plaque to fall sharply. Below a critical pH (approximately 5.5 for enamel), demineralisation occurs, whereby mineral ions (calcium and phosphate) that are part of the enamel and dentine structure are released. When the exposure to free sugars ceases, the pH slowly rises due to the buffering capacities of the saliva, and lost minerals can be redeposited back into the enamel structure, a process known as remineralisation. Essentially, the tooth structure is able to repair itself through the movement of calcium and phosphate back into the enamel and dentine tissues. However, if the acid attacks are prolonged or occur too frequently, the balance shifts towards demineralisation and a carious lesion can develop.

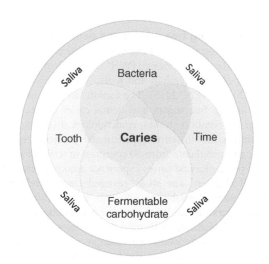

Figure 21.1 The Keyes diagram. *Source:* Keyes and Jordan (1963). Reproduced with permission of Elsevier.

This dynamic process is influenced by the presence of fluoride in the mouth (see Section 21.3: 'The role of fluorides in the prevention of dental caries'), the microbial composition of the plaque and the anatomy of the tooth. The pits and fissures on the occlusal (biting) surfaces of molars are the most susceptible; however, smooth surfaces can also be affected if caries activity is high. Another important factor is the quality and quantity of the saliva. A reduced salivary flow (xerostomia) is a side effect of some types of medication, as well as radiotherapy involving the salivary glands, and is associated with an increased caries risk. It is also a symptom of autoimmune disease resulting in Sjögren's syndrome.

Classification of sugars

There is some confusion among consumers and even health professionals regarding the cariogenicity (potential to induce caries) of different types of sugars. The classification developed by the UK Committee on Medical Aspects of Food Policy distinguished between intrinsic and extrinsic sugars. Intrinsic sugars are found inside the cell structure of unprocessed foods (i.e. whole fruits and vegetables). Extrinsic sugars are those not incorporated in the cell structure. These can be further divided into milk sugars (lactose) and non-milk extrinsic sugars (NMES). It is the NMES that are the major contributors to the development of dental caries. The UK Scientific Advisory Committee on Nutrition (SACN) has advised that the term NMES is replaced by 'free sugars'. Free sugars are defined as 'monosaccharides and disaccharides added to foods and beverages by the manufacturer, cook or consumer, and sugars naturally present in honey, syrups, fruit juices and fruit juice concentrates' (SACN, 2015; WHO, 2015). They do not include the sugars naturally present in whole fruits and vegetables, or milk and dairy products.

Evidence linking free sugars and dental caries

The evidence on the role of free sugars in the caries process has been extensively reviewed (WHO, 2003; Moynihan and Petersen, 2004; Moynihan and Kelly, 2014; Sheiham and James, 2014; SACN, 2015). The convincing collective evidence linking free sugars and dental caries comes from human intervention studies, epidemiological studies, animal studies and in-vitro experimental studies. Sreebny (1982) compared data from 60 countries in terms of sugar supply per capita and caries experience among 6- and 12-year-old children. The study revealed clear correlations between sugar availability and caries levels, which were especially pronounced for the permanent dentition. Several other population studies showed that changes in the availability of sugar were followed by changes in caries levels; for example, during and after the Second World War, and among Iraqi children before and after the introduction of United Nations sanctions (Takeuchi, 1961; Jamel et al.,

2004). Further, there are studies demonstrating that population subgroups who consume high amounts of sugar, such as confectionery industry workers and children taking sugar-based medicines, have higher average caries levels, while children whose sugar intake is low due to hereditary fructose intolerance experience low levels of caries (Moynihan and Petersen, 2004). Later studies that were undertaken in industrialised countries after the use of fluoride toothpaste became widespread tend to show weaker associations; however, there is still good evidence that exposure to fluorides does not eliminate the detrimental effect of a diet high in sugar, as shown recently in a large study among Australian children (Armfield et al., 2013).

Intervention studies on diet and caries are rare due to feasibility problems, as well as for obvious ethical concerns. In the 1940s and 1970s, studies were carried out in Sweden (the Vipeholm study) and Finland (the Turku study) that today are considered deeply unethical as they involved the prescription of a high-sugar diet, in the case of the Vipeholm study to vulnerable people living in a mental health institution. Both studies showed strong associations between sugar intake and caries increment (Gustafsson et al., 1953; Scheinin et al., 1976). More recently, food policies in nurseries that had a significant effect on reducing both the frequency and quantity of free sugars also led to a reduction in caries levels over an 18-month period (Rodrigues and Sheiham, 2000).

In summary, there is a wealth of evidence from a multitude of studies with different study designs and coming from different populations showing that free sugars are the most important aetiological factor in the development of dental caries.

Table 21.1 provides an illustrative list of foods and drinks containing free sugars.

Table 21.1 Examples of foods and drinks containing free sugars.

Table sugar (including brown sugar)
Confectionery
Cakes and biscuits
Buns and pastries
Sponge puddings and rice pudding
Sugared breakfast cereals
Sugared yoghurts and fromage frais
Jams and preserves
Honey
Ice cream
Dried fruit
Fruit in syrup
Sugared soft drinks
Fruit juice and smoothies (including freshly made)
Sugared milk drinks (e.g. hot chocolate)
Sugar-containing alcoholic beverages
Tomato ketchup

Frequency or amount of free sugars?

Both the total amount of free sugars and the frequency of their consumption play a role in the caries process, and it is not surprising that these factors are strongly related to each other. There is no agreed 'safe' amount of free sugars that can be consumed (Sheiham and James, 2015). Evidence from population studies showed that countries with free sugars intakes below 10 kg per person per year had the lowest caries levels. As already mentioned, the correlation between free sugars and caries is weaker among industrialised countries, where overall sugars consumption is very high with small between-country differences, and where the association is confounded by the exposure to fluorides (Moynihan and Petersen, 2004).

Owing to the nature of the caries process, the frequency with which free sugars are consumed is an important factor in the disease development (Beighton et al., 1996; Arcella et al., 2002; Moynihan, 2002; Harris et al., 2004). As has already been described, each time a sugary food or drink enters the mouth, the bacteria in the dental plaque produce acids, the pH drops rapidly and then slowly goes back up. The time it takes for the pH to recover depends on many other factors and varies considerably. The fall and recovery of the pH in dental plaque following an acid attack is visualised in the Stephan curve (Figures 21.2

and 21.3). The two examples show in simplified form what happens in the mouth when an individual consumes free sugars only at mealtimes (Figure 21.2) or frequently during the day (Figure 21.3). Because it takes time for the pH to recover, frequent sugary snacks result in prolonged acid attacks, leaving less time for remineralisation to occur. This means that the risk of developing caries becomes higher the more frequently sugary foods and drinks are consumed. The critical pH varies between individuals and is higher for dentine and root cement, making these structures even more susceptible. Also, compared with non-carious teeth, the plaque pH on the surface of carious teeth takes longer to recover to resting levels.

Free sugars and general health

The consumption of free sugars above recommended guidelines not only damages teeth but also adversely affects general health. Evidence is mounting that free sugars play a major role in the development of obesity and metabolic syndrome, thus increasing the risk of a wide range of chronic non-communicable diseases, such as diabetes and cardiovascular disease. A consistent link between intake of free sugars and increased body weight has been demonstrated in a recent meta-analysis of

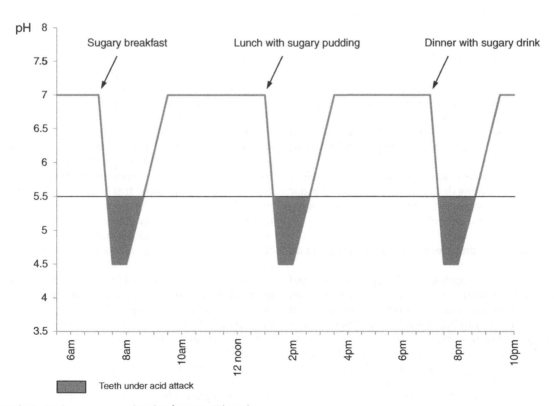

Figure 21.2 Stephan curve, example 1: less frequent acid attacks.

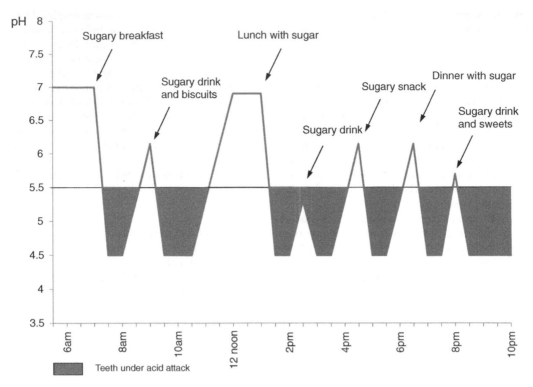

Figure 21.3 Stephan curve, example 2: frequent acid attacks.

randomised trials and prospective cohort studies that were published up to 2011 (Te Morenga *et al.*, 2013). Furthermore, there is convincing evidence that sugar-sweetened beverages, including fruit juice, are implicated in the development of obesity, type 2 diabetes, cardio-vascular disease and non-alcoholic fatty liver disease in both adults and children (Bray and Popkin, 2013; SACN, 2015).

A reduction in free sugars is therefore not only a priority for promoting dental health but is also of major public health importance for the prevention of obesity and the chronic diseases related to it.

Current patterns and trends in the consumption of free sugars

Free sugars are ubiquitous in today's middle- and high-income countries, while in low-income countries their consumption is fast increasing. In middle- and high-income countries, overall consumption has remained relatively stable over the past decades; however, the pattern of consumption has shifted from packaged table sugar to an increased consumption of hidden sugars in processed foods and drinks. The latest UK National Diet and Nutrition Survey reported average population intakes of NMES between 2008

and 2012 (Bates *et al.*, 2014). The figures show that mean intakes of NMES as a percentage of food energy far exceeded the current SACN guidelines in all age groups, and were highest among children and adolescents (Figure 21.4).

For children younger than 10 years, the main sources of NMES were sugary drinks (about 30%) and cereal products (25–30%). Children aged 11–18 years obtained 40% of their NMES intake from sugary drinks and about 20% from cereal products. It is worth noting that fruit juices alone made up 14% of the NMES intake in children under the age of 3 years. Table sugar, preserves and confectionery contributed an additional 20% to the NMES intake for children across all age groups (Bates *et al.*, 2014).

Hidden sugars in processed foods and drinks present a major challenge to consumers as it can often be very difficult to identify the quantity of sugars in these products due to confusing labelling information. Especially problematic is the targeting of children with foods and drinks that are marketed as 'healthy' products but are high in free sugars. For example, the average fruit smoothie consists of 12% of free sugars (*Which?*, 2012), while the sugar content of some breakfast cereals is as high as 40%.

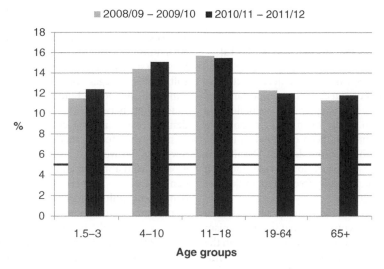

Figure 21.4 NMES intake in percentage food energy, by age group and years. NMES or free sugars intake should not exceed 5% of total dietary energy (represented by the thick black line). *Source:* Bates *et al.* (2014).

Intrinsic sugars in fresh fruits and vegetables, milk sugars and starches

Epidemiological studies on the association between the consumption of intrinsic sugars as present in whole fresh fruits and some vegetables have found that these are of low cariogenicity. On the contrary, fruits and vegetables are a very important part of a healthy diet because of the fibre and micronutrients they contain, and their consumption should be encouraged. Dried fruit and fruit juices, however, are cariogenic because their free sugar content is high, as the process of drying/juicing means that the cell structure has broken down and sugars are released (Moynihan and Petersen, 2004).

Milk (cows' milk as well as breast milk) contains milk sugar (lactose) and calcium, and these have been shown to be protective against caries rather than detrimental. Both sweetness and cariogenicity of lactose are very low (Moynihan and Petersen, 2004). A systematic review on breastfeeding and dental caries concluded that breast-feeding within the first year is not detrimental to teeth (Tham *et al.*, 2015).

The cariogenicity of starchy staple foods such as bread, rice and potatoes has been examined in several epidemiological studies and is considered minimal. Populations consuming diets that are high in starch but low in sugars have low caries levels, whereas a low-starch/high-sugars diet is associated with high levels of caries (Moynihan and Petersen, 2004). Starchy foods are, however, cariogenic when they also contain free sugars, as in cakes, biscuits and sugary cereals.

Protective foods and drinks

Foods which stimulate the secretion of saliva, as well as foods that contain high levels of calcium, are thought to have protective capacities against dental caries. These include cheese, cows' milk and all non-sugary foods that require significant chewing. Black and green teas without added sugar contain fluoride and polyphenols, which have also been shown to have caries-inhibiting effects.

Early childhood caries

Caries in the primary (baby) dentition is highly prevalent in both industrialised and developing countries. The presence of caries on at least one primary tooth in children under 6 years of age is defined by the American Academy of Pediatric Dentistry as early childhood caries (ECC). According to the British Association for the Study of Community Dentistry, the prevalence of ECC in the UK was about 40% in 2005, with severe forms being more prevalent in disadvantaged communities. The term 'severe ECC' is often used interchangeably with terms like 'rampant caries', 'nursing caries' or 'bottle caries', and refers to caries involving the smooth surfaces of primary teeth. Severe forms of ECC have a considerable impact on children's general health and well-being.

The most important risk factors related to ECC are inappropriate weaning practices, such as sweetened feeding bottles, particularly when used during the night, and high-frequency intake of sugary snacks and drinks (Harris *et al.*, 2004). Because many foods and drinks that are directly marketed at young children are very high in free sugars (García *et al.*, 2013), it is important that parents and carers know how to interpret the nutrition information on food labels.

The role of fluorides in the prevention of dental caries

While fluoride is strictly speaking not a dietary factor, its role in the prevention of dental caries is so important that it needs to be included in this chapter. The use of fluoride toothpaste is thought to be the main factor responsible for the caries decline that has been observed in industrialised countries over the past four decades. Despite this fall in caries levels, the exposure to fluoride does not eliminate the caries risk posed by free sugars in the diet (Moynihan and Kelly, 2014).

While all methods of fluoride delivery have systemic and topical effects, there is consensus that the mechanism of fluoride action is mainly topical. Fluoride present in the mouth reduces net demineralisation and enhances remineralisation of enamel. An antibacterial effect is often suggested but has so far only been demonstrated in laboratory research. Given the mechanism of fluoride action, the goal is to maintain a constant presence of low-concentration fluoride in the mouth, which is best achieved via the use of fluoride toothpaste. A Cochrane review of 70 trials estimated that the use of fluoride toothpaste reduces the caries incidence among children and adolescents by about a quarter (Walsh *et al.*, 2010). For young children whose permanent teeth are still developing (below age 6 years), a possible adverse effect associated with the use of fluoride toothpaste is dental fluorosis (mottling) due to the swallowing of excessive fluoride (Wong *et al.*, 2010). Public Health England recommendations for the use of fluoride toothpaste in children and adults are shown in Table 21.2 (PHE, 2014a).

Dental erosion

Dental erosion is the non-carious tooth surface loss that is caused by acids that are either intrinsic (produced in the body) or extrinsic (coming from the diet). The process of dental erosion does not involve bacteria. Sources of intrinsic acids are vomiting (e.g. in patients with bulimia nervosa) and gastro-oesophageal reflux. Dietary sources of acid are citrus fruits, fruit juices, soft drinks, vinegar and some alcoholic drinks, such as wine and 'alcopops'. Epidemiological surveys in the UK found that, between 1993 and 2013, the prevalence of dental erosion among children has slightly increased, possibly due to an increased consumption of acidic beverages. However, it is difficult to clinically distinguish erosion from abrasion and tooth wear. The prevalence of dental erosion in permanent teeth progressing into dentine or pulp, which is arguably of more clinical significance than enamel surface loss and can be measured more reliably, is very low and has been stable over time (Pitts *et al.*, 2015). It needs to be emphasised that while an excessive intake of acidic fruits has been linked to dental erosion, the risk is far outweighed by the health benefits of a diet high in fruits and vegetables. No conflicting messages should therefore be given to the public because of dental health concerns. Dental erosion is not currently thought to be a public health problem globally (Moynihan and Petersen, 2004).

Oral cancers

Oral cancer is one of the few conditions of the oral cavity that can be fatal. It includes cancer of the lip, tongue, mouth and pharynx. Oral cancer is one of the most prevalent cancers worldwide (approximately 400 000 new cases each year); however, there is a wide geographical variation in the incidence, with two-thirds of cases occurring in developing countries (Warnakulasuriya, 2009). In the UK each year around 7500 people are diagnosed with oral cancer and 2000 people die from the condition. In the past decade the incidence has risen by 33% and the condition increasingly affects middle-aged people (Cancer Research UK, n.d.).

The majority of oral cancers are preventable. The aetiology of oral cancer is multifactorial; however, it is well established that the most important risk factors are excess alcohol consumption, tobacco use (smoking or smokeless) and betel quid chewing. These risk factors may act separately or synergistically, meaning that the risk associated with alcohol abuse is amplified in people who are also smokers. Together, alcohol and tobacco products account for more than 80% of cases (Warnakulasuriya, 2009). A recent meta-analysis from 49 publications that included 18 000 oral cancer cases worldwide showed a direct dose–risk relationship between alcohol consumption and oral cancer (Turati *et al.*, 2013).

There is also convincing evidence for a protective effect of a diet high in fruits and vegetables. It is estimated

Table 21.2 Recommended fluoride concentrations in toothpastes for children and adults.

Age group	Recommendation
Children aged up to 3 years	Use only a smear of fluoridated toothpaste containing no less than 1000 ppm fluoride
Children aged 3–6 years	Use a pea-sized amount of fluoridated toothpaste containing more than 1000 ppm fluoride
Children from age 7 years and adults	Use fluoridated toothpaste containing 1350–1500 ppm fluoride

Source: PHE (2014a).

that each additional daily serving of fruits and vegetables reduces the risk for oral cancer by 25–50% (Pavia *et al.*, 2006).

Periodontal disease

Periodontal disease (inflammation of the supporting tissues around teeth) is the second most important oral health condition after dental caries. It mainly affects adults and older people, and is caused by bacteria in dental plaque. Susceptibility to periodontal disease among adults varies widely and is influenced by a range of genetic, behavioural and environmental risk factors, most notably smoking. Dietary risk factors include vitamin C deficiency, as well as low calcium and vitamin D levels (van der Velden *et al.*, 2011; Genco and Borgnakke, 2013).

21.4 Implications for action

Consensus dietary recommendations for the prevention of oral diseases

International and national health organisations have made consensus recommendations on diet and the prevention of oral diseases (WHO, 2003, 2015; Moynihan and Kelly, 2014; SACN, 2015). The robust scientific evidence linking dietary sugars to the development of dental caries, as well as unhealthy weight gain, have led SACN to recommend a halving of the previous recommendation on intakes of free sugars, from 10% to no more than 5% of total dietary energy for all age groups from 2 years upwards (SACN, 2015). This recommendation is in line with newer World Health Organization (WHO) guidelines and accepted by the UK Government (WHO, 2015). For the average adult, 5% of total dietary energy equates to approximately 25 g or six teaspoons per day.

Further, the consumption of fruits and vegetables should be increased to at least five portions per day (WHO, 2003).

Public health principles underpinning action on diet to promote oral health

As oral diseases are a classic public health problem, they require a public health solution. Dental treatment will never eradicate or control oral diseases. Instead, effective prevention is needed to achieve sustainable overall improvements in population oral health and a reduction in oral health inequalities. The core principles guiding public health action include the following:

- *Focus on the underlying determinants of oral diseases and oral health inequalities.* The consumption of free sugars, the main cause of dental caries, is influenced by a complex and interrelated array of biological, behavioural, social, environmental, economic and political factors. Focusing on behaviour change alone will not achieve sustained reductions in free sugars consumption. Most free sugars in the diet are now consumed via processed and manufactured foods and drinks. Sugary snacks and drinks are universally available and sold in supermarkets, shops and food stalls across the world in both urban and rural settings; they are a ubiquitous feature of the modern globalised world. The global food and drinks industry spends billions of dollars promoting and advertising their products in sophisticated marketing campaigns, often using the endorsement of film or music celebrities. In middle- and high-income countries, free sugars consumption is highest amongst poorer groups in the population and among adolescents and young people. Reducing free sugars consumption across the population therefore requires a coordinated strategic approach that addresses the underlying influences on free sugars intake to create a more supportive environment that promotes healthier nutrition (Watt and Rouxel, 2012). Traditionally, health professionals have focused their preventive efforts on particular diseases in a narrow and isolated fashion, mostly through the provision of specific health information aimed at changing a patient's behaviour. This individualistic approach is largely ineffective at achieving long-term improvements in health and may also increase inequalities, as the middle classes with access to support and resources are able to benefit the most from health advice (NICE, 2007). Public health policies need to recognise the common shared determinants of non-communicable diseases and implement integrated holistic strategies.

- *Work in partnership with different sectors and the community to promote oral health.* By acknowledging the wide and diverse underlying influences and determinants of chronic diseases, it is obvious that health professionals alone cannot achieve the desired changes in society. For example, doctors, dentists, pharmacists and nurses have limited influence over the marketing strategies of global corporations. It is therefore essential that health professionals work in a multidisciplinary way with other sectors and agencies who have more influence over the broader determinants of disease. Health professionals have a key role to play as health advocates ensuring that health concerns are raised onto the agenda of all relevant agencies and sectors.

  Community participation and involvement is also a core principle of public health practice. Change cannot be imposed on the public without their agreement and support. Draconian 'top-down' policies dictated by health bureaucrats are ineffective and just result in hostile responses from the public. Instead, working with patients, their families and the wider communities in developing policies that empower people to improve their health is a far more effective and sustainable approach.

- *Adopt a complementary range of strategies to achieve sustained and meaningful change.* The WHO Ottawa Charter remains a seminal policy document that outlines the need for a complementary range of health promotion strategies, including healthy public policy, creating supportive environments, strengthening community action, developing personal skills and reorienting health services to promote population health and reduce inequalities (WHO, 1986). This approach provides a wide range of opportunities to promote oral health through better nutrition. In essence, the Ottawa Charter seeks to enable individuals and communities to achieve better health through creating a more supportive environment for good health; in other words, through *making the healthy choices the easy choices*. Such an approach has been very successfully applied in the field of tobacco through the WHO Framework Convention on Tobacco Control, a global agreement on the adoption of a spectrum of policies and actions to reduce tobacco use.

Action at a clinical level

Primary dental care teams have regular and ongoing contact with a significant proportion of the general population. Unlike most other parts of the health-care system, otherwise 'healthy' adults, and a high proportion of children and adolescents, are routinely treated by dental staff. This provides an ideal opportunity for preventive input to promote both oral and general health. However, until recently, dentists have tended to concentrate very much on providing clinical treatment and have not been very actively engaged in a preventive agenda. This situation is now changing, partly in response to demands from patients for more preventive care, and as a result of government health policies that place greater emphasis on disease prevention. For example, Public Health England has published *Delivering Better Oral Health*, a preventive toolkit for dentists which aims to encourage dental teams to routinely offer preventive advice and support to their patients (PHE, 2014a). The evidence-based resource outlines how dental teams can provide preventive support in a range of relevant areas, including smoking cessation advice, alcohol support and dietary advice.

Dietary advice delivered by dental staff principally focuses on the importance of reducing both the frequency and amount of free sugars to prevent dental caries. This advice, however, should be tailored to the individuals' needs and circumstances. For example, diet advice for a mother and toddler would be very different from that for an older patient with dry mouth and at high risk of root caries. In all cases it is important to collect a detailed dietary history to establish a patient's pattern of free sugars consumption. This requires appropriate communication skills to gather the relevant information to help a patient reduce their free sugars intake. Of particular importance is establishing the number of intakes of foods and drinks per day that contain free sugars and whether these are consumed at a mealtime or as a snack. Based upon the information gathered from the diet history, patients should then be given tailored advice on practical ways of reducing their free sugars intakes. In particular, suggesting suitable and appealing alternative sugars-free snacks and drinks is important. It is essential, however, that any dietary advice given by dental staff is consistent with general healthy eating advice. In the past, conflicting and contradictory dietary messages have sometimes been delivered by different health professionals, which results in patients being confused and somewhat disillusioned. It is also important that other health professionals, such as general practitioners and health visitors, provide relevant dietary advice to promote the oral health of their patients. For example, consistent messages on complementary feeding practices and prescribing sugars-free medicines for both adults and children are both essential for caries prevention.

Action at a population level

From a public health perspective, although dietary advice offered by health professionals is important, such an approach alone has only limited scope in improving population health and in addressing inequalities (Stuckler *et al.*, 2012). Action to reduce free sugars consumption and promote healthy eating requires a coordinated food policy implemented at local, regional, national and international levels (PHE, 2014b). To be effective, food policies need to adopt a range of complementary intervention strategies and require a coalition of partners working together to achieve change, as illustrated in Figure 21.5 (Watt and Rouxel, 2012). Regulation and legislation are particularly important intervention strategies to promote good nutrition and a reduction in free sugars consumption across the population. In particular, stricter controls are needed on the food advertising and promotions targeting young children, most of which are for high-fat and high-sugar products. Tighter regulatory controls on the advertising, promotion and consistent labelling of sugary snacks and drinks, as well as processed foods, are urgently needed. Currently, the information provided on labels is confusing and often very misleading. To enable consumers to make informed food

Interventions \ Partners	Producers	Manufacturers	Caterers	Government (Local and National)	Media	Health Services	Public
Legislation & Regulation	*	*	*	*		*	
Substitution	*	*	*	*			
Fiscal change	*	*	*	*		*	
Organisational Change			*	*		*	*
Community Action		*	*	*	*	*	*
Education			*	*	*	*	*
Prevention				*		*	*

Figure 21.5 Food policy matrix. *Source:* Watt and Rouxel (2012). Reproduced with permission of BMJ Publishing Ltd.

choices, they require clear and understandable information on labels. A traffic light system highlighting whether the product has high, medium or low levels of sugars, fats and salt has been shown to be superior to other forms of labelling in tests of comprehension with consumers. In addition, consumers have difficulties interpreting label types that refer to portion sizes, especially when comparing different products (Malam *et al.*, 2009; Draper *et al.*, 2011).

In recent years, several influential health organisations have called for the use of fiscal measures to promote diet change. Particular interest has focused on placing a health tax on sugary drinks as a means of combating childhood obesity. Evidence indicates that a 20% increase in price would lead to a significant reduction in sugary drinks consumption (Ng *et al.*, 2012). It is also important to consider the use of price subsidies to promote healthier choices rather than only taxing the unhealthy options. Regulation, legislation and fiscal measures can be implemented at local, national and international levels to promote dietary change (PHE, 2014b). For example, local food policies can be developed in nurseries, schools, colleges and workplaces as part of a healthy settings initiative. To be successful it is essential that parents, students and workers are involved and consulted in the development and implementation of such policies.

21.5 Conclusions

Oral diseases, and in particular dental caries, are significant public health problems that affect a large proportion of the world's population. Dental caries, however, is largely preventable. The main risk factor for dental caries is the consumption of free sugars. Convincing scientific evidence from a multitude of different studies has highlighted that the amount and frequency of free sugars is associated with caries development. The consumption of free sugars is also linked to the development of obesity and a range of other metabolic conditions. Urgent action that includes a range of complementary public health strategies is now needed to create supportive environments to enable individuals to consume a diet low in free sugars.

References

Arcella, D., Ottolenghi, L., Polimeni, A. and Leclercq, C. (2002) The relationship between frequency of carbohydrates intake and dental caries: a cross-sectional study in Italian teenagers. *Public Health Nutrition*, 5, 553–560.

Armfield, J.M., Spencer, A.J., Roberts-Thomson, K.F. and Plastow, K. (2013) Water fluoridation and the association of sugar-sweetened beverage consumption and dental caries in Australian children. *American Journal of Public Health*, 103, 494–500.

Bates, B., Lennox, A., Prentice, A. *et al.* (eds), (2014) *National Diet and Nutrition Survey: Results from Years 1, 2, 3 and 4 (Combined) of the Rolling Programme (2008/2009–2011/2012).* Public Health England, London. https://www.gov.uk/government/uploads/system/uploads/attachment_data/file/310995/NDNS_Y1_to_4_UK_report.pdf (accessed 30 November 2016).

Beaglehole, R., Benzian, H., Crail, J. and Mackay, J. (2009) *The Oral Health Atlas. Mapping a Neglected Global Health Issue.* FDI World Dental Federation, Brighton.

Beighton, D., Adamson, A. and Rugg-Gunn, A. (1996) Associations between dietary intake, dental caries experience and salivary bacterial levels in 12-year-old English schoolchildren. *Archives of Oral Biology,* **41**, 271–280.

Benjamin, R.M. (2010) Oral health: the silent epidemic. *Public Health Reports,* **125**, 158–159.

Bray, G.A. and Popkin, B.M. (2013) Calorie-sweetened beverages and fructose: what have we learned 10 years later. *Pediatric Obesity,* **8**, 242–248.

Cancer Research UK (n.d.) *Oral cancer statistics.* http://www.cancerresearchuk.org/health-professional/cancer-statistics/statistics-by-cancer-type/oral-cancer (accessed 18 December 2016).

Draper, A.K., Adamson, A.J., Clegg, S. *et al.* (2011) Front-of-pack nutrition labelling: are multiple formats a problem for consumers? *The European Journal of Public Health,* **23** (3), 517–521.

García, A.L., Raza, S., Parrett, A. and Wright, C.M. (2013) Nutritional content of infant commercial weaning foods in the UK. *Archives of Disease in Childhood,* **98** (10), 793–797.

Genco, R.J. and Borgnakke, W.S. (2013) Risk factors for periodontal disease. *Periodontology 2000* **62**, 59–94.

Gustafsson, B.E., Quensel, C.-E., Lanke, L.S. *et al.* (1953) The Vipeholm dental caries study: the effect of different levels of carbohydrate intake on caries activity in 436 individuals observed for five years. *Acta Odontologica Scandinavica,* **11**, 232–364.

Harris, R., Nicoll, A.D., Adair, P.M. and Pine, C.M. (2004) Risk factors for dental caries in young children: a systematic review of the literature. *Community Dental Health,* **21**, 71–85.

Jamel, H., Plasschaert, A. and Sheiham, A. (2004) Dental caries experience and availability of sugars in Iraqi children before and after the United Nations sanctions. *International Dental Journal,* **54**, 21–25.

Keyes, P.H. and Jordan, H.V. (1963) Factors influencing the initiation, transmission, and inhibition of dental caries. In R.J. Harris (ed.), *Mechanisms of Hard Tissue Destruction.* Academic Press, New York; pp. 261–283.

Listl, S., Galloway, J., Mossey, P.A. and Marcenes, W. (2015) Global economic impact of dental diseases. *Journal of Dental Research,* **94**, 1355–1361.

Malam, S., Clegg, S., Kirwan, S. and McGinigal, S. (2009) *Comprehension and Use of UK Nutrition Signpost Labelling Schemes.* Food Standards Agency, London.

Marcenes, W., Kassebaum, N.J., Bernabé, E. *et al.* (2013) Global burden of oral conditions in 1990–2010: a systematic analysis. *Journal of Dental Research,* **92**, 592–597.

Moynihan, P.J. (2002) Dietary advice in dental practice. *British Dental Journal,* **193**, 563–568.

Moynihan, P.J. and Kelly, S.A.M. (2014) Effect on caries of restricting sugars intake: systematic review to inform WHO guidelines. *Journal of Dental Research,* **93**, 8–18.

Moynihan, P. and Petersen, P.E. (2004) Diet, nutrition and the prevention of dental diseases. *Public Health Nutrition,* **7**, 201–226.

Ng, S.W., Ni Mhurchu, C., Jebb, S.A. and Popkin, B.M. (2012) Patterns and trends of beverage consumption among children and adults in Great Britain, 1986–2009. *British Journal of Nutrition,* **108**, 536–551.

NICE (2007) *Behaviour Change: General Approaches.* Public Health Guideline PH6. National Institute of Health and Clinical Excellence, London. https://www.nice.org.uk/guidance/ph6 (accessed 18 December, 2016).

Pavia, M., Pileggi, C., Nobile, C.G. and Angelillo, I.F. (2006) Association between fruit and vegetable consumption and oral cancer: a meta-analysis of observational studies. *The American Journal of Clinical Nutrition,* **83**, 1126–1134.

PHE (2014a) *Delivering Better Oral Health: An Evidence-based Toolkit for Prevention.* Public Health England, London.

PHE (2014b) *Sugar Reduction: Responding to the Challenge.* Public Health England, London.

Pitts, N., Chadwick, B. and Anderson, T. (2015) *Children's Dental Health Survey 2013. Report 2: Dental Disease and Damage in Children. England, Wales and Northern Ireland.* Health and Social Care Information Centre.

Rodrigues, C.S. and Sheiham, A. (2000) The relationships between dietary guidelines, sugar intake and caries in primary teeth in low income Brazilian 3-year-olds: a longitudinal study. *International Journal of Paediatric Dentistry,* **10**, 47–55.

SACN (2015) *Carbohydrates and Health.* The Stationery Office, London.

Scheinin, A., Mäkinen, K.K. and Ylitalo, K. (1976) Turku sugar studies. V. Final report on the effect of sucrose, fructose and xylitol diets on the caries incidence in man. *Acta Odontologica Scandinavica,* **34**, 179–216.

Sheiham, A. and James, W.P. (2014) A new understanding of the relationship between sugars, dental caries and fluoride use: implications for limits on sugars consumption. *Public Health Nutrition,* **1**, 2176–2184.

Sheiham, A. and James, W.P. (2015) Diet and dental caries: the pivotal role of free sugars reemphasized. *Journal of Dental Research,* **94**, 1341–1347.

Sreebny, L.M. (1982) Sugar availability, sugar consumption and dental caries. *Community Dentistry and Oral Epidemiology,* **10**, 1–7.

Stuckler, D., McKee, M., Ebrahim, S. and Basu, S. (2012) Manufacturing epidemics: the role of global producers in increased consumption of unhealthy commodities including processed foods, alcohol, and tobacco. *PLoS Medicine,* **9**, e1001235.

Takeuchi M. (1961) Epidemiological study on dental caries in Japanese children, before, during and after World War II. *International Dental Journal,* **11**, 443–457.

Te Morenga, L., Mallard, S. and Mann, J. (2013) Dietary sugars and body weight: systematic review and meta-analyses of randomised controlled trials and cohort studies. *BMJ,* **346**, e7492.

Tham, R., Bowatte, G., Dharmage, S.C. *et al.* (2015) Breastfeeding and the risk of dental caries: a systematic review and meta-analysis. *Acta Paediatrica,* **104**, 62–84.

Turati, F., Garavello, W., Tramacere, I. *et al.* (2013) A meta-analysis of alcohol drinking and oral and pharyngeal cancers: results from subgroup analyses. *Alcohol Alcohol,* **48**, 107–118.

United Nations (2012) *Political Declaration of the High-level Meeting of the General Assembly on the Prevention and Control of Non-communicable Diseases.* United Nations, New York. http://www.who.int/nmh/events/un_ncd_summit2011/political_declaration_en.pdf?ua=1 (accessed 18 December 2016).

Van der Velden, U., Kuzmanova, D. and Chapple, I.L. (2011) Micronutritional approaches to periodontal therapy. *Journal of Clinical Periodontology,* **38** (Suppl 11), 142–158.

Walsh, T., Worthington, H.V., Glenny, A.M. *et al.* (2010) Fluoride toothpastes of different concentrations for preventing dental caries in children and adolescents. *The Cochrane Database of Systematic Reviews,* (1), CD007868.

Warnakulasuriya, S. (2009) Global epidemiology of oral and oropharyngeal cancer. *Oral Oncology,* **45**, 309–316.

Watt, R.G. and Rouxel, P.L. (2012) Dental caries, sugars and food policy. *Archives of Disease in Childhood*, **97**, 769–772.

Watt, R.G., Listl, S., Peres, M.A. and Heilmann, A. (eds) (2015) *Social Inequalities in Oral Health: From Evidence to Action*. UCL, London. http://media.news.health.ufl.edu/misc/cod-oralhealth/docs/posts_frontpage/SocialInequalities.pdf (accessed 18 December 2016).

Which? (2012) *Is Your Fruit Smoothie as Healthy as You Think?* http://www.which.co.uk/news/2012/12/is-your-fruit-smoothie-as-healthy-as-you-think-305688/ (accessed 18 December 2016).

WHO (1986), *Ottawa Charter for Health Promotion*. World Health Organization, Geneva.

WHO (2003) *Diet, Nutrition and the Prevention of Chronic Diseases*. WHO Technical Report Series 916. World Health Organization, Geneva.

WHO (2015) *Guideline: Sugars Intake for Adults and Children*. World Health Organization, Geneva. http://apps.who.int/iris/bitstream/10665/149782/1/9789241549028_eng.pdf?ua=1 (accessed 18 December 2016).

Wong, M.C., Glenny, A.M., Tsang, B.W. *et al.* (2010) Topical fluoride as a cause of dental fluorosis in children. *The Cochrane Database of Systematic Reviews*, (1) CD007693.

22
Mental Health and Cognitive Function

Iron
Paul A Sharp

Caffeine
Peter J Rogers

B Vitamins
Helene McNulty

Physical Activity
Kenneth R Fox

Iron

Key messages

- Imbalances in brain iron content at different life stages are related to impaired brain function.
- Iron deficiency in early childhood is common in the UK; approximately a quarter of children aged 18 months to 3.5 years have iron intakes below the lower reference nutrient intake, and a similar number have low serum ferritin.
- There is a critical window during which iron deficiency can adversely affect brain development and function.
- Iron-deficiency anaemia in early infancy is associated with poor neurological, cognitive, motor, psycho-social and behavioural

development; these effects can persist in the longer term even if iron nutrition is improved.
- The brain continues to accumulate iron during adulthood, and abnormally high amounts of iron have been detected in brain material from individuals with neurodegenerative disorders such as Alzheimer's and Parkinson's disease.
- It is unclear whether altered brain iron levels or its cellular distribution occur as a consequence of the disease process or whether it is a primary contributor to neurodegenerative pathology.

22.1 Introduction: iron accumulation in the brain

An adequate supply of iron is crucial for a number of biological functions including normal brain development and neuronal activity. There is now strong evidence that imbalances in brain iron content at different life stages are related to impaired brain function. Iron-deficiency anaemia in infancy is associated with impaired cognitive and psycho-motor development. In addition, there is a growing body of work indicating that excessive brain iron accumulation in later life may be associated with several neurodegenerative disorders.

Iron is found abundantly in oligodendrocytes, cells in the central nervous system that produce myelin, which forms the insulating sheath surrounding neurones and improves electrical conductivity. The regional distribution of iron in the brain is not uniform, and the highest levels in the adult brain are located within the structures that form the basal ganglia. These regions are important in the fine control of motor function and are rich in dopaminergic and serotoninergic neurones (Beard, 2003). Iron is an essential co-factor for the tryptophan and tyrosine hydroxylase enzymes which are involved in the synthesis of these neurotransmitters. Iron also accumulates within the hippocampus, which is involved in the control of spatial awareness. Iron-deficiency anaemia in infancy is linked to impaired development of both motor skills and spatial memory, highlighting the essential role of iron in these processes (Lozoff, 2007).

Cellular uptake of iron occurs via transferrin receptor 1. Oligodendrocytes and astrocytes synthesise and secrete the iron transport protein transferrin, which in turn binds iron entering the brain across the blood–brain barrier and the choroid plexus. Iron-loaded transferrin (the protein can accommodate two ferric ions) binds to its cell-surface receptor, transferrin receptor 1, and the receptor–ligand complex is endocytosed. At the acid pH of the intracellular endosome, iron is released from transferrin, exits the endosomal vesicle through the divalent metal transporter, DMT1, and is utilised by the cell for a number of metabolic processes.

22.2 Iron deficiency and cognitive development

Infants are born iron replete, and brain iron content is greatest at birth; however, levels decline during weaning, before increasing again during neuronal expansion and development in early infancy. This has raised the question of whether there is a critical window during which iron deficiency can adversely affect brain development and function. A number of studies have found that iron-deficiency anaemia in early infancy (6–24 months – a period which encompasses the neonatal growth spurt) is associated with poor neurological, cognitive, motor, psycho-social and behavioural development; and furthermore, these effects can persist in the longer term even if dietary intake levels are improved (Beard, 2003; Lozoff, 2007; Benton, 2008). In animal models these effects are directly related to poor myelination of neurones and changes in brain dopamine and iron levels (Beard, 2003).

In the UK the Scientific Advisory Committee on Nutrition (SACN, 2010) reviewed the evidence linking iron status and cognitive function and found that there is a strong association between iron-deficiency anaemia and poor cognitive development in children aged less than 3 years. However, there are insufficient data to support a direct link between iron deficiency and impaired cognitive or language development in older children. Furthermore, while there is compelling evidence that some of the developmental effects of iron-deficiency anaemia in early infancy are irreversible, it is apparent that there may be beneficial effects of iron therapy in anaemic older children (McCann and Ames 2007; SACN, 2010). A systematic review and meta-analysis of 14 randomised controlled trials in older children and adults found evidence that oral iron supplementation improved attention and concentration irrespective of baseline iron status and in anaemic children therapy also improved IQ scores (Falkingham et al., 2010).

Iron deficiency in early childhood is common in the UK. Data from the National Diet and Nutrition Survey (Bates et al., 2011) indicates that 12–24% of children aged 18 months to 3.5 years had iron intakes below the lower reference nutrient intake and 24–35% of children in the same age group had low serum ferritin (a marker of body iron levels). The socio-economic status of the family appears to be a major determinant of iron status. Lower iron status in infants was observed where the head of the household was unemployed and in households with low income. Maternal education and short-duration of (or never) breastfeeding are also associated with poor iron status (Thane et al., 2000). Department of Health guidelines recommend that, for healthy infants, breast milk or formula milk should provide adequate nutrition until 6 months of age. Early exposure to weaning foods with low iron bioavailability could adversely affect iron status in infants.

Studies in adolescents and adults have found that iron-deficiency anaemia is associated with tiredness, low mood, poor concentration and impaired memory (Bruner et al., 1996; Murray-Kolb and Beard, 2007; Murray-Kolb, 2011). In these groups, iron deficiency is closely associated with lower performance in a number of cognitive functions tests; however, attainment is improved by iron therapy. These studies suggest that the effects of iron deficiency on cognition are not limited to the developing infant brain.

The British Nutrition Foundation's (2013) *Nutrition and Development* report suggests that the developing fetus accumulates up to 2 mg iron per day during the final trimester of pregnancy. While the majority of this iron is utilised for production of haemoglobin, these high accretion rates may also impact on brain iron levels at birth, suggesting that maternal iron status in pregnancy might be an important criterion for subsequent neuronal development in the infant. A study in rural south-eastern China revealed that serum ferritin concentrations in mothers with very low iron status in late pregnancy are correlated with iron stores in the newborn infant (Shao *et al.*, 2012). Furthermore, a prospective cohort study in Finland found a direct positive association between maternal haemoglobin levels during pregnancy and the offspring's educational achievement in later life (Fararouei *et al.*, 2010). These findings suggest that iron therapy at late stages of pregnancy, particularly for those with low iron status, may be beneficial for the health and cognitive performance of the offspring. Currently, the UK does not provide universal iron supplementation for pregnant women as the physiological adaptations that take place during pregnancy and lactation should be sufficient to ensure that the supply of iron to the developing fetus is not compromised (SACN, 2010). However, the National Institute for Health Care Excellence in the UK does recommend that iron supplementation be considered for women with haemoglobin levels below 110 μg/L in the first trimester of pregnancy and below 105 μg/L at 28 weeks. In contrast, all pregnant women in the USA routinely receive 30 mg iron per day.

22.3 Iron and neurodegeneration

While there are noticeable changes in brain iron content during early life, it is important to recognise that the brain continues to accumulate iron during adulthood. There is increasing interest in monitoring iron levels and its distribution in different brain structures during ageing, and how this relates to health and cognitive changes in the elderly. Abnormally high amounts of iron have been detected in brain material from individuals with neurodegenerative disorders such as Alzheimer's and Parkinson's disease (Ward *et al.*, 2014). These changes in brain iron content and its cellular distribution are not related to dietary intake and more probably reflect perturbations in local iron homeostatic pathways. Presently, it is unclear whether the altered distribution of iron in the brain occurs as a consequence of the disease process or whether it is a primary contributor to neurodegenerative pathology.

It is intriguing to note a number of proteins implicated in neurodegenerative disease also appear to be involved in the movement of iron across cell membranes in the brain. For example, the amyloid precursor protein has been reported to interact with the iron exporter ferroportin to regulate the release of iron from cells (Wong *et al.*, 2014). Deficiency of the tau protein leads to the accumulation of toxic iron levels in neurones, indicating that it, too, plays a role in cellular iron homeostasis (Lei *et al.*, 2012). Other studies have found that alpha-synuclein (Davies *et al.*, 2011) and the prion protein (Singh *et al.*, 2013) can both function as ferric reductases and may therefore play a role in neuronal iron accumulation. Aberrant production of all of these proteins is linked to specific neuropathologies: amyloid precursor protein and tau are associated with the development of Alzheimer's disease; alpha-synuclein with a number of disorders, including Parkinson's disease; and prion protein with Creutzfeld–Jacob disease. The possible link between iron and Parkinson's disease is particularly intriguing since pathology is associated with impaired formation and activity of dopamine; as mentioned previously, iron is a crucial co-factor for dopamine production. It is therefore tempting to speculate that an imbalance in iron homeostasis, particularly within dopamine-rich regions of the brain, may be a risk factor for the development of neurodegenerative diseases.

In addition to Alzheimer's disease and Parkinson's disease, a number of other neurodegenerative disorders are characterised by increased iron deposition in specific regions of the brain. The potential pathogenic action of iron in these diseases is not defined; however, excess iron is known to lead to the production of reactive oxygen species, which damage cell membranes, generate cytotoxic aldehydes and promote the formation of protein adducts and aggregates, which characterise several neurodegenerative disorders (Ward *et al.*, 2014). There is currently substantial interest from the pharmaceutical industry in developing therapeutic iron chelators that can cross the blood–brain barrier and modify cellular iron levels for use as part of the treatment regimen for Alzheimer's disease and Parkinson's disease patients. Some of these compounds have already reached phase 2 clinical trials.

22.4 Summary

The current evidence suggests that maintaining brain iron levels within defined limits is important at all life stages. Further studies are required to determine how imbalances in iron homeostasis impact on educational performance in children and mental health in adolescence and early adulthood. With the increasing longevity of the global population, understanding the basis for alterations in brain iron accumulation and distribution during ageing and the subsequent consequences for the development and progression of neurodegenerative diseases is likely to be a major focus for future research.

References

Bates, B., Lennox, A., Prentice, A. and Swan, G. (eds) (2011) *National Diet and Nutrition Survey. Headline Results from Years 1 and 2 (Combined) of the Rolling Programme (2008/2009–2009/2010)*. https://www.gov.uk/government/publications/national-diet-and-nutrition-survey-headline-results-from-years-1-and-2-combined-of-the-rolling-programme-2008-9-2009-10 (accessed 18 December 2016).

Beard, J. (2003) Iron deficiency alters brain development and functioning. *Journal of Nutrition*, 133, 1468S–1472S.

Benton, D. (2008) Micronutrient status, cognition and behavioral problems in childhood. *European Journal of Nutrition*, 47 (Suppl 3), 8–50.

British Nutrition Foundation (ed.) (2013) *Nutrition and Development: Short and Long Term Consequences for Health*. Wiley-Blackwell, Chichester.

Bruner, A.B., Joffe, A., Duggan, A.K. *et al.* (1996) Randomised study of cognitive effects of iron supplementation in nonanaemic iron-deficient adolescent girls. *The Lancet*, 348, 992–996.

Davies, P., Moualla, D. and Brown, D.R. (2011) Alpha-synuclein is a cellular ferrireductase. *PloS One*, 6, e15814.

Fararouei, M., Robertson, C., Whittaker, J. *et al.* (2010) Maternal Hb during pregnancy and offspring's educational achievement: a prospective cohort study over 30 years. *British Journal of Nutrition*, 104 (9), 1363–1368.

Falkingham, M., Abdelhamid, A., Curtis, P. *et al.* (2010) The effects of oral iron supplementation on cognition in older children and adults: a systematic review and meta-analysis. *Nutrition Journal*, 9, 4.

Lei, P., Ayton, S., Finkelstein, D.I. et al. (2012) Tau deficiency induces Parkinsonism with dementia by impairing APP-mediated iron export. *Nature Medicine*, 18, 291–295.

Lozoff, B. (2007) Iron deficiency and child development. *Food and Nutrition Bulletin*, 28, S560–S571.

McCann, J.C. and Ames, B.N. (2007) An overview of evidence for a causal relation between iron deficiency during development and deficits in cognitive or behavioral function. *The American Journal of Clinical Nutrition*, 85, 931–945.

Murray-Kolb, L.E. (2011) Iron status and neuropsychological consequences in women of reproductive age: what do we know and where are we headed? *Journal of Nutrition*, 141, 747S–755S.

Murray-Kolb, L.E. and Beard, J.L. (2007) Iron treatment normalizes cognitive functioning in young women. *The American Journal of Clinical Nutrition*, 85 (3), 778–787.

SACN (2010) *Iron and Health*. TSO, London. https://www.gov.uk/government/uploads/system/uploads/attachment_data/file/339309/SACN_Iron_and_Health_Report.pdf (accessed 18 December 2016).

Shao, J., Lou, J., Rao, R. et al. (2012) Maternal serum ferritin concentration is positively associated with newborn iron stores in women with low ferritin status in late pregnancy. *Journal of Nutrition*, 142, 2004–2009.

Singh, A., Haldar, S., Horback, K. et al. (2013) Prion protein regulates iron transport by functioning as a ferrireductase. *Journal of Alzheimer's Disease*, 35, 541–552.

Thane, C.W., Walmsley, C.M., Bates, C.J. et al. (2000) Risk factors for poor iron status in British toddlers: further analysis of data from the National Diet and Nutrition Survey of children aged 1.5–4.5 years. *Public Health Nutrition*, 3, 433–440.

Ward, R.J., Zucca, F.A., Duyn, J.H. et al. (2014) The role of iron in brain ageing and neurodegenerative disorders. *The Lancet: Neurology*, 13 (10), 1045–1060.

Wong, B.X., Tsatsanis, A., Lim, L.Q. et al. (2014) β-Amyloid precursor protein does not possess ferroxidase activity but does stabilize the cell surface ferrous iron exporter ferroportin. *PLoS One*, 9 (12), e114174.

Caffeine

Key messages

- Caffeine is widely consumed, primarily in tea and coffee, which are major sources of fluid in the human diet worldwide. Dietary caffeine is associated with energy intake, primarily from added sugar (including in cola and 'energy' drinks) and milk.

- Caffeine increases wakefulness and anxiety, improves physical performance and decreases hand steadiness. It also increases blood pressure. With frequent consumption, tolerance develops to these effects to varying degrees.

- The almost complete tolerance to the effect on wakefulness means that frequent caffeine consumers are not more wakeful (and alert) overall than people who do not consume caffeine, and they risk sleepiness due to caffeine withdrawal.

- Frequent caffeine consumers are therefore 'dependent' on caffeine (they function below par without it); however, because caffeine does not have a strong positive reinforcing effect (it does not produce a 'high'), it poses a low risk of addiction.

- Although there is only partial tolerance to the blood-pressure-raising effect of caffeine, tea and coffee consumption are not associated with increased risk of hypertension, cardiovascular disease and early cognitive decline. This is possibly due to the protective effects of other compounds, including polyphenols, consumed in these beverages, which are not present in some other popular caffeine-containing products.

22.5 Introduction

Caffeine is a xanthine alkaloid occurring in a variety of plants. It is consumed by people worldwide, predominantly from tea and coffee (Grigg, 2003). It has significant physiological and behavioural effects, and as a 'dietary' constituent is associated with consumption of many other compounds naturally present in tea, coffee, chocolate and so on, and with the consumption of milk and sugar (the energy content of many popular café-prepared coffees exceeds 200 kcal). Caffeine-containing beverages, and especially tea, coffee and cola, are a major source of fluid in the human diet. The following sections review mainly the acute effects of consuming caffeine itself, but consideration is also given to longer term outcomes associated with consumption of caffeine-containing beverages.

22.6 Disposition, metabolism and physiological actions of caffeine

After drinking tea, coffee or other caffeine-containing beverage, caffeine is distributed rapidly throughout the body, reaching its highest concentration in the bloodstream and in the brain within 30–40 min (it also crosses the placenta into the fetus and amniotic fluid and appears in breast milk of caffeine-consuming mothers) (James, 1997). Behavioural effects are detectable within at least 10 min of consumption (Durlach, 1998). Caffeine and its metabolites, including the psychoactive metabolite paraxanthine, are then gradually eliminated from the body, mainly in the urine. For adults, the elimination half-life of caffeine (i.e. the time it takes for half of the caffeine consumed to be eliminated from the body) is around 3–6 h, and is longer during pregnancy and shorter in smokers (James, 1997). Liver enzymes involved in the metabolism of caffeine are induced by exposure to nicotine, and variation in activity of these enzymes is independently associated with caffeine intake (Amin et al., 2012).

In the amounts consumed in the diet, the physiological and behavioural effects of caffeine occur primarily via antagonism of the action of the neuromodulator adenosine at adenosine A_1 and A_{2A} receptors (Fredholm et al., 1999). These cell-surface receptors are distributed throughout the body, including the brain, and by blocking the action of endogenous adenosine, caffeine has cardiovascular, cerebrovascular, renal, psychomotor, psychostimulant and anxiogenic effects. As well as being involved in the regulation of sleep and wakefulness (Basheer et al., 2004), importantly adenosine plays a role in preventing cell damage during hypoxia and ischaemia (see later).

With exposure to caffeine, adjustments occur in adenosine signalling (James, 1997) that serve to counteract the effects of caffeine and, at least in part, maintain normal functioning. This, together with changes in neurotransmitter systems modulated by adenosine, underlies caffeine tolerance – drug tolerance refers to the loss of responsiveness that accompanies repeated exposure to the substance. The extent to which tolerance occurs is crucial in determining the various effects of frequent caffeine consumption – defined as >120 mg/day, equivalent to approximately at least one and a half cups of coffee or three cups of tea per day (Rogers et al., 2010).

22.7 Psychostimulant effects of caffeine

As humankind's favourite drug (judged by amount of frequency of consumption), caffeine is valued for its reputation as a mostly harmless psychostimulant. Indeed, its alerting effects, 'I can't start the day without a coffee,' and 'caffeine keeps me going when I begin to flag', provide an explicit motive for consuming caffeine. Accordingly, many double-blind, placebo-controlled studies have confirmed that caffeine, in doses relevant to dietary intakes, increases self-rated wakefulness (decreased sleepiness) and alertness (Rogers et al., 2013). Less straightforward is the observation that this effect appears not to represent a net benefit to the frequent caffeine consumer due to near complete tolerance to the wakefulness effect of caffeine (Table 22.1). As a result, even after overnight caffeine abstinence, wakefulness is decreased compared with that of non-caffeine consumers or long-term abstinent (former) caffeine consumers. On ingestion of caffeine, wakefulness increases, but not to above the level reported by non-consumers or former consumers (Rogers et al., 2013).

In non-consumers and very low caffeine consumers, caffeine increases wakefulness above 'baseline', but it also has a mild anxiogenic effect, as indicated by increases in self-rated 'jitteriness', 'anxiety', 'nervousness' and so on. Furthermore, this effect appears to offset the increase in wakefulness, such that these

Table 22.1 Summary of some of the effects of caffeine and the degree to which frequent caffeine consumers become tolerant to those effects.

	Effect	Tolerance
Wakefulness	Increased	Complete or near complete
Anxiety	Increased	Complete or near complete
Motor performance	Improved	Little or none
Hand steadiness	Decreased	Partial
Blood pressure	Increased	Partial

individuals are not made more mentally alert (defined as 'mentally alert', 'able to concentrate', 'attentive', 'observant'). In both frequent caffeine consumers and non-consumers the effects of caffeine on performance of tasks requiring sustained concentration and focussed attention parallel the effects of caffeine on mental alertness (Rogers et al., 2013). Finally, with frequent consumption there is complete or near-complete tolerance to the anxiogenic effect of caffeine, even in individuals genetically susceptible to caffeine-induced anxiety (Rogers et al., 2010) (Table 22.1).

22.8 Motor performance and tremor

Two highly reproducible effects of caffeine are an increase in motor performance and tremor (decrease in hand steadiness). Indeed, these effects were first demonstrated reliably over 100 years ago (Hollingworth, 1912) using tests in which participants were, respectively, required to tap a metal rod as quickly as possible on a metal surface and to hold a 2.5 mm diameter metal rod within a 6 mm hole in a brass plate (tremor was measured by contact between the rod and the perimeter of the hole). Both effects appear to be more strongly dose dependent than the effect of caffeine on mental alertness (which may be adversely affected by increased anxiety at high doses, as mentioned earlier). The motor effect of caffeine is consistent with extensive evidence of enhancement by caffeine of athletic performance, including an effect on muscular strength and endurance (Warren et al., 2010). Furthermore, it appears that while there is partial tolerance to the effect of caffeine on hand steadiness (P.J. Rogers, unpublished results), there is little or no tolerance to its effects on motor performance (Graham, 2001; James et al., 2011; Rogers et al., 2013) (Table 22.1). Central mechanisms are implicated in the motor effects of caffeine, as well as a direct effect on muscle (Graham, 2001; James et al., 2011; Rogers et al., 2013). An effect on adenosine modulation of activity of dopamine neurones located in motor control areas of the brain may also underlie the increase in tremor after caffeine, and may perhaps even help to explain the reported reduction in risk of Parkinson's disease associated with caffeine (coffee) consumption (Popat et al., 2011).

22.9 Blood pressure

Adenosine has a vasorelaxant effect and, accordingly, caffeine causes vasoconstriction and an increase in blood pressure via an increase in 'total peripheral resistance' (James et al., 2012). Contrary to a popular assumption,

caffeine does not reliably increase heart rate. The acute increase in blood pressure after consuming a single caffeine-containing beverage is typically ≥5 mmHg (James, 2004), and James makes a compelling case that frequent consumers do not become fully tolerant to this effect (Table 22.1). Partial tolerance is suggested by the observation that vasodilation leading to increased cerebral blood flow appears to be the cause of headache that occurs on withdrawal of caffeine in frequent caffeine consumers (Couturier et al., 1997).

22.10 Hypertension, vascular disease, stroke and dementia

The blood-pressure-raising effect of caffeine predicts that, in the longer term, caffeine consumption should increase risk of cardiovascular disease, stroke and cognitive decline (Stewart, 1999; James, 2004). It is reassuring, therefore, that tea and coffee consumption have not generally been found to be associated with these adverse effects (e.g. Mesas et al., 2011), or even a reduction in cardiovascular and/or cerebrovascular disease (Jarvis, 1993; Arts and Hollman, 2005; Cornelis and El-Sohemy, 2005; Ritchie et al., 2007). These findings suggest that other effects of tea and coffee must outweigh the consequences of the blood-pressure-raising effect of caffeine. For example, polyphenols present in tea, including catechin, may reduce risk via vasorelaxant effects, and effects on blood cholesterol, blood coagulation and inflammatory processes (Hodgson, 2006). Certain compounds, such as cafestol (the concentration of which is affected by brewing method) in coffee, may increase risk, but again, balancing this, chlorogenic acid and other phenols are thought to have beneficial effects (Cornelis and El-Sohemy, 2005). Furthermore, another risk factor for cognitive decline, type 2 diabetes (Stewart and Liolitsa, 1999), appears to be lowered by coffee intake (Natella and Scaccini, 2012), whether caffeine containing or decaffeinated (Bhupathiraju et al., 2013); and theanine, a nonproteinic amino acid that is structurally similar to glutamate, occurring in tea has been found to acutely oppose the blood-pressure-raising effect of caffeine (Rogers et al., 2008).

These observations suggest that the vehicle in which caffeine is consumed may be crucial, and this is borne out by the further findings that, in contrast to coffee, caffeinated and decaffeinated sugared cola consumption is associated with increased risk of type 2 diabetes (Bhupathiraju et al., 2013), and that sugared and 'diet' cola consumption is associated with increased risk of incident hypertension, whereas coffee consumption is associated with reduced risk of the same (Winkelmayer et al., 2005).

Finally, it is plausible that caffeine itself may exert a positive effect in relation to cognitive decline and dementia, a significant cause of which are transient ischaemic episodes linked to underlying vascular disease (atherosclerosis) (O'Brien *et al.*, 2004). Brain ischaemia is the loss of glucose and oxygen supply to the brain, and can lead to cell death. During ischaemia there is a large increase in extracellular adenosine that, acting via adenosine A_1 and A_{2a} receptors, helps to counter some of the key pathophysiological processes, including excitatory neurotransmitter release, that lead to ischaemic cell death (Fredholm *et al.*, 2005). It may be that frequent caffeine consumption sensitises the neuroprotective actions of adenosine (Rogers *et al.*, 2008).

22.11 Caffeine reinforcement, dependence and addiction

Caffeine provides a good illustration of the distinction between dependence and addiction. From the foregoing discussion it is apparent that frequent caffeine consumers are 'dependent' on caffeine in that they do not function 'normally' without it. Owing to tolerance, withdrawal from caffeine results in mild adverse effects, most noticeably sleepiness and headache, apparent after overnight caffeine abstinence and worsening over several days and then abating with ensuing readjustment of adenosine signalling. At the same time, caffeine poses only a very low risk of addiction. This is primarily because it does not have strong positive reinforcing effects; for example, consumption is not followed by a 'high'. Instead, on encountering caffeine for the first time there will be an increase in wakefulness and, if the dose is moderately high, an increase in anxiety. For the frequent (i.e. dependent) consumer taking their morning cup of tea or coffee there will be relief from mild withdrawal symptoms, which will (negatively) reinforce their habit (Rogers *et al.*, 1995). Notably, caffeine withdrawal, even when it is prolonged (e.g. the frequent consumer neglecting to drink coffee at weekends), is not associated with strong cravings or a compulsion to consume caffeine-containing products. This is confirmed by experiments in which participants have been required to abstain from caffeine for several weeks (e.g. Rogers *et al.*, 2005) and found this rather easy to do, and the observation that decaffeinated tea and coffee are enjoyed, whereas 'tobacco' without nicotine is not.

References

Amin, N., Byrne, E., Johnson, J. *et al.* (2012) Genome-wide association analysis of coffee drinking suggests association with *CYP1A1/CYP1A2* and *NRCAM*. *Molecular Psychiatry*, **17**, 1116–1129.

Arts, I.C.W. and Hollman, P.C.H. (2005) Polyphenols and disease risk in epidemiologic studies. *American Journal of Clinical Nutrition*, **81** (Suppl), 317S–325S.

Basheer, R., Strecker, R.E., Thakkar, M.M. and McCarley, R.W. (2004) Adenosine and sleep–wake regulation. *Progress in Neurobiology*, **73**, 379–396.

Bhupathiraju, S.N., Pan, A., Malik, V.S. *et al.* (2013) Caffeinated and caffeine-free beverages and risk of type 2 diabetes. *American Journal of Clinical Nutrition*, **97**, 155–166.

Cornelis, M.C. and El-Sohemy, A. (2005) Coffee, caffeine, and coronary heart disease. *Current Opinion in Lipidology*, **18**, 13–19.

Couturier, E.G.M., Laman, D.M., van Duijn, M.A.J. and van Duijn, H. (1997) Influence of caffeine and caffeine withdrawal on headache and cerebral blood flow velocities. *Cephalalgia*, **17**, 188–190.

Durlach, P.J. (1998) The effects of a low dose of caffeine on cognitive performance. *Psychopharmacology*, **140**, 116–119.

Fredholm, B.B., Bättig, K., Holmén, J. *et al.* (1999) Actions of caffeine in the brain with special reference to factors that contribute to its widespread use. *Pharmacological Reviews*, **51**, 83–133.

Fredholm, B.B., Chen, J.-F., Cunha, R.A. *et al.* (2005) Adenosine and brain function. *International Review of Neurobiology*, **63**, 191–270.

Graham, T.E. (2001) Caffeine and exercise. *Sports Medicine*, **31**, 785–807.

Grigg, D. (2002) The worlds of tea and coffee: patterns of consumption. *GeoJournal*, **57**, 283–294.

Hodgson, J.M. (2006) Effects of tea and tea flavonoids on endothelial function and blood pressure: a brief review. *Clinical and Experimental Pharmacology and Physiology*, **33**, 838–841.

Hollingworth, H.L. (1912) The influence of caffeine on motor and mental efficiency. *Archives of Psychology*, **22**, 1–166.

James, J.E. (1997) *Understanding Caffeine: A Biobehavioral Analysis*. Sage, Thousand Oaks, CA.

James, J.E. (2004) Critical review of dietary caffeine and blood pressure: a relationship that should be taken more seriously. *Psychosomatic Medicine*, **6**, 63–71.

James, J.E., Bloomer, R.J., Cox, G. *et al.* (2011) Caffeine and physical performance. *Journal of Caffeine Research*, **1**, 145–151.

James, J.E., Gregg, M.E.D., Matyas, T.A. *et al.* (2012) Stress reactivity and the hemodynamic profile–compensation deficit (HP–CD) model of blood pressure regulation. *Biological Psychology*, **90**, 161–170.

Jarvis, M.J. (1993) Does caffeine enhance intake above absolute levels of cognitive performance? *Psychopharmacology*, **110**, 45–52.

Mesas, A.R., Leon-Munõz, L.M., Rodriguez-Artalejo, F. and Lopez-Garcia, E. (2011) The effect of coffee on blood pressure and cardiovascular disease in hypertensive individuals: a systematic review and meta-analysis. *American Journal of Clinical Nutrition*, **94**, 1113–1126.

Natella, F. and Scaccini, C. (2012) Role of coffee in modulation of diabetes risk. *Nutrition Reviews*, **70**, 207–217.

O'Brien, J., Ames, D., Gustafson, L. *et al.* (2004) *Cerebrovascular Disease, Cognitive Impairment and Dementia*. Martin Dunitz, London.

Popat, R.A., van Den Eeden, S.K., Tanner, C.M. *et al.* (2011) Coffee, *ADORAA2A*, and *CYP1A2*: the caffeine connection in Parkinson's disease. *European Journal of Neurology*, **18**, 756–765.

Ritchie, K., Carrière, I., de Mendonça, A. *et al.* (2007) The neuroprotective effects of caffeine: a prospective population (the Three Cities Study). *Neurology*, **69**, 536–545.

Rogers, P.J., Richardson, N.J. and Elliman, N.A. (1995) Overnight caffeine abstinence and negative reinforcement of preference for caffeine-containing drinks. *Psychopharmacology*, **120**, 457–462.

Rogers, P.J., Heatherley, S.V., Hayward, R.C. *et al.* (2005) Effects of caffeine and caffeine withdrawal on mood and cognitive performance degraded by sleep restriction. *Psychopharmacology*, **179**, 742–752.

Rogers, P.J., Smith, J.E., Heatherley, S.V. and Pleydell-Pearce, C.W. (2008) Time for tea: mood, blood pressure and cognitive performance effects of caffeine and theanine administered alone and together. *Psychopharmacology*, **195**, 569–577.

Rogers, P.J., Hohoff, C., Heatherley, S.V. *et al.* (2010) Association of the anxiogenic and alerting effects of caffeine with *ADORA2A* and *ADORA1* polymorphisms and habitual level of caffeine consumption. *Neuropsychopharmacology*, **35**, 1973–1983.

Rogers, P.J., Heatherley, S.V., Mullings, E.L. and Smith, J.E. (2013) Faster but not smarter: effects of caffeine and caffeine withdrawal on alertness and performance. *Psychopharmacology*, **226**, 229–240.

Stewart, R. (1999) Hypertension and cognitive decline. *British Journal of Psychiatry*, **174**, 286–287.

Stewart, R. and Liolitsa, D. (1999) Type 2 diabetes mellitus, cognitive impairment and dementia. *Diabetic Medicine*, **16**, 93–112.

Warren, G.L., Park, N.D., Maresca, R.D. *et al.* (2010) Effect of caffeine ingestion on muscular strength and endurance: a meta-analysis. *Medicine and Science in Sports and Exercise*, **42**, 1375–1387.

Winkelmayer, W.C., Stampfer, M.J., Willett, W.C. and Curhan, G.C. (2005) Habitual caffeine intake and risk of hypertension in women. *Journal of the American Medical Association*, **294**, 2330–2335.

B Vitamins

Key messages

- Folate and vitamin B_{12} are important cofactors in one-carbon metabolism and are thus essential in brain health by providing methyl groups for numerous central nervous system methylation reactions involving neurotransmitter and membrane phospholipid synthesis and myelin methylation.
- The human *in utero* environment may influence brain health of the offspring in later life, through a phenomenon known as epigenetics, for which DNA methylation is an important mechanism of gene regulation. DNA methylation, in turn, is dependent on an adequate supply of folate and vitamin B_{12}. Whether maternal folate status during pregnancy can mediate health effects in the brain in childhood via changes in DNA methylation requires further study.

- Convincing evidence suggests that optimal folate and related B vitamin status can help in maintaining cognitive function in ageing, and that intervention to optimise biomarker status of B vitamins (though supplements or fortified foods) is likely to be most effective before overt signs of neurological disease have occurred, and in people with low B vitamin status.
- Folate deficiency is strongly associated with depression, but there is little evidence from randomised trials to prove a beneficial effect of folate and related B vitamins in the treatment of depression or in the maintenance of better mental health in the general population.

22.12 Introduction: B vitamins and the nervous system

Folate, vitamin B_{12} and vitamin B_6 play important roles in the nervous system at all ages, from neural development in early life through to the maintenance of mental health and cognitive function in later life. These vitamins are required for one-carbon metabolism. This involves the transfer and utilisation of one-carbon units in a number of important pathways involving amino acid metabolism, DNA and RNA biosynthesis, and methylation processes. The metabolism of homocysteine requires folate along with vitamin B_{12}, and to a lesser extent vitamin B_6 and vitamin B_2; when the status of these vitamins is low or deficient, plasma homocysteine concentration will invariably be elevated. There has been considerable interest in plasma homocysteine as a potential risk factor for cognitive dysfunction and other diseases of ageing. Whether homocysteine is a true disease risk factor remains unconfirmed; in any case however, its measurement provides a sensitive functional biomarker of folate and/or related B vitamin status. Plasma homocysteine shows significant lowering in response to B vitamin intervention.

Folate and vitamin B_{12} are required for the activity of methionine synthase, and therefore the synthesis of S-adenosylmethionine (SAM), which in turn provides methyl groups for numerous central nervous system methylation reactions involving neurotransmitter and membrane phospholipid synthesis and myelin methylation. With folate or vitamin B_{12} deficiency, the reduction in tissue levels of SAM will impair these methylation reactions. The reported neuropsychiatric effects of folate deficiency are remarkably similar to those described for vitamin B_{12} deficiency, and include cognitive decline, depression and peripheral neuropathy, although the latter is more commonly found in vitamin B_{12} deficiency (Reynolds, 2006). Vitamin B_6 plays an essential role in transamination and decarboxylation reactions, which in turn are involved in neurotransmitter synthesis, metabolism and release; deficiency of vitamin B_6 is associated with deficits in nerve conduction.

There is much interest in the potential roles of these B vitamins in the prevention of cognitive dysfunction and disorders of mood. The scope of this section is to focus on the relationship of folate and related B vitamins with cognitive function and mental health.

22.13 B vitamins and cognitive development in early life

Folate and related B vitamins are fundamental during brain development owing to their involvement in transcription, nucleotide synthesis, DNA integrity and methylation processes (Reynolds, 2006). In particular, both vitamins are essential in DNA methylation, which in turn is important in controlling gene expression. A new area of research suggests that the *in utero* environment can impact on DNA methylation patterns and in this way influence phenotype and health of the offspring in later life, through a phenomenon known as epigenetics, for which DNA methylation is an important mechanism of gene regulation.

The well-known roles of folate and vitamin B_{12} in DNA methylation provide a potential mechanism that underlies fetal programming. Furthermore, there is recent evidence from a human study suggesting that maternal folate exposure after 12 weeks' gestation may influence gene-specific DNA methylation in the offspring (Haggarty et al., 2013). Whether folate supplementation during pregnancy can mediate cognitive health effects in childhood via changes in DNA methylation, however, remains to be confirmed, but this is an exciting area of emerging scientific interest.

22.14 B vitamins and cognitive function in ageing

Cognitive dysfunction in ageing ranges from mild memory loss to dementia, the latter referring to a state where the decline in memory and thinking are sufficient to impair functioning in daily living. Among the modifiable risk factors that potentially contribute to a greater than expected rate of cognitive decline with advancing age, there is considerable evidence linking suboptimal status of folate or vitamin B_{12}, and/or elevated homocysteine concentrations, with cognitive dysfunction. Homocysteine concentrations are typically higher in patients with Alzheimer's disease (the most common form of dementia), and are strongly related to the rate of cognitive decline in patients with mild cognitive impairment and confirmed Alzheimer's disease. Some large observational studies implicate low folate status in this relationship, whereas other evidence supports a role for low vitamin B_{12}. Evidence from observational studies suggesting a role for B vitamins and other potential nutritional factors, however, can be complicated by the fact that poor diet may be both a cause and a consequence of impaired cognitive function. Only randomised trials can confirm whether a causative relationship exists.

Several randomised controlled trials have investigated the potential benefits of B vitamin supplementation on cognitive function, but many of these were of insufficient duration or sample size to provide clear evidence, while others intervened in patients with confirmed Alzheimer's disease where a beneficial effect is highly unlikely. One notable trial of healthy older adults in New Zealand reported no benefit of high dose combined folic acid/ vitamin B_{12}/vitamin B_6 for 2 years on any cognitive function parameter examined (McMahon et al., 2006), whereas another similar study in the Netherlands showed that supplementation with folic acid alone for 3 years significantly improved a number of cognitive parameters, including memory, information-processing speed and sensorimotor function (Durga et al., 2007). An important difference between these two studies was baseline folate status, which tended to be far lower in the Dutch trial, perhaps demonstrating that any benefit of folic acid on cognitive function arises through correction of suboptimal folate status, whereas providing additional folic acid to those whose status is already optimal may have no effect on cognitive outcomes. Of note, more recent randomised trials, showing that combined B vitamin intervention prevented cognitive decline in free-living older adults with depressive symptoms, or improved cognitive performance in participants with mild cognitive impairment, provide convincing evidence that low B vitamin status is causatively linked with cognitive dysfunction in ageing. These positive trial findings from questionnaire-based assessment of cognitive performance have been very substantially underpinned by the recent work of Smith and colleagues showing that B vitamin intervention slowed the rate of global and regional brain atrophy in participants with mild cognitive impairment but without dementia (Smith *et al.*, 2012; Douaud *et al.*, 2013).

Thus, optimal B vitamin status may help to maintain cognitive function in ageing. However, published trials have typically intervened at extremely high vitamin doses. Further evidence is clearly required to investigate the effects (and interactions) of these vitamins at typical exposure levels achievable through dietary means.

22.15 B vitamins and mental health

It is well recognised that B vitamin deficiencies can manifest with significant neurological and neuropsychiatric disturbances. Apart from memory deficits and cognitive dysfunction, depressive symptoms are well described in both folate and vitamin B_{12} deficiency, though depression is reported to be more than twice as common in folate deficiency as in vitamin B_{12} deficiency (Reynolds, 2006).

Depression is the most frequent psychiatric disease. Numerous observational studies show a strong association between folate deficiency and depression, with a reported one-third of depressed patients showing low red cell folate concentrations (Reynolds, 2006; Stanger *et al.*, 2009). Likewise, psychiatric disorders are frequently found in patients diagnosed with megaloblastic anaemia due to folate deficiency. Furthermore, folate deficiency can affect the duration and clinical severity of depression, and is associated with poorer response to antidepressant medication. Low concentrations of vitamin B_6, which acts as a cofactor in the metabolism of tryptophan and serotonin, have also been linked with symptoms of depression. Despite the strong association of folate deficiency with depression, relatively few randomised trials have been performed to investigate the effect of folate intervention on mood disorders.

There is insufficient evidence at this time to evaluate the impact of folate, vitamin B_{12} or vitamin B_6 in relation to other common psychiatric diseases, such as schizophrenia and bipolar disorder.

Folate and related B vitamins and their potential preventative effects in relation to a range of neuropsychiatric diseases have been extensively reviewed by an expert panel elsewhere (Stanger *et al.*, 2009).

22.16 Dealing with low B vitamin status and related public health challenges

It is clear that folate and vitamin B_{12} both play essential roles in relation to the brain, but the interaction between them is complex. There is some (though not consistent) evidence that high folic acid intake may potentially lead to an exacerbation of vitamin B_{12} deficiency and an increased risk of cognitive impairment in older people with low vitamin B_{12} status. This potential concern will need some consideration in relation to emerging food policy, given that there is a high prevalence of food-bound vitamin B_{12} malabsorption found generally in older people (leading to poor status even with good dietary vitamin B_{12} intakes), and mandatory folic acid fortification is now in place in over 80 countries worldwide.

Assessing the vitamin B_{12} status of populations in relation to health outcomes is important, however, and it remains to be determined which vitamin B_{12} status assay (or combination of assays) provides the best predictive value for brain function. Along with the more established assays, plasma vitamin B_{12} and homocysteine, potentially more sensitive status biomarkers include methylmalonic acid and holotranscobalamin. The latter represents the fraction of total plasma vitamin B_{12} bound to the transport protein transcobalamin, and is thus the metabolically active vitamin fraction. Many published studies, however, have relied on plasma vitamin B_{12} as the sole measure of vitamin B_{12} status, whereas those studies that have used alternative tests, or two or more bioassays in combination, are generally more supportive of a role for vitamin B_{12} in relation to brain health.

22.17 Conclusions

Folate and vitamin B_{12} interact closely in one-carbon metabolism and are essential for methylation reactions in brain function. They may, therefore, have overlapping roles in the prevention of disorders of central nervous system development, and mood disorders and cognitive dysfunction in older people. Further evidence is clearly required to provide a better understanding of the effects (and interactions) of these vitamins, and to confirm whether improving B vitamin status will have a role in preventing cognitive impairment and dementia. Given that there are potentially harmful effects of folic acid at high exposure levels in those with low vitamin B_{12} status, future trials should investigate the potential benefits of these vitamins at nutritional levels rather than at pharmacological doses far in excess of dietary recommendations. For governments worldwide considering such public health policy issues, there is a need for a balanced approach and an emphasis on maintaining an optimal status of both folate and vitamin B_{12} throughout life.

References

Douaud, G., Refsum, H., de Jager, C.A. *et al.* (2013) Preventing Alzheimer's disease-related gray matter atrophy by B-vitamin treatment. *Proceedings of the National Academy of Sciences of the United States of America*, **110**, 9523–9528.

Durga, J., van Boxtel, M.P.J., Schouten, E.G. *et al.* (2007) Effect of 3-year folic acid supplementation on cognitive function in older adults in the FACIT trial: a randomised, double blind, controlled trial. *The Lancet*, **369**, 208–216.

Haggarty, P., Hoad, G., Campbell, D.M. *et al.* (2013) Folate in pregnancy and imprinted gene and repeat element methylation in the offspring. *The American Journal of Clinical Nutrition*, **97**, 94–99.

McMahon, J.A., Green, T.J., Skeaff, C.M. *et al.* (2006) A controlled trial of homocysteine lowering and cognitive performance. *The New England Journal of Medicine*, **354**, 2764–2772.

Reynolds, E. (2006) Vitamin B12, folic acid, and the nervous system. *The Lancet: Neurology*, **5**, 949–960.

Smith, A.D., Smith, S.M., de Jager, C.A. *et al.* (2010) Homocysteine-lowering by B vitamins slows the rate of accelerated brain atrophy in mild cognitive impairment: a randomized controlled trial. *PLoS One*, **5** (9), e12244.

Stanger, O., Fowler, B., Piertzik, K. *et al.* (2009) Homocysteine, folate and vitamin B12 in neuropsychiatric diseases: review and treatment recommendations. *Expert Review of Neurotherapeutics*, **9**, 1393–1412.

Physical Activity

Key messages

- Physical activity reduces the risk of depression, cognitive decline, dementia and Alzheimer's disease.
- Physical activity can be effective in the treatment of depression, and can be helpful in the management of illnesses such as schizophrenia and anxiety disorders.
- Physical activity helps people feel better in terms of improved mood and sense of well-being, and stress and anxiety reduction. It also helps people feel better about themselves, as indicated by increased levels of confidence, physical self-perceptions and to a lesser extent self-esteem.
- Given levels of mental illness and increasing prominence of diseases involving cognitive decline, physical activity can play an increasing role in prevention and treatment. It also is an important strategy for improving well-being and quality of life.

22.18 Introduction

The case for physical activity and health has largely been established through its effectiveness in preventing and treating diseases such as cardiovascular disease, diabetes, some cancers and, to a lesser extent, obesity (Lee *et al.*, 2012). Recently, the value of physical activity in helping people maintain good mental health and well-being has been recognised (Penedo and Dahn, 2005). This is a complex area of health, and the evidence is best viewed in terms of (a) prevention of mental illness, (b) treatment of mental illness and (c) general benefits for mental well-being or 'feeling good'.

22.19 Physical activity and the prevention of mental illness

Mental illness is widespread, with clinical depression predicted to be the most debilitating of modern diseases across the world by 2020 (WHO, 2002). Within any year, one in four adults in the UK visit their doctor with a mental health problem, such as sleeplessness, stress and anxiety, as well as depression (https://www.mentalhealth.org.uk/publications/fundamental-facts-about-mental-health-2015). Other serious diseases commonly termed severe and enduring mental illness (SEMI) also seems to be on the increase. Furthermore, as people live longer and the sector of society who are older than 70 years increases, the prevention of cognitive decline, dementia and Alzheimer's disease has become critical if health and social services are to cope.

Evidence, largely derived through prospective cohort studies using large samples of the population, is emerging that physical activity in middle to later years can have an important effect on reducing risk of several of these debilitating mental diseases. Several studies show, for example, that those who maintain physical activity in later years are subsequently 20–30% less likely to suffer clinical depression (Teychenne *et al.*, 2008; Mammen and Faulkner, 2013). A similar finding is seen with the prevention of dementia and Alzheimer's disease, where over 40 studies now indicate substantial reductions in risk for those who are physically active in middle and older years (Hamer and Chida, 2009). An exciting new area of research is the impact of physical activity on brain function. Recent studies with older adults, including some with existing dementia, are showing positive changes such as growth of the hippocampus, which is the memory centre of the brain (Erikson *et al.*, 2010). This is backed up by studies which show improvements in several aspects of cognitive function with exercise. The mechanisms for this very positive effect of exercise are not clear and might include improved blood supply, neurogenesis or improved neural efficiency (Ahlskog *et al.*, 2011), and teams of researchers using functional magnetic resonance imaging scanning techniques are busy trying to identify them.

It is more difficult to study the prevention of SEMI, as these disorders are less prevalent in the population and are often accompanied by chaotic lifestyles, so the impact of physical activity has not been widely studied.

22.20 Physical activity and the treatment of mental illness and disorders

Many forms of mental illness are widespread, and effective treatments are needed. The most widely used approach by doctors involves medication, although for some conditions, such as mild to moderate depression, cognitive behaviour therapy is increasing in prominence. Definitions of depression range from episodes of unhappiness that affect most people from time to time, to persistent low mood and inability to continue work. If such feelings persist over time, they may be classified as 'clinical' and may be classed as mild, moderate or severe. Several reviews of randomised controlled trials have been conducted to assess the effectiveness of physical activity to reduce depression and its recurrence (Lawlor and Hopker, 2001; Brosse *et al.*, 2002; Barbour *et al.*, 2007). On the whole, there is a general acceptance that physical activity is an effective treatment, and indeed this idea is supported by the National Institute for Clinical Excellence and Mental Health Foundation. However, the more sceptical reviewers are less optimistic. A recent attempt in the UK to add physical activity to usual care in primary care settings increased activity in depressed patients, but this did not result in greater reductions in depression than the control group (who also increased in activity) (Chalder *et al.*, 2012). Clearly, physical activity works for some depressed patients, and future research is needed to identify who is most likely to benefit.

The effectiveness of activity to treat anxiety-related problems is also difficult to estimate. Presenting symptoms for a person with a clinical level of anxiety might include fear, worry, inappropriate thoughts or inappropriate actions. Diagnosis might include phobias (such as agoraphobia), panic attacks, schizophrenia, obsessive–compulsive disorder and stress disorders (such as post-traumatic stress). Some symptoms are enduring and others intermittent, and sufferers often lead chaotic lives. However, attempts are being made with some degree of success at local level to involve people with SEMI in sports activities such as football, swimming and badminton. Qualitative research indicates that participants find the programmes helpful in the management of their conditions (Hodgson *et al.*, 2011). Recently, governments have been asking researchers and local care authorities to develop effective programmes for dementia and Alzheimer's sufferers, and several programmes are currently being evaluated. There is also enough evidence to encourage general practitioners to recommend activity for improving sleep, and there is also some evidence that physical activity can help improve the lives of recovering alcoholics and substance abusers.

22.21 Psychological well-being and physical activity

The effect of physical activity on mental well-being or positive mental health has been studied for some time and has been summarised by Biddle *et al.* (2000), and more recently by Biddle and Mutrie (2008). There is population-based cross-sectional evidence indicating that those who are active are happier, have higher levels of subjective well-being and life satisfaction, and lower levels of stress than those who are low in activity. The immediate impact of an exercise session on mood, state anxiety and subjective well-being has been established through hundreds of controlled trials. There is little doubt that, at least in the short term, exercise in forms as diverse as swimming, walking, jogging, weight training, competitive sports, yoga, gardening or dancing generally has positive effects. A small number of studies have also shown that lunchtime activity improves mood and well-being at work in the afternoons. Teachers also claim that activity at school also improves children's mood and concentration in class, although this has not been fully confirmed through rigorous research.

In the longer term, exercise programmes have been shown through randomised controlled trials to reduce trait anxiety, improve various aspects of subjective well-being and also help people feel better about themselves and their bodies. Physical self-perceptions involve feelings of physical attractiveness, confidence and competence, and these consistently improve with increased levels of exercise and improved fitness (Fox, 2000). This finding remains even in the absence of weight loss. The effect generalises to global feelings of worth or self-esteem in some people, particularly those initially with low self-esteem.

The effects of activity on psychological well-being therefore help people feel well and can clearly improve quality of life.

22.22 How do we make a difference?

These benefits of physical activity for prevention and treatment of mental illness and improved psychological well-being are summarised in UK (Department of Health, Physical Activity, Health Improvement and Protection, 2011) and American physical activity guidelines (Physical Activity Guidelines Writing Group, 2008). The recommended amounts of physical activity are primarily based on the effects seen for all-cause mortality, cardiovascular disease, diabetes and some cancers that require upgrading of elements of the metabolic systems of the body. Producing recommendations for optimal amounts of physical activity for mental health is more challenging.

The mechanisms underpinning effects of physical activity and mental illnesses, disorders, or even daily fluctuations in mood, anxiety and sense of well-being are far from fully understood. They are likely to involve some combination of metabolic, circulatory and endocrinological changes, depending on the particular mental state or condition. This means that identification of a generalised dose of exercise that is optimally beneficial is unlikely. The optimal amount and type of activity will depend on the preferences and characteristics of the individual, their past experiences, with activity, as well as the setting in which it takes place. Well-designed research, for example, has shown improvements in mood with 10-min walks (Ekkekakis et al., 2000). On the other hand, increased circulation to the brain through moderate to vigorous activity seems important for cognitive benefit. It is prudent, therefore, to provide a more facilitative approach to activity for mental health, allowing the individual to have choice of mode and intensity.

Furthermore, feeling healthier and better about oneself are consistent reasons provided for continuing with an activity, and long-term adherence to activity programmes is critical if participants are to experience all the benefits of preventing physical and mental disease. Mental effects are therefore central to the whole physical activity–health relationship and should be the primary consideration in the design and delivery of physical activity interventions to improve public health.

References

Ahlskog, J.E., Geda, Y.E., Graff-Radford, N.R. and Petersen, R.C. (2011) Physical exercise as a preventive or disease-modifying treatment of dementia and brain aging. *Mayo Clinic Proceedings*, **86** (9), 876–884.

Barbour, K.A., Edenfield, T.M. and Blumenthal, J.A. (2007) Exercise as a treatment for depression and other psychiatric disorders: a review. *Journal of Cardiopulmonary Rehabilitation and Prevention*, **27** (6), 359–367.

Biddle, S.J.H. and Mutrie, N. (2008) *Psychology of Physical Activity: Determinants, Well-being Interventions*, 2nd edn. Routledge, London.

Biddle, S.J.H., Fox, K.R. and Boutcher, S.H. (eds) (2000) *Physical Activity and Psychological Well-being*. Routledge, London.

Brosse, A.L., Sheets, E.S., Lett, H.S. and Blumenthal, J.A. (2002) Exercise and the treatment of clinical depression in adults. *Sports Medicine*, **32**, 741–760.

Chalder, M., Wiles, N.J., Campbell, J. *et al.* (2012) Facilitated physical activity as a treatment for depressed adults: randomised controlled trial. *BMJ*, **344**, e2758.

Department of Health, Physical Activity, Health Improvement and Protection (2011) *Start Active, Stay Active: A Report on Physical Activity for Health from the Four Home Countries' Chief Medical Officers*. https://www.gov.uk/government/uploads/system/uploads/attachment_data/file/216370/dh_128210.pdf (accessed 10 December 2016).

Ekkekakis, P., Hall, E.E., van Landuyt, L.M. and Petruzzello, S.J. (2000) Walking in (affective) circles: can short walks enhance affect? *Journal of Behavioral Medicine*, **23** (3), 245–275.

Erikson, K.I., Voss, M.W., Prakash, R.S. *et al.* (2010) Exercise training increases size of hippocampus and improves memory. *Proceedings of the National Academy of Sciences of the United States of America*, **108**, 3017–3022.

Fox, K.R. (2000) Self-esteem, self-perceptions and exercise. *International Journal of Sport Psychology*, **31**, 228–240.

Hamer, M. and Chida, Y. (2009) Physical activity and risk of neurodegenerative disease: a systematic review of prospective evidence. *Psychological Medicine*, **39**, 3–11.

Hodgson, M.H., McCullough, H.P. and Fox, K.R. (2011) The experiences of people with severe and enduring mental illness engaged in a physical activity programme integrated into the mental health service. *Mental Health and Physical Activity*, **4** (1), 23–29.

Lawlor, D.A. and Hopker, S.W. (2001) The effectiveness of exercise as an intervention in the management of depression: systematic review and meta-regression analysis of randomised controlled trials. *BMJ*, **322**, 763–767.

Lee, I.-M., Shiroma, E.J., Lobelo, F. *et al.* (2012) Effect of physical inactivity on major non-communicable diseases worldwide: an analysis of burden of disease and life expectancy. *The Lancet*, **380** (9838), 219–229.

Mammen, G. and Faulkner, G. (2013) Physical activity and the prevention of depression: a systematic review of prospective studies. *American Journal of Preventive Medicine*, **45**, 649–657.

Penedo, F.J. and Dahn, J.R. (2005) Exercise and well-being: a review of mental and physical health benefits associated with physical activity. *Current Opinion in Psychiatry*, **18**, 189–193.

Physical Activity Guidelines Writing Group (2008) *2008 Physical Activity Guidelines for Americans: Be Active, Healthy, and Happy!* US Department of Health and Human Services, Washington, DC.

Teychenne, M., Ball, K. and Salmon, J. (2008) Physical activity and likelihood of depression in adults: a review. *Preventive Medicine*, **46** (5), 397–411.

WHO (2002) *World Health Report 2002: Reducing Risks, Promoting Healthy Life*. World Health Organization, Geneva.

Part Four

Environmental Factors

23
Obesogenic Neighbourhood Food Environments

Amelia A Lake, Tim G Townshend, and Thomas Burgoine

Key messages

- Food environments shape our dietary behaviours.
- The mechanisms by which food environments influence our dietary behaviours are complex and difficult to measure.
- Food environments include the retail environment, foods available at home, the policy environment, residential neighbourhoods, schools and workplaces.
- A geographic information system (GIS) can help us to understand the relationships between individuals and their food environments.

- GIS measures of food outlet 'exposure' are only as reliable as the data on which they are based, and the theoretical frameworks that underpin their use.
- Policies to address obesogenic environments through urban planning are being developed, but as yet their effectiveness is unproven.

23.1 Introduction to obesogenic environments and the concept of the food environment

Obesogenic environments have been defined as 'the sum of influences that the surroundings, opportunities, or conditions of life have on promoting obesity in individuals or populations' (Swinburn and Egger, 2002). Obesogenic environments are related to both energy intake and energy expenditure. This chapter will focus on the energy intake aspects of the obesogenic neighbourhood food environment, sometimes referred to as the 'foodscape'. Alongside the exponential increase in the prevalence of overweight and obesity worldwide, the food environment has also changed dramatically in recent decades. In the UK there has been the rise of the large supermarkets, accompanied by the demise of smaller, independent grocery shops, the increase in out-of-town retailers and the increased availability of foods designed to be consumed outside of the home (Burgoine *et al.*, 2009).

Food choice and eating behaviours are influenced by multiple factors. The relationship between the food environment and obesity is complex (Foresight, 2007),

and is likely to be influenced by other individual and social factors. While there is little research linking food access with obesity as an outcome measure (White, 2007), understanding the relationship between what we eat and the environmental context in which these food choices are made is essential to the development of long-term obesity prevention strategies (Holsten, 2009).

The food environment constitutes any opportunity to obtain food and includes physical, socio-cultural, economic and policy influences at both micro– and macro-levels (Townshend and Lake, 2009). The broader food environment includes the home food environment, food policies and school food policies in addition to the neighbourhood food environment. Glanz *et al.* (2005) have conceptualised the food environment to incorporate four different elements (Figure 23.1); community (type and location of food outlets); consumer (availability of healthy options, price, promotion and nutritional information); organisational (home, school and workplace); and informational (media and advertising).

The neighbourhood food environment, which is focused on in this chapter, is usually a mixture of retail outlets, from small convenience stores to supermarkets, as well as restaurants and takeaway ('fast food') outlets.

Public Health Nutrition, Second Edition. Edited by Judith L Buttriss, Ailsa A Welch, John M Kearney and Susan A Lanham-New.
© 2018 by The Nutrition Society. Published 2018 by John Wiley & Sons, Ltd.
Companion website: www.wiley.com/go/buttriss/publichealth

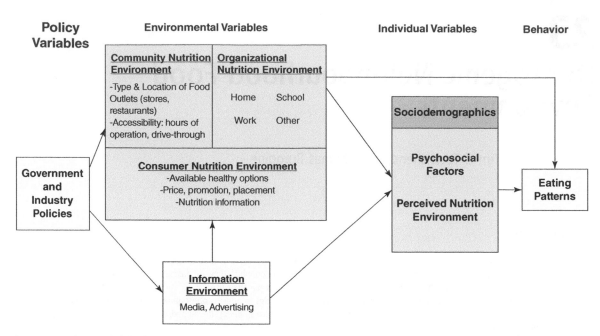

Figure 23.1 The model of the food environment as conceptualised by Glanz *et al.* (2005). *Source*: Glanz *et al.* (2005). Reproduced with permission of SAGE Publications.

The neighbourhood food environment influences individual food choice and food intake through the concept of food *access*. The seemingly simple concept of access has been explored by Charreire *et al.* (2010) and Caspi *et al.* (2012), who have suggested use of Penchansky and Thomas's (1981) five dimensions as a theoretical

Table 23.1 A framework for exploring the food environment.

Availability	The number and density of different types of food outlets near an individual, usually measured by classifying, counting and describing food outlets)
Accessibility	The distance to the nearest food outlet, or to different types of food outlet, usually measured using geographic information systems (GISs)
Affordability	Food prices and perceptions of food prices, which can be measured using in-store audits of identified items and surveys of individuals
Acceptability	Individuals' perceptions of the ability of local food outlets to meet their needs and standards, often measured by responses from individuals or in-store food quality audits
Accommodation	The ability of food outlets to accept and adapt to local needs, for example with respect to opening times and payment methods, usually measured by surveys of food outlets and individual responses

Source: Penchansky and Thomas (1981). Reproduced with permission of Wolters Kluwer Health Inc.

framework for exploring the food environment, which are *availability*, *accessibility*, *affordability*, *acceptability* and *accommodation* (see Table 23.1).

In terms of the availability and accessibility of food outlets, research not only identifies the types of outlets in a given environment, but also the spatial configuration of these outlets. A 'concentration' effect has been observed, for example, whereby fast food outlets tend to cluster in more deprived areas of England and Scotland (Macdonald *et al.*, 2007). The clustering of food outlets around schools has also been discussed in both the UK and international literature, as well as at local authority level (see Section 23.4). There is also an interest in the difference between urban and rural settings, with a need for researchers and policy makers to be context specific when dealing with issues of neighbourhood food exposure and diet.

Despite being a relatively new field of research, interest in the influence of the food environment on eating behaviours and its relationship with outcome measures such as dietary intake and adiposity has increased rapidly.

23.2 Eating behaviours and how the food environment influences diet and obesity

While individual foods are not labelled obesogenic, we have a good understanding of which types of food are implicated in causing ill health or excess weight gain.

Availability of low-fat milk relative to high-fat milk in a store

Purchases of low-fat milk relative to high-fat milk

Consumption of low-fat milk relative to high-fat milk

Fat content of the diet of store customers

Population-level disease related to fat in the diet

Figure 23.2 Lytle (2009) causal model linking an environmental attribute with population-level disease. *Source*: Lytle (2009). Reproduced with permission of Elsevier.

This is why some local authorities are proposing limits to fast food outlets (see Section 23.4) or some cities, such as New York, have proposed and implemented legislation around the size of soft drinks, trans fat and nutritional labelling.

Individual preferences drive food choice and eating behaviours; yet, more recently, there has been a growing interest in how the environment might influence dietary intake. However, to date there has been a lack of research on the mechanisms by which food environments influence diet (Caspi *et al.*, 2012). There is a need to better understand *which* factors and *how* these factors influence individual food behaviour and ultimately energy balance and obesity. The Lytle (2009) causal model (Figure 23.2) illustrates how the availability of a food, in this case low-fat versus high-fat milk, may influence population-level health outcomes.

It is hypothesised that the food environment influences our dietary behaviours and subsequently health. Being able to *measure* dietary behaviour is essential to understanding behaviour in relation to the food environment. As well as being able to define and describe the food environment (see Section 23.3), the accurate assessment of food intake is important.

Food is consumed in a range of locations, from within the home, within institutions (school, workplace etc.) and elsewhere. Recently, there has been an increase in consumer demand for convenience in eating and an increase in eating outside of the home (The Strategy Unit, Cabinet Office, 2008). Food and beverages consumed outside of the home are associated with higher energy intakes than foods prepared at home (Lachat *et al.*, 2012). Evidence indicates that dietary behaviours are an important contributing factor to socio-economic inequalities in overweight and

obesity (Giskes *et al.*, 2010). These factors all point to the importance of exploring the food environment in relation to dietary intake and obesity.

When reviewing the evidence it is important to bear in mind that there are differences in international contexts (both cultural and physical) in relation to food environment studies (Townshend and Lake, 2009). The USA and UK, for example, are vastly different in terms of their populations, the density of their populations and, therefore, the spatial patterning of food outlets (Beaulac *et al.*, 2009). More broadly, many studies tend to focus on food environments surrounding residential addresses rather than taking into account other environments, such as work (Burgoine and Monsivais, 2013), where individuals are likely to obtain food. Such residentially based research does not take into account the dynamic nature of an individual's food environment exposure on a day-by-day basis (e.g. around their workplace, their commuting routes, leisure activities). Studies tend to be cross-sectional in nature, and longitudinal studies are rare.

Diet as an outcome measure

The infancy of this field is illustrated by the fact that Giskes *et al.* (2007), in a systematic review (1980–2004), did not find a study that clearly showed how the environment might influence the intake of energy and dietary fat. However, the literature has moved rapidly. Since then, Caspi *et al.*'s (2012) systematic review of local food environments and diet (to March 2011) reported 38 studies. Most of these studies (16 out of 38) used short instruments assessing consumption patterns of specific foods (fruit and vegetable intake or fast food) rather than complete dietary records. The questions were similar to food frequency questionnaires in nature and focused on food groups rather than individual foods. Most studies used GIS assessments of neighbourhoods in combination with food frequency questionnaires or other brief tools. Fruits and vegetables were the most common outcome measure (26 out of 38 studies). Their review of 38 studies found moderate evidence to support an association between food environments and diet and/or health (Caspi *et al.*, 2012). However, the evidence for an association between fast food availability and consumption was equivocal. This could be due to a number of factors, from the dominance of fast food in the food environment, to individual preferences or to the methods used (see Section 23.3).

Adiposity as an outcome measure

The broad review of economic and social determinants of obesity by Black and Macinko (2008) (to March 2007) explored other neighbourhood characteristics as well as the food environment. Across the 37 studies they reviewed, they found economic and social deprivation was associated with increased obesity. They reported that there was inconsistency in the results regarding the availability of healthy versus unhealthy food in relation to obesity.

Holsten's (2009) systematic review (in 2006) examined adiposity as an outcome measure in relation to the community or consumer food environment, as defined by the Glanz model (Figure 23.1). While seven studies were reported, they used different methods of measuring the food environment throughout. For example: number of outlets per capita, proximity to various food outlets, assessed in multiple ways and analyses of food price data. In view of the mixture of methods used, it is hardly surprising that the results were also mixed.

More recently, the longitudinal Framingham Study Cohort of 3113 subjects was used to explore body mass index in relation to driving distance between residential address and the nearest fast food restaurant or food store. They reported that for every 1 km increase in driving distance to the closest fast food restaurant, body mass index decreased by 0.11 units in the overall sample and 0.19 units among women (Block et al., 2011). Although cross-sectional in study design, a recent analysis of home, work and commuting takeaway food access for 5442 adults in Cambridgeshire (UK), found that those with the greatest overall access were nearly twice as likely to be obese, relative to those with the least access (Burgoine et al., 2014).

Implications

Dietary behaviours are an important contributing factor to socio-economic inequalities in overweight/obesity (Giskes et al., 2010). Evidence indicates that, globally, more deprived neighbourhoods have less access to healthy food (Black et al., 2014), which is likely to result in less healthy diets. It is a logical assumption that the food available within a neighbourhood environment will influence dietary intake and ultimately adiposity. However, the broad range of methodological approaches, the resultant nature of the evidence and its limitations make it difficult to draw strong policy conclusions.

23.3 Defining spatial access to food outlets

Introduction to geographic information systems

A GIS represents a powerful tool for computerised mapping. However, its true capabilities lie with the integration of layers of spatial data and the resulting synthesis of new information, which often constitutes the basis of further analyses. For example, in food environment research, through combining spatial information on the locations of food retailers and study participants, inferences have been drawn regarding how spatial access to food is related to dietary and health outcomes (see Section 23.2 'Diet as an outcome measure' and 'Adiposity as an outcome measure'). This notion of a geographic approach to exposure assessment is not new, and can be traced back to the 19th century when John Snow mapped cases of cholera by hand, subsequently relating them to the contaminated Broad Street water pump.

This section describes a range of commonly used GIS approaches to objectifying food outlet access within the community nutrition environment (Glanz et al., 2005). We also detail the data sources used to underpin these assessments. We aim to show that, despite increased user friendliness, GIS metrics remain only as reliable as the data on which they are based and the theoretical frameworks underpinning their use.

Food environment data for use in geographic information system research

Secondary data, commonly used in food environment research, allow large studies to be conducted over wide geographic areas, with potential for increased generalisability in findings. Studies involving primary data collection are usually much more limited in scope. A number of sources can provide business names and locations for food outlets of all types (however, none provide the *trading* locations of mobile vendors). Examples of datasets commonly used include: commercial sources (e.g. Ordnance Survey Points of Interest in the UK; InfoUSA and Dun & Bradstreet in the USA), telephone directories (e.g. Yellow Pages and yell.com in the UK, held digitally by Experian as part of their National Business Database), company websites (for fast food chains, major supermarkets, etc.) and data freely acquired from local authority food premises registers. There are pros and cons associated with the use of each dataset. Large commercial datasets are readily available, but are often expensive; company websites are accurate, but incomplete; telephone directories from previous years are useful for building historic food outlet databases, but are either expensive or inaccessible; council data require resource-intensive data collection and preparation (Burgoine, 2010), but offer the most complete records (Lake et al., 2010).

A complete food outlet database will help to ensure that faithful exposure estimates are derived. Data need to be sensitive (a high proportion of food outlets on the ground need to be present in the dataset) and precise (a high proportion of food outlets in the dataset need to be present on the ground); and unbiased in these regards across key divides, such as between urban and rural areas, types of food outlet and across socio-economic divisions. For example, datasets may not fully represent the availability of small, ethnic food outlets, therefore biasing further analyses through underestimating food access for groups that rely upon this type of food store (Odoms-Young *et al.*, 2009). Accurate classifications of outlet type are also necessary, but whether such accuracy can be achieved using secondary data is questionable (Lake *et al.*, 2012). Primary data collection permits auditing of within-store characteristics, thereby informing store type classification. Numbers of cash registers have been used to differentiate supermarkets from grocery stores (Powell *et al.*, 2011); metres of shelf length devoted to healthy foods have also been measured (Farley *et al.*, 2009). Food outlet classification systems also vary between studies; proprietary (such as the 21-point classification system developed by Lake *et al.* (2010)) and adopted systems (such as those self-selected by business owners in commercial listings) have been applied and utilised. Labelling food outlets as 'healthy' or 'unhealthy' is problematic, due to the mix of products sold within most stores, but is often done (Kelly *et al.*, 2011).

Geographic coordinates are required to position a feature in geographic space. These coordinates are rarely provided with food outlet data; however, other information can be geocoded (the process of obtaining geographic coordinates from geographic data). For example, street address data can be geocoded manually or using GIS software. Reducing geocoding error relies on the accuracy of the street networks' address attributes, and of the network being correctly positioned in geographic space. One study showed positional errors ranging from 38 to 75 m (Zandbergen and Green, 2007). Further error can be introduced through low geocoding match rates (the proportion of addresses successfully geocoded); for example, due to spelling mistakes in addresses and use of colloquial place names. Match rates may also differ systematically, introducing bias; for example, they may be lower in rural areas (Hay *et al.*, 2009). Postcodes, common in UK data, can be geocoded automatically using online services such as GeoConvert (http://geoconvert.mimas.ac.uk/). Full UK postcodes contain roughly 15 addresses, so while they are less precise than street addresses, in most cases they provide an acceptable level of spatial accuracy.

How can we use geographic information systems to assess neighbourhood exposure to the foodscape?

With regard to metrics of spatial food outlet access, measures of density or proximity, or both, have mostly been used to date in the literature (Thornton *et al.*, 2011). However, there are myriad choices regarding how each of these constructs is operationalised.

Food outlet density

The density of food outlets in an area is a measure of intensity, designed to reflect the number of outlets to which an individual is exposed, and potentially related to diet through offering a greater number of locations from which to purchase food. The complexity in estimating density largely stems from the need to define neighbourhoods – the 'containers' within which density can be calculated. Classically, pre-existing administrative boundaries, such as census tracts or zip codes, have been used. This approach is particularly useful in ecological (area-level) studies because individual-level data are not required. This said, these boundaries have also found use in individual-level studies, where individuals are assigned to their respective administrative areas, which are assumed to be their 'neighbourhoods'. Either way, these boundaries usually offer convenient, complementary data availability; for example, census data are available at the ward level in the UK. However, these boundaries were created for another purpose, and may no longer represent meaningful divides between neighbourhoods. Researchers should anticipate errors-in-variables bias vis-à-vis heterogeneity in food access within these boundaries (Fortney *et al.*, 2000), and while reducing boundary sizes may increase within-area homogeneity, the border-crossing 'edge effect' (Lawson *et al.*, 1999) – that is, the likelihood that an individual will cross the boundary of their designated neighbourhood to utilise the facilities of an adjacent one – increases. Moreover, the selection of areal units almost certainly invokes the modifiable areal unit problem (MAUP) (Fotheringham and Wong, 1990). Specifically, the MAUP 'scale' effect, attributed to selecting boundaries of a different size – for example, smaller lower super output areas (LSOAs) or larger middle super output areas (MSOAs) – and 'zoning' effect, attributed to study area division with the same (or similar) number of boundaries, but positioned differently; for example, MSOAs and electoral wards (Flowerdew *et al.*, 2008). Figure 23.3 illustrates how patterns of food outlet access differ when using LSOAs ($n = 366$), MSOAs ($n = 75$) and electoral ward ($n = 124$) boundaries in Cambridgeshire, UK. Remember that the same food outlet location database underpins each of these patterns. The potential effects of the MAUP can be evaluated through such sensitivity analyses, although it cannot be solved.

Recently, as our understanding of the need for 'person-based' exposure has grown (Kwan, 2009), alongside GIS advances, the creation of bespoke neighbourhood

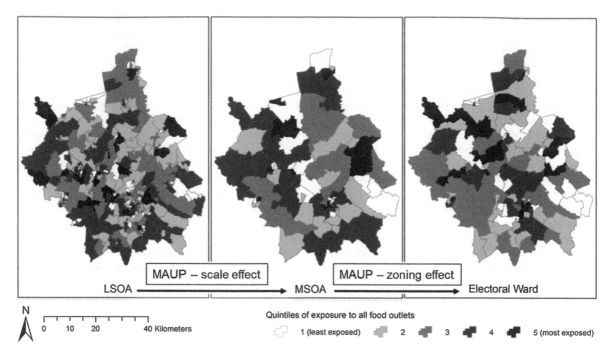

Figure 23.3 MAUP 'scale' and 'zoning' effects upon quintiles of food outlet density in Cambridgeshire, UK. © Crown Copyright/database right 2013. An Ordnance Survey/EDINA supplied service. We are grateful to Cambridgeshire local councils for supplying food outlet location data.

boundaries around locations of individuals has become more commonplace. Once participants have been mapped, and a theoretically relevant size of neighbourhood determined, such as the distance one could walk in 10 minutes, neighbourhood 'buffers' are created using a GIS. However, the size of neighbourhoods created has ranged from 400 to 3000 m, since little consensus exists on how far people are actually willing to travel for food (Smith *et al.*, 2010), nor how this distance might differ between individuals. Further, food outlets even marginally beyond the neighbourhood boundary make no contribution to density, raising the issue of the 'local trap' (Cummins, 2007). Moreover, studies have defined neighbourhood extent using Euclidean distance ('straight line', 'circular', 'as the crow flies'), or distance along the street network (based on a least-cost algorithm), which may limit comparability between studies (Burgoine *et al.*, 2013). Variations of these techniques, including the 'sausage' buffer (see Forsyth *et al.* (2012) for details), have also been proposed. Figure 23.4 illustrates how an individual is differentially 'exposed' to fast food outlets (counts shown per panel), contingent on the choices made with respect to GIS technique and scale parameters.

Density can be calculated when neighbourhoods have been defined. Where neighbourhood size remains

constant (e.g. when buffering individuals using 1000 m Euclidean radii throughout), counts of food outlets are appropriate, allowing comparable exposures between neighbourhoods. Where neighbourhood size varies (e.g. when using administrative areas), counts are inappropriate as the number of outlets present is likely to vary according to an underlying distribution (e.g. population). The normalisation of counts into rates, per population (e.g. per 1000 people) or per square unit of area (e.g. per square kilometre), is commonplace.

Food outlet proximity

Proximity is usually the distance or estimated travel time to one's nearest food outlet. The assumption is that distance/time is inversely related to utilisation, such that food outlets close by are more accessible and therefore more often used than those farther away – this is Tobler (1970)'s *first law of geography*, which states that 'everything is related to everything else, but near things are more related than distant things'. GIS approaches to calculating proximity have employed Euclidean, Manhattan (distance along a grid-like network, measured at right angles, sometimes referred to as city block distance) and street network distances or times. GIS software packages allow for sophisticated estimates of proximity

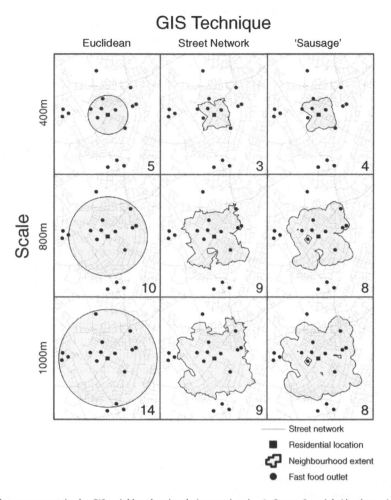

Figure 23.4 Food outlet exposure varies by GIS neighbourhood technique and scale. © Crown Copyright/database right 2013. An Ordnance Survey/EDINA supplied service. We are grateful to Cambridgeshire local councils for supplying food outlet location data.

along street networks; time measures can account for speed by transport mode, accounting for speed limits, while both time and distance measures can account for one-way streets, turn restrictions and topography (rivers, mountains, etc.). Measures of access are not constrained by user- or administratively-defined neighbourhood definitions (except where proximity is calculated from the centre of these boundaries in ecological research) and, as such, do not suffer from border-crossing effects. However, edge effects near study area margins may be important. An individual's nearest food outlet may lie outside the study area, yet because the data in this area may be incomplete, not collected or unavailable, the individual's most proximal food outlet *within* the study area would be incorrectly identified instead. Suggested

solutions include the use of internal or external 'guard areas' (van Meter *et al.*, 2010). Densities, as described here within neighbourhood 'containers', do not 'borrow' information from beyond their boundaries, and therefore do not suffer from study area edge effects.

Summary and future directions

Using a GIS to estimate food outlet access, with a view to capturing exposure 'truth' (White *et al.*, 2008) is not straightforward. While this was not a comprehensive review of all GIS approaches, it is clear that however a GIS is used, the researcher is a 'critical agent' and is central to the research process, and to some extent, therefore, the results obtained. The ontic fallacy describes an unquestioning acceptance of our representation of reality as *the* reality (Leszczynski, 2009); this is a dangerous presumption.

Going forward, whatever the definition of neighbourhood, no matter how nuanced the proximity metric, focusing solely on the place of residence, as many studies tend to do, is problematic because people will travel beyond these thresholds into wider 'activity spaces', and probably into radically different food environments (Burgoine and Monsivais, 2013). These non-residential exposures may be as or more important to food purchasing behaviours than those in residential neighbourhoods. Participatory GIS, interactive web-mapping tools such as VERITAS (Chaix *et al.*, 2012), wearable camera technologies such as SenseCam, global positioning systems (GPS) devices, and even travel diary data represent the next generation of technologies with the potential to capture overall access to food outlets. Nevertheless, objective exposure does not necessarily equal utility. Subjective perceptions of neighbourhood and competing economic and social constraints, among others, all combine to determine the potential influence of the food environment, beyond simply its spatial configuration.

23.4 Urban planning and health in the UK

Introduction

As stated in Section 23.3 'Introduction to geographic information systems', in the 19th century it was discovered that by mapping out urban health problems they could be related to the living conditions in towns and cities. Overcrowding and pollution created ideal situations for epidemics, such as cholera. These were in part tackled by public health legislation, which set out standards for decent housing and sanitation. To an extent, therefore, urban planning was a reaction to the health problems of the rapidly industrialising city. As the 20th century progressed, the foci of the disciplines of public health and urban planning diverged. However, more recently there has been recognition that contemporary health issues, such as rises in obesity, while very different from the infectious diseases of the 19th century, may well be linked to the way we have planned our towns and cities in recent times (Townshend, 2010).

To this end, there has been an increased emphasis on the need for local authorities to consider the relationship between planning the built environment and impacts on health. In March 2012 a new National Planning Policy Framework (NPPF) for England was launched. While its key aim was to reduce complexity in the planning system, from a health perspective an entire section of the policy is dedicated to promoting 'healthy communities' (Department for Communities and Local Government, 2012). While this is not the first national planning policy document to include health aims, the prominence given to health is significant.

Local planning policy initiatives to controlling takeaway hot food outlets

Local planning authorities (LPAs) have to draw up plans and policies for their local area in response to the NPPF. In doing so, LPAs must consider the health status and needs of the local population. Key health priorities for planning policies may be identified, for example, by working with health professionals – for example, those taking a lead role on obesity prevention – and through the creation of local 'health and wellbeing boards'. (The Health and Social Care Act 2012 established 'health and wellbeing boards' in upper tier local authorities as fora where leading health and care professionals work together to improve the health and well-being of their local population and reduce health inequalities though more joined up thinking and strategy making. See DoH (2012) for more information.)

It is likely, therefore, that more and more LPAs will develop planning policies that directly address health issues. While recognising that takeaway food availability is only one environmental factor implicated in the obesity crisis (and currently, as stated in Section 23.1 'Introduction to geographic information systems', perhaps the least evidenced by research), planning policies that attempt to control their proliferation have already been developed. They therefore provide an example of how urban planning may contribute to tackling the obesity crisis. A review by Dr Foster Intelligence (2011) found four main approaches taken by LPAs:

1. *Only allowing takeaway outlets in specified areas.* This approach means defining only certain locations (e.g. existing shopping areas) where further takeaway outlets are deemed acceptable; paradoxically, this may introduce issues of *concentration* and *clustering*.

2. *Restricting concentration and clustering.* If a location is deemed suitable, local authorities can seek to restrict the number of takeaway outlets in a row (e.g. to two, or three) or the percentage of frontage (ground floor use facing the street) given over to takeaways (e.g. 5% has been used).

3. *Restricting proximity to other uses.* This means setting out buffer zones (e.g. 400 m) around land uses such as

schools, parks and children's centres, where the development of takeaway outlets is forbidden (as noted in Section 23.1, there has been a focus on research on environments surrounding schools in particular).

4. *Clamping down on 'back door' applications.* Fast food outlets have their own 'classification' in UK planning terms – referred to as 'A5' Hot Food Takeaways. Unscrupulous developers can sometimes try to circumvent takeaway restrictions by opening outlets under different classifications, primarily 'A3' Restaurants and Cafes, where the intention is that food will be primarily consumed on the premises. This might be done by adding in a nominal seating area on plans submitted to the LPA, for example.

In addition, some LPAs have sought to charge a levy, or fee, where planning permission is granted for a new takeaway, with funds raised going to initiatives to tackle childhood obesity; for example, improving green spaces to encourage physical activity. A further approach would be to only grant planning permission to businesses reaching certain nutritional standards with the products they sell. However, it is doubtful if this latter approach could be applied with current planning legislation. Approaches 1–3 in particular speak to emerging evidence surrounding the potential impacts of increased spatial access to takeaway food outlets.

Case study: London Borough of Barking and Dagenham

The London Borough of Barking and Dagenham has high rates of childhood obesity. The 2009–2010 National Child Measurement Programme showed obesity rates for the borough of 14% for children aged 4–5 years, and 24% for children aged 10–11 years. The Childhood Obesity Task Force, formed by the local authority and the NHS, identified the planning system as a 'key tool' in tackling obesity (Barking and Dagenham NHS, 2010: 9). In 2010 the borough adopted a Supplementary Planning Document (SPD), 'Saturation Point – Addressing the Health Impact of Hot Food Takeaways'. (An SPD forms part of the council's Local Development Framework; that is, the portfolio of local planning policies. SPDs must be taken into consideration when determining planning applications.) This guidance includes recommendations for a combination of approaches, including exclusion zones for new takeaways within 400 m of a primary or secondary school, and restricting clustering, meaning no more than 5% of the units within a shopping centre, or frontage (row of shops) may be A5 hot food takeaways; no more than two takeaways may be located next to each other; and there should be no less than two non-A5 units between a group of hot food takeaways. In addition, where hot food

takeaways are deemed appropriate a £1000 levy will be charged for obesity amelioration initiatives.

The policy has been tested since its adoption. In a high-profile case the LPA refused permission for a well-known pizza chain to open a premises in a prime retail location because it exceeded both the percentage of shop frontage allowed for takeaway usage and because it was within the 400 m takeaway exclusion zone surrounding a primary school (which had also been awarded Healthy School status). The case went to appeal, but was dismissed. In rejecting the appeal, the planning inspector in charge of the case gave significant weight to policy that restricted takeaways on prime retail frontage. (Anyone who has a planning permission refused by the LPA may appeal that decision to the Planning Inspectorate – a central government department. A planning inspector will be appointed, if appropriate, who will review all relevant evidence in the case. They may uphold a decision, or overturn it, dependant on their findings.) They gave less weight to issues pertaining to health and well-being, though they did note the SPD was a 'material consideration'. In other words, it was taken into account in the decision-making process, though the importance attached to the guidance was unclear. Not all cases have been successfully defended by the LPA. In another case where a takeaway was refused solely on the basis of being within a 400 m exclusion zone round a primary school, the case was subsequently overturned on appeal. The inspector noted that there were a number of hot food outlets on routes around the school, presenting opportunities for fast food purchase. The inspector was not convinced that this particular location would attract pupils from the identified school, whether accompanied by their parents, or not. The Barking and Dagenham example remains the most tested guidance to date and has been widely cited by other authorities seeking to impose their own restrictions.

Other examples of planning appeals and guidance

So far, the evidence from appeals elsewhere is mixed. In 2012, Hammersmith and Fulham successfully defended a decision to refuse the conversion of a convenience store to a takeaway, arguing it would undermine the vitality and viability of a parade of shops. However, a planning inspector overturned Islington's decision to refuse the conversion of a former public house to a takeaway restaurant, despite its proximity (130 m) to a primary school and concerns about the health of local school children. While noting the borough had a high rate of childhood obesity, the inspector reasoned that primary school children using the takeaway would be accompanied by an adult who would be able to 'guide food choices', while the premises would also offer a 'balanced nutritional menu' (Development Control Services Ltd, 2012b). Similar reasoning was also used by an Inspector, who overturned a decision in South Yorkshire to refuse a fried chicken restaurant and drive through just 40 m away from a primary school. The Inspector concluded that since children would be unlikely to travel to and from the school unaccompanied and were not able to leave the school at lunchtime, she did not consider that the development would jeopardise local healthy eating initiatives (Development Control Services Ltd, 2012a).

The Greater London Authority has also raised concerns about the effectiveness of current planning policies. In their 'Takeaways Toolkit' (Mayor of London, 2012), the authority suggests that 400 m (based on 10 min walking time) exclusion zones around secondary schools may not be effective if students are prepared to walk further than this to purchase food at lunchtimes. Moreover, in London, transport is free for school children, so they may also take a bus to access takeaway food outlets. These practical examples illustrate the kinds of problem inherent in trying to delineate neighbourhood food environments, as discussed in Section 23.4 'Local planning policy initiatives to controlling takeaway hot food outlets'. A further problem is that many non-A5 businesses (e.g. local corner shops) sell, amongst other things, relatively cheap, energy-dense foods, and it is impossible to control these with the same planning restrictions. Neighbourhood plans, where the community themselves have a greater say in what is developed in their local area, also present opportunities for improving health. (The Localism Act, 2011, introduced new 'neighbourhood plans'. The plans can be prepared by two types of body: town and parish councils or 'neighbourhood forums' – community groups that take the lead in areas without parishes. It is the role of the local planning authority to agree who should be in the neighbourhood forum in such areas.) By working with communities the problems caused by the proliferation of takeaways may become more embedded in the public consciousness and resistance to further development might emerge from within the local population themselves.

Summary: opportunities and limitations

Local planning policies that aim to contribute to the fight against obesity are in their infancy. Opinion among academics and policy makers is that planning does have a key role in creating built environments that enable people to make healthier choices about their lifestyle. This includes choices around food consumption. However, the aforementioned example concerning the constrained development of takeaway premises demonstrates that developing planning policies that restrict unhealthy options are by no means straightforward. Policies that encourage healthier behaviour, such as only granting planning permission for premises that reach certain nutritional standards, may be even more complex and require substantive changes to legislation.

Urban planning is a process based in legislation, and evidence to support planning decisions needs to hold up to legal scrutiny. At present, the evidence around food environments is likely not robust enough for this purpose. Furthermore, the modern planning system has been largely developed without having health impacts as a central focus.

More broadly, there are likely to be other ways in which urban planning can help towards addressing the obesity crisis. Creating environments that encourage people to undertake physical activity is the most obvious way; however, in relation to food environments, enabling urban food production through providing space for community gardens and allotments, for example, may be fruitful avenues for investigation. Moreover, exploiting the benefits of GISs as outlined in Section 23.3 may well help to both develop the evidence base and the delivery and monitoring of future policies.

23.5 Conclusions

'Reliable' measures of the food environment have been described as the 'foundation' of research that will help to inform obesity-related policy (McKinnon et al., 2009). A broad evidence base is required, ranging from spatial analyses to within-store audits, alongside individual- and neighbourhood-level data (Caspi et al., 2012). Tackling the obesogenic environment, and specifically the food environment, requires a multidisciplinary approach (Lake et al., 2010) and joined-up thinking from across professions and sectors. While policy changes in relation to the food environment have been implemented, evidence for such changes remains inconclusive. This is a challenging area of research with the potential to influence population health.

Acknowledgements

Amelia A. Lake is supported by Fuse, the Centre for Translational Research in Public Health – a UK Clinical Research Collaboration (UKCRC) Public Health Research Centre of Excellence. Thomas Burgoine is supported by the Centre for Diet and Activity Research (CEDAR), a UKCRC Public Health Research Centre of Excellence. Both centres receive funding from the British Heart Foundation, Cancer Research UK, Economic and Social Research Council, Medical Research Council, National Institute for Health Research and the Wellcome

Trust, under the auspices of the UK Clinical Research Collaboration. This funding is gratefully acknowledged.

The digital maps used hold Crown copyright from EDINA Digimap, a JISC supplied service.

References

Barking and Dagenham NHS (2010) *Saturation Point: Addressing the Health Impacts of Hot Food Takeaways: Supplementary Planning Document.* London Borough of Barking and Dagenham, London.

Beaulac, J., Kristjansson, E. and Cummins, S. (2009) A systematic review of food deserts, 1966–2007. *Preventing Chronic Disease*, 6, A105.

Black, C., Moon, G. and Baird, J. (2014) Dietary inequalities: what is the evidence for the effect of the neighbourhood food environment? *Health & Place*, 27, 229–242.

Black, J.L. and Macinko, J. (2008) Neighborhoods and obesity. *Nutrition Reviews*, 66, 2–20.

Block, J.P., Christakis, N.A., O'Malley, A.J. and Subramanian, S.V. (2011) Proximity to food establishments and body mass index in the Framingham Heart Study Offspring Cohort over 30 years. *American Journal of Epidemiology*, 174, 1108–1114.

Burgoine, T. (2010) Collecting accurate secondary foodscape data: a reflection on the trials and tribulations. *Appetite*, 55, 522–527.

Burgoine, T. and Monsivais, P. (2013) Characterising food environment exposure at home, at work, and along commuting journeys using data on adults in the UK. *The International Journal of Behavioral Nutrition and Physical Activity*, 10, 85.

Burgoine, T., Lake, A.A., Stamp, E. *et al.* (2009) Changing foodscapes 1980–2000, using the ASH30 Study. *Appetite*, 53, 157–165.

Burgoine, T., Alvanides, S. and Lake, A.A. (2013) Creating 'obesogenic realities'; do our methodological choices make a difference when measuring the food environment? *International Journal of Health Geographics*, 12, 1–9.

Burgoine, T., Forouhi, N.G., Griffin, S.J. *et al.* (2014) Associations between exposure to takeaway food outlets, takeaway food consumption, and body weight in Cambridgeshire, UK: population based, cross sectional study. *BMJ*, 348, g1464.

Caspi, C.E., Sorensen, G., Subramanian, S.V. and Kawachi, I. (2012) The local food environment and diet: a systematic review. *Health & Place*, 18, 1172–1187.

Chaix, B., Kestens, Y., Perchoux, C. *et al.* (2012) An interactive mapping tool to assess individual mobility patterns in neighbourhood studies. *American Journal of Preventive Medicine*, 43, 440–450.

Charreire, H., Casey, R., Salze, P. *et al.* (2010) Measuring the food environment using geographical information systems: a methodological review. *Public Health Nutrition*, 13, 1773–1785.

Cummins, S. (2007) Commentary: investigating neighbourhood effects on health – avoiding the 'local trap'. *International Journal of Epidemiology*, 36, 355–357.

Department for Communities and Local Government (2012) *National Planning Policy Statement.* Department for Communities and Local Government, London.

Development Control Services Ltd (2012a) Healthy Eating Initiatives not Undermined by Fast Food Restaurant. http://www.dcservices.co.uk/healthy-eating-initiatives-not-undermined-fast-food-restaurant/article/1112566 (accessed 19 December 2016).

Development Control Services Ltd (2012b) *No Link between Childhood Obesity and Takeaway Food.* http://www.dcservices.co.uk/no-link-childhood-obesity-takeaway-food/article/1138305 (accessed 19 December 2016).

DoH (2012) *A short guide to health and wellbeing boards.* Department of Health. http://webarchive.nationalarchives.gov.uk/20130805112926/http://healthandcare.dh.gov.uk/hwb-guide/ (accessed 19 December 2016).

Dr Foster Intelligence (2011) *Tackling the Takeaways: A New Policy to Address Fast-Food Outlets in Tower Hamlets.* NHS Tower Hamlets, London.

Farley, T.A., Rice, J., Bodor, J.N. *et al.* (2009) Measuring the food environment: shelf space of fruits, vegetables, and snack foods in stores. *Journal of Urban Health: Bulletin of the New York Academy of Medicine*, 86, 672–682.

Flowerdew, R., Manley, D.J. and Sabel, C.E. (2008) Neighbourhood effects on health: does it matter where you draw the boundaries? *Social Science and Medicine*, 66, 1241–1255.

Foresight (2007) *Tackling Obesities: Future Choices – Project Report*, 2nd edn. Government Office for Science, London.

Forsyth, A., van Riper, D., Larson, N. *et al.* (2012) Creating a replicable, valid cross-platform buffering technique: the sausage network buffer for measuring food and physical activity built environments. *International Journal of Health Geographics*, 11, 3–9.

Fortney, J., Rost, K. and Warren, J. (2000) Comparing alternative methods of measuring geographic access to health services. *Health Services and Outcomes Research Methodology*, 1, 173–184.

Fotheringham, A.S. and Wong, D.W.S. (1990) The modifiable areal unit problem in multivariate statistical analysis. *Environment and Planning A*, 23, 1025–1044.

Giskes, K., Kamphuis, C.B., van Lenthe, F.J. *et al.* (2007) A systematic review of associations between environmental factors, energy and fat intakes among adults: is there evidence for environments that encourage obesogenic dietary intakes? *Public Health Nutrition*, 10, 1005–1017.

Giskes, K., Avendaňo, M., Brug, J. and Kunst, A.E. (2010) A systematic review of studies on socioeconomic inequalities in dietary intakes associated with weight gain and overweight/obesity conducted among European adults. *Obesity Reviews*, 11, 413–429.

Glanz, K., Sallis, J.F., Saelens, B.E. and Frank, L.D. (2005) Healthy nutrition environments: concepts and measures. *American Journal of Health Promotion*, 19, 330–333.

Hay, G., Kypri, K., Whigham, P. and Langley, J. (2009) Potential biases due to geocoding error in spatial analyses of official data. *Health & Place*, 15, 562–567.

Holsten, J.E. (2009) Obesity and the community food environment: a systematic review. *Public Health Nutrition*, 12, 397–405.

Kelly, B., Flood, V.M. and Yeatman, H. (2011) Measuring local food environments: an overview of available methods and measures. *Health & Place*, 17, 1284–1293.

Kwan, M.-P. (2009) From place-based to people-based exposure measures. *Social Science and Medicine*, 69, 1311–1313.

Lachat, C., Nago, E., Verstraeten, R. *et al.* (2012) Eating out of home and its association with dietary intake: a systematic review of the evidence. *Obesity Reviews*, 13, 329–346.

Lake, A.A., Burgoine, T., Greenhalgh, F. *et al.* (2010) The foodscape: classification and field validation of secondary data sources. *Health & Place*, 16, 666–673.

Lake, A.A., Burgoine, T., Stamp, E. and Grieve, R. (2012) The foodscape: classification and field validation of secondary data sources across urban/rural and socio-economic classifications. *The International Journal of Behavioral Nutrition and Physical Activity*, 9, 3–12.

Lawson, A.B., Biggeri, A. and Dreassi, E. (1999) Edge effects in disease mapping. In A.B. Lawson, A. Biggeri, D. Bohning *et al.* (eds), *Disease Mapping and Risk Assessment for Public Health*. John Wiley & Sons Ltd, Chichester.

Leszczynski, A. (2009) Poststructuralism and GIS: is there a 'disconnect'? *Environment and Planning D: Society and Space*, **27**, 581–602.

Lytle, L.A. (2009) Measuring the food environment: state of the science. *American Journal of Preventive Medicine*, **36**, S134–S144.

Macdonald, L., Cummins, S. and Macintyre, S. (2007) Neighbourhood fast food environment and area deprivation – substitution or concentration? *Appetite*, **49**, 251–254.

Mayor of London (2012) *Takeaways Toolkit: Tools, Interventions and Case Studies to Help Local Authorities Develop a Response to the Health Impacts of Fast Food Takeaways*. Greater London Authority/Chartered Institute of Environmental Health, London. https://www.london.gov.uk/sites/default/files/takeawaystoolkit. pdf (accessed 19 December 2016).

McKinnon, R.A., Reedy, J., Morrissette, M.A. *et al.* (2009) Measures of the Food environment: a compilation of the literature, 1990–2007. *American Journal of Preventive Medicine*, **36**, S124–S133.

Odoms-Young, A.M., Zenk, S.N. and Mason, M.M. (2009) Measuring food availability and access in African-American communities: implications for intervention and policy. *American Journal of Preventive Medicine*, **36**, S145–S150.

Penchansky, R. and Thomas, J.W. (1981) The concept of access: definition and relationship to consumer satisfaction. *Medical Care*, **19**, 127–140.

Powell, L.M., Han, E., Zenk, S.N. *et al.* (2011) Field validation of secondary commercial data sources on the retail food outlet environment in the US. *Health & Place*, **17**, 1122–1131.

Smith, G., Gidlow, C., Davey, R. and Foster, C. (2010) What is my walking neighbourhood? A pilot study of English adults' definitions of their local walking neighbourhoods. *The International Journal of Behavioral Nutrition and Physical Activity*, **7**, 34.

Swinburn, B. and Egger, G. (2002) Preventive strategies against weight gain and obesity. *Obesity Reviews*, **3**, 289–301.

The Strategy Unit, Cabinet Office (2008) *Food: An Analysis of the Issues*. http://webarchive.nationalarchives.gov.uk/+/http:/www. cabinetoffice.gov.uk/media/cabinetoffice/strategy/assets/food/ food_analysis.pdf (accessed 19 December 2016).

Thornton, L.E., Pearce, J.R. and Kavanagh, A.M. (2011) Using geographic information systems (GIS) to assess the role of the built environment in influencing obesity: a glossary. *The International Journal of Behavioral Nutrition and Physical Activity*, **8**, 71.

Tobler, W.R. (1970) A computer movie simulating urban growth in the Detroit region. *Economic Geography*, **46**, 234–240.

Townshend, T.G. (2010) What role can urban planning and transportation policy play in the prevention of obesity? In D. Crawford, R.W. Jeffery, K. Ball and J. Brug (eds), *Obesity Epidemiology: from Aetiology to Public Health*. Oxford University Press, Oxford.

Townshend, T.G. and Lake, A.A. (2009) Obesogenic urban form: theory, policy and practice. *Health & Place*, **15**, 909–916.

Van Meter, E.M., Lawson, A.B., Colabianchi, N. *et al.* (2010) An evaluation of edge effects in nutritional accessibility and availability measures: a simulation study. *International Journal of Health Geographics*, **9**, 1–30.

White, E., Armstrong, B.K. and Saracci, R. (2008) *Principles of Exposure Measurement in Epidemiology: Collecting, Evaluating, and Improving Measures of Disease Risk Factors*. Oxford University Press, Oxford.

White, M. (2007) Food access and obesity. *Obesity Reviews*, **8**, 99–107.

Zandbergen, P.A. and Green, J.W. (2007) Error and bias in determining exposure potential of children at school locations using proximity-based GIS techniques. *Environmental Health Perspectives*, **115**, 1363–1370.

24

The Wider Environment and its Effect on Dietary Behaviour

Bridget Benelam and Judith L Buttriss

Key messages

- Around the world, government-led initiatives, such as development of food-based dietary guidelines, are designed to encourage appropriate dietary patterns and to promote positive behaviour change.
- Campaigns have raised the profile of the need to reduce intakes of some dietary components, such as saturated fat and salt, and most recently sugars, or to increase intakes of fruits and vegetables or fish. There are examples of where these have been successful in part, in particular with regard to salt reduction and increasing fruit and vegetables.
- Also important are cultural factors and attitudes to environmental issues and sustainable sourcing of foods, education and income.
- Recently, attention has focused on the price of food and drinks, promotions, advertising and choice in portion size and healthier options.

- There is also growing interest in whether or not fiscal policies such as taxation may influence purchasing and consumption behaviour.
- Nutrition labelling has become a legal requirement in Europe, providing details to support consumer choice, and legislation exists to control the use of nutrition and health claims.
- Social and health marketing, such as the UK Government's Change4Life campaign, have increasingly been used to promote healthy eating and healthy lifestyles.
- The effects of these many factors can be supportive, detrimental or additive in achieving positive dietary change and in supporting appropriate dietary behaviour, and it is increasingly recognised that there is no silver bullet when it comes to driving positive behaviour change; a multifaceted approach is needed.

24.1 Introduction

This chapter will look at the effects of the wider environment on eating behaviour and how these may be influenced beneficially. In this chapter, a number of examples from the UK are used to illustrate the various ways in which the wider environment, including UK Government policies, can influence dietary behaviour. Also see Chapters 23 and 26.

24.2 Government-led initiatives and policy

For many decades, government policies around the world have aimed to shape population eating habits to encourage adequate nutrient intakes and good health. A historical example is the policy put in place during World War II in the UK to help ensure the nation's nutrition (British Nutrition Foundation, n.d. https://www.nutrition.org.uk/nutritioninthenews/wartimefood/warnutrition.html). In this section, some examples of recent UK Government initiatives will be discussed.

Food-based dietary guidelines

For several decades, the Eatwell Guide, formerly the Eatwell Plate and prior to that the Balance of Good Health, has formed the basis of food-based dietary advice in the UK, and similar guidance exists in many other counties, as discussed in Chapter 8, and is updated from time to time, as has happened recently in the USA (USDA, 2015) and the UK – see later and Buttriss (2016a). The Eatwell Guide

Public Health Nutrition, Second Edition. Edited by Judith L Buttriss, Ailsa A Welch, John M Kearney and Susan A Lanham-New.
© 2018 by The Nutrition Society. Published 2018 by John Wiley & Sons, Ltd.
Companion website: www.wiley.com/go/buttriss/publichealth

has described the proportions that different food groups should contribute to the diet and has been widely used in schools, often alongside the '8 Tips for Healthy Eating' from Public Health England, and is accompanied by other messages to promote healthy eating, such as choosing wholegrains or potatoes with skins to increase fibre intake, choosing lean cuts of meat and reduced-fat dairy foods to reduce saturated fat intake and checking food labels.

In 2011, to understand whether food-based dietary advice influenced eating behaviour, the Food Standards Agency's (FSA's) 'Food and You' survey investigated consumer attitudes to healthy eating (Prior *et al.*, 2011). The survey comprised over 3000 face-to-face interviews with adults aged ≥16 years (no upper age limit was applied) across the UK. Samples in Scotland and Northern Ireland were boosted to enable more detailed analysis at a country level. The majority of respondents rated a variety of factors as important for a healthy lifestyle: 99% said eating fruit and vegetables was very or fairly important, 94% said that eating less salt was important and 92% said that limiting foods high in saturated fat was important. About a fifth of respondents were able to identify the types and proportions of foods needed for a healthy balanced diet (based on the Eatwell Guide). Almost 1 in 10 (9%) correctly stated that the maximum daily intake of salt for an adult was 6 g. The survey also asked about intakes of other nutrients, such as total fat, saturated fat and calories. Over half (55%) agreed they do not need to make changes to the food they eat as it is already healthy enough. Nevertheless, almost three-fifths (57%) reported having made a change to their diet in the previous 6 months. The most common changes were eating more fruit and vegetables (28%) and eating smaller portions of food (25%). The most common reason respondents gave for changing their diet was to lose or maintain weight (mentioned by 33% of respondents who had made changes to their diet) and to be more healthy (18%).

Respondents were asked what difficulties they would have, if any, if they tried to eat more healthily. The main difficulties reported were the cost of eating more healthily (12% of respondents mentioned this) and time constraints (8%). Almost a quarter (23%) said they would not have any difficulties (Prior *et al.*, 2011).

This study suggests that UK consumers are aware of some of the healthy eating messages put forward by the Government and others, although the messages are not always well understood; in particular, most people did not recall the proportions of the Eatwell Guide. However, measuring the effect these messages have on dietary behaviour is not straightforward. The UK National Diet and Nutrition Survey (NDNS) monitors food consumption in the UK and calculates average nutrient intakes. Results suggest that, in recent years, saturated fat, sodium

and non-milk extrinsic sugars intakes have fallen (although these are still above recommended levels) (Bates *et al.*, 2014). Information on trends in fruit and vegetables intake can be found in Section 24.2: 'The 5-A-DAY campaign'.

The Family Food Survey (Defra, 2015a) measures UK household food and drinks purchases, used as a proxy for consumption, and provides reliable information on trends. It has also been used to compare proportions of current food and drink purchases (as a proxy for consumption) with the proportions suggested by the Eatwell Guide, shown in Figure 24.1 (Defra, 2015a).

This comparison suggests that UK households are not purchasing foods in line with the proportions of the Eatwell Guide, with starchy foods and fruit and vegetables representing a smaller proportion than recommended and the proportion of foods and drinks high in fat and/or sugars much higher than recommended. While these data do not measure what people are actually eating, the figure does suggest that dietary patterns in the UK are not currently in line with that suggested by the Eatwell Guide.

A review of the UK guide has recently taken place in light of new UK recommendations on carbohydrates (particularly sugars and fibre) (SACN, 2015) and also to assess its continued relevance as a healthy eating tool. This work was supported by consumer research to review various aspects of the visual presentation, and also by extensive dietary modelling using linear programming techniques applied to data from the NDNS. For a summary, see Buttriss (2016a) and Scarborough *et al.* (2016).

Examples of Government campaigns

The 5-A-DAY campaign

The 5-A-DAY campaign was started in the 1990s by the Department of Health, and 5-A-DAY is perhaps the most widely recognised public health nutrition message in the UK, as evidenced by the Food and You survey mentioned earlier, where 99% of respondents mentioned that eating more fruit and vegetables is important for a healthy lifestyle.

The Family Food Survey, conducted annually for over 60 years, is an invaluable source of trend data, using household purchases as a proxy for consumption. It reveals that over the period 1975 to date, purchases of fruits and vegetables (excluding potatoes) rose, peaking around 2005–2006. It has been suggested that the subsequent decline was initially triggered by the economic climate at the time. Overall, fruit and vegetable purchases were 10% lower in 2014 than at their peak in 2007; a 5.2% fall for vegetables and 14% for fruit (including fruit juice). The decline in purchases of vegetables is mainly attributed to fresh vegetables, which account for roughly 70% of all vegetable purchases. In lower income households, purchases are typically lower and the decline over

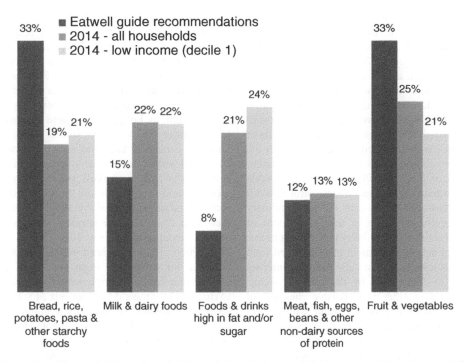

Figure 24.1 Comparison of food and drink purchases in UK households with the Eatwell Guide recommendations. *Source*: Defra (2015a).

the past decade has been greater. Averaged across all households, purchases equate to 3.9 5-A-DAY portions per day, but for the 10% of households with the lowest income this falls to 3.0. The Health Survey for England shows a similar trend: consumption of fruit and vegetables by adults peaked in 2006 and levels have dropped since. Again, higher consumption was associated with higher income, and vice versa: 30% of men and 35% of women in the highest income quintile had consumed five or more portions on the previous day compared with only 19% of men and 23% of women in the lowest quintile. The same pattern was seen in children.

Using Family Food data from 2011, estimates show that in 2012 an average of £66 per household per week was spent on food and drink; £9 of this food and drink was avoidable waste, £1.84 (20%) of which was fresh fruit, vegetables and salad. This wasted food is estimated to have provided more than 13 billion 5-A-DAY portions of fruit and vegetables (Defra, 2015b).

According to the NDNS, which measures consumption rather than purchases, only 30% of adults, 10% of boys and 7% of girls aged 11–18 years are reaching the 5-A-DAY target (Bates *et al.*, 2014); there is clearly some progress needed before this target is met. An evaluation of the impact of the 5-A-DAY programme between 2002 and 2006, which took into account the effect of changes in prices, concluded that the campaign had increased

fruit and vegetable consumption by between 0.2 and 0.7 portions per day (average 0.3), depending on the income group (Capacci and Mazzocchi, 2011).

In 2003, funding was granted to the 5-A-DAY local community initiative. Sixty-six primary care trusts in the UK worked for 2 years across local communities to address local barriers and contribute to increasing consumption of fruit and vegetables, to increase awareness and knowledge, change attitudes and beliefs and to increase access to fruit and vegetables. Activities included home delivery services, improving transport to local markets, voucher schemes, media campaigns, growing and cookery skills, and promoting networking among existing healthy food groups. Evaluation of the project found that it resulted in greater levels of improvement in awareness and understanding of the issues and implications of eating fruit and vegetables than in improvements in overall consumptions levels. Consumption levels showed signs of increase, but this was not statistically significant compared with control groups. These results highlight the difficulty in encouraging changes to dietary behaviours, even when intervening to support such changes (TNS Social, 2006).

Salt programme

The campaign to encourage UK consumers to reduce their intake of salt began in 2003 and included the setting of salt reduction targets for the food industry and a Government-funded public awareness campaign. An evaluation of the campaign activities suggested that substantial reductions (up to 70%) in sodium content of some foods had been achieved, and evaluation of the FSA's consumer campaign showed increased awareness of the benefits of reducing salt intake on health, with 43% of adults in 2009 claiming to have made a special effort to reduce salt in their diet compared with 34% of adults in 2004, before the campaign commenced (Wyness *et al.*, 2012). The responsibility for salt reduction transferred to the Department of Health in 2009 and the large-scale Government-funded consumer awareness campaign did not continue. However, work with the food industry continued under the umbrella of the Department of Health's Public Health Responsibility Deal, which monitored progress in salt reductions in manufactured food categories against targets, and has also more recently set targets for salt in foods sold by the catering sector. Urinary sodium data (the most reliable measure of salt intakes) has shown a reduction in salt intakes between 2000–2001 and 2014 from 9.5 g to 8.0 g per day. Urinary sodium analysis data reported in 2014 found that men and women had a mean estimated intake of 9.1 g per day and 6.8 g per day respectively (Bates *et al.*, 2016). It is not clear whether the driver for this reduction has been changes in consumer behaviour or simply the gradual reductions in salt content of many widely eaten foods, or a combination of the two. It has been suggested that reformulation is the more likely explanation, and so the strategy of 'health by stealth', whereby changes are unannounced, may be more effective than attempting to encourage widespread changes in behaviour in the population.

Sugars reduction

Concern about intake of free sugars in relation to health has increased considerably in recent years, fuelled by recommendations to restrict intakes from SACN (2015) and WHO (2015). Free sugars are defined as including all monosaccharides and disaccharides added to foods by the manufacturer, cook or consumer, plus sugars naturally present in honey, syrups and unsweetened fruit juices. Under this definition, lactose (milk sugar) when naturally present in milk and milk products and sugars contained within the cellular structure of foods (particularly fruits and vegetables) are excluded. Intakes in teenagers and young adults are three times the 5% energy recommendation adopted by the UK Department of Health in 2015 and, on average, intakes in all other age/sex groups are above 10% energy. In October 2015, Public Health England published a report on the evidence for action on sugar reduction, advising on actions that could be implemented (PHE, 2015), refer to chapter 17 for more details. See Box 24.1. For a summary, see Buttriss (2016b). Subsequently, a number of these levers have been included in the government's childhood obesity plan published in summer 2016 (https://www.gov.uk/government/uploads/system/uploads/attachment_data/file/546588/Childhood_obesity_2016__2__acc.pdf).

Public Health England (2015) emphasised that it is unlikely that a single action alone would be effective in reducing sugar intakes. Their analysis of the evidence suggested that a broad, structured approach, involving restrictions on price promotions and marketing, product reformulation, portion size reduction and price increase on products considered to be less healthy, implemented in parallel, is likely to have a more universal effect on reducing sugar intake. Positive

---

Box 24.1 Actions proposed by Public Health England in relation to sugar reduction

1. Reduce and rebalance the number and type of price promotions in all retail outlets, including supermarkets and convenience stores and the out-of-home sector (including restaurants, cafes and takeaways).
2. Significantly reduce opportunities to market and advertise high-sugar food and drink products to children and adults across all media, including digital platforms and through sponsorship.
3. The setting of a clear definition for high-sugar foods to aid with actions 1 and 2. Currently, the only regulatory framework for doing this is via the Ofcom nutrient profiling model, which would benefit from being reviewed and strengthened.
4. Introduction of a broad, structured and transparently monitored programme of gradual sugar reduction in everyday food and drink products, combined with reductions in portion size.
5. Introduction of a price increase of a minimum of 10–20% on high-sugar products through the use of a tax or levy such as on full-sugar soft drinks, based on the emerging evidence of the impact of such measures in other countries.
6. Adopt, implement and monitor the government buying standards for food and catering services across the public sector, including national and local government and the NHS to ensure the provision and sale of healthier food and drinks in hospitals, leisure centres and other related settings.
7. Ensure that accredited training in diet and health is routinely delivered to all of those who have opportunities to influence food choices in the catering, fitness and leisure sectors and others within local authorities.
8. Continue to raise awareness of concerns around sugar levels in the diet to the public, as well as health professionals, employers, the food industry and so on, encourage action to reduce intakes and provide practical steps to help people lower their own and their family's sugar intake.

changes to the food environment (e.g. public-sector food procurement, provision and sales of healthier foods) as well as information and education are also needed to help support people in making healthier choices. Furthermore, success will depend on the engagement of a wide range of people and organisations. Rather than relying on provision of choice to drive behaviour change, Public Health England stressed the need to reduce sugar levels in food and drinks through reformulation and portion size reduction.

Secondary analysis conducted by Public Health England of data from the NDNS considered the impact of decreasing the amount of sugar coming from the key foods and drinks contributing to current intakes. It was concluded that a 50% reduction in the average sugar content of key food groups would reduce mean sugar intake to about 9% of energy for adults (from 12%) and about 10% for teenagers and children (from around 15% for both groups). This level of change in diet would bring intakes of 'free' sugars close to the previous recommendation of 10% of total dietary energy, but intakes would still be twice the new <5% energy recommendation, suggesting that more dramatic changes in food choice and/or further reformulation would be required.

Reformulation: opportunities and challenges

Whilst there is potential to decrease sugars substantially in some categories (e.g. soft drinks), technical issues exist for others, especially baked goods such as biscuits because of the functional and structural roles sugar plays. Furthermore, in dry foods such as breakfast cereals, sugar will be replaced by other ingredients that also contribute energy (even dietary fibre provides 2 kcal/g), and so calorie contribution is unlikely to fall substantially even if the ingredients used as replacers are higher in dietary fibre. In addition, there are legal constraints, such as compositional directives that curtail the extent to which composition can be changed (e.g. for chocolate) and, for example, energy content has to be reduced by at least 30% before artificial sweeteners can be used (e.g. in soft drinks), making gradual reductions in sugar more challenging.

Although it would seem logical that taste preference for sugar can be adapted over time (e.g. by gradual reduction, as with salt) there is currently limited evidence in this area of research. However, randomised controlled trials in children and adults suggest that replacing foods and drinks sweetened with sugar with those containing no–/low-calorie sweeteners can be useful in weight management. A recent meta-analysis of randomised controlled trials reported that the use of low-calorie sweeteners does not increase energy intake or body weight when compared with groups receiving either sugar-sweetened or non-caloric (e.g. water) alternatives (see Rogers *et al.* (2016) for further information).

Public Health England reported that evidence does not support the view that sugar is addictive in the same way that some drugs can be (PHE, 2015).

24.3 Income, price, marketing, promotions, portion size and fiscal strategies

Income

The Low Income Diet and Nutrition Survey provides nationally representative evidence on the eating habits, nourishment and nutrition-related health of people on low income in the UK (Nelson *et al.*, 2007). Although it is often assumed that the diets of those on low incomes are poorer across the board, for many foods, the types and quantities eaten by people on low income appeared similar to those of the general population. In this survey, those on low income were less likely to eat wholemeal bread and vegetables. They tended to drink more soft drinks (not diet drinks) and eat more processed meats, whole milk and sugar. Intakes of saturated fat, non-milk extrinsic sugars and sodium were above recommended levels, but were not significantly different to the general population. Intakes of fibre and fruit and vegetables were below recommendations, but again were similar to those in the general population. Large percentages (62% of men and 63% of women) were overweight or obese, in about the same proportion as in the population at large (Nelson *et al.*, 2007). Also see Chapter 8.

Data from the Health Survey for England suggest that there is a social gradient to obesity. For adults, those in the lowest income households and most deprived areas were most likely to be obese. This relationship was particularly strong among women: 31% of women in the fifth of households with lowest income were obese, double the rate of the fifth of women in households with highest incomes (15%). The equivalent figures for men were 30% and 23%. This relationship was also seen in children. Among children aged 2–15 years, levels of obesity were highest in the lowest quintile of household income (22% of boys and 21% of girls) compared with those in the highest quintile (7% and 6% respectively) (HSCIC, 2014). The same trends are evident in the child measurement programme (https://www.noo.org.uk/NCMP).

The Marmot review of health inequalities in England reported that not only was there a 7-year difference in life expectancy between those living in the richest neighbourhoods versus those living in the poorest, but also the difference in disability-free life expectancy was 17 years (Marmot *et al.*, 2010). So, not only do those in poorer areas have shorter lives, but they also spend more of their life in ill health. Nutrition is only one of a number of potential contributing factors to these differences in health outcomes, but tackling the social gradient in health behaviours is highlighted in the report as being a key to reducing health inequalities.

Food prices

Price is consistently cited as a key driver of food choice (Defra, 2014). According to the UK Family Food Survey 2013 (Defra, 2014), food prices rose significantly from September 2007 and peaked in February 2009. In 2013, food prices were 12% higher than in 2007 in real terms, although since 2014 food price inflation appears to have fallen. Consumer response to higher food prices may vary; people may simply spend more, buy less of certain products or 'trade down', choosing cheaper versions of a given product type. Between 2007 and 2013, households tended to trade down on cereals, biscuits and cakes, pork, fish, butter, sweets and chocolates. They also tended to buy more butter and eggs and less beef, lamb, fish, tea, potatoes, fruit and alcoholic drinks. People spent more on cereals, poultry, butter, cheese, eggs, coffee and hot drinks, soft drinks and on sugar and preserves.

In terms of the quantities of food purchased, purchases of various household foods are on clear short-term downward trends since at least 2010, including carcase meat and meat products, potatoes (driven by a decline in purchases of fresh potatoes), bread and beverages. Eggs are on a short-term upwards trend since 2010 (Defra, 2014). While overall purchases of fruit and vegetables reduced between 2010 and 2013, consumers spent somewhat more on fresh and processed fruit and vegetables. The amount of food eaten out has declined since 2001, with decreases in many categories; nevertheless, meals eaten out still account for one in six meals.

According to the Family Food Survey, these trends in purchases translated into a decline in total energy intake from all food and drink, especially in lower income households, a decreased intake of non-milk extrinsic sugars (recently replaced with the term 'free sugars') and sodium. Fibre intakes have also declined since 2010. It is not possible to determine the extent of the effect of food prices on these trends, but the survey data showed a more pronounced decline in energy intakes starting in 2007 when food prices rose. It is possible that reductions in fibre intakes could be related to decreases in purchases of fresh potatoes and fruit and vegetables.

Price promotions

Public Health England reports that price promotions in Britain are the highest in Europe, accounting for 40% of expenditure on food and drink taken home, which is twice the level in Germany, France and Spain. A typical household would have to spend 16% more (or an extra £630 a year) in order to buy their annual selection of promoted items at full price (PHE, 2015).

The impact on purchases of price promotions (temporary price reduction, multi-buy and extra free) of high-sugar foods has been explored using Kantar Worldpanel data from the past 2 years (from a continuously reporting panel of 30 000 British shoppers). Promotions appealed to all demographic groups, and while promotions make products cheaper, they also tended to encourage people to buy more. The analysis indicated that promotions lead to expansion of all food and drink categories, not just switching from one brand to another, and encourage people to buy and spend more overall. It was estimated that 22% more food and drink was purchased as a result of promotions. Higher (total) sugar items were more likely to be promoted and at a greater discount than non-high-sugar items; promotions were estimated to account for 35% of total sugars purchases and, for many categories, were largely incremental. Over the 2-year study period, it was estimated that 8.7% of 'sugars' taken home was an incremental consequence of purchases being on promotion, with 6.1% of total take-home sugars coming from the higher sugar categories (PHE, 2015). On the basis of this it was hypothesised that a saving of 6.1% in sugar volumes might be achieved if the level of promotions in higher sugar categories was reduced to zero, and this equates to an average of about 7.4 g of total sugars a day per person. In considering the implications of this analysis, it is important to note that it proved necessary to use on-pack total sugars declarations (which include sugars from fruit, vegetables and milk) rather than values for free sugars specifically.

Box 24.2, derived from the Public Health England analysis published in 2015, summarises findings for a number of marketing approaches (PHE, 2015).

The effect of portion size

A recent Cochrane review (Hollands et al., 2015) of 72 randomised controlled trials provides the most conclusive evidence so far that efforts to reduce the size, availability and appeal of larger sized portions, packages and tableware has the potential to reduce the amounts of food selected and consumed. The review found that people consistently ate more food or drank more non-alcoholic drinks when offered larger sized portions, packages or tableware than when offered smaller sized versions. The size of the effect was judged to be small to moderate among both children and adults. It was not clear from the available evidence whether this effect was maintained over time, but should this be shown to be the case it would equate to around a 12–16% change in

---

Box 24.2 Key considerations arising from Public Health England's review of the health and behavioural impacts of marketing strategies

- Promotion can impact on high-sugar food preference, purchase and consumption, although the current evidence base is strongly focused on children.
- TV advertising remains a popular food marketing channel, and evidence suggests it has potential to influence preference for, or intake of, high-sugar products. However, independent research suggests that current UK broadcast regulations – see PHE (2015: Annex 3, Table 1) – are not strong enough to reduce children's exposure to unhealthy food advertising (See Section "Advertising").
- Digital marketing strategies are rapidly growing and are a potentially influential area, given the highly immersive and interactive nature of these approaches. However, this remains an underresearched field, with current research evidence focusing on advergaming, which was found to significantly influence intake of, or preference for, high-sugar foods in school-age children.
- Understanding the behavioural and health impacts of new digital marketing strategies is essential, given they differ in approach to most traditional marketing strategies, therefore introducing a number of new concerns that may require additional regulatory consideration.
- Sponsorship is recognised as an emerging marketing strategy; yet despite many high-profile sponsorship deals in the UK, there remains a lack of evidence as to the diet–and health-related impacts of this approach.
- Price discounting can promote the sales of less healthy food; however, more research is required to understand the broader implications of discounting on overall dietary intake and impact across different demographic groups.
- Character branding can be an effective strategy to market high-sugar foods to young children, and while current regulations prevent the use of the approach to young school-age children, they may still be susceptible to products branded for wider appeal.
- Altering portion size can influence sugar intake; however, it is important to consider the impact of possible counter marketing or compensatory behaviours to any size regulation.
- Supermarket placement may influence high-sugar purchases; however, evidence is limited (one study identified in Public Health England's review) and lacks further detail on consequential health and behavioural impacts.

Source: PHE (2015: Annex 3, p. 10).

---

average daily energy intake from food among UK adults. The effect was smaller in children, although they still responded in a similar manner to larger portions.

This evidence suggests that policies and practices that successfully reduce the size, availability and appeal of large portions, packages, individual units and tableware – inside and outside the home – can contribute to meaningful reductions in the quantities of food and non-alcoholic beverages selected and consumed, at least in the short term, and the effect probably is not limited to specific population groups, although it is noteworthy that few studies considered socio-economic status. With the exception of age, the Cochrane review found no evidence to support claims that the effects of exposure to different portion sizes varied between men and with a different body mass index (BMI), or between those with different baseline levels of dietary restraint, dietary disinhibition or hunger. By contrast, differences regarding gender and BMI were found in a review by Zlatevska et al. (2014).

Hollands et al. (2015) did find evidence that the effect of portion size on consumption may be moderated by the type of food, with the relationship specifically being characterised by the 'healthiness' and energy density; larger effects were reported in studies that manipulated these characteristics.

The review lists possible interventions as regulations and legislative frameworks or voluntary agreements with the food industry to decrease portion size, reducing

default serving sizes of energy-dense foods and drinks or providing smaller plates and so on, and various 'choice architecture' interventions in restaurants and supermarkets. The choice architecture interventions include decreased availability of larger portions, packages or tableware sizes, placing larger portions further away from purchasers, and demarcation of single portion sizes in packaging through wrapping or a visual cue.

There are a number of examples where food companies have already taken steps to reduce portion size, for example, calorie caps on confectionery and smaller bag sizes for savoury snacks. In the evidence package on sugars reduction published by Public Health England in October 2015, emphasis was placed on the role of portion size manipulation, alongside product reformulation in reducing energy intake (PHE, 2015).

Apart from approaches that seek to directly alter the availability or cost of larger sizes, Hollands et al. (2015) found only limited and equivocal evidence for the effectiveness of initiatives that aim to educate people about appropriate portion sizes but suggest that this does not rule out a potential role for social marketing campaigns.

In summary, Hollands et al. (2015) estimated that elimination of larger portion sizes could reduce energy intake by up to 16% in adults, and a cap on portion sizes has been suggested as a way to reduce sugar and energy intake, pointing to the example of reduction in size of some chocolate bars to limit calories per bar (PHE, 2015).

Fiscal policies such as food taxation

Food taxes are increasingly being discussed as a potential policy measure in the UK to reduce free sugars intake, particularly in relation to sugars and sugars-sweetened beverages. While one effect of such measures would be to raise tax revenues that could be ring-fenced for public health initiatives (there are very few examples where this has been done), discussions on food taxes generally focus on their potential to change behaviour within populations. Much of the evidence for the potential effect of food taxes on consumer behaviour and health comes from economic modelling of the impact higher prices might have on consumer purchasing and consumption habits. One such study investigated the potential impact of a 20% tax on sugars-sweetened soft drinks to change purchase and consumption levels of these drinks and the impact this could have on energy intake, body weight and obesity prevalence in the UK (Briggs *et al.*, 2013). It was assumed that the projected reduction in sugars-sweetened soft drink consumption would translate into an equivalent reduction in total energy intake and body weight. Based on these calculations, this 20% tax was estimated to reduce the number of obese adults in the UK by 1.3% (or 180 000 people) and the number who are overweight by 0.9% (or 285 000 people). Although these small percentages represent large numbers of people within a population, with approximately 65% of adults in the UK either overweight or obese, these estimated effects might not have a significant impact on UK obesity prevalence. The authors noted that the predicted revenue generated (estimated as £276 million) could be used to increase NHS funding during a period of budget restrictions or to subsidise foods with health benefits, such as fruit and vegetables. But few governments have used the revenue in this way.

Denmark introduced a tax on foods high in saturated fat and had also proposed introducing a tax on sugars-sweetened foods and drinks. However, the fat tax was repealed after 15 months as it proved very unpopular and politically difficult to justify. There was evidence of stockpiling of food before the tax was introduced, and people switching to discount stores to buy the taxed products or travelling to neighbouring countries to shop. The planned sugar tax was then not introduced, and so it is not possible to draw conclusions on the efficacy of food taxes in changing dietary behaviour from the Danish experience. However, a number of countries have now introduced taxes, generally on sugars-sweetened beverages, including Hungary, France, Mexico and some states in the USA.

These initiatives are discussed in detail in an annex to the evidence package on sugar reduction strategies published by Public Health England in October 2015 (PHE, 2015). The report concludes that early data from five countries (Norway, Finland, Hungary, France and Mexico) show a reduction in sales of drinks classified as soft drinks/sugar-sweetened beverages, following implementation of a tax.

A recent 10% tax on sugars-sweetened beverages in Mexico (from January 2014) is reported to have resulted in an average reduction in purchases of 6% in 2014, with a 9% decline in lower socio-economic households. Overall, the data from the 11 studies were considered relatively consistent, suggesting taxes on high-sugar foods and drinks reduce purchases, at least in the short term. However, the evidence is reported to be of moderate quality, and no evidence of sustained effects has been published to date. Public Health England concluded that the effect appears to be proportional to the size of the tax implemented but that there is no evidence of the long-term effects of sugar taxes on the nutritional quality of the diet or health, or the impact on different population groups. Modelling suggests taxes need to be set at a relatively high level (around 10–20%) to have an effect on purchases, consumption and population health. In Spring 2016, a levy on sugar sweetened soft drinks was announced in the UK; this is due to come into effect in 2018 (https://www.gov.uk/government/publications/soft-drinks-industry-levy/soft-drinks-industry-levy).

Advertising

There has been much debate about the effect of advertising on food choice, particularly in relation to children. In 2007, regulations were brought in by Ofcom to prevent advertising of high-fat, –sugar or –salt (HFSS) foods during children's television programmes in the UK. A nutrient profiling system, developed by the FSA in consultation with a panel of experts, is used to classify foods as to whether they can or cannot be advertised to children (sometime referred to as the 'Ofcom model'). Ofcom's principal aim has been 'to reduce the exposure of children to HFSS advertising, as a means of reducing opportunities to persuade children to demand and consume HFSS products'. When the exposure to advertising in 2009 (when the Ofcom regulations were fully in place) was compared with 2005, it was estimated that, overall, children saw around 37% less HFSS advertising: younger children (4– to 9-year-olds) saw 52% less; older children (10– to 15-year-olds) saw 22% less (Ofcom, 2010).

However, owing to the multifactorial nature of influences on eating habits, it is not possible to extrapolate from these data to any changes in children's eating behaviour. In its review of the effect of advertising on childhood obesity (Ofcom, 2004), Ofcom cited the following influences on children's food choices, of which advertising is only one part:

- psychosocial factors (e.g. food preferences, meanings of food, and food knowledge);
- biological factors (e.g. heredity, hunger and gender);
- behavioural factors (e.g. time and convenience, meal patterns, dieting);

- family (e.g. income, working status of mother, family eating patterns, parental weight, diet and knowledge);
- friends (e.g. conformity, norms and peer networks);
- schools (school meals, sponsorship, vending machines);
- commercial sites (fast food restaurants, stores);
- consumerism (youth market and pester power);
- media (food promotion, including television advertising).

The debate on the influence of and controls on advertising continues, with some suggesting that controls on advertising of HFSS foods should be extended to cover programmes typically watched by families and online marketing to children. See Boxes 24.1 and 24.2 for some of Public Health England's conclusions in the evidence package on sugars reduction published in October 2015 (PHE, 2015).

In 2016, following a consultation, new rules were announced for nonbroadcast adverts (e.g. on websites) for products high in fat, sugar and salt. From July 2017, these will be subject to a new framework of restrictions based on the nutrient profiling approach used for TV adverts. The restrictions will be applied if more than 25% of the audience are children. Furthermore, Public Health England is undertaking a review of the nutrient profiling model that is used currently, to align it with new recommendations on free sugars and dietary fibre. A consultation is due to take place in the latter half of 2017.

Location of food outlets

This topic, the built environment, is primarily addressed in Chapter 23. There is limited evidence that there may be interactions between the availability and accessibility of food outlets at a neighbourhood level and development of obesity. In a study of over 200 children, Jennings *et al.* (2011) showed that availability of food outlets classified as BMI-healthy (supermarkets, fruit and veg shops) was favourably associated with measures of obesity and dietary intake. Conversely, availability of outlets classified as BMI-unhealthy (fast food and takeaway shops) was adversely associated with both weight status and food intake. A greater understanding of such relationships may be important in targeting policies and interventions to reduce childhood obesity, not only at an individual level but also by identifying and overcoming neighbourhood barriers to choosing and purchasing healthier foods.

24.4 Cultural-, environmental- and school-related influences

Trends in meal patterns

It has been suggested that snacking (eating between main meals) has increased in prevalence over the last three to four decades and now makes a significant contribution to average daily energy intake. This could be influenced by the wider environment in terms of increased availability of snack foods and foods to be eaten on the go, and also by changes to lifestyles for some people where traditional meal patterns may be less applicable. In the USA, it has been reported that adoption of a snacking dietary pattern (defined as one or more snacks per day, with snacks being defined as food intake >15 min after a meal) has increased from 71% and 74% in 1977–1978 to 97% and 98% in 2003–2006 for adults ($n = 44\,754$) and children aged 2–18 years ($n = 31\,337$) respectively. The different datasets also showed an increase in the contribution of snacks to total energy intake between 1977–1978 and 2003–2006, from 18% to 24% in adults and from 20.5% to 27% in children (Piernas and Popkin, 2010a,b). In addition, the number of eating and drinking occasions has been reported to have increased in American children from 3.9 per day in 1977–1978 to 5.1 per day in 2005–2010 ($n = 33\,635$) and has been proposed to be one of the main contributors to the increase in total energy intake observed over the past 30 years in the USA (Duffey and Popkin, 2013). In contrast, within the UK, evidence is mixed as to whether snacking has increased (Adams *et al.*, 2005; Kerr *et al.*, 2009). It is possible that interpretation of the evidence base is complicated by the variety of definitions of snacking in use (Miller *et al.*, 2013). Within some countries, the perception that snacking and eating occasions have increased over the past few decades has coincided with an increase in the proportion of the population who is overweight or obese and it has been suggested that the energy density of snack foods has increased (de Graaf, 2006). However, for many countries, including the UK, the evidence that snacking has increased is lacking and it may well be 'eating on the go' linked to an increased pace of life rather than snacking per se that is increasing (Miller *et al.*, 2013).

Given the number of meals consumed outside the home, it is interesting to note that much of the improvement in the nutrition of young children is attributed to meals taken outside the home whilst at school and in childcare (see Chapter 11).

Sustainability and environmental concerns

The Foresight (2011) report, *The Future of Food and Farming*, warned that 'without change, the global food system will continue to degrade the environment and compromise the world's capacity to produce food in the future, as well as contributing to climate change and the destruction of biodiversity'. It is recognised that there are numerous challenges in addressing this scenario as it sits within the context of a need to produce more food, linked to the growing global population expected to exceed 9 billion by 2050 (Foresight, 2011) and increases in life expectancy, the associated increased requirement for water and energy, the environmental impact of climate change, and the need for resilience in the face of the effects on the global food system of the threat of extreme weather. The amount of land available for conventional food production may also be compromised as urban areas expand to house the growing population. Furthermore, although in broad terms the characteristics of a more sustainable food supply are recognised and can be linked inversely to greenhouse gas emissions associated with food production (Garnett, 2014), the detail of what this means in practice is yet to be settled.

It has been predicted that, by 2030, the world will need to produce about 50% more food than it does currently in order to feed its population and to provide 30% more fresh water (Population Institute, 2010). There is a strong positive relationship between the level of income and the consumption of animal protein, with the consumption of meat and milk increasing at the expense of staple plant-derived foods. Therefore, increasing prosperity in growing world economies will also bring increased demand for meat and dairy foods. The Food and Agriculture Organization of the United Nations predicts that, by 2050, the expanded world population will be consuming two-thirds more animal protein, with meat consumption rising nearly 73% and dairy product consumption growing by 58% over current levels (FAO, 2013). This trend will put increased pressure on global food availability as production of these foods requires more natural resources than staple crops such as wheat and rice. The emission of greenhouse gases is also greater.

The UK produces less than 60% of its food, importing the remainder from over 180 countries (FSA, 2016). But the food supplies that we rely on may not be sustainable in the future if the predicted changes in climate occur and as demand for food globally increases as population rises and becomes more prosperous. Overconsumption and waste exacerbate the situation by placing unnecessary pressure on the food system.

In this context it is important to understand the public's priorities and expectations and how consumers might respond to messages designed to encourage more sustainable dietary patterns, the dietary substitutions that might emerge and the impact of these on the overall nutritional quality of diets. Surveys suggest that consumers lack an understanding of the principles of sustainability from a dietary perspective. In a Public Dialogue on food system challenges and possible solutions, conducted by the consumer organisation *Which?* in association with the Government Office for Science, participants' initial priorities emerged as quality, price and health. Even when pressed to consider wider issues, the environment was low down the list. However, once participants became more informed about the interactions between food production, water shortage and climate change, they developed a strongly held view that the challenges to the food system can only be addressed if all the parties – farmers, manufacturers, retailers, caterers, governments and consumers – play their part. The need to raise awareness about the challenges to the food system amongst consumers was an essential requirement (*Which?* and Government Office for Science, 2015).

Research from the FSA (2016) builds on this work, finding that people are not yet used to thinking globally about food but recognise the importance of the challenges faced. Participants were surprised and concerned to realise that they knew so little about the complex global food system, but there was a strong desire to know more about the processes that bring food to their tables. Four key themes were identified:

1. Convenience versus connection with how food is produced and, associated with this, loss of cooking skills and food traditions and increased waste.
2. Health and quality versus price, with concern that healthy food may become a luxury.
3. The need for information, education and transparency (e.g. about the provenance of food).
4. Need for more visibility from Government regarding its role in protecting consumer interests, and participants expected global governments to work together cooperatively to address the global challenges facing the food supply.

About 30% of all global greenhouse gas emissions are derived from food production. Two-thirds of this is associated with farming and land usage, and the remaining third occurs in the supply chain beyond the farm gate and in the home (see Figure 24.2).

Livestock makes one of the largest contributions to greenhouse gas emissions in the UK, and discussions on sustainable diets often suggest that meat and dairy product consumption should be reduced. However, the realities are often not as simple as they are portrayed in the consumer media because of the global nature of trade in meat and dairy products and differences in the sustainability of production practices. Also important to consider is the nature of the substitutions made when diets change. There is a paucity of evidence on this topic, although a recent review has begun to summarise worldwide evidence on food substitution (Green *et al.*, 2013) and this has been taken into consideration in an investigation of the potential to reduce greenhouse gas emissions whilst still achieving nutritional recommendations (Green *et al.*, 2015). If average diets conformed to World Health Organization recommendations, associated greenhouse gas emissions would be reduced by 17%. Further reductions could be achieved, but reductions beyond 40% through dietary change alone will be

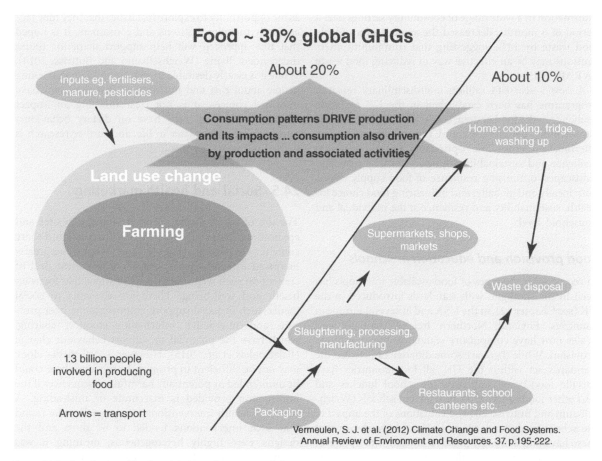

Figure 24.2 Contribution of food to global greenhouse gas emissions.

unlikely without radically changing current consumption patterns and potentially reducing the nutritional quality of diets (Green *et al.*, 2015). It was also shown that modest health benefits could be achieved without the need to resort to an extreme diet (Milner *et al.*, 2015)

Fish is also often under scrutiny from a sustainability viewpoint. There are a number of initiatives that aim to help consumers and retailers make more informed choices about the fish they purchase. For example, the Marine Conservation Society consumer guide *Good Fish Guide* (http://www.goodfishguide.org) and the blue Marine Stewardship Council ecolabel, which appears on certified fish products in the UK (http://www.msc. org). Some retailers are also 'choice editing', meaning that endangered fish species are not available for purchase in their stores.

As a starting point, until the evidence gaps are filled, analysis of the greenhouse gas emissions of different foods in the diet has suggested that moving towards a healthy varied diet, as depicted in the UK Government's

Eatwell Guide, will help reduce greenhouse gas emissions associated with the diet and improve the health of the UK population (Scarborough *et al.*, 2016; see also Cobiac *et al.*, 2016) .

As a means of addressing sustainability concerns, food waste reduction is an issue that consumers could immediately embrace to improve the sustainability of the food supply. Research by the Waste and Resources Action Programme (WRAP) in 2012 suggested that avoidable household food waste had already been cut by 21% since 2007, saving UK consumers almost £13 billion over the 5 years to 2012 (WRAP, 2013a). However, despite this significant drive to reduce food waste, UK households in 2012 were still throwing away 4.2 million tonnes of household food and drink annually – the equivalent of six meals every week for the average UK household. The *Love Food Hate Waste* (LFHW) campaign, delivered by WRAP, is a consumer-focused initiative encouraging the reduction of avoidable food waste. An intervention undertaken in West London, delivering LFHW information in a wide range of community settings over a period of 6 months, decreased the amount of avoidable food waste by 14%, suggesting that community interventions may be an effective way of reducing food waste (WRAP, 2013b).

A new 5-year £14 million interdisciplinary research programme has been established in the UK to tackle resilience in the food system, co-designed by relevant UK Government departments and research councils. The interlinked themes are: optimising the productivity, resilience and sustainability of agricultural systems and landscapes; optimising resilience of food supply chains both locally and globally; and influencing food choice for health, sustainability and resilience at the individual and household level.

Food provision and education in schools

In recent years the types of food available in schools has been in the spotlight, with standards introduced in the UK (see Chapter 12), in the USA and in several European countries. England, Northern Ireland, Scotland and Wales now have compulsory standards governing food provision. While there are some differences between the standards set within the UK, all four countries have specific food-based standards for school lunches and also other foods and drinks provided in schools (Weichselbaum and Buttriss, 2014). Evaluations of the impact of the school food standards in England have shown that these have had a broadly positive impact, with uptake of lunches increasing and the nutrient content of the lunches provided and the food choices made by pupils improving (Weichselbaum and Buttriss, 2014). This suggests that modifying the food environment in schools can improve the diets of schoolchildren.

As well as the provision of food in schools, education about food, cooking, diet and health in schools is increasingly high on the agenda in many countries, especially in the context of rising levels of childhood obesity and risk of non-communicable disease in later life. Food and diet may feature in a range of subjects taught in schools, from the basics of metabolism and digestion in a science lesson, to the social and financial aspects of food in subjects including personal development, plus specialist lessons on food science and on food preparation in food technology. For example, in English secondary schools, food is taught through three main areas of learning: learning for life at work (food technology); science and technology (science); and learning for life and work (personal development). Food technology is compulsory for all secondary school-aged pupils (ages 11–14 years), and is taught through three themes: healthy eating, home and family life, and independent living. The concept is to help all young people learn practical skills in food safety and preparation, as well

as the opportunity to explore real issues that they may face as family members, citizens and consumers. It is hoped that this approach will help support them for future independent living (Weichselbaum and Buttriss, 2014). While it is clearly desirable to educate children and young people about diet and nutrition so that they can make informed choices, it is not clear how big an impact education at school may have on dietary behaviours during childhood or later in life, and further research is needed to investigate this.

24.5 Social and health marketing

The use of social media, in other words web sites and applications ('apps') that enable users to create and share content or to participate in social networking, has greatly increased in recent years, and there is a great deal of content on such web sites and applications that focus on health and well-being. There are elements to social media, such as social support, empowerment, peer pressure and interactive information–emotion sharing, which have the potential to support behaviour change (Balatsoukas et al., 2015). However, social media alone may not be sufficient to promote health, and there could be unintended or potentially harmful consequences if the information provided is inaccurate or misleading. A review of health interventions using social media found that such interventions tended to be short and the designs were highly heterogeneous, meaning it was not possible to draw broad conclusions about the efficacy of such approaches (Balatsoukas et al., 2015). The use of such technologies for health promotion is still relatively recent, and more research will be needed in order to determine the more effective ways to use social media to encourage health-related behaviour change.

In response to concerns about rising rates of childhood obesity, a social (or health) marketing campaign Change4Life was launched by the Department of Health in 2009, with the aim to improve eating and physical activity habits in families and support long-term health. The programme was evaluated in 2010, 1 year after the 'launch (DH, 2010). At this stage, the outcomes measured related to awareness of the campaign; for example, recognition of the campaign logo by the key target audience (mothers of children under 11 years), responses to surveys undertaken by the campaign, sign up to the campaign and the percentage of those who signed up who were still engaged with the campaign 6 months later. In all cases, the targets for these outcomes were exceeded. Although measures of behaviour change were not included at this stage, self-reports from families involved in Change4Life suggested they were taking on suggestions from the campaign such as swapping sugar-sweetened drinks for sugar-free ones, eating five portions of fruit and vegetables a day and consuming appropriate portion sizes.

An evaluation of the campaign questionnaire and the effect of personalised feedback provided in a 'Family Information Pack' was undertaken during 2009–2010, with families recruited from primary schools across England, with a mixture of social and demographic characteristics. Outcome measures were awareness of the campaign, attitudes and intention to change, and adult and child behaviours, in relation to key behaviours targeted by *Change4Life*. Although awareness of the campaign was high at baseline, responses to the questionnaire were low in number and the evaluation found little impact on attitudes or behaviours (Croker *et al.*, 2012). Again, this highlights the challenge in translating public health messages into behaviour change in populations.

Public Health England, in its analysis of drivers for sugar reduction, noted that health marketing such as *Change4Life* is an important enabler but that it generally only has short-term effects and tends to help those who are already engaged with health and may therefore widen health inequalities (PHE, 2015).

24.6 Food labelling

Back and front of pack labelling on packaged foods

Nutritional labelling in the UK is controlled by EU regulations. The European (EU) Food Information Regulation (FIR) came into force in December 2011 and applies to all member states. The new regulation serves to draw together existing general food labelling and nutrition labelling legislation and aligns it with recent developments in food information. It has also simplified certain aspects to improve clarity, and therefore aid consumer understanding. There was a 3-year transitional period to implement the legislation, giving companies until December 2014 to comply with the changes to packaging. Mandatory provision of back of pack nutrition information on pre-packaged foods applied from 13 December 2016 (although companies already providing nutrition information had to change to the new format from December 2014). The information has to be presented per 100 g/mL and can additionally be presented per portion. The following needs to be included in the back of pack declaration: energy value (in kilojoules and kilocalories), and amount in grams of fat, saturated fat, carbohydrate, sugars, protein and salt. Further information can be included, but is not compulsory, for monounsaturated fat, polyunsaturated fat, starch, fibre, vitamins or minerals. For vitamins and minerals, a

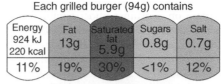

Each grilled burger (94g) contains

Energy 924 kJ 220 kcal	Fat 13g	Saturated fat 5.9g	Sugars 0.8g	Salt 0.7g
11%	19%	30%	<1%	12%

of an adult's reference intake
Typical values (as sold) per 100g: Energy 966kJ / 230kcal

Figure 24.3 'Hybrid' front of pack labelling scheme.

minimum amount (15% of the nutrient reference value) has to be present per 100 g of food before the nutrient may be added to the list. Nutrition or health claims are also covered by legislation (see later), and if a claim is made on the packaging then the nutrient in question must be declared as part of the back of pack information.

For consumers in the UK, where back of pack nutrition labels are used almost universally on packaged foods, the introduction of compulsory back of pack nutrition labelling may not make much practical difference. However, elsewhere in Europe, where nutrition labelling provision has sometimes been less evident, the difference may be more noticeable.

Repetition of information about certain nutrients from back of pack labelling on the front of packaging is allowed on a voluntary basis. This information must comprise: energy value (kilojoules and kilocalories) alone or energy plus the amounts of fat, saturated fat, sugars and salt per portion, no additions are allowed. In the UK, Government guidelines on a consistent 'hybrid' front of pack labelling scheme exist and have been widely implemented, combining reference intakes–previously guideline daily amounts (GDAs) – and colour coding with high, medium or low text (see Figure 24.3) (DH, 2013). Other European countries also have national schemes; for example, the Swedish keyhole mark and introduction of schemes is under consideration in others (e.g. France).

Effect on dietary behaviour of nutrition labelling on packaged foods

The aim of providing nutrition information on food packaging is to inform consumers and, in the context of wider information provision on healthy diets, to encourage choice of healthier options. Clearly, to have any impact on food choices, people must first be aware of and read the nutrition label. However, there is little published information about the actual use of nutrition labels by consumers in the real world.

Assuming that the label is read, the information provided needs to be easily understood if it is to be of use. Studies in the UK have investigated consumer understanding of front of pack label information using different labelling formats. The FSA commissioned consumer research on consumer understanding and use of front of pack labelling (Malam *et al.*, 2009), comparing labels using GDAs, traffic light labelling and hybrid schemes that combined the two. Comprehension was generally high (58–71%) and two schemes stood out as being best understood: a front of pack label combining text (the words high, medium, low), traffic light colours and percentage GDA (70%), and a label combining text and traffic light colours (71%). Shoppers who used front of pack labels valued them but reported that, when making purchasing decisions, this nutrition information was competing with other factors such as price, branding and other label information such as organic or healthy range labels. Those who had an interest in healthy eating were more likely to use front of pack labels but they were less likely to be used once the shopper felt confident that they now knew whether or not a product is healthy. Conversely, those who were not interested in healthy eating tended not to use labels and some actually avoided them because they perceived front of pack labelling as an unwelcome attempt to control their behaviour.

Since this research was conducted, the presence of front of pack labelling has become widespread in the UK and a uniform presentation is encouraged by the Government, but it remains the case that more needs to be done to establish use of nutrition labelling as an effective tool to encourage healthier food and drink choices.

Nutrition and health claims

Nutrition and health claims in Europe are controlled by the European Commission's (EC) Regulation No 1924/2006. This covers claims about what a food contains (e.g. statements such as 'high in fibre' or 'low in fat') and about the health effect of foods (e.g. 'Beta-glucans contribute to the maintenance of normal blood cholesterol levels'). The regulation sets out the approval process for claims, and a list of both accepted and rejected health claims has been published.

An FSA review reported that consumers may find it difficult to distinguish between nutrition and health claims, particularly if the consumer is already familiar with a nutrient–disease relationship (Food Standards Agency, 2007). The regulation states that the beneficial effects expressed in the claim must be understood by an average consumer, with an average consumer defined as 'reasonably well informed and reasonably observant and circumspect' (EC, 2007). Research suggests that consumers perceive a product to be of greater benefit and are more likely to pay attention to the claim if it relates to a health concern they are familiar or associated with; for example, a consumer with a history of high blood cholesterol levels may pay more attention to a related

claim (Dean *et al.*, 2007; Leathwood *et al.*, 2007; Nocella and Kennedy, 2012).

Consumers appeared to prefer short adjectives (e.g. low, free) as they are easier to understand than long, complicated words, and too much information on pack can lead to claims being disregarded (Food Standards Agency, 2007). The majority of research investigating consumer understanding of claims was carried out prior to the EC regulation coming into force. This must be taken into account when looking at the research, as it may not be appropriate to extrapolate findings to current claims that are being communicated in the context of the regulation. Understanding of claims is influenced by consumers' familiarity with food products and ingredients (Food Standards Agency, 2007; Nocella and Kennedy, 2012). The increase in the prevalence of products containing stanols and sterols has rapidly increased, leading to a greater consumer familiarity with these products and thus potentially a better understanding of associated claims. This must be acknowledged when considering older research into claims on these products. However, there do seem to be some consistent findings with respect to topics consumers find confusing and barriers and aids to understanding claims. Research suggests that consumers are often confused by inconsistent terminology of nutrients, and can struggle to differentiate between terms such as salt and sodium; calories, kilojoules and energy; lactose and dairy; and sugar and carbohydrates. Consumers seem to be confused by technical terms and put off by worrying words such as cancer and cardiovascular disease. Qualifiers (e.g. may and can) are seen to weaken the claim; 'may' more so than 'can'. On the other hand, consumers seem to consider and understand brief claims better than longer claims, and positive claims that mention good health are preferred by consumers compared with claims that mention poor health. Some research suggests that consumer evaluation of health claims is in part determined by the perceived healthiness of a base food product (e.g. yogurts are perceived healthy by women). In this way, some health claims combine better with certain food products because these messages link the beneficial component with specific products.

In summary, nutrition and health claims may influence consumers' food choices, but more research is needed, especially in the context of more recent regulation, to establish how this works in practice. A summary of the processes in place for establishing the validity of health claims and some of the challenges encountered in the implementation of the regulation can be found in Buttriss (2015) and guidance on the process for applying for an EU health claim is available as an output of the EU funded BACCHUS (Beneficial effects of dietary bioactive peptides and polyphenols on cardiovascular health in humans) project (www.bacchus-fp7.eu).

Out-of-home calorie labelling

While nutrition labelling has been a feature on prepacked foods for some time in the UK, until recently there was little or no information about the nutritional content of foods eaten outside the home available to consumers.

On average in the UK, one in every six meals is eaten out of home; if snacks are added in, men consume about a quarter of their calories when eating out and women a fifth. Therefore, the choices that are made when eating away from home could have a significant impact on energy intakes.

The provision of nutrient information on foods sold outside the home presents a challenge as many foods are not prepacked. This means that careful thought is needed on how and where to provide the information to allow it to be easily seen and read. For this reason, generally labelling of foods eaten outside the home is typically restricted to calorie content. New York City was one of the first places to implement widespread calorie labelling in chain restaurants, and this is now provided in many outlets in the UK either via menus or menu boards, point of choice or via a web site. In evaluating the effects of calorie labelling on consumer choices, some studies have found that diners chose dishes with significantly fewer calories, while other studies have found no significant differences (Block and Roberto, 2014). These inconsistencies may be due to differences in the study design, but it appears that the benefits of the scheme are not clear in the data currently available.

24.7 Impact of fortification/supplementation

Policies on fortification of foods differ from country to country. Many countries have some level of mandatory fortification, often to replace nutrients lost during food processing. For example, in the UK there is mandatory fortification of non-wholemeal flour (and hence bread) with iron, thiamin, niacin and calcium, in part to replace the losses of these nutrients during milling.

Voluntary fortification of foods by manufacturers is also common in some food categories. and voluntary fortification, in Europe, is controlled by European regulations that specify the specific formulations that can be added and the minimum levels allowed. Both mandatory and voluntary fortification can have significant effects on nutrient intakes within populations. For example, in the UK, white bread provides about 10% of iron and calcium intakes, nutrients that are added via mandatory fortification (Bates *et al.*, 2014). Data from Ireland suggest that about 67% of the adult population consume foods that have been voluntarily fortified and that these foods make a relatively large contribution to micronutrient intakes compared with the proportion of energy they provide. For example, fortified foods contributed 4% energy intake for men and 5% for women but provided 16% and 19% of iron intakes in men and women respectively (Hennessy *et al.*, 2013).

Ready-to-eat breakfast cereals are one of the most widely consumed fortified foods, and a number of studies have looked at their impact on micronutrient intakes and status. A study using 2000–2001 NDNS data showed that consumption of breakfast cereals by adults resulted in micronutrient intakes that were 30–90% higher than when a non-cereal breakfast was consumed (Gibson and Gunn, 2011).

Vitamin D status is of particular concern in Europe (Spiro and Buttriss, 2014) and in many countries around the world (see Chapters 8, 10 and 20), and although supplements have been advocated for vulnerable groups for some time, uptake has generally been poor. Vitamin D is unique among the vitamins as, for most people, the main source is through the action of UVB sunlight on the skin. Natural food sources are limited (e.g. eggs, oily fish and meat), and so intake from these is on average only about 3–5 µg/day in adults (SACN, 2016). In recognition of recent evidence of low vitamin D status in a substantial proportion of the population and because of the limited use of supplements in the UK, there is growing interest in fortification of foods with vitamin D as a means of addressing low vitamin D status. A systematic review of intervention studies using foods fortified with vitamin D found that these increased serum vitamin D in a dose-dependent manner (Black *et al.*, 2012). Further details on vitamin D, including information on fortification strategies, can be found in a series of papers on vitamin D available at http://bit.ly/1nTb56p.

Another nutrient of interest in this context is folic acid, supplementation with which is recommended for women of childbearing age, although uptake is relatively low (see Chapters 8 and 10). In North America and many other parts of the world, flour is fortified with this vitamin, but the practice has yet to be adopted in Europe.

24.8 Conclusions

Many factors in the wider environment affect dietary behaviour. These include government policy and initiatives; cultural factors, attitudes to environmental factors and sustainable sourcing of foods, education and income; price of food and drinks, promotions, advertising, and choice in portion size and healthier options. There is also growing interest in whether or not fiscal policies such as taxation may influence purchasing and consumption behaviour. In recent years, nutrition labelling has become a legal requirement in Europe, providing details to support consumer choice, and campaigns on salt and sugars, for example, have provided a rationale to change dietary behaviour. Social and health marketing have increasingly been used to promote healthy eating. The effects of these many factors can be supportive or detrimental in achieving positive dietary change and in supporting appropriate dietary behaviour, and it is increasingly recognised that there is no silver bullet when it comes to driving positive behaviour change; a multi-faceted approach is needed.

References

Adams, J., O'Keeffe, M. and Adamson, A. (2005) Change in snacking habits and obesity over 20 years in children aged 11 to 12 years. Project NO9 019 (Jan–Sept 2005). Final report to the Food Standards Agency.

Balatsoukas, P., Kennedy, C.M., Buchan, I. et al. (2015) The role of social network technologies in online health promotion: a narrative review of theoretical and empirical factors influencing intervention effectiveness. *Journal of Medical Internet Research*, **17** (6), e141.

Bates, B., Cox, L., Maplethorpe, N. et al. (2014) *National Diet and Nutrition Survey: Assessment of Dietary Sodium Adults (19 to 64 years) in England*. https://www.gov.uk/government/uploads/system/uploads/attachment_data/file/509399/Sodium_study_2014_England_Text_final.pdf

Bates, B., Lennox, A., Prentice, A. et al. (eds) (2014) *National Diet and Nutrition Survey: Results from Years 1, 2, 3 and 4 (Combined) of the Rolling Programme (2008/2009-2011/2012)* Public Health England, London. https://www.gov.uk/government/uploads/system/uploads/attachment_data/file/310995/NDNS_Y1_to_4_UK_report.pdf (accessed 30 November 2016).

Black, L.J., Seamans, K.M., Cashman, K.D. et al. (2012) An updated systematic review and meta-analysis of the efficacy of vitamin D food fortification. *Journal of Nutrition*, **142**, 1102–1108.

Block, J.P. and Roberto, C.A. (2014) Potential benefits of calorie labeling in restaurants. *JAMA*, **312** (9), 887–888.

Briggs, A.D., Mytton, O.T. and Kehlbacher, A. (2013) Overall and income specific effect on prevalence of overweight and obesity of 20% sugar sweetened drink tax in UK: econometric and comparative risk assessment modelling study. *BMJ*, **347**, f6189.

British Nutrition Foundation (n.d.) *How the War Changed Nutrition: From There to Now*. https://www.nutrition.org.uk/nutritioninthenews/wartimefood/warnutrition.html (accessed 20 December 2016).

Buttriss, J.L. (2015) Nutrition and health claims in practice. *Nutrition Bulletin*, **40**, 211–222.

Buttriss, J. (2016a) The Eatwell Guide refreshed. *Nutrition Bulletin*, **41** (2), 135–141.

Buttriss, J.L. (2016b) Sugars – part of a bigger picture? *Nutrition Bulletin*, **41**, 78–86.

Capacci, S. and Mazzocchi, M. (2011) Five-a-day, a price to pay: an evaluation of the UK program impact accounting for market forces. *Journal of Health Economics*, **30** (1), 87–98.

Cobiac et al. (2016) http://journals.plos.org/plosone/article?id=10.1371/journal.pone.0167859; https://www.abdn.ac.uk/staffnet/documents/Carbon_Trust_Final_report.pdf Carbon Trust 2016

Croker, H., Lucas, R. and Wardle, J. (2012) Cluster-randomised trial to evaluate the 'Change for Life' mass media/social marketing campaign in the UK. *BMC Public Health*, **12**, 404.

Dean, M., Shepherd, R., Arvola, A. et al. (2007) Consumer perceptions of healthy cereal products and production methods. *Journal of Cereal Science*, **46**, 188–196.

Defra (2014) *Family Food 2013*. Department for Environment, Food and Rural Affairs, London. https://www.gov.uk/government/uploads/system/uploads/attachment_data/file/385694/familyfood-2013report-11dec14.pdf (accessed 21 December 2016).

Defra (2015a) *Family Food 2014*. Department for Environment, Food and Rural Affairs, London. https://www.gov.uk/government/uploads/system/uploads/attachment_data/file/485982/familyfood-2014report-17dec15.pdf (accessed 20 December 2016).

Defra (2015b) *Food Statistics Pocketbook 2014*. Department for Environment, Food and Rural Affairs, London. https://www.gov.uk/government/uploads/system/uploads/attachment_data/file/423616/foodpocketbook-2014report-23apr15.pdf (accessed 20 December 2016).

De Graaf C. (2006) Effects of snacks on energy intake: an evolutionary perspective. *Appetite*, **47**, 18–23.

DH (2010) *Change4Life – One Year On*. Department of Health. http://webarchive.nationalarchives.gov.uk/20130107105354/http://www.dh.gov.uk/prod_consum_dh/groups/dh_digitalassets/@dh/@en/documents/digitalasset/dh_115511.pdf (accessed 21 December 2016).

DH (2013) Guide to Creating a Front of Pack (FoP) Nutrition Label for Pre-packaged Products Sold through Retail Outlets. https://www.gov.uk/government/publications/front-of-pack-nutrition-labelling-guidance#history (accessed 21 December 2016).

Duffey, K.J. and Popkin, B.M. (2013) Causes of increased energy intake among children in the U.S., 1977–2010. *American Journal of Preventive Medicine*, e1–e8.

EC (2007) Regulation (EC) No 1924/2006 of the European Parliament and of the Council of 20 December 2006 on nutrition and health claims made on foods. *The Official Journal of the European Union*, **L12/18** http://eur-lex.europa.eu/LexUriServ/LexUriServ.do?uri=OJ:L:2007:012:0003:0018:EN:PDF.

FAO (2013) *Tackling Climate Change through Livestock: A Global Assessment of Emissions and Mitigation Opportunities*. Food and Agriculture Organization of the United Nations, Rome. http://www.fao.org/3/i3437e.pdf (accessed 21 December 2016).

Food Standards Agency (2007) *Review and Analysis of Current Literature on Consumer understanding of Nutrition and health Claims Made on Food*. Food Standards Agency, London.

Foresight (2011) *The Future of Food and Farming: Challenges and Choices for Global Sustainability*. Final Project Report. The Government Office for Science, London.

FSA (2016) *Our Food Future*. Food Standards Agency. https://www.food.gov.uk/news-updates/campaigns/ourfoodfuture (accessed 21 December 2016).

Garnett, T. (2014) *What is a Sustainable Healthy Diet? A Discussion Paper*. Food Climate Research Network. http://www.fcrn.org.uk/sites/default/files/fcrn_what_is_a_sustainable_healthy_diet_final.pdf (accessed 21 December 2016).

Gibson, S.A. and Gunn, P. (2011) What's for breakfast? Nutritional implications of breakfast habits: insights from the NDNS dietary records. *Nutrition Bulletin*, **36** (1), 78–86.

Green, R., Cornelsen, L., Dangour, A.D. et al. (2013) The effect of rising food prices on food consumption: systematic review with meta-regression. *BMJ*, **346**, f3703.

Green, R., Milner, J., Dangour, A.D. et al. (2015) The potential to reduce greenhouse gas emissions in the UK through healthy and realistic dietary change. *Climatic Change*, **129**, 253–265.

Hennessy, A., Walton, J. and Flynn, A. (2013) The impact of voluntary food fortification on micronutrient intakes and status in European countries: a review. *Proceedings of the Nutrition Society*, **72**, 433–440.

Hollands, G.J., Shemilt, I., Marteau, T.M. *et al*. (2015) Portion, package or tableware size for changing selection and consumption of food, alcohol and tobacco. *The Cochrane Database of Systemic Reviews*, (9) CD011045.

HSCIC (2014) *Health Survey for England – 2013*. Health and Social Care Information Centre. http://www.hscic.gov.uk/catalogue/PUB16076 (accessed 20 December 2016).

Jennings, A., Welch, A., Jones, A.P. *et al*. (2011) Local food outlets, weight status, and dietary intake: associations in children aged 9–10 years. *American Journal of Preventive Medicine*, **40**, 405–410.

Kerr, M.A., Rennie, K.L., McCaffrey, T.A. *et al*. (2009) Snacking patterns among adolescents: a comparison of type, frequency and portion size between Britain in 1997 and Northern Ireland in 2005. *The British Journal of Nutrition*, **101**, 122–131.

Leathwood, P.D., Richardson, D.P., Sträter, P. *et al*. (2007) Consumer understanding of nutrition and health claims: sources of evidence. *The British Journal of Nutrition*, **98**, 474–484.

Malam, S., Clegg, S., Kirwan, S. *et al*. (2009) *Comprehension and Use of UK Nutrition Signpost Labelling Schemes*. Food Standards Agency. http://webarchive.nationalarchives.gov.uk/20131104005023/http://www.food.gov.uk/multimedia/pdfs/pmpreport.pdf (accessed 21 December 2016).

Marmot, M., Allen, J., Goldblatt, P. et al. (2010) Fair Society, Healthy Lives: The Marmot Review. Strategic Review of Health Inequalities in England Post-2010. http://www.instituteofhealthequity.org/projects/fair-society-healthy-lives-the-marmot-review/fair-society-healthy-lives-full-report (accessed 20 December 2016).

Miller, R., Benelam, B., Stanner, S. and Buttriss, J.L. (2013) Is snacking good or bad for health: an overview? *Nutrition Bulletin*, **38** (3), 302–322.

Milner *et al* (2015) http://bmjopen.bmj.com/content/5/4/e007364.

Nelson, M., Erens, B., Bates, B. *et al*. (2007) *Low Income Diet and Nutrition Survey*, vol. 3, TSO, London.

Nocella, G. and Kennedy, O. (2012) Food health claims – what consumers understand. *Food Policy*, **37**, 571–580.

Ofcom (2004) *Childhood Obesity – Food Advertising in Context. Children's Food Choices, Parents' Understanding and Influence, and the Role of Food Promotion*. http://stakeholders.ofcom.org.uk/binaries/research/tv-research/report2.pdf (accessed 20 December 2016).

Ofcom (2010) HFSS Advertising Restrictions. Final Review. http://stakeholders.ofcom.org.uk/binaries/research/tv-research/hfss-review-final.pdf (accessed 20 December 2016).

PHE (2015) *Sugar Reduction: From Evidence into Action*. Public Health England, London. https://www.gov.uk/government/publications/sugar-reduction-from-evidence-into-action (accessed 20 December 2016).

Piernas, C. and Popkin, B.M. (2010a) Snacking increased among U.S. adults between 1977 and 2006. *The Journal of Nutrition*, **140**, 325–332.

Piernas, C. and Popkin, B.M. (2010b) Trends in snacking among U.S. children. *Health Affairs*, **29**, 398–404.

Population Institute (2010) *2030: The 'Perfect Storm' Scenario*. https://www.populationinstitute.org/external/files/reports/The_Perfect_Storm_Scenario_for_2030.pdf (accessed 21 December 2016).

Prior, G., Hall, L. Morris, S. and Draper, A. (2011) *Exploring Food Attitudes and Behaviours in the UK: Findings from the Food and You Survey 2010*. https://www.food.gov.uk/sites/default/files/food-and-you-2010-main-report.pdf (accessed 20 December 2016).

Rogers, P.J., Hogenkamp, P.S., de Graaf, C. *et al*. (2016) Does low-energy sweetener consumption affect energy intake and body weight? A systematic review, including meta-analyses, of the evidence from human and animal studies. *International Journal of Obesity*, **40** (3), 381–394.

Sadler, K., Nicholson, S. and Steer, T. (2001) National Diet and Nutrition Survey – Assessment of Dietary Sodium in Adults (aged 19 to 64 years) in England, 2011. Department of Health, London. http://webarchive.nationalarchives.gov.uk/20130402145952/https://www.wp.dh.gov.uk/transparency/files/2012/06/Sodium-Survey-England-2011_Text_to-DH_FINAL1.pdf (accessed 20 December 2016).

SACN (2015) *Carbohydrates and Health*. TSO, London. https://www.gov.uk/government/uploads/system/uploads/attachment_data/file/445503/SACN_Carbohydrates_and_Health.pdf (accessed 20 December 2016).

SACN (2016) *Vitamin D and Health*. https://www.gov.uk/government/uploads/system/uploads/attachment_data/file/537616/SACN_Vitamin_D_and_Health_report.pdf (accessed 21 December 2016).

Scarborough *et al*. (2016) http://bmjopen.bmj.com/content/6/12/e013182.full? keytype=ref&ijkey=Uo55Bu2X5HD3ukv

Spiro, A. and Buttriss, J.L. (2014) Vitamin D: an overview of vitamin D status and intake in Europe. *Nutrition Bulletin*, **39**, 322–350.

TNS Social (2006) Evaluation of the 5 a Day Programme. Final Report. https://biglotteryfund.org.uk/-/media/Files/Research%20Documents/er_eval_5aday_final_report.pdf (accessed 20 December 2016).

USDA (2015) *Dietary Guidelines for Americans 2015–2020*, 8th edn. US Department of Agriculture, Washington, DC. http://health.gov/dietaryguidelines/2015/guidelines/ (accessed 11 December 2016).

Weichselbaum, E. and Buttriss, J.L. (2014) Diet, nutrition and schoolchildren: an update. *Nutrition Bulletin*, **39** (1), 9–73.

Which? and Government Office for Science (2015) Food System Challenges: Public Dialogue on Food System Challenges and Possible Solutions. http://www.which.co.uk/documents/pdf/food-system-challenges—public-dialogue-on-food-system-challenges-and-possible-solutions-445299.pdf (accessed 21 December 2016).

WHO (2015) *Guideline: Sugars Intake for Adults and Children*. World Health Organization, Geneva. http://apps.who.int/iris/bitstream/10665/149782/1/9789241549028_eng.pdf?ua=1 (accessed 20 December 2016).

WRAP (2013a) Household Food and Drink Waste in the United Kingdom 2012. http://www.wrap.org.uk/sites/files/wrap/hhfdw-2012-main.pdf.pdf (accessed 21 December 2016).

WRAP (2013b) Household Food Waste Prevention Case Study: West London Waste Authority in Partnership with Recycle for London. http://www.wrap.org.uk/sites/files/wrap/West%20London%20LFHW%20Impact%20case%20study_0.pdf (accessed 21 December 2016).

Wyness, L.A., Buttriss, J.L. and Stanner, S.A. (2012) Reducing the population's sodium intake: the UK Food Standards Agency's salt reduction programme. *Public Health Nutrition*, **15** (2), 254–261.

Zlatevska, N., Dubelaar, C. and Holden, S.S. (2014) Sizing up the effect of portion size on consumption: a meta-analytic review. *Journal of Marketing*, **78** (3), 140–154.

Part Five

Public Health Nutrition Strategies and Approaches

25

Global and National Public Health Nutrition Approaches

Francesco Branca[1] and Cassandra H Ellis

Key messages

- Malnutrition is an imbalance in energy, protein and/or other nutrient intake and is used to refer to both undernutrition and overweight, although it is more commonly associated with undernutrition.
- Most countries are affected by multiple nutrition challenges. This is commonly referred to as the multiple burden of malnutrition.
- Malnutrition is multifactorial. A sustainable solution requires a multisectorial approach with an understanding of the scope of the problem, why it needs tackling and how each sector can play a role in combating malnutrition.
- There has been a global shift from communicable to non-communicable disease in the past 30 years, with cardiovascular diseases

accounting for the greatest number of deaths from non-communicable disease.
- Public policies are needed to address the causal factors leading to malnutrition. Civil society can also play an important role. A suitable accountability mechanism needs to be put in place.
- Through global actions plans and targets, progress is being made to reduce malnutrition, although progress is not consistent and rates are still disproportionately high in sub-Saharan Africa and parts of Asia.

25.1 Introduction

The focus of global public health nutrition is to prevent disease, promote well-being and protect health, which is not solely remaining disease free. The World Health Organization (WHO) describes health as 'a state of complete physical, mental and social well-being, and not merely the absence of disease or infirmity'. To achieve this, good nutrition is vital. However, poverty, drought, wars or political agendas can affect access to enough safe, nutritious food to fulfil individual requirements. At the other end of the scale, access to food 24/7, a shift towards knowledge-based economies and food becoming a cheap commodity can lead to overweight and its related comorbidities (see Chapters 23 and 24 for more information on the impact of the environment on health).

Malnutrition refers to both undernutrition and overweight, and can be considered as an imbalance in energy,

protein and/or other nutrient intake. Undernutrition can take the form of stunting, a reduction in linear growth of children, and wasting, having lower than normal weigh for height. A diet deficient in vitamins or minerals can also cause micronutrient malnutrition, or 'hidden hunger'.

Both undernutrition and overweight have an impact on population health and are a strain on health-care systems. Most countries are affected by a combination of nutrition challenges, previously referred to as the double burden of undernutrition and obesity or sometimes as the multiple burden of malnutrition, when we want to highlight the presence of micronutrient malnutrition.

Global nutrition frameworks are required to tackle malnutrition in all its forms. Global nutrition policies, strategic documents and target setting provide guidance for individual countries to create national policy to reduce the burden of non-communicable disease (NCD) using regionally relevant strategies. These

---

[1] *Disclaimer:* The named authors alone are responsible for the views expressed in this publication.

Public Health Nutrition, Second Edition. Edited by Judith L Buttriss, Ailsa A Welch, John M Kearney and Susan A Lanham-New.
© 2018 by The Nutrition Society. Published 2018 by John Wiley & Sons, Ltd.
Companion website: www.wiley.com/go/buttriss/publichealth

strategies and interventions must ensure they reach vulnerable groups such as the poor, malnourished and food insecure. Childhood malnutrition is of particular concern as it affects growth and ability to contribute to the community; therefore many intervention strategies and reduction targets focus on improving child malnutrition.

Organisations such as the WHO, the Food and Agriculture Organization of the United Nations (FAO) and United Nations Children's Fund (UNICEF) are involved in funding research, carrying out nutrition surveillance, policy implementation and target setting. Local government organisations are responsible for setting regional policy, implementation and monitoring.

25.2 The scope for global public health nutrition approaches: global nutrition challenges

Quantifying the burden of disease

In 1990, the Global Burden of Disease study provided the first comparative assessment of mortality at a global and national level, providing a comprehensive examination of the state of the world's health (Murray and Lopez, 1996) – see http://www.who.int/healthinfo/global_ burden_disease/publications/en/for links to more recent Global Burden of Disease reports. Analysis of the global burden of disease identified childhood underweight as the leading factor of death and disability; maternal and child undernutrition contributed to 11% of the global burden of disease. The international community acknowledged this scandalous primacy and included a goal to eradicate extreme hunger and poverty in the 2000 Millennium Declaration (United Nations General Assembly, 2000). More specifically, the target was to halve the proportion of people who suffer from hunger between 1990 and 2015; the prevalence of underweight children under 5 years of age was selected as an indicator.

By 2010, childhood undernutrition had dropped to eighth in the most important factors contributing to the burden of death and disability. However, it remained the main contributor in sub-Saharan Africa. Globally, the death toll attributable to maternal and child undernutrition had decreased to 6.7% of the global burden of disease and accounted for 1 400 000 deaths. Rates continued to decrease, and by 2015 there were 156 million children under the age of 5 years classed as stunted and 50 million had acute malnutrition. Conversely, 42 million were overweight or obese (UNICEF–WHO–The World Bank, 2016).

By 2015, despite remarkable progress all over the world, the leading risks contributing to NCD still varied greatly by region. The 1990 malnutrition reduction target had not been achieved in sub-Saharan Africa (32% stunting rate) and southern Asia (25% stunting rate), and global childhood overweight rates had risen by 10 million cases. Additionally, nearly 2 billion adults aged 18 years and above were overweight (39% of the world adult population) and more than half a billion (13%) were obese (WHO, 2014a) (Figure 25.1).

Global risk of nutrition-related disease

Almost no country in the world is exempt from some form of malnutrition, and diet-related health conditions are still dominating the rank of the global health risk (WHO, 2009). In 2010, high blood pressure became the leading risk factor for poor health for the first time, with 1.7 million annual deaths from cardiovascular disease associated with high sodium intake alone. Other nutrition-related risk factors in the top 20 included high body mass index (BMI), high fasting blood glucose, high total cholesterol and dietary risk factors (diet low in fruits, vegetables, whole grains, nuts and n-3 fatty acids, and high in sodium).

To quantify this burden of disease, the WHO calculates disability-adjusted life years (DALYs). One DALY can be considered as 1 year of healthy life lost. The sum of these years lost across the population can be used to measure the gap between current health status and the ideal health situation (where the entire population lives to an advanced age, free of disease and disability). By 2012, ischaemic heart disease was the leading global risk, accounting for 6.0% of DALYs. High BMI accounted for 3.8% of DALYs (3.4 million deaths), while poor diet and physical inactivity accounted for 10% of DALYs. Three of the top six causes of DALYs related to coronary heart disease, showing a shift away from communicable disease, to NCD. Other nutrition deficiencies, such as vitamin A, zinc and iodine deficiency, rated lower, accounting for less than 0.8% DALYs each. However, micronutrient deficiencies are a particular concern for at-risk groups such as pregnant and lactating women and infants, as discussed in Chapter 10.

With an estimate that 90% of deaths from NCDs, under the age of 70 years old, could be prevented through lifestyle changes to reduce risk factors, the 66th World Health Assembly (WHA) endorsed the WHO Global Action Plan for the Prevention and Control of NCDs 2013–2020 (WHO, 2013a). This was created in parallel to the global nutrition targets (Box 25.1) to create a world free of the avoidable burden of NCDs. The Global Action Plan offered a paradigm shift by providing a road map and menu of policy options established through nine voluntary targets (including three diet-related targets). The *Global Status Report* (WHO, 2014a) provided an

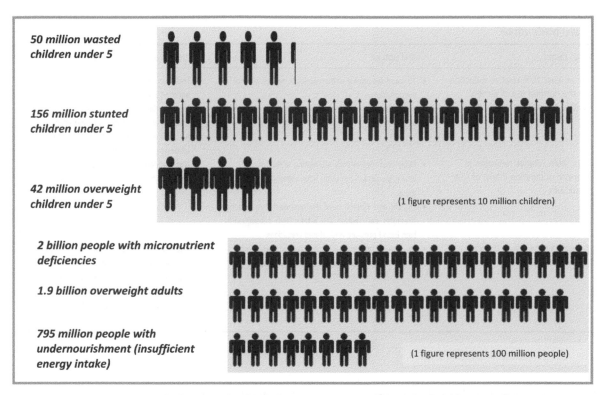

Figure 25.1   Global scale of different forms of malnutrition – Modified from IEG 2015 with data from WHO-UNICEF-World Bank 2016.

update on current NCD status focused on the nine voluntary targets. Uptake of the nutrition targets and the target measurement can be found in Table 25.1.

The *Global Nutrition Report* (UNICEF–WHO–World Bank, 2016) is a comprehensive report on all forms of malnutrition in all countries and measured progress of both sets of targets. The 2016 report takes a holistic approach to malnutrition, considering the roles of government, food systems, climate change and accountability. The report combined the global estimates on child malnutrition developed by WHO, UNICEF and the World Bank Group, 2016 with other sources and provided an overview on the global scale of malnutrition (Figure 25.1).

Box 25.1   Global nutrition targets set by the World Health Assembly in 2012

In response to the multiple burden of malnutrition, the WHA (their role is discussed in Section 25.3: 'The World Health Assembly') established six global nutrition targets to guide improvements of global nutrition by 2025, as part of a comprehensive implementation plan for maternal, infant and young child nutrition (WHO, 2014b).

Global target 1: A 40% reduction in the number of children under 5 years who are stunted by 2025; from 171 million estimated in 2010 to approximately 100 million by 2025.
Global target 2: A 50% reduction of anaemia in women of reproductive age by 2025; from 29.4% estimated in 2012 to 14.7% by 2025.
Global target 3: A 30% reduction of low birth weight by 2025; from a 2012 baseline of 15% to 10%.
Global target 4: No increase in childhood overweight by 2025, keeping global prevalence to 6.7%.
Global target 5: Increase exclusive breastfeeding rates in the first 6 months to at least 50% by 2025; from the 2006–2010 estimate of 37%.
Global target 6: Reduce childhood wasting to less than 5%; from the 8.6% estimate in 2010.

Progress data are collected on five of the six global nutrition targets (reduction in low birth weight not collected), but the availability of the data is uneven. In 2015, of the 74 countries which provided data, 70 were on track to meet at least one target. Kenya was the only country on track to meet all five targets. For a full breakdown of country progress, refer data from the Global Nutrition Report (Independent Expert Group, 2016).

Table 25.1 Voluntary nutrition targets, measurements and uptake of the *Global Action Plan for the Prevention and Control of Noncommunicable Diseases* (WHO, 2013a).

Global target	Global uptake	Target measurements
Two: at least 10% relative reduction in the harmful use of alcohol within the national context.	• 76 countries have a written policy to reduce alcohol consumption. • 160 countries have age limits imposed on buying alcohol.	• Total alcohol consumption per capita (in people aged ≥15 years). • Age-standardised prevalence of heavy episodic drinking among adolescents and adults. • Alcohol-related morbidity and mortality among adolescents and adults.
Four: 30% relative reduction in mean population intake of salt/ sodium.	• Many countries already attempting to reduce salt intake, particularly through reformation of processed foods. • The UK and Finland have demonstrated that national strategies can reduce salt intake and, subsequently, high blood pressure and related conditions.	• Age-standardised mean population intake of salt (sodium chloride), in grams per person per day.
Seven: halt the rise in diabetes and obesity.	• No data on progress so far, but agreed that obesity must be targeted through a multisectorial approach.	• Age-standardised prevalence of raised blood glucose/diabetes in adults. • Age-standardised prevalence of overweight and obesity in adults. • Prevalence of overweight and obesity in adolescents.

25.3 Global policy fora discussing public health nutrition

To address nutrition challenges, multiple sectors must be coherently developing policies that are explicitly aimed at improving people's nutritional status. The terms 'nutrition sensitive' and 'nutrition driven' have been used to indicate these programmes which help scale up nutrition-specific policies and interventions. Action is required in all sectors, particularly across the food system. Collaborative approaches from production to consumer are needed, including education, social protection and environmental policy (as outlined in Chapter 24). The engagement of multiple actors in addition to governments has been considered a necessary step to ensure full alignment of the resources to improve nutrition. This must include civil society, academia and the private and not for profit sectors.

At global level, formal discussions of nutrition priorities and policies have taken place in three member state bodies, the WHA, the Committee for Food Security and the United Nations General Assembly (UNGA). The greatest level of integration and the broadest scope was achieved with the Second International Conference on Nutrition (ICN2) held in 2014 (discussed in detail within: 'Shifting the focus to noncommunicable disease').

The World Health Assembly

The WHA is the highest body discussing health matters. It meets annually in Geneva to discuss major public health issues, make global health policy decisions and guide the work of the WHO. The WHA makes formal decisions or 'resolutions'. The first meeting of the WHA was in 1948 and had 55 member states. In 2016, the WHA held its 69th Assembly and had grown to 194 member states.

Nutrition has been a concern of the WHA since its very beginning, with concerns focused on severe acute malnutrition in the early years. In 1949 the WHA called for the establishment of national nutrition committees, in collaboration with the WHO and FAO (Resolution WHA 2.13). More than 20 years later, the WHA discussed the outcomes of the World Food Conference (Resolution WHA 28.42), which also focused on eradicating malnutrition, declaring every man, woman and child had the right to be free from hunger. At that time, the WHA recognised the importance of good infant and child nutrition and identified that the global decline in breastfeeding rates worldwide was, in part, due to the aggressive marketing of infant formula, particularly in developing countries. As a response, the WHA adopted The International Code of Marketing Breast-milk Substitutes under Resolution 34.22 in 1981.

In addition to the code, other WHA highlights are the endorsement of the WHO/UNICEF (2003) *Global*

Box 25.2 The infant and young child feeding strategy

The infant and young child feeding strategy was jointly developed by the WHO and UNICEF with the aim of improving infant nutrition, health and growth through optimal feeding practices (WHO/UNICEF, 2003). The strategy is based on scientific and epidemiological evidence and is intended as a guide for action on feeding practices. It provides guidelines for intervention, promotes best practice through supporting mothers and families, and outlines key stakeholders and accountable organisations.

As well as reiterating the importance of good feeding practice, the strategy was designed to strengthen commitment to established initiatives, particularly the Code of Marketing of Breast-milk Substitutes (1981), the Innocenti Declaration on the Protection, Promotion and Support of Breastfeeding (1990), and the Baby Friendly Hospital Initiative (1991). It aims to build upon these, emphasising the need for comprehensive guidelines to promote and support appropriate infant feeding, promote exclusive breast feeding for 6 months and improve complementary feeding practise with support for using local foods, food fortification and micronutrient supplementation, while protecting breastfeeding from commercial influences.

In particular, it highlights the importance of feeding infants and young children in difficult circumstances, such as HIV, malnutrition or emergency situations. It emphasises the role of health services engagement, pre-service education and in-service training to maximise skills during difficult situations.

The strategy outlines interventions to promote and support infant and child feeding, highlighting the importance of investing in this area to ensure children develop to their full potential. It provides 'governments and society's other main agents with both a valuable opportunity and a practical instrument for rededicating themselves, individually and collectively, to protecting, promoting and supporting safe and adequate feeding for infants and young children'.

Strategy on Infant and Young Child Feeding (Box 25.2), and the endorsement of the *Comprehensive Implementation Plan on Maternal, Infant and Young Child Nutrition* (WHO, 2014b) (Box 25.3). The latter includes the addition of maternal nutrition and focuses on a life-course approach. It also establishes the six global nutrition targets (Box 25.1), providing a more comprehensive scope to nutrition policies. The implementation plan expanded and updated previous policy documents on infant and young child nutrition and complemented the diet and physical activity strategy (DPAS) (WHO, 2004) that had been developed specifically to address diet-related NCDs. The implementation plan flagged the importance of addressing nutrition in sectors other than health. It considered agriculture and food production, trade, education and information, labour and social protection, and the environment, recommending that other policy fora involving those sectors be engaged to make recommendations.

In 2016, the WHA discussed recommendations on marketing complementary foods, recognising that the inappropriate promotion of baby foods favours the establishment of unhealthy diets in the early years of life. A second related area of interest has been micronutrient malnutrition, and particularly iodine deficiency disorders and vitamin A deficiency (as discussed in Chapter 9).

The WHA is also a forum for integration of related health agendas. Policy discussions on maternal and infant nutrition have influenced health and social policies directed to women and children. The global strategy for women's, children's and adolescents health (2016–2030) gives greater attention to nutrition interventions (Box 25.4).

Box 25.3 WHA's *Comprehensive Implementation Plan on Maternal Infant and Young Child Nutrition*

The WHA's Comprehensive Implementation Plan on Maternal Infant and Young Child Nutrition (WHO, 2014b) provides guidance on how to design national nutrition policies and recommends to:

1 create a supportive environment for the implementation of comprehensive nutrition policies;
2 include all effective health interventions in national nutrition plans;
3 stimulate development policies and programmes outside the health sector that recognise and include nutrition;
4 provide sufficient human and financial resources for the implementation of nutrition interventions;
5 monitor and evaluate the implementation of policies and programmes.

Effective nutrition interventions during the life course have been evaluated by *The Lancet* series on maternal and child undernutrition (*Lancet*, 2008, 2013). The WHO is continuously reviewing the evidence on direct nutrition interventions and has been developing guidelines on effective programmes to achieve nutrition outcomes. The WHO has also established the e-Library of Evidence of Nutrition Actions (eLENA) that includes all researched interventions and the underlying evidence (discussed in detail in Section 25.5).

Box 25.4 Case study: the human rights approach

'No woman, child or adolescent should face a greater risk of preventable death because of where they live or who they are' (United Nations Secretary-General, Ban Ki-moon).

The Every Woman Every Child strategy (http://www.everywomaneverychild.org/) was launched in 2010 during the UN Millennium Development Goals summit. It is a unique global movement putting into action the Global Strategy for Women's, Children's and Adolescents' Health. The strategy sets out a vision for every women, child and adolescent to realise their right to health and to be able to fully contribute to thriving, sustainable societies by 2030. It calls for national and international action by governments, the private sector and civil society to address the health challenges facing women, children and adolescents globally.

There are three overarching objectives of the strategy: (1) survive by ending preventable deaths; (2) thrive through ensuring health and well-being; (3) transform through enabling environments.

The health of these vulnerable groups is viewed as critical to human development and progress; therefore, the strategy aims to provide the opportunity to improve their health, and consequently the lives, of all people. This provides a high return on national investment with the strategy directly impacting the attainment of the Sustainable Development Goals.

At a regional level there are many documents reflecting local priorities, but all must be substantially aligned to global strategies and the Sustainable Development Goals. A recent paper in the British Medical Journal (Temmerman *et al.*, 2015) highlighted important gains since the launch of the Every Women Every Child strategy whilst suggesting that the human rights based approach should underpin any future government strategy to ensure continued progress.

The global strategy for women's, children's and adolescents' health has now aligned its time frame and vision with that of the Sustainable Development Goals (2016–2030) (https://sustainabledevelopment.un.org/?menu=1300).

Shifting the focus to non-communicable disease

In recognition of the increasing burden of NCDs, DPAS (WHO, 2004) was endorsed by WHA in 2004. DPAS addresses the two main risk factors of NCDs (i.e. diet and physical activity) and made the following recommendations:

- to reduce trans fatty acids and salt;
- to restrict availability of energy dense foods and high calorie non-alcoholic beverages;
- to increase availability of healthier foods including fruits and vegetables.

The DPAS indicated the following policy priorities:

- to practice responsible marketing of unhealthy foods to children;
- to make healthy options available and affordable;
- to provide simple, clear and consistent food labels that are consumer friendly;
- to reshape industry to introduce new products with improved nutritional value;
- to make physical activity accessible in all settings.

A follow-up to DPAS was the approval of a WHO set of recommendations on marketing foods and beverages to children, aimed to guide efforts in designing, and/or strengthening, existing policies on food marketing to children in order to reduce the impact of marketing foods high in saturated fats, trans-fatty acids, free sugars or salt.

The WHA has been discussing broader nutrition policy issues since the First International Conference on Nutrition in 1992 when it endorsed the World Declaration and Plan of Action for Nutrition. They urged its implementation, particularly by incorporating nutrition objectives in national development programmes. In 2015, the WHA endorsed the outcome of the ICN2 and called for the implementation of food and nutrition policies across the health sector, the food system, education and the environment. The acknowledgement of the intersectoral nature of public health nutrition challenged the WHA to establish connections with other sectoral nutrition fora such as the Committee for Food Security.

In 2016, the WHA discussed the Commission on Ending Childhood Obesity (WHO, 2016). The commission was established to guide the WHO response to the obesity epidemic and recommended a suite of interventions to effectively prevent and treat childhood and adolescent obesity. The commission promotes healthy foods, discourages unhealthy eating and promotes physical activity to fight sedentary habits. The commission also called for appropriate guidance on obesity and NCD prevention in preconception and antenatal care, and the provision of family-based, multicomponent, lifestyle weight management services for children and young people who are obese.

The Committee for Food Security

In 1974, the Committee on World Food Security (CFS) (http://www.fao.org/cfs/en/) was established in the United Nations (UN) system recognising the need for an intergovernmental body to review food security policies. Hosted by the FAO, the CFS was later reformed in

2009 to maximise stakeholder input. The vision of the reformed CFS was to be an international inter-governmental platform for all stakeholders to work together to ensure food security and nutrition for all. The High Level Panel of Experts on Food Security and Nutrition (HLPE) was created to provide independent, evidence-based analysis and advice. The findings from the HLPE are used as the basis for CFS policy discussion.

The CFS reform document states that 'CFS strives for a world free from hunger where countries implement the voluntary guidelines for the progressive realisation of the right to adequate food in the context of national food security' and that CFS 'constitutes the foremost inclusive international and intergovernmental platform for a broad range of committed stakeholders to work together in a coordinated manner and in support of country-led processes towards the elimination of hunger and ensuring food security and nutrition for all human beings'. The landmark document agreed by the reformed CFS was the *Global Strategic Framework for Food Security & Nutrition (GSF)* (Committee for World Food Security, 2013) – see Box 25.5.

In 2015, a work stream on nutrition was established. The CFS will work as a forum for policy convergence work on nutrition and food systems, aiming to: formulate policy recommendations, international strategies, voluntary guidelines, principles and other policy frameworks; share lessons and good practices that are relevant to CFS work on nutrition and food systems; report on the implementation of the ICN2 recommendations for sustainable food systems promoting healthy diets; raise awareness of CFS stakeholders in nutrition. In addition, CFS is committed to include a nutrition lens in other policies, such as the GSF.

CFS is also recognising the need for multisectoral collaboration on nutrition, to bring agriculture, food security, nutrition and health together and is working towards the establishment of a two-way communication between CFS and WHO/FAO. Good governance and coordination between stakeholders are key requisites in the fight against hunger and malnutrition. This should be through strategies, programmes, policies and funding with cross-sectorial government support to implement the right-to-food guidelines. Brazil have been pioneers in implementing the right to food through government and civil society collaboration (see Box 25.6).

The United Nations General Assembly

UNGA is the most important forum for inter-governmental policy discussions. While nutrition issues have not been prominent in the plenary discussions, they have been considered in the Convention of the Right of the Child (A/RES/44/25), in the United

---

Box 25.5 *The Global Strategic Framework for Food Security & Nutrition (GSF)*

The GSF was created as an overarching framework and reference document in response to rising hunger and unconnected governance on nutrition and food security around the world (Committee for World Food Security, 2013). The GSF was initiated by the CFS to provide guidance, strategy and action on nutrition policy. The focus of the GSF is the importance of coherence across all sectors which have an impact on food security.

The GSF looks to strengthen coordination between a wide range of stakeholders to improve global food security. Serving as a reference document to guide countries to improve nutrition, the GSF is described as a 'living document' which is flexible and can be adjusted as priorities change. The framework emphasises the role of country ownership and the responsibility of individual governments in combating food security and malnutrition. It serves as an essential tool for policy makers and stakeholders involved in nutrition and food security at a global, regional and country level.

When creating the GSF, all prior recommendations and frameworks were considered to reflect the current state of the evidence based on cross-country consensus (with input from CFS stakeholders).

The GSF uses a twin-track approach which strives for a comprehensive approach to address food security and malnutrition. This approach consists of (a) direct action to immediately tackle hunger for the most vulnerable groups who are unable to meet food and nutrition requirements and (b) medium-/long-term actions to build resilience and address the root causes of hunger focusing on sustainable agricultural, food security, nutrition and rural development programmes, including the continued realisation of the right to adequate food. Linkages between the tracks is vital to connect the immediate and long term interventions. For example, social protection can form the bridge between humanitarian aid in crisis and long-term investment into infrastructure.

The framework highlights the importance of investing in small-scale food producers, as these play a central role in feeding the community. It pays particular attention to the role of women food producers who need specific policies and support. This includes actions to increase food production and availability using coordinated approaches to reducing price volatility, as this has a greater effect on high-risk groups.

Action must be taken to improve nutrition. Measures should be taken to strengthen dietary diversity and improve healthy eating, ensuring access to food does not negatively affect intake and dietary composition. These nutrition interventions should include education, labelling and information involving all relevant stakeholders. The nutritional needs of vulnerable groups must be addressed. Breastfeeding should be encouraged and promoted in line with the International Code of Marketing of Breast-milk Substitutes (see Section 25.3: 'The World Health Assembly').

Box 25.6 Brazil – Zero Hunger (Fome Zero): a government and civil society collaborative success story

In 2002, as part of his inauguration speech, Brazilian President Luis Inacio Lula de Silva, declared he would eradicate hunger and poverty in Brazil. In 2003, at a time when 40% of the population reported food insecurity, the Zero Hunger strategy was implemented (da Silva *et al.*, 2011). The aim of the strategy was to tackle food and nutrition insecurity across Brazil's 11 million poor families. As part of the strategy, the National Council on Food and Nutrition Security (CONSEA) was established as an advisory board to the president, to develop policies and strategies to guarantee the right to food. The board, chaired by a civil society representative, comprised two-thirds civil society and one-third government officials.

Through a combination of government funding and community-based interventions, Zero Hunger has taken 14 million Brazilians out of extreme poverty and Brazil achieved the Millennium Development Goal target of reducing hunger by half, well before the 2015 deadline. Individuals have been empowered through training, community engagement, social inclusion and price regulation. Governments were made accountable for the right to food.

Taking the human rights perspective, Zero Hunger successfully implemented 52 programmes, including:

- Bolsa Familia – a family allowance system.
- National School Feeding Programme – uses local small-scale farming to provide 47 million children with school meals.
- Support for small-scale food producers – based on credit, insurance and technical support.
- Food acquisition programme – for family farmed products.

In 2009, the National School Feeding Programme was passed as law. In 2010, the right to food was included in the constitution as a basic human right. By 2011, decentralised CONSEAs had been formed in all of Brazil's 27 states responsible for establishing guidelines for implementing the National Policy on Food and Nutrition Security. Owing to its widespread success, Zero Hunger has provided a conceptual framework for initiatives throughout the rest of Latin America, Asia and Africa.

Nations Millennium Declaration (A/RES/55/2), in the Political Declaration of the High-level Meeting of the General Assembly on the Prevention and Control of Non-communicable Diseases (A/RES/66/2), and most recently in the 2030 Agenda for Sustainable Development (https://sustainabledevelopment.un.org/?menu=1300) (A/70/L1).

In 2015, UNGA approved the 2030 Agenda for Sustainable Development: a plan of action for people, the planet and for prosperity. Nutrition appears as a powerful driver of sustainable development. It is explicitly mentioned in the second goal to 'end hunger, achieve food security and improved nutrition, and promote sustainable agriculture'. Nutrition also has a role to play in achieving other goals of the 2030 Agenda for Sustainable Development, such as the goals related to poverty, health, education, gender, work, growth, inequality and climate change. To achieve the good health and well-being goal, good nutrition throughout the life course is needed, particularly to reduce maternal mortality, end newborn and child mortality, and end premature mortality from NCD. Optimum nutrition is required to achieve social development (particularly education and gender equality) and economic development goals (particularly labour force and productivity). Improved eating patterns would also allow substantial environmental benefits, through sustainable and climate smart food production. Furthermore, nationally appropriate social protection systems (Target 1.3) would benefit nutrition. Overall, the 2030 Agenda for Sustainable

Development looks to end malnutrition, address nutritional needs throughout the life course and provide access to safe, healthy and sustainable food.

Food security matters have been discussed in the Economic and Financial Committee. The 2014 report of the Secretary General of the UN on agriculture development, food security and nutrition highlighted the double burden of malnutrition and called for the need to address the different dimensions of malnutrition. In 2015, the UNGA has endorsed the International Conference on Nutrition outcomes and in 2016 the UNGA declared a decade of action on nutrition. This effectively has created a new multisectoral Forum on public health nutrition.

The Second International Conference on Nutrition (ICN2)

Recognising the need for collaborative, multisectoral approaches, the WHO and FAO convened the ICN2 in 2014. Building on the 1992 International Conference on Nutrition which focused efforts on reducing hunger, malnutrition and micronutrient deficiency, ICN2 recognised the new dimension to malnutrition: obesity and diet-related NCDs. World leaders made commitments to tackle malnutrition in all its forms and committed to fix the global food system so everyone has access to safe, healthy and affordable diets.

The Rome Declaration (FAO and WHO, 2014) was the outcome document of ICN2. The declaration considers the 'broken' food system. It reviews the challenges of providing food security for a growing population whilst recognising the complexity of malnutrition. The document sets out a vision for 'a world with coherent policies to promote a diversified, balanced and healthy diet at all stages of life, with national health systems integrating nutrition, coordinated action among different actors and sectors, empowerment of consumers, and policies that pay special attention to women'.

In particular, the Rome Declaration recommends a set of policy and programme options designed to create an enabling environment to improve nutrition. These options cut across all sectors, including sustainable food systems, international trade and investment, nutrition education, sanitation and accountability. Members of FAO and WHO have committed themselves, inter alia, to the following commitments:

- to increase investments for effective interventions and actions to improve diets;
- to develop coherent policies from production to consumption and across relevant sectors to provide year-round access to food that meets nutrition requirements;
- to raise the profile of nutrition within relevant national strategies, policies, action plans and programmes, and align resources accordingly;
- to strengthen human and institutional capacities to address all forms of malnutrition;
- to strengthen and facilitate contributions by all stakeholders to improve nutrition and promote collaboration within and across countries;
- to develop policies, programmes and initiatives for ensuring healthy diets throughout the life course;
- to empower people to make informed choices about food products for healthy dietary practices and appropriate infant and child feeding practices;
- to implement the commitments through the Framework for Action, a set of voluntary policy and strategy options to create an enabling environment to improve nutrition.

The United Nations Conference on Climate Change

The UN Conference on Climate Change (COP21), in 2015, presented an opportunity for those involved in nutrition and climate change to work together to advance their overlapping agendas. The Paris Agreement recognised the priority of safeguarding food security and ending hunger, and the vulnerabilities of food production systems to the adverse impacts of climate change. It called for the adoption of measures to reduce greenhouse gas emissions in a manner that does not jeopardise food production. The agreement highlighted the importance of the co-benefits of mitigation actions for adaptation, health and sustainable development. However, no clear mention was made in the agreement on the need to modify the diet to reduce the impact on environment.

25.4 Role of non-government actors in nutrition

The implementation of such complex agendas spanning several sectors requires the engagement of other actors as well as governments. Such actors may act in the interest of specific groups they represent or in public interest. However, whilst there is general recognition that there is a need for multi-stakeholder engagement, the nature of these specific roles is highly controversial.

The private sector has a primary responsibility for the food that reaches our tables, but there are several actors in the food system: primary producers – farmers, fishermen, livestock farmers; food manufacturers; food distributors; and food retailers. Political choices and investments at each stage of the food system affects availability, cost and product appeal to consumers. Consumer demand is not only linked to personal preference, it is heavily influenced by commercial variables and expectation of profit by company shareholders. For example, highly processed products are better suited to a global food system and allow greater financial returns. Additionally, standardised products sold in large fast food chains can be better marketed and have greater taste and quality control. Trade liberalisation has been associated with an increase in the risk of nutrition-related NCDs, as large multinationals have seen major financial returns in expanding their markets to low- and middle-income countries. (Stuckler et al., 2012).

In the past, food manufacturers and distributors have paid more attention to the safety of products, in part due to regulations, although more recently the potential positive or negative health impacts of food have focused more on nutrient composition. The concept of 'functional' food – that is, a food that can improve physiological function or even protect from disease – has been the focus of considerable industry interest, supported by legislation (e.g. in Europe) that is recognising the right to make claims over those characteristics. Food manufacturers and distributors have been responding to consumer requests for products containing less sugar, fat and salt by reformulating products. The reformulation of food products has been encouraged by public policies, introducing taxation and/or warning consumers through colour-coded labels on products which are high in fat, sugar and salt (see Chapter 24). Food manufacturers can also influence food habits by redesigning portion sizes and providing information to consumers on the product packs. The nutrition labelling of products, including nutrients to be included, the position on the pack and the reference to population needs (e.g. through the use of colour codes) is broadly debated and considered by the regulation of Codex Alimentarius (see Chapter 5 for more information).

In some instances, food companies have offered to provide nutrition education to consumers or support government initiatives to address malnutrition through corporate social responsibility schemes. However, these approaches have been criticised as giving rise to conflicts of interest.

Civil society can perform an important role in improving nutrition in a variety of roles. They represent citizens in policy dialogue, advocate for the establishment of policies and programmes, monitor the commitments of policy makers and other actors and assist governments in the delivery of services. Public-interest non-governmental organisations include organisations defending consumers' rights, organisations protecting human rights and international aid organisations.

Whilst the 2030 Sustainable Development Agenda calls for collaboration across all actors in society, the establishment of partnerships was also characteristic of the Millennium Development Goals. To achieve Millennium Development Goals to reduce child mortality and improve maternal health, The Partnership on Maternal, Newborns and Child Health was established as an alliance of more than 720 member organisations, across seven constituencies: academic, research and teaching institutions; donors and foundations; health-care professionals' associations; multilateral organisations; non-governmental organisations; partner countries; and the private sector.

In nutrition, an example is that of the Scaling Up Nutrition (SUN) movement (http://scalingupnutrition.org/). The SUN movement was launched in September 2010. SUN brings together representatives from governments, civil society, the UN, donors, businesses and researchers with a core focus on empowering women. SUN countries are collectively aiming to reach the WHA global targets. Countries joining are asked to commit to nutrition at the highest political level through four strategic processes: (a) sustained political commitment and establishment of functioning multistakeholder platforms; (b) endorsement of national nutrition policies that incorporate best practices; (c) alignment of actions across sectors and among stakeholders through high-quality and well-costed country plans based on agreed results frameworks; (d) increased resources for nutrition and demonstration of results. In December 2016, 57 countries were members of the SUN movement.

25.5 Effective policies and effective interventions

The World Health Organization guideline process

Nutrition interventions are vital for addressing nutritional challenges at a population and individual level. Interventions focus on high-risk groups and major areas of concern, and include health promotion and disease prevention. One of the WHO core functions is the development of global guidelines for nutrition intervention. This is a rigorous process which ensures guidelines are based on scientific evidence. To ensure transparency of development and best practice, the WHO have created the *WHO Handbook for Guideline Development* (WHO, 2012), which considers internal and external stakeholders, regular review throughout the planning stage and a public call for input (Figure 25.2).

The global guidelines produced by the WHO to inform the guidance on how local policy can improve nutritional status throughout the life cycle provide a framework for country-specific policies to be developed and implemented. To disseminate these guidelines, eLENA (http://www.who.int/elena/about/guidelines_ process/en/) was created as a single point of reference. This provides a suite of nutrition actions alongside the latest recommendations, scientific evidence and expert commentary. eLENA aims to support countries in implementing nutrition interventions, guide local policy development and inform programme design.

When creating guidelines, the WHO adopts the life-cycle approach. This recognises the unique nutritional needs of individuals at varying stages: from conception to infancy, childhood to adulthood and through to old age. Each stage has different nutrition requirements. To address these stages, in particular the key development stages, the WHO has created over 150 nutrition actions, divided into key life stages, of evidence-based guidelines to inform local nutritional intervention.

The implementation of successful interventions

A successful intervention must address the multiple burden of malnutrition, and caution must be taken not to replace one burden with another. An effective intervention should be multilevel, reaching vulnerable populations by providing adequate food environment, education, promotion and social welfare support. Throughout all stages of planning, implementation and evaluation, there must be accountability across

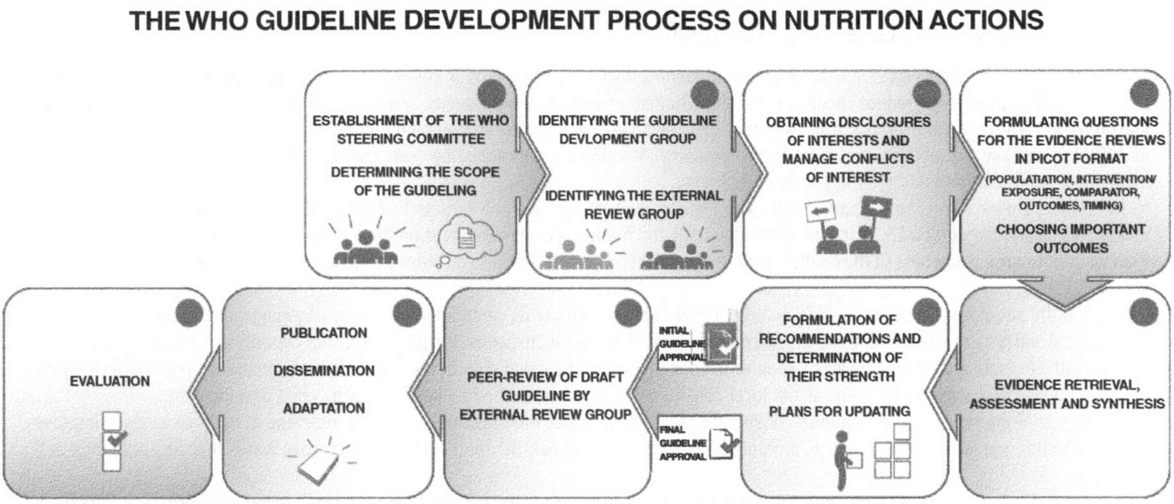

THE WHO GUIDELINE DEVELOPMENT PROCESS ON NUTRITION ACTIONS

Figure 25.2 Overview of the WHO guideline development process. Taken from: Zamora *et al.* (2015).

all levels. The following considerations need to be made:

1. Risk groups must be identified – who is at risk, where do they live, what are the determinants of the risk, how many people are affected and what are the causes. The correct type of intervention must be identified to promote health and prevent disease. Which intervention will best affect change and reach the target population.
2. Cost–benefit analysis must be undertaken through systematic analysis of the strengths and weaknesses of the intervention, ensuring that the benefit of any given intervention is greater than the cost. Economic modelling should also be used to inform planning decisions.
3. Key stakeholders must be identified during the planning process. A good intervention should be multi-factorial and engage multilevel stakeholders to ensure it reaches vulnerable populations (i.e. farmers), distributers, commerce, health practitioners and the local community through education and promotion. See Box 25.7 for an example of a successful intervention with multifactorial stakeholder collaboration.
4. Community engagement is key. On a local level, cultural sensitivities must be taken into consideration and interventions must align with cultural values.
5. Once implemented, ongoing promotion and communication are key to maximise engagement.
6. When setting interventions and programmes, evaluation methods must be built in using systematic processes to monitor efficacy. There must be scope to modify the intervention where necessary.

7. Programmes should be effective in the long term and must not cause harm.
8. Where appropriate, successful interventions can be translated into national policy and legislation (see Box 25.6 on the Zero Hunger policy in Brazil).

25.6 Developing national nutrition policies and programmes

Whilst global policy documents indicate priorities, decisions must be made nationally giving consideration of the epidemiological patterns, the country's political and administrative characteristics, as well as the existing capacities and the presence and commitment of national actors and development partners. Individual countries must be responsible for their own target and priority setting (see Box 25.8 for an example). Nutrition plans should consider direct interventions, usually delivered through the health sector, or nutrition sensitive interventions, delivered through agriculture and social protection.

In 2009–2010 the WHO conducted a global nutrition policy review (WHO, 2013) to which 119 member states responded. Most countries indicated they had established policies and programmes to tackle undernutrition, obesity and diet-related NCDs, infant and young child feeding and vitamin and mineral malnutrition. However, the review emphasised that policies were often not officially adopted, were of variable quality and did not have adequate budgets and resources. Often, policies were lacking operational plans and programmes of

Box 25.7 Intervention case study: The Healthy Growth Project

The Healthy Growth Project (http://www.who.int/nutrition/healthygrowthproj/en/) is a collaborative project coordinated by the WHO to promote healthy growth and reduce childhood stunting. Stunted growth and development causes a child to be short for their age and have impaired cognitive, motor and language development. This can have a large impact on the community, as children are at greater risk of obesity and disease and are less able to contribute to the economy. Stunting can be caused by poor maternal nutrition, poor feeding practices, inadequate sanitation and water supply or food insecurity.

The project's main aim is to support countries to implement stunting reduction targets to contribute to the achievement of the WHA stunting reduction target (Box 25.1). It aims to develop tools and frameworks to make stunting the primary measure on undernutrition rather than weight, to raise awareness about the relationship between stunting and NCD, and to increase understanding of the link with obesity in later life.

Because the aetiology of stunting is multifactorial, the project promotes cross-sectorial approaches, engaging stakeholders at a national, sub-national and grassroots level, encouraging accountability at all intervention stages. The project calls for capacity building and political will through infrastructure and policy implementation at the national level. The foundation of the project focuses on the importance of caregiver education and community engagement as the local community has been identified as key to healthy child development.

The project promotes global and national collaborations, using combined multifactorial actions to intervene at multiple levels to improve maternal health, improve feeding practice, promote healthy diets, strengthen the food system and improve water supplies, sanitation and hygiene.

To ensure efficacy, the project recommends setting goals and targets to allow for performance tracking. Regular monitoring is encouraged, and modifications should be made accordingly. Stakeholders should be regularly updated throughout the programme to ensure collaboration continues.

Box 25.8 *Recipe for a Healthier Diet*

An example of a multisectoral plan to improve diet is the *Recipe for a Healthier Diet*, an action plan developed by the Norwegian Government with a vision to improve public health through a healthy diet (Ministry of Health and Care Services, 2007). The plan aimed to help people choose healthy diets, facilitate good meals in kindergartens, schools and among the elderly, and increase knowledge about food, diet and nutrition.

The plan was a collaboration across 12 ministries (labour and social inclusion; children and equality; finances; health and human services; local government and regional development; culture and church affairs; agriculture and food; environment; trade and industry; fisheries and coastal affairs, education and research, foreign affairs).

Included in the plan were 73 measures across 10 key areas, including: communicating about food and diet; encouraging the production of healthy foods and meals; promoting the consumption of fruit and vegetables and fish; promoting good nutrition since birth; providing healthy meals in kindergartens, schools and the workplace; improving nutrition through health and social services; strengthening research and monitoring. The document also gave consideration to the administrative and financial implications as well as follow-up evaluation to continue to monitor dietary change.

The efficacy if the plan was evaluated by the WHO and a comprehensive report published (WHO, 2013c). The general findings were:

- The nutrition policy had increased knowledge of nutrition and health in the population.
- Dietary patterns had shifted with a reduction in fat intake and increased fruit and vegetable intake.
- Authorities viewed the plan as a supportive tool for initiating and implementing nutrition-related activities.
- Aggressive marketing campaigns of foods high in fat, salt and sugar are negatively impacting the diets of the younger generation.

Whilst the report acknowledges room for improvement in some areas, it highlights that the plan should be seen as an example of good practice in the application of the WHO Health 2020 policy framework.

work, were missing clear goals, targets, timelines or deliverables, did not specify roles and responsibilities, and did not envisage an evaluation. Second, the review identified challenges in governance. Many countries did not have intersectoral coordination mechanisms placed at a high level, such as a prime minister's or president's office, or a planning commission. Third, countries were not implementing a comprehensive package of interventions at different stages of the life course and not all eligible beneficiaries were reached. Furthermore, the quality of implementation was variable. Fourth, the human and financial resources were often inadequate. Fifth, the nutrition surveillance systems in place were insufficient in relation to the list of indicators, the level of disaggregation and the frequency of reporting.

To help improve nutrition policy development, the WHO has developed tools that may help formulating policies, such as the landscape analysis of stakeholders' commitment and capacity to scale up evidence-informed interventions (http://www.who.int/nutrition/landscape_analysis/en/), or the OneHealth tool (http://www.who.int/choice/onehealthtool/en/) to facilitate strategic planning through cost effectiveness analysis. The WHO has also established GINA, a global database on the implementation of nutrition actions (http://www.who.int/nutrition/gina/en/), which includes policy documents and implemented programmes from over 170 countries so that good practices can be better identified.

25.7 Conclusions

On 1 April 2016, UNGA adopted resolution 70/259 entitled 'United Nations Decade of Action on Nutrition (2016–2025)'. The UN has declared decades to call the international attention on major development topics since the 1970s, but only two are specifically named 'decades of action' (water and road safety) to highlight the determination to translate into concrete action the political commitment made. With the decade of action on nutrition there is an expectation that governments and other actors publicly announce which recommendations of the ICN2 they are going to implement and when, so that public accountability mechanisms could be built. This is an unprecedented opportunity for public health nutrition: the directions of change are clear and broadly accepted; there is an understanding of the broad range of sectors and actors needed; high-level commitments have been made and accountability mechanisms are in place. Public health leadership is necessary to ensure that serious change happens, for the sake of people's and the planet's health.

References

Committee for World Food Security (2013) *Global Strategic Framework for Food Security & Nutrition (GSF)*, version two. http://www.fao.org/fileadmin/templates/cfs/Docs1213/gsf/GSF_Version_2_EN.pdf (accessed 22 December 2016).

Da Silva, J.G., Del Grossi M.E. and de França, C.G. (eds) (2011) *The Fome Zero (Zero Hunger) Program: The Brazilian Experience*. Ministry of Agrarian Development, Brasília. http://www.fao.org/docrep/016/i3023e/i3023e.pdf (accessed 22 December 2016).

FAO and WHO (2014) *Rome Declaration on Nutrition*. http://www.fao.org/3/a-ml542e.pdf (accessed 22 December 2016).

Independent Expert Group (2016) *Global Nutrition Report 2015: Actions and Accountability to Advance Nutrition and Sustainable Development*. International Food Policy Research Institute, Washington, DC. http://ebrary.ifpri.org/utils/getfile/collection/p15738coll2/id/130354/filename/130565.pdf (accessed 22 December 2016).

Lancet (2008) Maternal and child undernutritionrrdrr. *The Lancetrrdrr*. http://wwwrrdrr.thelancetrrdrr.com/series/maternal-and-child-undernutrition (accessed 22 December 2016).

Lancet (2013) Maternal and child nutrition. *The Lancet*. http://www.thelancet.com/series/maternal-and-child-nutrition (accessed 22 December 2016).

Ministry of Health and Care Services (2007) *Recipe for a Healthier Diet. Norwegian Action Plan on Nutrition (2007–2011)*. https://www.regjeringen.no/globalassets/upload/hod/dokumenter-fha/sem/kostholdsplanen/is-0238-kortversjon-eng.pdf (accessed 22 December 2016).

Murray, C.J.L. and Lopez, A.D. (eds) (1996) *Global Burden of Disease: A Comprehensive Assessment of Mortality and Disability from Diseases, Injuries, and Risk Factors in 1990 and Projected to 2020*. The Global Burden of Disease and Injury 1. Harvard School of Public Health, Boston, MA.

Stuckler, D., McKee, M., Ebrahim, S. and Basu, S. (2012) Manufacturing epidemics: the role of global producers in increased consumption of unhealthy commodities including processed foods, alcohol, and tobacco. *PLoS Medicine*, **9** (6), e1001235.

Temmerman, M., Khosla, R., Bhutta, Z.A. and Bustreo, F. (2015) Towards a new global strategy for women's, children's and adolescents' health. *BMJ*, **351**, h4414.

UNICEF–WHO–The World Bank (2013) *2012 Joint Child Malnutrition Estimates – Levels and Trends*. http://www.who.int/nutrition/publications/jointchildmalnutrition_2016_estimates/en/ (accessed 22 December 2016).

UNICEF–WHO–World Bank Group (2015) *Levels and Trends in Child Malnutrition. UNICEF–WHO–World Bank Group Joint Child Malnutrition Estimates. Key Findings of the 2015 Edition*. UNICEF/WHO/World Bank, New York/Geneva/Washington, DC. http://www.who.int/nutgrowthdb/jme_brochure2015.pdf?ua=1 (accessed 22 December 2016).

United Nations General Assembly (2000) *Millennium Declaration*. http://www.un.org/en/development/devagenda/millennium.shtml (accessed 22 December 2016).

WHO (2004) *Global Strategy on Diet, Physical Activity and Health*. http://apps.who.int/iris/bitstream/10665/43035/1/9241592222_eng.pdf?ua= (accessed 10 January 2017).

WHO (2009) *Global Health Risks: Mortality and Burden of Disease Attributable to Selected Major Risks*. World Health Organization, Geneva. http://www.who.int/healthinfo/global_burden_disease/GlobalHealthRisks_report_full.pdf (accessed 22 December 2016).

WHO (2012) *WHO Handbook for Guideline Development*. World Health Organization, Geneva. http://apps.who.int/iris/bitstream/10665/75146/1/9789241548441_eng.pdf?ua=1 (accessed 22 December 2016).

WHO (2013a) *Global Action Plan for the Prevention and Control of Noncommunicable Diseases 2013–2020*. World Health Organization, Geneva. http://apps.who.int/iris/bitstream/10665/94384/1/9789241506236_eng.pdf (accessed 22 December 2016).

WHO (2013b) *Global Nutrition Policy Review: What Does It Take to Scale Up Nutrition Action?* World Health Organization, Geneva. http://apps.who.int/iris/bitstream/10665/84408/1/9789241505529_eng.pdf (accessed 22 December 2016).

WHO (2013c) *Evaluation of the Norwegian Nutrition Policy with a Focus on the Action Plan on Nutrition 2007–2011*. WHO Regional Office for Europe, Copenhagen. http://www.euro.who.int/__data/assets/pdf_file/0003/192882/Evaluation-of-the-Norwegian-nutrition-policy-with-a-focus-on-the-Action-Plan-on-Nutrition-20072011.pdf (accessed 22 December 2016).

WHO (2014a) *Global Status Report on Noncommunicable Diseases 2014*. World Health Organization, Geneva. http://apps.who.int/iris/bitstream/10665/148114/1/9789241564854_eng.pdf (accessed 22 December 2016).

WHO (2014b) *Comprehensive Implementation Plan on Maternal, Infant and Young Child Nutrition*. World Health Organization, Geneva. http://apps.who.int/iris/bitstream/10665/113048/1/

WHO_NMH_NHD_14.1_eng.pdf?ua=1 (accessed 22 December 2016).

WHO (2016) *Report of the Commission on Ending Childhood Obesity.* World Health Organisation Geneva. http://apps.who.int/iris/bitstream/10665/204176/1/9789241510066_eng.pdf (accessed 22 December 2016).

WHO/UNICEF (2003) *Global Strategy for Infant and Young Child Feeding.* World Health Organization, Geneva. http://apps.who.int/iris/bitstream/10665/42590/1/9241562218.pdf (accessed 22 December 2016).

Zamora, G., Meneses, D., De-Regil, L.M., Neufeld, L., Peña-Rosas, J.P. and Sinisterra, O. (2015) Consideraciones sobre el uso de las directrices de nutrición de la OMS para la implementación de intervenciones eficaces y seguras (Considerations on the development of the World Health Organization's nutrition guidelines and their implementation). *Archivos Latinoamericanos de Nutrición.* **65** (1), 1–11.

26
Developing Strategies in the Community

Janet E Cade, Charlotte EL Evans, and Jayne Hutchinson

Key messages

- Community dietary behaviour change interventions can be delivered through whole community actions or individual-level approaches, which could include personalised nutrition linked to genetic status.
- Levels of intervention range from regulation, eliminating choice through to 'nudging' behaviour.
- The Nuffield Bioethics ladder and a taxonomy of interventions are available to help explore different levels of intervention.
- Features of successful community interventions include community capacity building and advocacy.
- Features of successful individual interventions based on psychological theories include components related to improving self-efficacy: goal setting, self-monitoring and self-reinforcement.

- Measuring success can be achieved through randomised controlled trials; where this is not practical or possible, standard evaluation frameworks exist.
- The majority of dietary interventions are based on a 'one-size-fits all' approach. Nutritional genomics allows advice to be tailored to an individual.
- Personalised nutrition could be based on either genotype (which is the set of genes that a person carries) or phenotype (which is the individual's characteristics linked to their genotype and environment).

26.1 Introduction to the chapter

This chapter explores the different levels at which public health strategies aim to influence dietary behaviour that can be defined and developed within the community. This includes strategies at the group or population level, such as changes to the physical environment, including 'nudges', individual approaches (such as the use of social norms in weight loss programmes) and 'personalised' nutrition (which can take an individual's genetic predisposition into account).

26.2 Group or population approaches

Theory behind group strategies

Behaviour is affected by a multitude of factors, many of which can be described as environmental factors rather than those attributable to an individual. Dietary behaviour is no exception, and the Foresight map of factors affecting the risk of obesity (http://www.shiftn.com/

obesity/Full-Map.html) clearly demonstrates the many areas where we can intervene at a population level, such as in food production and the environment, to improve dietary intake and reduce risk of obesity and other important diet-related non-communicable diseases (NCDs).

The Nuffield Bioethics ladder (Figure 26.1) has been used to help policy makers consider the degree of intervention needed to ensure it is proportionate in terms of how much evidence is available, and weighed against the potential financial consequences and interference in people's lives. The ladder of intervention recognises that doing nothing is an active decision, and this is the first rung of the ladder. Eliminating choice is the highest rung and is reserved for policies where there is strong evidence that the interference is worth it on balance.

The concepts in the ladder have been further developed to support the design of public health initiatives and are linked to the degree to which the intervention will have an impact on the individual either consciously or unconsciously. A taxonomy of different types of

Public Health Nutrition, Second Edition. Edited by Judith L Buttriss, Ailsa A Welch, John M Kearney and Susan A Lanham-New.
© 2018 by The Nutrition Society. Published 2018 by John Wiley & Sons, Ltd.
Companion website: www.wiley.com/go/buttriss/publichealth

| Eliminate choice |
| Restrict choice |
| Guide choice by disincentives |
| Guide choice by incentives |
| Guide choice by changing the default policy |
| Enable choice |
| Provide information |
| Do nothing |

Figure 26.1 Nuffield Bioethics ladder of intervention.

intervention has been developed by the House of Lords, Science and Technology Select Committee; this has been adapted for public health dietary behaviour change interventions, shown in Table 26.1. This table has a range of options from regulation with elimination or restriction of choice at one end of the spectrum to choice architecture interventions including nudges at the other end.

A similar approach has been taken by the UK Health Forum, who identified six different areas for action when considering dietary behaviour change in relation to sugar reduction policies (Mwatsama and Landon, 2014). The six themes are set out in Table 26.2 and begin with producing and importing less, through to recommending less, and ultimately changing what we consume. Dietary factors associated with health outcomes where this type of intervention could be applied include the reduction of trans and saturated fats, free sugars, salt and alcohol. Complex interventions may tackle more than one of these areas of action, while other interventions focus on one particular area. Themes 1–4 concentrate on national policy, while community-based interventions target specific subgroups of the population and take place at a regional level. National policies can be mandatory (and therefore law) or can be voluntary. Change in national policy can only take place with consistent support across a wide range of stakeholders, including public support. Themes 5 and 6 relate more closely to individual approaches discussed later in this chapter.

National regulation

An example of where regulation has been introduced to improve dietary behaviour is the school meal system in England. New food and nutrient standards were introduced by law into all schools in England in 2006–2008 to reduce intake of poor-quality food such as fatty meats, fried foods and sweetened drinks, and to ensure children only had access to good quality food, including fruits and

Table 26.1 Taxonomy of different types of public health diet behaviour change interventions.

Intervention category	Regulation		Financial policies		Non-financial policies		Choice architecture including 'nudges' (environment in which choices are made)		
	Remove choice	Restrict choice	Disincentives	Incentives	Incentives and disincentives	Persuasion	Provision of information	Changes to physical environment	Use of social norms and salience
Example of policy interventions	Prohibiting goods or services (e.g. banning trans fats)	Restricting options available to individuals (e.g. only fruit for break at schools)	Making behaviour more costly (e.g. taxation of high-fat or -sugar foods)	Make behaviour financially beneficial (e.g. tax breaks on fruit and vegetables)	Reward or penalise behaviour (e.g. free bicycles for travel to work)	Persuade individuals (e.g. counselling services or marketing campaigns)	Providing information (e.g. leaflets; web sites; front of pack nutrition labelling; calorie information on menus)	Altering environment (e.g. removing confectionery from checkout aisles; restricting advertising of high-fat, -salt, -sugar foods)	Changing default option (e.g. providing salad as default side dish) Provide information about what others are doing (e.g. about own calorie intake compared with others)

Source: based on House of Lords Science and Technology Committee (2011: Table 1).

Table 26.2 Six potential areas for action for changing population diet.

Theme 1 Produce or import less	Theme 2 Use less	Theme 3 Sell less	Theme 4 Marketing codes	Theme 5 Recommend less	Theme 6 Eat less
Review market	Reformulation	Taxes	Marketing tax deductibility	Food-based dietary guidelines	Front of pack labelling
Health impact assessment	Substitution	Portion sizes	Health and nutrition claims	Social marketing campaigns	Health warnings
		In store promotions		Education	Menu labels

Source: based on Mwatsama and Landon (2014).

vegetables and low-fat dairy foods. Published surveys of lunchtime intake have reported improved intakes from school meals compared with intakes before standards were introduced, and also compared with packed lunches. A large survey of packed lunches reported that only 1% met the food-based standards introduced for school meals (Evans *et al.*, 2010).

Legal regulation is not always necessary. Sometimes voluntary codes of practice agreed within the food industry are sufficient to improve health, although these are often backed up with the threat of regulation if voluntary action is not sufficient. An example of this is the Responsibility Deal in England. This has worked successfully with reducing salt consumption by approximately 10% to date. Food manufacturing companies are encouraged to sign up to the Responsibility Deal pledges (https://responsibilitydeal.dh.gov.uk/). Many food manufacturers have signed up and have duly reformulated foods to reduce salt intake across a wide range of foods. Assessments of salt intake using 24-h urinary sodium measures by the national diet and nutrition surveys report that adult salt intakes reduced from 9.5 g in 2000–2001 to 8.6 g in 2008 across England (Wyness *et al.*, 2012). During the same period, blood pressure has also reduced across the country. Although these are promising results, the impact is likely to be smaller than if regulation had been introduced. Nevertheless, voluntary action can be a useful measure either on its own or as a prerequisite to regulation when more support is needed.

Disincentives at a national level

Recently, taxes on high-fat or -sugar foods have been introduced in different countries in order to change behaviour. In the USA, many states have instigated a 10 or 20% tax on sugar-sweetened beverages with an aim to reduce sales of drinks and ultimately to reduce obesity rates (http://www.uconnruddcenter.org/). In 2014, Mexico introduced a levy of 1peso per litre on sugary drinks, equivalent to a tax of approximately 10%.

Evaluation of the levy reported reductions in purchasing and consumption of sugary drinks but longer term evaluation is needed to measure reductions in prevalence of obesity (Colchero *et al.*, 2016). In 2016, the World Health Organization recommended that countries introduce a 20% sugar sweetened beverage tax to reduce consumption of sugary drinks and reduce risk of obesity and type 2 diabetes (http://www.who.int/dietphysicalactivity/publications/fiscal-policies-diet-prevention/en/) and this was followed by action from the British government. A levy on producers and importers is planned for April 2018 in the UK at two different levels; a lower levy for drinks exceeding 5g sugar per 100mls and a higher levy for drinks exceeding 8g sugar per 100mls (https://www.gov.uk/government/publications/soft-drinks-industry-levy). Australia is also considering the introduction of a tax on drinks. Further evaluations of these taxes are needed to clarify the impact of this type of intervention.

Nudging

The definition of nudging is 'any aspect of the choice architecture that alters people's behaviour in a predictable way without forbidding any options or significantly changing their economic incentives'. Improving healthier choices through nudging (as opposed to regulation) is a relatively new concept (Marteau *et al.*, 2011). Conversely, nudging people in other directions has been used by advertisers and retailers selling confectionery and snacks for many years; for example, the placement of confectionery in more accessible locations in supermarkets, such as checkouts or ends of aisles. Behaviour-change specialists realise that many of the decisions made that affect health are automatic decisions that use little cognitive capability and are more affected by the environment rather than conscious decisions. Buying the chocolate bar means that immediate pleasure wins over long-term weight loss goals. Nudging in the right direction has the potential to play a role in improving our health. If effective, it means that governments can regulate less. Nudging would be found on the Nuffield

Bioethics ladder on the 'change default setting' rung. For instance, this would include making stairs rather than the lift the obvious choice, or making the salad rather than chips the default choice on a menu. In addition, nudging can include providing information on others' healthy behaviour (social norm feedback) or peer modelling of the behaviour.

The environment is important, and it may be easier to nudge in the 'wrong' direction rather than nudging in the 'right' direction. For example, the immediate pleasure of a chocolate bar placed at the checkout compared with a special offer on fruit. However, there are some interventions where nudging has been reported to be effective. Examples include placing fruit instead of confectionary near the cash register and serving food on smaller plates and drinks in smaller cups to reduce portion size. There is very little research that has evaluated interventions using nudging techniques to date. It may still be necessary to use legislation in conjunction with nudging in order to reduce marketing to children or to ban confectionery from checkouts.

Role of public health nutritionists

Registered public health nutritionists (www.association fornutrition.org) can play a key role in planning public health programmes either through strategic long-term planning over several years or short-term project management. The aim of most programmes is to improve dietary quality and consequently risk of non-communicable disease in populations with the poorest diets, which is determined through a needs assessment. Public health nutritionists working at a national or regional level can be involved in introducing in new regions or populations established programmes that have already been developed and evaluated, such as the conversion of the NHS Expert Patient Programme specifically for people with diabetes, as well as development of new programmes.

Public health nutritionists are most likely to be involved at regional or community level rather than nationally. Interventions to change behaviour through changing the environment are increasingly complex, as it becomes clear that there are no easy solutions.

Group or population approaches to change dietary behaviour involve intervention at one or more different points that impact on the availability, accessibility or desirability of a particular dietary behaviour. Government programmes have mainly concentrated on providing information which is low on the ladder of intervention and has little impact. More sophisticated community programmes have intervened at a higher level, such as 'enabling choice' or even 'restricting choice', to increase the chances of improving dietary behaviour.

Developing strategies in the community

Public health strategies to improve dietary behaviour tend to be defined as complex interventions. The Medical Research Council has defined a complex intervention as having a range of interacting components. They may also have a number of behaviours targeted for change by those receiving the intervention. The components usually include behaviours, parameters of behaviours (e.g. frequency, timing), and methods of organising and delivering those behaviours (e.g. type(s) of practitioner, setting and location). It is not easy to precisely define the 'active ingredients' of a complex intervention. Some highly complex interventions, such as the Sure Start intervention, which supports families with young children in deprived communities, is built around a set of individually complex interventions. A summary of key elements of a complex intervention is shown in Box 26.1.

New interventions or programmes should be based on the most up to date available evidence and be tested initially using a pilot study before moving to a full experimental study. For large projects it is useful to have a health education planning model; many of these are available, but they are mostly US based (Edelstein, 2010). The National Institutes of Health in the USA has a useful resource on 'Making Health Communication Programs Work' (http://www.cancer.gov/pinkbook) which provides details of how planning models have been based in large programmes. Evaluation of new programmes is covered in Chapter 28.

Community programmes to improve nutritional behaviour in children

Community programmes targeting children are usually based around schools, and less commonly the home

---

Box 26.1 What makes an intervention complex?

- Number of interacting components within the experimental and control interventions.
- Number and difficulty of behaviours required by those delivering or receiving the intervention.
- Number of groups or organisational levels targeted by the intervention.
- Number and variability of outcomes.
- Degree of flexibility or tailoring of the intervention permitted.

Source: Craig *et al.* (2008).

environment. Attending school until late adolescence is a legal requirement for most countries, and therefore school-based research provides an opportunity to target a representative section of the population. Programmes aimed at children in low-income families focus on schools in more deprived areas of the country, usually in larger cities. Many school-based programmes have successfully improved dietary quality (as well as physical activity), but few programmes have reported a significant reduction in body mass index (BMI) – compared with control schools. In a Cochrane review (Waters *et al.*, 2011) it was reported that the most successful school-based programmes to reduce the risk of obesity were those that included the following components:

- a school curriculum that includes healthy eating, physical activity and body image;
- increased sessions for physical activity and the development of fundamental movement skills throughout the school week;
- improvements in nutritional quality of the food supply in schools;
- environments and cultural practices that support children eating healthier foods and being active throughout each day;
- support for teachers and other staff to implement health promotion strategies and activities (e.g. professional development, capacity building activities);
- parent support and home activities that encourage children to be more active, eat more nutritious foods and spend less time in screen-based activities.

The authors of the review recommended that these components should be 'embedded within health, education and care systems to achieve long term sustainable impacts'. The World Health Organization is active in encouraging schools to become health-promoting schools.

Community programmes to improve nutritional behaviour in adults

Development of community programmes targeting adults with the aim of reducing obesity is more diverse and more complex than for children. Unlike children, adults may attend a range of places during the day, including working at home. Groups of adults representative of the whole community are more difficult to locate easily for recruitment into programmes. Instead, community programmes are usually based around a workplace or a community centre with a sports, religious or social focus. Whereas most of the interventions in children aim to restrict or even eliminate the opportunities to choose poor-quality food (or not choose healthy food), the main aim of adult interventions is to facilitate healthy choices.

Interventions in the work place have been reviewed and conclude that worksite interventions achieve modest improvements in weight and BMI, in the region of 1.5 kg and $0.5 \, kg/m^2$ respectively (Anderson *et al.*, 2009). Most of the studies in the review included individual informational and behavioural strategies to change diet and physical activity. However, fewer studies in the review actually changed the work environment by improving the quality of food served in the cafeteria, reducing vending machines or increasing exercise facilities to help employees make healthy choices. Employers can offer vegetables or salad as the default in the canteen so that employees have to ask not to have the vegetables. Other actions employers can make are subsidising healthy foods low in fats and sugars and high in vegetables or offering reward schemes for choosing healthy behaviours. In some of the programmes, lowering blood pressure was the main aim rather than weight loss. In a community setting such as a worksite with a diverse population of normal, overweight and obese individuals, choosing an outcome other than weight can ensure that all employees stay engaged whatever their weight status. High blood pressure has been identified as one of the most important risk factors for CVD, and modest reduction in all, except those with the lowest blood pressure, can improve health, making it a high priority in many populations.

The importance of the food environment on risk of obesity has been reviewed (see Chapters 23 and 24 for more information); this identified important associations with the food environment and weight status but not with dietary behaviour (Giskes *et al.*, 2010). Nearly all the studies in this review were cross-sectional in nature, so only measured current behaviour; however, weight status may be a stronger indicator of long-term behaviour rather than current behaviour. Most of the studies looked at associations between accessibility factors and obesity risk. For fruit and vegetable consumption, access to supermarkets or takeaways was not associated with consumption. However, greater access to takeaway food and less access to supermarkets was associated with higher BMI. Those living in more deprived neighbourhoods were more likely to be overweight or obese and less likely to have regular eating patterns.

Features of successful community programmes

There is growing evidence of the independent impact of the environment on health and obesity risk in communities, and this is an area where we expect to see more research in the future. Already we have seen councils in England take action to reduce the number of takeaway outlets in some areas.

Community capacity building

In order to change the environment that we live in and make healthier choices easier it is important that knowledge and decision making are at least partly in the hands of the community and not just in the hands of specialists in government and health. Ensuring that this happens is known as capacity building and is likely to increase the effectiveness of community-based programmes to tackle obesity or other health outcomes. Capacity building is relatively new in interventions to reduce obesity but is becoming more common. The term capacity building is now included in the World Health Organization health promotion glossary. An example is the EPODE prevention programme in France. Most people recognise that there is a childhood obesity problem, but to bring about change communities must be able to look at the causes and the solutions at a local level in order to design a plan of action. Community leaders need to be identified and the programme tailored to the needs of the community. In general, capacity-building effectiveness has not often been evaluated, and it is unclear why some programmes work and others do not. The community capacity index (CCI) published by the Centre for Primary Health Care in Brisbane (Bush *et al.*, 2002) provides a tool to assess effectiveness in different capacity building domains.

Advocacy

Successful behaviour change cannot happen without advocacy. Advocacy is defined as 'a process to overcome structural barriers to change the legislative, fiscal, physical and social environment in which individuals' knowledge and attitudes are developed and expressed, and in which behaviour change can take place' (Chapman and Lupton, 1994).

Advocacy needs action from all organisations that are involved with the public health issue, including the media, who provide access to information about those that are making or influencing decisions. Views need to be heard from all sides, including nutrition and medical experts, as well as those who are threatened by policies to reduce obesity in order for effective policies to be planned.

Examples of community programmes

Example 1: school meal standards in England

What happened?
Food- and nutrient-based standards were introduced to schools between 2006 and 2009. These standards were legal requirements for all non-fee-paying schools and were included in the quality reports from individual schools. A change of government gave schools the choice to be academies with more independence. These schools did not have to adhere to the school meal standards. In 2014 the School Food Plan was produced with new simplified standards that were food based, not nutrient based.

What made it happen?
The School Meal Review Panel was convened with support from the government in 2005. This panel included representatives from a range of stakeholders in education, catering and nutrition and produced the food- and nutrient-based standards. The School Food Plan was led by restaurateurs with input from education, health and catering and introduced to new academies, but existing academies could still serve what they chose.

Capacity building
Little community capacity building was planned with the original change in school food policy. Some parents were against the idea of restricting choice of school meals, and much of this was hyped up in the media. Many school caterers complained that the extensive nutrient standards (13 nutrients plus energy) were complicated and required complex menu planning and expensive software.

Advocacy
Many stakeholders were involved in the production of the School Food Plan, which built on existing standards and simplified them to ensure users could understand, afford and follow the new standards.

Outcomes
Evaluation of the school food standards found that, compared with 2004, catering provision at lunchtime was healthier. In 2011, foods promoted by the new standards, such as compliant drinks, fruit juice, vegetables and salad, water and starchy food not cooked in oil, were offered more regularly than they had been in 2004. Foods with less healthy nutrient profiles, such as condiments, starchy food cooked in oil, non-permitted drinks, confectionery and non-permitted snacks, were offered less regularly in 2011 compared with 2004 (http://www.childrensfoodtrust.org.uk/blog/research-subject/impact-of-standards/).

Example 2: improving the food environment in Wigan, an area with high obesity rates in England

What happened?
The Healthy Business Award run by Wigan Council aimed to improve the nutritional profile of food available to those with very poor diets, including takeaways and care homes. The aims were to reduce salt, eliminate trans fats, reduce fats, reduce the energy density of food, increase fruit and vegetables and increase fibre intake. One hundred and fifty-five businesses were involved in the programme over 3 years.

What made it happen?

Wigan Council was commissioned by the regional NHS to improve the quality of food available to the poorest and hard to reach in the area. The healthy business team worked with other stakeholders, such as the University of Leeds, to reduce the fat content of pies. Businesses were made aware of the marketing advantage of offering healthy food which was affordable to the business and the consumer.

Capacity building

Local businesses were encouraged to get involved and to change their practices.

Advocacy

A range of specialists were involved, including nutritionists and food safety, trading standards, food science and catering. Media articles were published with case studies of businesses that had successfully received the Healthy Business Award and businesses who had increased profits after they had received the award.

Outcomes

An evaluation of a number of businesses taking part in the Healthy Business Award scheme found that revised menus had no impact on consumer choice or cost; and customer choices were closer to nutritional guidelines for a single meal (Dag *et al.*, 2011).

26.3 Individual approaches

The distinction between community-based and individual approaches may in some cases be a difficult one to make. For example, the school-based approaches described earlier may intervene at the whole school level in terms of school meals or policies or may directly influence the individual child or parent. This section aims to draw out some specific aspects related to intervention at the individual level.

Theory behind individual strategies

There are many different theories which have been developed to support individual dietary behaviour change. These come from a range of disciplines, including psychology, sociology and behavioural economics. Each behavioural change theory or model focuses on a range of different factors to explain behavioural change. The health belief model (or health action model) states that individuals change their health-related behaviour in response to the perceived severity of the risk to their health. The relapse prevention model promotes longer term healthy behaviour by distinguishing between lapses

and relapses to encourage individuals to maintain healthy lifestyles. The I-change model, the integrated model for explaining motivational and behavioural change, is derived from the attitude–social influence–self-efficacy model. This is an integration of Ajzen's theory of planned behaviour, Bandura's social cognitive theory, Prochaska's transtheoretical model (stages of change), the health belief model and goal setting theories. Elements of these theories – such as self-efficacy (which is an individual's belief of their own ability to perform a demanding or challenging task), outcome expectations, self-regulation, goal setting and attitudes – are common to several of the theories.

Social marketing is a further approach that has been applied to dietary behaviour. This uses a marketing approach to achieve specific behavioural goals and is the theoretical basis behind the Change4Life programme. Change4Life is the first national social marketing campaign to tackle the causes of obesity in England, which started in 2009. Change4Life aims to help families and middle-aged adults make small, sustainable improvements in diet, activity levels and alcohol consumption. For example, it provides tips to support 'five-a-day', another Department of Health (UK) initiative to increase fruit and vegetable consumption. Social marketing provides a framework for behaviour change and applies techniques from commercial sector marketing. These theories are also used and applied in development of community-based interventions described earlier.

Maintenance of positive dietary behaviour change is challenging. Dietary risk factors and physical inactivity account for 10% of global disability adjusted life years. A high calorie intake is associated with overweight and obesity. Intake of saturated fatty acids is strongly associated with increased coronary heart disease incidence and mortality. A high daily intake of fruits and vegetables promotes health. Evaluation of Change4Life found that people struggled to sustain dietary change, particularly in the face of an adverse environment. Improving dietary behaviour and maintaining improved intake is a longstanding challenge for public health. Thus, practical and effective strategies to achieve and maintain positive dietary behaviour for individuals are needed. The application of an effective theory base to the development of an intervention can increase the chances of the intervention being successful.

Measuring success

Although a systematic review of randomised controlled trials of an intervention would provide the strongest evidence of effectiveness, in many cases these studies would be too expensive to conduct or not practical.

Therefore, in order to measure success of behavioural interventions, a standard evaluation framework (SEF) for dietary, weight management and physical activity interventions has been developed (http://www.noo.org.uk/core/frameworks). The SEFs aims to describe and explain information to be collected in evaluation of an intervention aiming to improve dietary intake or associated behaviour. It is aimed at interventions that work at individual or group level, not at population level. This new approach was necessary due to a lack of high-quality evidence on the effectiveness of interventions. The SEF provides guidance on the following areas:

- how to identify appropriate dietary outcomes for evaluating different types of intervention;
- how to define suitable measures for different types of dietary outcome;
- how to approach the challenges of assessing and measuring dietary intake and diet-related behaviour.

Features of successful individual strategies

As linked to the theories noted earlier, most successful individual diet behaviour change or weight loss strategies have a number of particular components (Michie et al., 2009). These include self-efficacy strategies, where an individual is supported to believe that they can achieve the desired changes. This can be encouraged by goal setting; for example, aiming to eat an extra portion of fruit per day. All individuals will face barriers to their desired behaviour change. These barriers will vary from person to person, but could include concerns about cost, availability and views of others. Self-monitoring allows individuals to monitor their progress towards their goals on a regular basis. Interventions that combined self-monitoring with at least one other technique derived from control theory have been shown to be more effective than the other interventions. Dietary intake monitoring has been shown to be effective in relation to weight loss, particularly using a smartphone app such as My Meal Mate (Carter et al., 2013). Self-reinforcement of goals and intentions is another important aspect relating to individual rewards supporting motivation for change. For example, in long-term weight control, an individual's intrinsic motivations, such as enjoyment for regular physical activity, play a more important role than focusing on changes in body weight and diet-related changes. A systematic review of potential mediators of energy-balance-related behaviour found limited high-quality research (van Stralen et al., 2011). However, self-efficacy and intention may be useful mediators of physical activity; there was also some indication that attitude, knowledge and habit strength were mediators of dietary behaviour intentions.

A number of specific behavioural strategies have been recommended for cardiovascular risk factor reduction in adults in the USA (Artinian et al., 2010). These have been summarised in Box 26.2 and link to elements from the theory base.

Cost-effectiveness is inevitably also important when considering development and delivery of interventions. There is a range of existing commercial or primary-care-led weight reduction programmes aimed at the individual. Results of a randomised controlled trial of six different weight management programmes found that commercially available approaches were more cost-effective and cheaper than primary-care-based services led by specialist staff.

Examples of individual interventions

Intervention to support weight loss: My Meal Mate

An intervention delivered by smartphone could be a convenient, potentially cost-effective and wide-reaching weight management strategy. A smartphone app intervention, My Meal Mate, was developed using an evidence-based behavioural approach. The app incorporated goal setting, self-monitoring of diet and activity, and feedback via weekly text message. The app was tested in a sample of 128 overweight volunteers, randomised to receive a weight management intervention delivered either by smartphone app, web site or paper diary. Mean weight change at 6 months was −4.6 kg (95% confidence interval −6.2 to −3.0) in the smartphone app group (Carter et al., 2013). This was higher than the other groups, showing the potential for this type of individualised intervention.

Using social marketing to change individual dietary behaviour: Change4Life

This social marketing campaign started in the UK in 2009, supports the overall Healthy Weight, Healthy Lives strategy aiming to reduce obesity rates. Change4Life initially focused on families with children aged 5–11 years who were at greatest risk of becoming overweight or obese. The elements of this campaign included:

- Targeting individuals most in need of help. In this case, it is adults whose attitudes and behaviours placed their children most at risk of excess weight gain.
- Providing insight into why those individuals behaved in this way.
- Creating a communications campaign to change attitudes.
- Providing 'products' (such as handbooks, questionnaires, wall charts, web content) that people could use to help them change.
- Signposting people to services (such as breastfeeding cafés, accompanied walks, free swimming and cookery classes).

Box 26.2 Recommendations for counselling individuals to promote dietary and physical activity changes to reduce CVD risk

Level of evidence A: data derived from multiple randomised clinical trials.
Level of evidence B: data derived from a single randomised trial or non-randomised studies.
Cognitive-behavioural strategies for promoting behaviour change

- Design interventions to target dietary and physical activity (PA) behaviours with specific, proximal goals (goal setting). (Level of evidence: A)
- Provide feedback on progress toward goals. (Level of evidence: A)
- Provide strategies for self-monitoring. (Level of evidence: A)
- Establish a plan for frequency and duration of follow-up contacts (e.g. in person, oral, written, electronic) in accordance with individual needs to assess and reinforce progress toward goal achievement. (Level of evidence: A)
- Utilise motivational interviewing strategies, particularly when an individual is resistant or ambivalent about dietary and PA behaviour change. (Level of evidence: A)
- Provide for direct or peer-based long-term support and follow-up, such as referral to ongoing community-based programmes, to offset the common occurrence of declining adherence that typically begins at 4–6 months in most behaviour-change programs. (Level of evidence: B)
- Incorporate strategies to build self-efficacy into the intervention. (Level of evidence: A)
- Use a combination of two or more of the above strategies (e.g. goal setting, feedback, self-monitoring, follow-up, motivational interviewing, self-efficacy) in an intervention. (Level of evidence: A)

Intervention processes and/or delivery strategies

- Use individual- or group-based strategies. (Level of evidence: A)
- Use individual-oriented sessions to assess where the individual is in relation to behaviour change, to jointly identify the goals for risk reduction or improved cardiovascular health, and to develop a personalised plan to achieve it. (Level of evidence: A)
- Use group sessions with cognitive-behavioural strategies to teach skills to modify the diet and develop a PA programme, to provide role modelling and positive observational learning, and to maximise the benefits of peer support and group problem solving. (Level of evidence: A)
- For appropriate target populations, use internet- and computer-based programmes to target dietary and PA change; evidence is less for targeting PA alone; adding a form of E-counselling improves outcomes. (Level of evidence: B)

Source: based on Artinian *et al.* (2010).

- Bringing together a range of organisations, including the commercial sector, who used their influence to change behaviour.

The idea was that the programme should be more than just provision of information, which we know is not particularly effective. Evaluation at year 1 found that 'brand awareness' was high and positive; in addition, mothers claimed to have made changes to their children's behaviours as a result. However, actual impact on dietary behaviour was not assessed directly.

Complex interventions designed for the individual will require input from a range of disciplines, including epidemiology, psychology, public health, environmental planners and others. A good starting point is to learn from existing research that has been summarised in systematic reviews. These can point to the appropriate theory base and practical elements for success. Intervention design should include understanding of how the intervention will result in behaviour change through conscious or unconscious actions. Tailoring of the

initiative to the individual is required and may depend on a range of social, environmental and lifestyle factors.

26.4 Omics approaches (stratified or 'personalised' nutrition)

Background

Currently, the majority of dietary advice is based on population guidelines using a one-size-fits-all approach. Some recommended nutrient intakes and other nutritional advice are stratified, based, for example, on age, gender, pregnancy status or BMI, but only a small proportion of advice is currently personalised through the use of clinical measures. However, since the sequencing of the human genome, the recent growth in knowledge of gene–nutrient interactions has the potential to increase the effectiveness and availability of personalised nutrition. The relatively new and expanding field of nutritional genomics includes nutrigenomics, which studies how specific food and nutrients affect gene expression: not only how food affects the genome, but also how it affects the expression of messenger RNAs (transcriptomics), proteins (proteomics) and metabolites (metabolomics). Also included in the field of nutritional genomics is nutrigenetics, which explores how gene variation (single nucleotide polymorphism) can affect a body's response to diets and nutrients thereby potentially resulting in an increased or decreased disease risk compared to people who do not have the gene variation. Single nucleotide polymorphisms can result in altered end products of gene expression; that is, proteins such as enzymes with altered structure and function.

Personalised nutrition could be based on either genotype, which is the set of genes that a person carries, or phenotype, which is the individual's characteristics linked to their genotype and environment.

Examples of personalised nutrition

There are well-documented examples of nutrigenetics effects on human health. A classical gene mutation, such as phenylketonuria, has been known for many years. People with mutations in the enzyme phenylalanine hydroxylase cannot metabolise foods containing the amino acid phenylalanine and must alter their diet to minimise consumption. With modern genomic data, gene mutations with less severe effects are being explored to determine whether dietary practices can be more closely personalised to individual genetic profiles. Riboflavin supplementation can reduce blood pressure in hypertensive individuals with the methylenetetrahydrofolate reductase (MTHFR) 677TT genotype. Folic acid supplementation may be beneficial for carriers of C677T and A1298C polymorphisms in the *MTHFR* gene because these are associated with impaired folate metabolism and cardiovascular disease risk. Further examples are discussed in more detail below.

Genotype: haemochromatosis
Haemochromatosis, an autosomal recessive disease that is characterised by progressive iron overload, is an example of how a single gene variation can affect an individual's response to diet. Two common mutations of the *HFE* gene have been linked to hereditary haemochromatosis: C282Y and H63D. Cade *et al.* (2005), for instance, observed that postmenopausal women eating a diet rich in haem iron and who carried two C282Y mutations (homozygotes) had the highest serum ferritin concentrations compared with those who carried other combinations. C282Y homozygote individuals are advised to eat less meat, particularly beef and lamb, which contain the highest levels of the easily absorbed

haem iron. Left unchecked, progressive iron overload will eventually lead to organ failure, diabetes and early death. This is a clear example of the benefits and effectiveness of genetic-based personalised nutritional advice that is currently utilised. It is set within the general population-based dietary advice that, conversely, encourages the intake of iron to prevent deficiency. Furthermore, postmenopausal women carrying only one copy of the C282Y mutation (and particularly compound heterozygotes, i.e. C282Y/H63) may have higher than average iron absorption and could be advised to reduce their iron intake; high levels of iron storage, even within the normal range, may predispose individuals to many chronic diseases, including heart disease, diabetes and some cancers.

Phenotype: caffeine metabolism
Differences in an individual's phenotype rather than their genotype may be used for providing nutritional advice. An example is the individual variation in caffeine metabolism and its effect on fetal growth restriction during pregnancy. Currently, the general advice to pregnant women is to reduce their caffeine consumption during pregnancy because caffeine consumption has been independently associated with increased risk of fetal growth restriction. However, evidence from measuring the half-life of caffeine in saliva shows that women with a faster compared with a slower caffeine clearance could be at greater risk of giving birth to babies whose growth is restricted (CARE Study Group, 2008). The amount of caffeine available to both the mother and the fetus depends on the enzyme cytochrome P450 1A2 (CYP1A2), the principal enzyme involved in caffeine metabolism that is absent in the placenta and the fetus. Although genetic differences are likely to be involved, pregnant women would only need to undergo caffeine metabolism tests rather than a genetic test, especially since environmental factors such as nicotine intake also influence caffeine metabolism. Test results providing evidence of faster metabolism of caffeine are likely to have a greater influence on pregnant women to reduce their caffeine intake than the general advice given to all women, though, as yet, such tests are not utilised.

Nutrigenomics: apolipoprotein E
Nutrigenomic-based personalised nutrition has the potential to be more effective at preventing polygenic NCDs, such as CVD, cancer and obesity than population-based guidance. For instance, it has been shown that individuals with the E4 genotype of apolipoprotein E, which has been associated with a higher risk of heart disease than the wild-type genotype, have a much larger and beneficial response to low-fat diets in relation to

circulating lipids implicated in the development of heart disease (Lovegrove and Gitau, 2008).

Genetic tailoring of diets

Future research may help to classify individuals into those that are likely to respond well to certain diets. Preliminary research has shown that diets tailored to genes involved in metabolism can aid weight loss in obese individuals, though larger randomised trials on this are required. A large European trial, Food4Me, did not find that knowledge of phenotype or genotype affected dietary behaviour.

Incorporating individuals' food preferences is likely to improve acceptance of a new personalised diet; therefore, individuals could also be tested for genetic differences in taste. Genetic differences in sensitivity to bitter taste and to sweetness have been found; advice on food preparation to improve the palatability of healthy foods perceived as bitter could be provided within tailored diets. For instance, there are common *TAS2R38* haplotypes that influence the ability to taste phenylthiocarbamide, propylthiouracil as well as thiocyanates found in brassica vegetables such as Brussels sprouts and broccoli. Higher intakes of these vegetables have also been linked to decreased cancer risks, and although sensitivity to bitter taste may reduce the intake of these there is no conclusive evidence that genetic *sensitivity to bitter taste* is associated with increased cancer, or BMI and adiposity.

Since NCDs are usually associated with a variety of genes, involving complex interactions between genes and the environment, the use of nutritional genomics and its solutions are likely to be complex and difficult to apply. It may be too early to evaluate the potential effectiveness of nutritional genomics for reducing NCDs.

Application of personalised nutrition to the population at large

Regulation and ethics

A number of factors need to be in place or considered before the broad application of personalised nutrition to the population at large is likely to occur. These factors include regulations and ethical considerations. Regulations should cover nutrigenomic testing providers and their claims, and new functional food products and related claims, as well as the privacy and storage of genetic data (Camp and Trujillo, 2014). Social and ethical considerations include unequal access to personalised nutrition, possible pressure on people to use the service, and the psychological cost of genetic testing. Some countries already have more developed strategies in relation to some of these issues than other countries. In 2004, the European scientific community established

the Nutrigenomics Organisation (NuGo) to pull together multidisciplinary scientific knowledge, to develop and validate research tools, and amongst other things to educate health-care practitioners. Since then, similar organisations around the world have been established.

Despite advances in knowledge, it may be some years before the evidence base is sufficiently robust to provide nutrigenomic-based personalised nutrition in the market place to the population at large. Current promotion on a wide scale is likely to be premature and open to exploitation by private companies directly targeting the general public, who could be misled. Private companies abandoned personalised nutrition marketing strategies in the UK after organised consumer opposition took place. However, nutrigenomic tests are currently marketed in the USA through health practitioners as well as directly to consumers online. New functional foods are also marketed in the USA. Functional foods often incorporate bioactive compounds, such as epigallocatechin-3-gallate, a potent antioxidant. These compounds could interact with genetic polymorphisms. An individual's genotype may prevent them deriving significant benefit from an increased intake of such foods, and some who may be disadvantaged. Owing to previous health scares, including those relating to genetically modified crops, many people, especially in Europe, mistrust new foods. Some proactive consumers may be willing to pay directly for personalised nutrition services and products whether or not claims are endorsed or regulated by official bodies. Clear regulation is needed, not only to protect the consumer, but also to promote trust in personalised nutrition services and products.

Because of its individualism, personalised nutrition is most likely to be taken up privately, and inequality of access to the services and products is likely to result. Although some polymorphisms may be common enough for nutritional advice to be provided at a stratified level and for functional food products to be mass produced, equitable access to these may still be an issue. Strategies to encourage and enable poorer and less proactive individuals to access personalised nutrition services and products may be needed if there are clear benefits for the individual and society in using the services.

Individuals' engagement with genetic testing

Once the evidence base and regulations are in place, the uptake of personalised nutrition in the wider community is likely to depend on an individual's willingness to be genetically tested. Success will depend on their motivation to adhere to nutritional advice based on their genetic test results. Sufficient self-efficacy and/or social support will be needed to help maintain adherence to advice. Diets tailored to genetic taste preferences may also help here. Research reviewed from a number of countries indicates a large proportion of individuals are willing to be genetically tested for the prevention of diseases (48–85%) (Fallaize et al., 2013), though this is likely to be considerably lower when cost to the individual is taken into account. Out of six European countries, the UK was most willing to be genetically tested for personalised nutrition. Fallaize et al. (2013) concluded that research findings indicated individuals with personal experience of genetic diseases (e.g. within the family) were more likely to be willing to undergo genetic testing, and therefore were possible targets for personalised nutrition services. Such individuals may also be more motivated to comply with nutritional advice based on their genetic test results, especially if there is evidence that diet can reduce disease risk and their genetic predisposition is not seen as fatalistic. Although the uptake of personalised nutrition may be more likely for proactive individuals with heightened perceived susceptibility to disease, they may not represent a large proportion of the population to produce a large overall reduction in disease risk. Nevertheless, even a 1% reduction in relative risk of CVD in England and Wales, for instance, has been estimated to save the UK National Health Service £30 million per year (Barton et al., 2011).

Privacy was found to be a particular concern relating to genetic testing in the USA, especially surrounding potential misuse of genetic information that may impact the cost and provision of insurance policies and may impact acquisition of jobs (Morren et al., 2007). Other concerns researched related to whether or not to inform family members. Some individuals may react in a fatalist manner to results and not alter their eating habits. Alternatively, genetic results may cause distress and anxiety if pre- and post-test counselling are not provided, and if the advised increased risks cannot be effectively reduced. Nutrigenomic testing may create large numbers of worried-well, and its psychological effects may be burdensome; the resulting stress may even promote disease. Therefore, future research should compare the psychological impact from different methods of delivering nutrigenomic-based personalised nutrition.

Education and communication

Evidence-based education of health practitioners, dietitians and nutritionists in this new area of health is needed for it to be successful on a wide scale. Communication to the general public should help to develop confidence in personalised nutrition, without confusing and weakening current population public health messages, which will remain important. In the past, media reporting of conflicting associations between nutrition and disease risk from individual studies has confused and/or disillusioned a large portion of the general public, who now mistrust nutritional information. Information can be delivered more directly to the general public through face-to-face contact with health-care professionals or via the internet by private companies supplying direct-to-consumer testing. Face-to-face counselling, pre- and post-testing, reduces financial viability compared with direct-to-consumer delivery. Costs are minimised in the latter by utilising self-administered genetic swabs, results from which can be interpreted and then fed back to the individual by mail, electronically or by telephone. Future research could compare the effectiveness of different methods of delivery on dietary change and disease prevention (Fallaize et al., 2013). Consumers may be suspicious about the commercial interest of private companies, and believe they may be motivated more by financial gain than by health promotion. However, the 2013 Fallaize review also reports a lack of knowledge of genetic testing amongst health-care professionals and of gene–diet interactions amongst dietitians. The European Nutrigenomics Organisation has started to address this issue by providing training courses. Also the European Food4Me project (http://www.food4me.org/) has researched best practice communication strategies.

Nutritional genomics is a promising field of research that has the potential to reduce NCDs through personalised nutritional advice based on knowledge of genetic–environment interactions, though it is too early to evaluate its effectiveness. In addition to the growth of a robust evidence base, clear strategies regarding education of professionals and regulation of services and products need to be developed further before widespread uptake is promoted.

26.5 Overall conclusion

Public health nutrition strategies designed to deliver improved dietary behaviour for the community can be created and delivered at a number of levels. At one end of the spectrum, legislation eliminating choice is possible; at the other end of the spectrum, 'nudges' can support individual behaviour change. In addition, the emerging field of nutritional genomics will allow tailoring of individual dietary interventions to focus on those who are likely to benefit the most from particular recommendations. Evaluation of different approaches is needed to determine effectiveness and ensure that health inequalities are not widened.

References

Anderson, L.M., Quinn, T.A., Glanz, K. et al. (2009) The effectiveness of worksite nutrition and physical activity interventions for controlling employee overweight and obesity: a systematic review. *American Journal of Preventive Medicine*, **37**, 340–357.

Artinian, N.T., Fletcher, G.F., Mozaffarian, D. *et al.* (2010) Interventions to promote physical activity and dietary lifestyle changes for cardiovascular risk factor reduction in adults: a scientific statement from the American Heart Association. *Circulation*, **122**, 406–441.

Barton, P., Andronis, L., Briggs, A. *et al.* (2011) Effectiveness and cost effectiveness of cardiovascular disease prevention in whole populations: modelling study. *BMJ*, **343**, d4044.

Bush, R., Dower, J. and Mutch, A. (2002) *Community Capacity Index Manual*, Version 2. Centre for Primary Health Care, Brisbane. http://equalityandsafetyforwomen.org.au/wp-content/uploads/2015/08/Community-Capacity-Index-Manual.pdf (accessed 10 January 2017).

Cade, J.E., Moreton, J.A., O'Hara, B. *et al.* (2005) Diet and genetic factors associated with iron status in middle-aged women. *The American Journal of Clinical Nutrition*, **82**, 813–820.

Camp, K.M. and Trujillo, E. (2014) Position of the Academy of Nutrition and Dietetics: nutritional genomics. *Journal of the Academy of Nutrition and Dietetics*, **114**, 299–312.

CARE Study Group (2008) Maternal caffeine intake during pregnancy and risk of fetal growth restriction: a large prospective observational study. *BMJ*, **337**, a2332.

Carter, M.C., Burley, V.J., Nykjaer, C. and Cade, J.E. (2013) Adherence to a smartphone application for weight loss compared to website and paper diary: pilot randomized controlled trial. *Journal of Medical Internet Research*, **15** (4), e32.

Chapman, S. and Lupton, D. (1994) *The Fight for Public Health: Principles and Practice of Media Advocacy*. BMJ Publishing Group, London.

Colchero, M.A., Popkin, B.M., Rivera, J.A., Ng, S.W. (2016) Beverage purchases from stores in Mexico under the excise tax on sugar sweetened beverages: observational study. *BMJ*, **352**, h6704.

Craig, P., Dieppe, P., Macintyre, S. *et al.* (2008) Developing and evaluating complex interventions: the new Medical Research Council guidance. *BMJ*, **337**, a1655.

Dag, N., Grime, J., Lang, L. and Orfila, C. (2011) Evaluation of the Healthy Business Award (HBA): improving the accessibility of healthy foods in Wigan borough. *Proceedings of the Nutrition Society*, **70** (OCE4), E167.

Edelstein, S. (2010) *Nutrition in Public Health*. Jones & Bartlett Learning, Sudbury, MA.

Evans, C.E., Greenwood, D.C., Thomas, J.D. and Cade, J.E. (2010) A cross-sectional survey of children's packed lunches in the UK: food- and nutrient-based results. *Journal of Epidemiology and Community Health*, **64** (11), 977–983. [Erratum in *Journal of Epidemiology and Community Health* (2010), **64**(12), 1105.]

Fallaize, R., Macready, A.L., Butler, L.T. *et al.* (2013) An insight into the public acceptance of nutrigenomic-based personalised nutrition. *Nutrition Research Reviews*, **26**, 39–48.

Giskes, K., Avendano, M., Brug, J. and Kunst, A.E. (2010) A systematic review of studies on socioeconomic inequalities in dietary intakes associated with weight gain and overweight/obesity conducted among European adults. *Obesity Reviews*, **11**, 413–429.

House of Lords Science and Technology Select Committee (2011) *2nd Report of Session 2010–12: Behaviour Change*. The Stationery Office, London.

Lovegrove, J.A. and Gitau, R. (2008) Personalized nutrition for the prevention of cardiovascular disease: a future perspective. *Journal of Human Nutrition and Dietetics*, **21**, 306–316.

Marteau, T.M., Ogilvie, D., Roland, M. *et al.* (2011) Judging nudging: can nudging improve population health? *BMJ*, **342**, d228.

Michie, S., Abraham, C., Whittington, C. *et al.* (2009) Effective techniques in healthy eating and physical activity interventions: a meta-regression. *Health Psychology*, **28**, 690–701.

Morren, M., Rijken, M., Baanders, A.N. and Bensing, J. (2007) Perceived genetic knowledge, attitudes towards genetic testing, and the relationship between these among patients with a chronic disease. *Patient Education and Counseling*, **65**, 197–204.

Mwatsama, M. and Landon, J. (2014) *Options for Action to Support the Reduction of Sugar Intakes in the UK*. UK Health Forum, London.

Van Stralen, M.M., Yildirim, M., te Velde, S.J. *et al.* (2011) What works in school-based energy balance behaviour interventions and what does not? A systematic review of mediating mechanisms. *International Journal of Obesity*, **35**, 1251–1265.

Waters, E., de Silva-Sanigorski, A., Hall, B.J. *et al.* (2011) Interventions for preventing obesity in children. *The Cochrane Database of Systematic Reviews*, (2), CD001871.

Wyness, L.A., Butriss, J.L. and Stanner, S.A. (2012) Reducing the population's sodium intake: the UK Food Standards Agency's salt reduction programme. *Public Health Nutrition*, **15**, 254–261.

27
Dietary Change and Evidence on How to Achieve This

Janice L Thompson

Key messages

- Dietary intake involves a complex set of behaviours that include not only personal food choices, but also social, cultural, financial and environmental factors that influence food consumption.
- To effectively change dietary behaviours, the factors influencing dietary intake of individuals and populations must be understood.
- Behaviour change theories and models are used to explain and predict behaviours, and are also used as a framework to develop effective intervention strategies.
- The most common behaviour change theories and models that have been used in examining dietary behaviour include social cognitive theory, theory of planned behaviour, the trans-theoretical model, and ecological models.

- Both individual and upstream approaches can be used to change dietary behaviours.
- Evidence indicates that the most effective strategy in changing dietary behaviour of individuals is self-monitoring, combined with at least one of four other self-regulation strategies, including intention formation, specific goal setting, feedback on performance and review of behavioural goals.
- The UK salt reduction strategy is an example of an effective upstream approach, resulting in a decline in salt intake from 9.5 g/day in 2000–2001 to 8.1 g/day in 2011.

27.1 Introduction to the chapter

The consumption of a healthy diet is recognised as a key factor in the prevention and treatment of chronic diseases such as cardiovascular disease, type 2 diabetes, obesity, osteoporosis and some cancers (Joint WHO/FAO Expert Consultation, 2003). The overarching characteristics of a healthy diet include adequacy, moderation, balance and variety. A plethora of research studies have identified fruits, vegetables, pulses and whole grains and foods low in total and saturated fats, salt and added sugars as specific dietary components that promote and optimise health.

Despite the recognised benefits of consuming a healthy diet, existing evidence suggests that individuals and populations do not consistently consume diets that meet current health promotion recommendations. For instance, recent evidence from the National Diet and Nutrition Survey conducted in the UK indicates that only 30% of adults (19–64 years) and 41% of older adults

(65 years and older) consumed at least five portions of fruits and vegetables per day, while intakes of saturated fat and non-milk extrinsic sugars exceeded daily recommended values in all age groups (Bates et al., 2014). In addition, excessive energy intake (above that of energy expenditure) due to the consumption of fast foods, sugared soft drinks and other energy-dense, nutrient-poor foods is consistently identified as a major contributor to the burgeoning global obesity epidemic (Schulze et al., 2004; Drewnowski and Darmon, 2005; Rosenheck, 2008). Although public health campaigns (such as the UK's Change4Life) have been delivered in an attempt to promote the consumption of a healthy diet, current national dietary trends draw into question the effectiveness of this approach at a population level.

Dietary intake involves a complex set of behaviours that include not only personal food choices, but also social, cultural, financial and environmental factors that influence food consumption (see Chapter 24). In order to change dietary intake, and ensure that healthy changes

Public Health Nutrition, Second Edition. Edited by Judith L Buttriss, Ailsa A Welch, John M Kearney and Susan A Lanham-New.
© 2018 by The Nutrition Society. Published 2018 by John Wiley & Sons, Ltd.
Companion website: www.wiley.com/go/buttriss/publichealth

can be sustained, there is a critical need to understand what drives the dietary intake behaviours of both individuals and populations, and then to use this understanding to develop and implement effective behaviour change approaches.

The main aim of this chapter is to examine what is currently known about dietary-change strategies, and to present evidence of the effectiveness of the various approaches that have been implemented. In order to better understand the rationale for implementing these strategies and the issues affecting their potential effectiveness, this chapter begins with a brief review of select behavioural theories and models underpinning efforts to more fully understand and change dietary intake behaviours.

27.2 Behaviour change theories and models

There are numerous psychological behaviour change theories and models that have been used to explain, predict and subsequently change various health-related behaviours. Behaviour change theories are typically used to examine and predict behaviours of individuals, and are also used as a framework to develop effective intervention strategies. This section provides a brief overview of the theories and models most commonly applied to changing dietary behaviour. These include social cognitive theory (SCT), theory of planned behaviour (TBP), the trans-theoretical model (TTM) and ecological models.

Social cognitive theory

SCT (Bandura, 1986) emphasises the concept of *reciprocal determinism*, which refers to the interaction between people and their environments (Table 27.1). In SCT, human behaviour is proposed to be a result of the constant interaction between a person and the influences of their environment. The focus of SCT is on a person's potential to alter and construct their environments to suit their needs, both individually and via collective action by working with others in organisations and systems to change environments. These interactions can subsequently benefit the individual and larger groups. In addition to reciprocal determinism, the constructs of SCT include (McAlister *et al.*, 2008):

- outcome expectations – a person's beliefs about the likelihood and value of the consequences of behaviours;
- observational learning – learning to perform a new behaviour through example, such as peer modelling;

- collective efficacy – a person's beliefs about the ability of a group to perform actions together to result in desired outcomes;
- incentive motivation – using or misusing rewards and punishments to change behaviour;
- facilitation – providing resources or altering the environment to make behavioural changes easier to implement;
- self-efficacy – a person's confidence that they can take action to change their behaviour;
- self-regulation – controlling oneself through self-monitoring, goal-setting, self-reward and garnering of social support; and
- moral disengagement – a psychological process by which a person finds justifications for the harmful effect of their behaviour on themselves and others by convincing themselves that ethical and moral standards do not apply to them.

Theory of planned behaviour

TPB (Ajzen, 1991) asserts that the primary determinant of an individual's behaviour is *behavioural intention* (Table 27.1). Further, TPB states that the constructs that determine behavioural intention are attitude, subjective norms and perceived control. Within TPB, attitude is determined by a person's beliefs about the outcomes of performing a particular behaviour, balanced with an evaluation of these outcomes. Subjective norms are comprised of normative beliefs (i.e. whether key individuals approve or disapprove of engaging in a particular behaviour) balanced with the person's motivation to comply with the beliefs and expectations of those key individuals. Perceived control takes into account factors beyond a person's control that can affect intention and behaviour. It includes the person's beliefs about control and barriers and facilitators affecting behaviour change, balanced with perceived power about how these factors promote or inhibit their ability to change behaviour (Montaño and Kasprzyk, 2008).

Trans-theoretical model

As the name specifies, TTM (DiClemente and Prochaska, 1982) is not a theory per se, but a model; models are frameworks that draw on various theories as a means to enhance our understanding of behaviours within specific contexts (Table 27.1). TTM is also referred to as the stages of change model, as it uses *stages of change* to integrate principles across various psychotherapy and behaviour change theories to enhance our understanding of a person's readiness to change their behaviour. The constructs of TTM include (Prochaska *et al.*, 2008):

Table 27.1 An overview of theories and models most commonly applied to changing dietary behaviour of individuals.

Theory or model	Reference	Description	Key constructs	Behaviour change strategies or techniques commonly applied from these theories/models
SCT	Bandura, (1986)	Assumes behaviours occur in a reciprocal model in which personal factors, environmental influences, and behaviour constantly interact	• Reciprocal determinism • Outcome expectations • Observational learning • Collective efficacy • Incentive motivation • Facilitation • Self-efficacy • Self-regulation • Moral disengagement	• Demonstration and modelling • Skill development • Social support • Goal setting • Reinforcement • Self-monitoring • Rewards and incentives
TPB	Ajzen (1991)	Assumes the best predictor of behaviour change is behavioural intention, which is determined by attitude and social norms regarding the behaviour	• Attitude • Subjective norms • Perceived behavioural control	• Skill development • Social support • Modelling • Reinforcement
Trans-theoretical model	DiClemente and Prochaska (1982)	Uses stages to integrate processes of change across various psychotherapy and behaviour change theories	• Stages of change • Processes of change • Decisional balance • Self-efficacy	• Dependent upon individual's stage of change. Includes: • Skill development • Demonstration and modelling • Reinforcement • Self-monitoring • Goal setting • Social support

- stages of change – pre-contemplation, contemplation, preparation, action, maintenance and termination;
- processes of change – includes consciousness raising, self-re-evaluation, environmental re-evaluation, stimulus control, dramatic relief, self-liberation, helping relationships, counterconditioning, reinforcement management and social liberation;
- decisional balance – the pros and cons of changing one's behaviour; and
- self-efficacy.

Although SCT, TPB and TTM are commonly used as theoretical frameworks in the development of dietary change interventions, minimal detail is reported in published lifestyle intervention studies as to how theoretical constructs are used to inform intervention development, if and how constructs are used to evaluate intervention implementation, and the link between constructs and behavioural outcomes. This information is important to assist researchers, health educators and programme planners in developing a structured process by which they can apply the constructs of a theory (or theories) when they design and deliver an intervention, and also to provide a road map to allow for the evaluation of how theoretical constructs may or may not contribute to changes in behaviours. By doing so, the success or failure of a given intervention can be examined to determine if the causes may be a result of issues with implementation (e.g. fidelity to the delivery plan) or related to the theory itself (e.g. inappropriate theory selection).

Helitzer et al. (2008) addressed this important gap in the literature by describing in detail the development of a planning evaluation methodology for assessing the contribution of SCT to a diabetes prevention intervention targeting American Indian women. The intervention targeted reducing consumption of dietary fat and added sugars, increasing consumption of fruits and vegetables, increasing physical activity, getting and giving support to achieve lifestyle changes, and sustaining healthy changes over the longer term. A theory matrix was developed for each behaviour, and all SCT constructs were covered in the intervention curriculum at least once for each behaviour. This paper provides useful tools and processes that can be applied to the development, delivery and evaluation of any behaviour change intervention.

Based on existing literature, it is more common for researchers to select constructs from one or more theories that they believe are particularly salient to their participants and the behaviour changes they hope to achieve, instead of using a single theory (and all of its constructs) as a framework for intervention development. One example of this approach is a study conducted by Carpenter et al. (2004), in which select constructs from SCT and TTM were used to develop and deliver a randomised, controlled pilot study to determine the effect of a lifestyle education intervention on improving dietary intake in healthy adults. The stages of change construct from TTM was used to design the intervention and informed participant recruitment, with eligible adults being those in the early stages of change (pre-contemplation, contemplation or preparation) for at least two of four dietary goals, including reducing dietary fat, increasing consumption of whole grains, increasing intake of calcium-rich foods and increasing consumption of fruit and vegetables. The SCT constructs included in the dietary education curriculum were self-efficacy, self-regulation and outcome expectations. With this approach the researchers selected the theories and constructs that they felt were most appropriate for their target audience and had the highest likelihood of resulting in successful dietary change.

Ecological models

Although the theories previously described recognise the influences of factors external to the individual, their application to date has predominantly focused on factors more proximal to the actions of the individual. Much of the published behaviour change research does not focus on analysing the significance of, or evaluate attempts to, change, the social, cultural, economic and environmental factors that may be key determinants of health behaviours in both individuals and communities. This limitation has been highlighted as a major factor contributing to the failure of examining the role of these external influences in contributing to health inequalities (Taylor et al., 2006). A more detailed discussion of the limitations of existing theories and models is provided later in this section.

To provide a framework that allows for the examination of broader social, environmental and policy-related influences on behaviour change and to develop more comprehensive intervention approaches that target these influences, ecological models have been developed. The basic premise of these models is that there are multiple levels of influence on behaviour – these include not only intrapersonal influences (e.g. biological and psychological), but also interpersonal (social and cultural), organisational (e.g. worksite or school), community-level factors, the physical environment and public policy.

Sallis et al. (2008) have proposed four core principles of ecological models of health behaviour.

1. Specific health behaviours are influenced by factors across multiple levels: intrapersonal, interpersonal, organisational, community, and public policy.
2. The various influences on behaviours interact across these levels.

3. Ecological models should be specific to each behaviour of interest, and should be capable of identifying the influences that are most relevant at each level.
4. Interventions that should be most effective in changing behaviour are those that address issues at multiple levels (referred to as 'multi-level interventions').

Numerous ecological models have been developed for health behaviours, such as smoking cessation, physical activity and dietary intake. The two models discussed here are illustrative examples of those used to examine factors that influence dietary behaviours, and are thus factors deemed to be important targets for change. These two models are the family ecological model (Davison and Campbell, 2005), and an ecological framework of multiple influences on what people eat (Story *et al.*, 2008).

Figure 27.1 illustrates the family ecological model as originally developed by Davison and Campbell (2005).

This model was developed to account for family-associated factors that affect parenting, specific to nutrition and physical activity behaviours that are associated with obesity risk. The model illustrates the effort to move away from emphasising the individual child as the focal point of interventions and instead focuses on the family. The inner circle summarises the influences of parents on children's behaviours, while the outer circles represent contextual domains that influence these behaviours, such as family demographics, characteristics of the child, organisations and community, and the influences of policy and the media.

This model has recently been examined for its applicability and appropriateness in 84 low-income families. Davison *et al.* (2012) used qualitative and quantitative measures to assess parents' cognitions and behaviours related to the diet, physical activity and screen-viewing behaviours of their children. They then mapped the

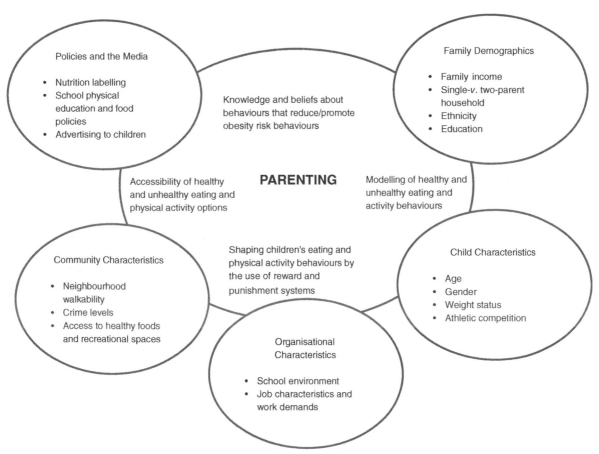

The original Family Ecological Model. From: Davison KK, Campbell K. Opportunities to prevent obesity of children within families: an ecological approach. In: D. Crawford and R. Jeffery, eds. 2005. *Obesity Prevention and Public Health*. Oxford: Oxford University Press. pp. 207-230.

Figure 27.1 The original family ecological model. *Source*: Davison and Campbell (2005).

results onto the constructs highlighted in the family ecological model. The findings from this study provided support for the validity of the model, as the constructs outlined in the model were found to be important influences amongst the families participating in the study. However, a number of limitations in the model were identified, including the inability of the construct 'family demographics' to adequately reflect the breadth of various factors occurring within families. Additionally, the authors state that while the model provided a great deal of valuable information about families and family life, it was less helpful in guiding intervention development, delivery and evaluation. In response to these findings, this model has been revised to address these limitations (see Figure 27.2). Research is now needed to test this revised model in various family populations to determine its utility for designing, implementing and evaluating family-based interventions.

Story et al. (2008) developed a framework outlining the multiple influences that affect what people eat (Figure 27.3). In this model, individual or personal factors include demographic and biological factors, in addition to skills, attitudes, knowledge and beliefs. Environmental influences more proximal to the individual are separated into 'social' factors (such as family, friends and peers) and 'physical' settings (such as worksites, schools, supermarkets and restaurants). Macrolevel factors, also referred to as 'upstream' factors, include both environmental and policy-related factors. Although these factors are considered to be more distal to the individual, their impact on what people eat can be quite powerful. These include food pricing, food and beverage marketing strategies, and societal/cultural norms related to food choice; arguably, in many cases these factors can override an individual's best intentions to change dietary behaviours.

To date, this model has been promoted as a framework to guide policy decisions and promote environmental changes that result in making it easier for people and communities to eat more healthfully. As an example, it has been adapted and combined with other existing models by the US Department of Agriculture and US Department Health and Human Services (2010) into a social ecological framework for nutrition and physical activity decisions. However, at the time this chapter was written, there were no published studies examining the validity and appropriateness of this proposed model in the development, implementation and evaluation of dietary interventions.

Limitations of behaviour change theories and models

There are a number of limitations regarding the research that has been conducted examining behaviour change theories and models and their application to dietary behaviours. While existing research identifies associations between theoretical constructs and certain dietary behaviours, there is little evidence indicating exactly *which* of the multitude of constructs and factors examined are the most influential in determining an individual's dietary behaviours or in changing their dietary behaviours, and no insights are offered into how dietary behaviour change can be most effectively facilitated (Taylor et al., 2006).

In regard to ecologic models, very few have been tested for their validity and evaluated for their applicability across various target populations. In addition, it is recognised that upstream factors are difficult to measure, and intervening to change physical and social environments is quite challenging (Story et al., 2008). Thus, there is currently little evidence to support or refute the role that ecologic models play in effectively changing dietary behaviours.

Another major limitation of the research focusing on the testing of behaviour change theories is that the majority of research is predominantly conducted in white or Caucasian populations, and also within 'individualistic' communities and societies. 'Individualistic' societies are those in which individuals believe that their life belongs to them, and that she or he has a right to live their life as they see fit within the values of personal choice. 'Collectivist' societies are those in which individuals believe that their life belongs to a broader group or society, and that she or he must sacrifice or disregard personal goals and values to support the broader group. Thus, we know little about if, and how, behaviour change theories and dietary behaviour change strategies apply to ethnically and culturally diverse individuals and communities.

27.3 Strategies used to change dietary behaviours and food intake

There is a substantial body of literature examining efforts to change dietary behaviours and food intake in adults. The vast majority of studies have focused on trying to change behaviours of individuals; fewer studies have examined upstream approaches designed to change food environments at a community or population level. Both of these types of approaches, and evidence of their effectiveness, are discussed in this section.

Individual approaches and evidence of effectiveness

The large number of intervention studies published, the diversity of approaches used in the design and delivery of

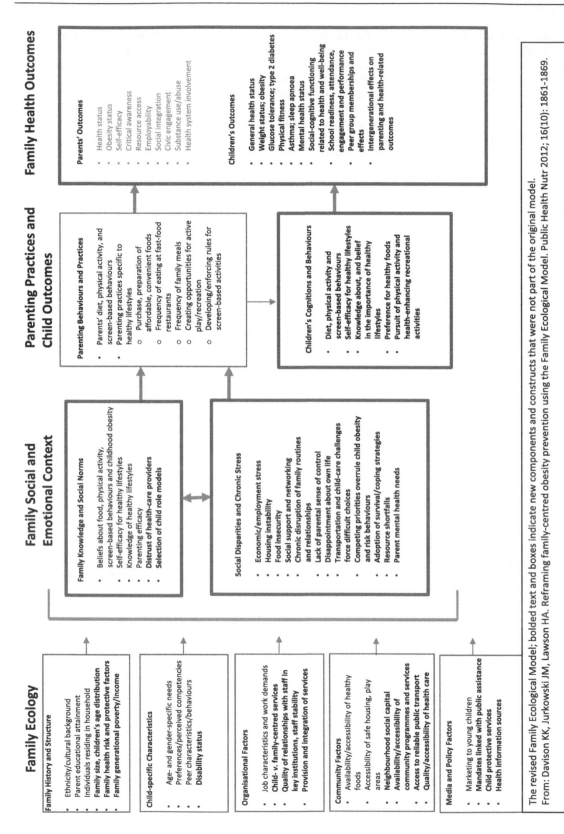

Figure 27.2 The revised family ecological model; bolded text and boxes indicate new components and constructs that were not part of the original model. *Source: Davison et al. (2012).*

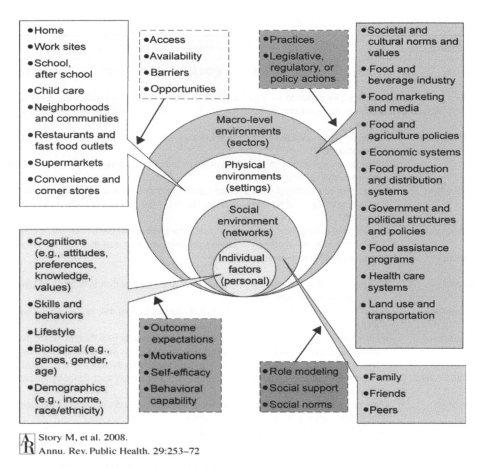

Story M, et al. 2008.
Annu. Rev. Public Health. 29:253–72

Figure 27.3 An ecological framework depicting the multiple influences on what people eat.

dietary behaviour change interventions, and the relatively small effect observed in many intervention studies make it challenging to identify which dietary behaviour change approaches are most effective in individuals. Michie *et al.* (2009) addressed these challenges by using the sophisticated techniques of meta-analysis and meta-regression to examine the extensive existing literature to provide a comprehensive classification of the content of healthy eating interventions into component techniques, and subsequently determine which strategies are most effective in changing dietary behaviour. They focused on 'active interventions', or those that directly engaged with participants in changing their behaviours, and did not include any evidence from 'passive interventions', or those that only provide information or advice. Studies were included in the analysis if they involved adults 18 years and older, used experimental or quasi-experimental designs, and employed dietary measures that were objective, standardised or derived using validated self-report measures. Additionally, interventions had to use

cognitive or behavioural change strategies. Studies were excluded if they examined pregnant or recently postnatal women, athletes, people already involved in another intervention (such as weight loss programmes), people living in an institutional setting, or people with mental or physical health problems. A total of 53 studies met the inclusion criteria.

Table 27.2 lists the strategies most frequently implemented in the dietary change interventions included in the analyses (Michie *et al.*, 2009) and provides an example of how each strategy can be used to change a particular dietary behaviour (in this case, reducing saturated fat intake). These strategies are based on constructs from various behaviour change theories, including TPB and SCT. Interventions typically used more than one behaviour change technique, with an average of six techniques used per intervention. Modes of delivery included one-to-one individual consultations and group sessions, with delivery being done by either clinically trained health professionals (e.g. dietitian or nurse),

Table 27.2 Common strategies used in dietary change interventions.

Behaviour change strategy	Practical example of applying strategy
Provide information on consequences	Providing information on how consuming a diet high in saturated fat increases one's risk for heart disease
Prompt intention formation	Encouraging the person to set a goal or define an action, such as 'I will reduce my intake of full-fat cheese'
Prompt barrier identification	Identify barriers to reducing intake of foods high in saturated fat, and planning ways to overcome these barriers
Provide general encouragement	Praising the person for making efforts to reduce their saturated fat intake, even if target goals have not been achieved
Provide instruction	Tell the person actions they can take to reduce their saturated fat intake, including reducing consumption of red meats and full-fat dairy products
Prompt specific goal setting	Involves detailed planning of what a person can do to reduce saturated fat intake – for example, 'I will reduce my intake of full-fat cheese to one ounce, two times per week at home during evening meals with my family"
Prompt review of behavioural goals	Reviewing and reconsidering previously set goals – for example, the person may find it difficult to reduce their intake of full-fat cheese to two ounces per week, and may reset their goal to four ounces per week
Prompt self-monitoring of behaviour	Keeping a diet diary to document food intake
Provide feedback on performance	Providing feedback on whether the person has been able to reduce their total intake of saturated fat as a result of their dietary changes
Provide contingent rewards	Provide verbal praise and encouragement when the person achieves their goals for reducing saturated fat intake
Teach to use prompts/cues	Teach the person to identify environmental cues that can remind or help them to reduce their saturated fat intake, such as no longer purchasing full-fat cheese to reduce its availability in the home, and when buying pre-prepared foods read food labels to only select foods that are low in saturated fat
Agree to a behavioural contract	Agreement to reduce saturated fat intake is manifest in a written contract signed by the participant and witnessed by intervention deliverer
Use of follow-up prompts	Contacting the person again after the intervention is completed to discuss whether they are continuing to meet their goals in reducing saturated fat intake
Provide opportunities for social comparison	Facilitate opportunities for the person to observe the performance of non-experts in changing their saturated fat intake, such as using a video or group class approach where others illustrate how they have reduced their saturated fat intake
Plan social support/social change	Prompt the person to consider how their partner, who prepares most of the meals at home and does the food shopping, can provide support in reducing saturated fat intake, such as no longer buying full-fat cheese and avoiding using full-fat cheese in recipes or as a snack
Relapse prevention	Following initial changes that have resulted in reducing consumption of full-fat cheese, help the person identify situations that may result in them relapsing and readopting their intake of cheese, and assist them in developing a plan for avoiding or managing these situations
Motivational interviewing	Prompt the person to provide self-motivating statements and evaluations of their full-fat cheese intake to minimise their resistance to change – for example, the dietitian expresses empathy regarding the barriers to reducing cheese intake as expressed by the client and encourages the client to reflect on these challenges and prompt self-motivating statements that will support the client in reducing cheese intake

Sources: Abraham and Michie (2008) and Michie *et al.* (2009).

non-clinically trained health professionals (e.g. health educator), or non-professionals (e.g. non-clinically trained research staff). Settings of delivery included workplaces, primary care and community, with studies being conducted in the USA, UK or other European country, Australasia, Japan or Canada.

The results of meta-regression confirmed that participants that received behaviour change interventions experienced better outcomes than those in a control group. The effect size for improved outcomes was considered small, but in the range typically observed in psychological interventions. Additionally, analyses indicated that the most effective strategy in changing dietary behaviour was self-monitoring, combined with at least one of four other self-regulation strategies, including intention formation, specific goal setting, feedback on performance and review of behavioural goals. Interestingly, design factors such as duration of the intervention, mode of delivery, the person delivering the intervention, the setting for delivery and the target population were not associated with intervention effectiveness.

Upstream approaches and evidence of effectiveness

Upstream approaches are those applied at the macro-level, focusing on targeting changes at environmental and policy levels. As discussed earlier, making changes to social and physical environments and governmental policy can be quite challenging. However, there are some examples of upstream approaches targeting dietary behaviour change, such as the UK Department of Health's 'Change4Life' campaign, mandatory menu-labelling in restaurants in New York City, USA, and the UK salt reduction strategy. Owing to its well-documented evolution and evidence of effectiveness, the UK salt reduction strategy is the focus of discussion in this section.

The UK is recognised as a global leader in reducing the salt intake of the population (for more information on the relationship between salt and cardiovascular disease, see Chapter 16). These efforts started in 1991, and have continued to evolve to the present day. The World Action on Salt & Health (http://www.worldactiononsalt.com/worldaction/europe/54026.html) provides a timeline of key milestones in the UK's salt reduction strategy:

- In 1991, the Committee on Medical Aspects of Food and Nutrition Policy (COMA) set dietary reference values for salt and other nutrients. This is followed by a second report in 1994 examining the relationship between salt intake and risks for hypertension and cardiovascular disease, with recommendations given that salt intake should be reduced from 9 g/day to 6 g/day through reducing an individual's use of salt in cooking and at the table, and also through voluntary reductions made by the food and catering industries.
- In 1996, the Chief Medical Officer (CMO) refused to endorse the recommendations to reduce salt intake, prompting a group of scientific experts to set up an action group called Consensus Action on Salt and Health dedicated to reaching a consensus with the food industry and Government over the harmful effects of salt and reducing the amount of salt in the diet.
- In 2001, the CMO agreed to support a national salt target of no more than 6 g/day, which led to the Food Standards Agency (FSA) committing to a nationwide salt reduction initiative in 2002 – this commitment resulted in subsequent public health campaigns, including 'Sid the Slug', 'Check the Label' and 'Is Your Food Full of It?'
- In 2003, the Scientific Advisory Committee on Nutrition published a report emphasising that the evidence linking salt with hypertension is even stronger than it was when the original COMA report was released in 1994, leading to a call to reduce salt intake to below 6 g/day and further highlighting that, in addition to

individuals reducing their salt intake, the food and catering industries also need to play a key role in reducing the salt content of foods. That same year, a paper was published in the journal *Hypertension* (He and MacGregor, 2003) providing evidence that even greater health benefits will result from reducing salt intake to 3 g/day.

- In 2005, the World Action on Salt and Health was set up to implement salt reduction strategies worldwide.
- In 2010, the World Health Organization, the FSA, experts from 33 countries, key non-governmental organisations and the food industry held a meeting in which worldwide salt reduction was recognised as being as important to health as smoking cessation. In the same year, salt reduction commitments were secured in the UK from key catering and food manufacturers.
- In 2012, the Department of Health reported that salt intakes in the UK have declined from 9.5 g/day in 2000–2001 to 8.1 g/day in 2011.

This timeline provides an example of an effective upstream approach that moves beyond attempting to change individual behaviour by changing food environments and national policy. Although the target of consuming less than 6 g/day of salt has not yet been reached in the UK, the Department of Health continues its promotion of reducing salt intake through the New Salt Strategy released in 2013. This strategy aims to revise salt reduction targets for industry to encourage reformulation of recipes, push the catering and take-away sectors to set maximum targets for salt in sandwiches and chips, and to get more food industry companies to pledge their commitment to the new salt reduction strategy.

27.4 Advantages and limitations of individual approaches and upstream approaches

There are advantages and limitations to both individual and upstream approaches to changing dietary behaviour. Individual approaches can be specifically tailored to individuals and select target groups, taking an individual's knowledge, skills, motivation, key influences and health status into consideration. In addition, individual approaches can lead to the acquisition of knowledge and development of skills that can help individuals overcome barriers so they can consistently engage in healthy lifestyle behaviours. Additional limitations of individual approaches are that they can be relatively time, labour and resource intensive, and there is limited evidence of their cost-effectiveness.

Another limitation of individual approaches is that we know very little about how healthy eating behaviour change interventions can be best delivered within ethnic minority groups. The importance of cultural tailoring of interventions, and guidance on how to culturally tailor interventions, has been highlighted in previous research (Netto *et al.*, 2010; Barrera *et al.*, 2012). However, employing a mixed-methods evidence synthesis of the adaptation of health promotion interventions to meet the needs of ethnically minority communities, Liu *et al.* (2012) found scant evidence on the effectiveness of culturally tailored healthy eating interventions compared with standard (non-tailored) interventions. These researchers concluded that there is evidence that culturally adapting interventions can increase salience, acceptability and uptake; however, there is insufficient evidence of the effectiveness and cost-effectiveness of culturally tailored interventions compared with standard interventions.

One of the advantages of upstream approaches is that they have the potential to result in population-wide dietary behaviour change. If sustained, these changes can reduce morbidity and premature mortality resulting from chronic diseases, and substantially reduce healthcare costs. Another advantage is that they do not exclusively depend upon the ability of individuals to change their behaviour: as demonstrated by the UK salt reduction strategy, dietary changes can occur through implementing changes in food industry practices and national policies, in addition to targeting behaviours of individuals. One of the limitations of upstream approaches is that they can be very challenging to implement, as they demand sustained commitment across a wide range of sectors (such as local, regional and national policy makers, transport, urban design and planning, food and beverage industries, and local businesses). This is a likely contributor to the fact that there is limited systematic evidence examining the effectiveness of upstream approaches on changing dietary behaviours. Another limitation is that the benefits or successes of upstream approaches may not be observed for a relatively long period of time. To track their effectiveness, regular surveillance of dietary intake is required in a representative sample of the population. This requires political and financial commitment over the long term. Despite the limitations highlighted here for both types of approaches, it can be argued that successful long-term dietary change is more likely to occur through the implementation of effective individual *and* upstream approaches.

27.5 Conclusions

Behaviour change theories and models are tools that are necessary in enhancing our understanding of the factors that affect the dietary intake of individuals and populations. They also serve as frameworks for the development of effective interventions targeting dietary change. Much of the existing literature has focused on changing the behaviour of individuals. The most effective behaviour change strategies identified for individuals include self-monitoring combined with at least one of four other self-regulation strategies, including intention formation, specific goal setting, feedback on performance and review of behavioural goals. Upstream approaches to changing behaviour involve trying to effect change at the environmental and policy levels. An example of an effective upstream approach is the UK salt reduction strategy, which has led to a reduction in salt intake at the population level over a 10-year period. To be effective, upstream approaches demand a long-term commitment across a wide range of sectors. Although changing dietary behaviours of individuals and populations is not necessarily easy, there is evidence that changes can be achieved through the implementation of theoretically derived interventions amongst individuals and at the population level.

References

Abraham, C. and Michie, S. (2008) A taxonomy of behavior change techniques used in interventions. *Health Psychology*, **27**(3), 379–387.

Ajzen, I. (1991) Theory of planned behaviour. *Organizational Behavior and Human Decision Processes*, **50**, 179–211.

Bandura, A. (1986) *Social Foundations of Thought and Action: A Social Cognitive Theory*. Prentice Hall, Englewood Cliffs, NJ.

Barrera Jr, M., Castro, F.G., Strycker, L.A. and Toobert, D.J. (2013) Cultural adaptations of behavioral health interventions: a progress report. *Journal of Consulting and Clinical Psychology*, **81**(2), 196–205.

Bates, B. Lennox, A., Prentice, A. *et al.* (eds) (2014) *National Diet and Nutrition Survey: Results from Years 1-4 (Combined) of the Rolling Programme 2008/09-2011/12. Executive Summary*. https://www.gov.uk/government/uploads/system/uploads/attachment_data/file/310997/NDNS_Y1_to_4_UK_report_Executive_summary.pdf (accessed 02 February 2017).

Carpenter, R.A., Finley, C. and Barlow, C.E. (2004) Pilot test of a behavioral skill building intervention to improve overall diet quality. *Journal of Nutrition Education and Behavior*, **36**, 20–26.

Davison, K.K. and Campbell, K. (2005) Opportunities to prevent obesity of children within families: an ecological approach. In D. Crawford and R. Jeffery (eds), *Obesity Prevention and Public Health*. Oxford University Press, Oxford; pp. 207–230.

Davison, K.K., Jurkowski, J.M. and Lawson, H.A. (2012) Reframing family-centred obesity prevention using the family ecological model. *Public Health Nutrition*, **16**(10), 1861–1869.

DiClemente, C.C. and Prochaska, J.O. (1982) Self change and therapy change of smoking behavior. A comparison of processes and change in cessation and maintenance. *Addictive Behaviors*, 7, 133–142.

Drewnowski, A. and Darmon, N. (2005) The economics of obesity: dietary energy density and energy cost. *The American Journal of Clinical Nutrition*, **82**(1), 265S–273S.

He, F.J. and MacGregor, G.A. (2003) How far should salt intake be reduced? *Hypertension*, **42**, 1093–1099.

Helitzer, D., Peterson, A.B., Thompson, J. and Fluder, S. (2008) Development of a planning and evaluation methodology for assessing the contribution of theory to a diabetes prevention lifestyle intervention. *Health Promotion Practice*, **9**, 404–414.

Joint WHO/FAO Expert Consultation (2003) *Diet, Nutrition and the Prevention of Chronic Diseases*. WHO Technical Report Series 916. World Health Organization, Geneva. http://www.who.int/dietphysicalactivity/publications/trs916/en/gsfao_introduction.pdf (accessed 24 December 2016).

Liu, J.J., Davidson, E., Bhopal, R.S. *et al.* (2012) Adapting health promotion interventions to meet the needs of ethnic minority groups: mixed-methods evidence synthesis. *Health Technology Assessment*, **16**, (44).

McAlister, A.L., Perry, C.L. and Parcel, G.S. (2008) How individuals, environments, and health behaviors interact: social cognitive theory. In K. Glanz, B.K. Rimer and K. Viswanath (eds), *Health Behavior and Health Education: Theory, Research and Practice*, 4th edn. Jossey-Bass, San Francisco, CA; pp. 169–188.

Michie, S., Abraham, C., Whittington, C. *et al.* (2009) Effective techniques in healthy eating and physical activity interventions: a meta-regression. *Health Psychology*, **28**(6), 690–701.

Montaño, D.E. and Kasprzyk, D. (2008) Theory of reasoned action, theory of planned behavior, and the integrated behavioral model. In K. Glanz, B.K. Rimer and K. Viswanath (eds), *Health Behavior and Health Education: Theory, Research and Practice*, 4th edn. Jossey-Bass; San Francisco, CA; pp. 67–96.

Netto, G., Bhopal, R., Lederle, N. *et al.* (2010) How can health promotion interventions be adapted for minority ethnic communities? Five principles for guiding the development of behavioural interventions. *Health Promotion International*, **25**(2), 248–257.

Prochaska, J.O., Redding, C.A. and Evers, K.E. (2008) The trans-theoretical model and stages of change. In K. Glanz, B.K. Rimer and K. Viswanath (eds), *Health Behavior and Health Education: Theory, Research and Practice*, 4th edn. Jossey-Bass, San Francisco, CA; pp. 97–121.

Rosenheck, R. (2008) Fast food consumption and increased caloric intake: a systematic review of a trajectory towards weight gain and obesity. *Obesity Reviews*, **9**(6), 535–547.

Sallis, J.F., Owen, N. and Fisher, E.B. (2008) Ecological models of health behavior. In K. Glanz, B.K. Rimer and K. Viswanath (eds), *Health Behavior and Health Education: Theory, Research and Practice*, 4th edn. Jossey-Bass, San Francisco, CA; pp. 465–485.

Schulze, M.B., Manson, J.E., Ludwig, D.S. *et al.* (2004) Sugar-sweetened beverages, weight gain, and incidence of type 2 diabetes in young and middle-aged women. *JAMA*, **292**, 927–934.

Story, M., Kaphingst, K.M., Robinson-O'Brien, R. and Glanz, K. (2008) Creating healthy food and eating environments: policy and environmental approaches. *Annual Review of Public Health*, **29**, 253–272.

Taylor, D., Bury, M., Campling, N. *et al.* (2006) *A Review of the Health Belief Model (HBM), the Theory of Reasoned Action (TRA), the Theory of Planned Behaviour (TPB), and the Trans-Theoretical Model (TTM) to Study and Predict Health Related Behaviour Change.* https://www.nice.org.uk/guidance/ph6/resources/behaviour-change-taylor-et-al-models-review2 (accessed 11 January 2017).

US Department of Agriculture and US Department of Health and Human Services (2010) *Dietary Guidelines for Americans, 2010*, 7th edn. US Government Printing Office, Washington, DC. https://www.cnpp.usda.gov/sites/default/files/dietary_guidelines_for_americans/PolicyDoc.pdf (accessed 28 December 2016).

28
Evaluation of Public Health Nutrition Interventions and Policies

Ailsa A Welch and Richard PG Hayhoe

Key messages

- Nutrition is one of the key behavioural determinants of health. Thus, measuring the impact of interventions to improve food intakes and rates of obesity is important.
- The types of study design for evaluation may be based on more pragmatic options than randomised controlled trials (RCTs) and include process evaluation, impact evaluation and outcome evaluation. These newer types of study design – 'realistic study designs', 'process evaluation' and 'natural experiments' – are beginning to be accepted as alternatives to the traditional gold standard of RCTs.

- Evaluation tools for assessing dietary intakes and body composition, and for statistical analysis of results arising from evaluations, are described.
- Practical recommendations include ensuring sufficient funding is available to cover the cost of the evaluation, involving an academic institution in the design and performance of the evaluation process where possible, integrating evaluation into the commissioning cycle of all public health nutrition programmes, setting up of structured data collection databases, and publication in peer-reviewed journals where possible.

28.1 Introduction: background

Global rates of obesity have almost doubled world-wide, since 1980, with 11% of men and 15% of women obese (WHO, 2014). Within England the most recent statistics indicate that 67% of men and 57% of women are either overweight or obese (HSCIC, 2015). In children, an estimated 6.3% worldwide are overweight or obese. In the UK, 9.5% of children who start school are obese, with a rise in prevalence to 19.1% in year 6 (Lifestyles Statistics Team, 2015). With the well-established link between obesity, poor health outcomes, non-communicable chronic diseases (including diabetes, cardiovascular disease and cancer) and all-cause mortality, public health interventions to tackle the problem of obesity are essential. Furthermore, despite the coherence in the dietary recommendations for consumption of fruits and vegetables and the health benefits on outcomes for chronic diseases and mortality, only approximately a quarter of people in the UK consume the recommended intake of five portions of fruits and vegetables a day, with even

fewer children (16%) reaching this target (Lifestyles Statistics Team, 2015). Moreover, other dietary guidelines for foods and nutrients (e.g. for dietary fibre (non-starch polysaccharides), oily fish and iron) within the UK are only partially reached (Bates *et al.*, 2014).

With such important problems in public health nutrition there are a number of local and national health improvement initiatives designed to treat or reduce the prevalence of obesity and improve dietary intakes (particularly of fruits and vegetables) in the population. It is also important to understand whether health improvement interventions are effective, and there are compelling reasons to evaluate the success of public health interventions because evaluation provides evidence to influence future practice and policy. Evidence from evaluations may be used to continue or discontinue intervention programmes and, more importantly, to recommend service improvements that can be implemented during the course of a public health intervention. Evaluation can 'increase the quality and effectiveness of any initiative by contributing to the processes of its

Public Health Nutrition, Second Edition. Edited by Judith L Buttriss, Ailsa A Welch, John M Kearney and Susan A Lanham-New.
© 2018 by The Nutrition Society. Published 2018 by John Wiley & Sons, Ltd.
Companion website: www.wiley.com/go/buttriss/publichealth

planning, development and implementation' (Rootman *et al.*, 2001). The outcome of evaluations provides information for public health practitioners to inform future work. The results of evaluations are relevant for planning and to inform development of policy at local and national levels. Other reasons for evaluation include understanding whether the investment in resources, both human and financial, results in effective outcomes from public health initiatives. Finally, the results from evaluation provide the evidence base for future public health interventions.

This chapter covers aspects of evaluation that relate to either health promotion, health improvement or public health interventions in nutrition, including obesity (termed public health interventions or programmes from here on). Evaluation can be either quantitative or qualitative and can be carried out in a range of health improvement programmes, particularly in individual and setting-based interventions, which is the main focus of the material we provide in this chapter. Some of the content of this chapter is based on our practical experience on a long-term project working within academia alongside public health colleagues (within a primary care trust and subsequently the local authority). We have provided guidance which we hope will be useful to those who are new to the field of evaluation for public health nutrition interventions. We have covered styles and designs of evaluations, study design, tools for assessment, statistical methods and ethical issues. We have also highlighted resources and web sites that can be used for further information and have provided examples of successful evaluations for interventions in public health nutrition, such as those designed to treat or reduce obesity or to increase fruit and vegetable consumption.

28.2 Evaluation design

Evaluation design may vary considerably depending on the specifics of the programme being evaluated and the aims to be addressed. Nevertheless, programme evaluations may be categorised into three principal types: process, impact and outcome. For the effective evaluation of a particular programme, evaluators may use more than one type as appropriate.

Fundamental to all evaluations are the following components:

- *A clearly defined objective.* This will help to focus the evaluation and guide what measures are used.
- *A distinct target population.* Defining the target population is essential in order to set boundaries for the evaluation.
- *Appropriate methodology.* The information to be collected for the evaluation needs to be defined and the

methods for gathering this information decided. This may involve designing and testing data collection instruments before the full evaluation is carried out.
- *Data collection, data processing and analysis.* Data collected using appropriate methodology must be collated and processed into a suitable format before analysis may take place.
- *An evaluation report.* Once all other components have been completed, the report can be written using the results of the data analysis, interpreting and putting the results into context, and drawing conclusions.

Process evaluation

Process evaluation focuses on the procedures involved in programme delivery and whether the implementation went according to plan. This type of evaluation should be begun soon after programme implementation and monitored regularly throughout its duration. Appropriate methods include observation, interviews and analysis of programme activity to answer a number of questions, such as:

- How was the programme provided?
  - Were there any significant barriers to effective provision?
- What population groups and how many individuals were reached by the programme?
  - How does this compare with the planned activity and target group?
- What was the quality of the service according to participants?

Answering these questions will give valuable information about the provision of the programme, allowing both positive and negative aspects of programme provision to be identified and recommendations made for potential improvements to address any problems. It is possible that some of these issues would be generalisable if the programme were implemented elsewhere, although it is likely that most will be unique to the local delivery team, population, and location.

Impact evaluation

Impact evaluation assesses the immediate effects of the intervention on participants and other stakeholders. Baseline data should be collected at the start of the programme, and compared with data collected at follow-up time-points during service delivery. What changes have occurred as a result of the programme which would be expected to influence the programme-relevant health outcomes? These might include:

- increased knowledge;
- changes in attitudes, beliefs, and behaviour.

Using impact evaluation at an early stage of the programme can guide service development if the expected changes are not evident. Data at different time-points are critical to this type of evaluation process, in order to be able to monitor change. This monitoring of data will be highly informative to the programme funders or commissioners, and will influence early decisions as to whether to continue funding.

Outcome evaluation

The distinction between impact and outcome evaluations of public health programmes may be confused as they both typically assess the effects of an intervention on health and health behaviours. However, the distinction is based on different scales and timelines of these effects. Outcome evaluation assesses the longer term effects of the intervention (e.g. changes in risk factors, morbidity, mortality, disability, functional independence, equity and quality of life) that have occurred as a result of the intervention. For nutritional and weight management interventions these may include reduced prevalence of obesity, reduced morbidity (hospital admission rates) and reduced mortality from obesity and cardiovascular disease. Some of these data may be available from existing sources (e.g. local authority data, GP practice data, hospital episode statistics, national surveys – including the National Diet and Nutrition Survey and the Health Survey for England), as well as locally commissioned surveys.

Evidence from outcome evaluation should help inform future funding and commissioning decisions, and may contribute to the evidence base used for the introduction of specific health policies. Indeed, although outcome evaluations are often particularly informative for other areas and applications, the specific type of study design used may have implications for the acceptability of the results for publication in peer-reviewed literature. Evaluation of public health interventions often requires a pragmatic approach to collecting data using relatively basic resources, while ensuring there is minimal influence on intervention content and participation. Unfortunately, some journals are less prepared than others to publish findings of evaluations using 'observational' study designs rather than randomised controlled trials (RCTs). Nevertheless, evaluators should always strive to disseminate their findings as widely as possible.

Typical non-RCT options are outlined as follows:

- *Post-intervention study.* Measurements are taken at the end of the intervention period. This is the least reliable study design option as it can only provide a 'snapshot' of the situation following the intervention. Effects cannot be causally attributed to the intervention.

- *Paired pre- and post-intervention study.* Measurements are taken from the same population or individuals at the start of the intervention and at completion. Allows change to be assessed, but causality cannot be ascertained since there is no control of possible contributing factors. Additional time-points during and post-intervention may also be used to give an indication of interim and longer term changes respectively.

- *Non-paired pre- and post-intervention study.* Measurements are taken both at the start of the intervention and at completion, but from a different population or individuals. Allows change to be assessed, but any differences between pre- and post-intervention study groups may be responsible for differences in outcomes observed. These may be statistically adjusted for, but causality cannot be proven.

Economic evaluation

Incorporating some simple cost analyses is particularly useful for outcome evaluations, as this will allow comparison with other programmes that have undergone economic evaluation and may, therefore, be used to justify the continuation or discontinuation of a programme. However, full economic evaluation of a public health programme is likely to require specialist knowledge or engagement of a health economics team.

Summary

Design of public health evaluation studies is highly situation dependent and is influenced by a multitude of factors, including timescale, funding and availability of data. RCTs are regarded as the gold standard for research evidence, with pre- and post-intervention measurements from participants randomised to intervention or control groups providing reliable evidence of the effects of a particular programme. Given the nature of public health nutrition interventions, and the vulnerability of the target populations, RCTs may be difficult to achieve both in practical and ethical terms. However, there is ongoing discussion regarding the utility and effectiveness of RCT study design for public health interventions, with alternative study designs such as 'realistic study designs', 'process evaluation' and 'natural experiments' being suggested (Bonell *et al.*, 2012; Craig *et al.*, 2012; Moore *et al.*, 2014). Indeed, the importance of process evaluation should not be underestimated as it can provide invaluable information regarding the implementation and delivery of public health interventions (e.g. school-based nutrition promotion) (Steckler *et al.*, 2003; Volpe *et al.*, 2013), while realistic study design has also been discussed for health promotion evaluation in schools (Pommier, 2010). Natural experiments have been used extensively in the past in epidemiology, where naturally occurring variations in exposure have been available for comparison – for example, John Snow's seminal investigation of a cholera outbreak in London (Snow, 1855) – and this type of study design also has a place in public health evaluation of nutritional interventions. For example, the Norwegian School Fruit Scheme has been evaluated as a natural experiment with different groups generated 'naturally' by differing availability of the scheme at schools and changes to the scheme from subsidised to free fruit provision (Øvrum and Bere, 2013).

28.3 Data collection tools and their validation

A fundamental consideration when choosing impact measurement tools or questionnaires is whether the tool measures what it was intended to measure. For example, in the case of a food frequency questionnaire, do the data accurately reflect actual dietary intake? Published questionnaires will normally have undergone some form of validation process. However, the validation may not necessarily translate directly for use in a different population group. For example, a validated adult questionnaire is unlikely to be suitable for children, and may also pose difficulties for adult populations with low levels of literacy or education. The National Obesity Observatory documents provide a list of some of the more common questionnaires used in weight management interventions, together with the population groups for which they have been validated; see Box 28.1 for links. Please also see Chapters 3 and 4. However, it may be necessary to consider piloting a questionnaire when the population group to be studied has not previously been included in a validation process.

Box 28.1 Evaluation resources

National Obesity Observatory: standard evaluation frameworks

The Public Health England National Obesity Observatory has published evaluation guidance in the form of standard evaluation frameworks for 'weight management interventions', 'physical activity interventions' and 'dietary interventions'. These make recommendations for the structure and content of an evaluation, subdivided into essential and desirable criteria for data collection.
   http://www.noo.org.uk/core/frameworks

National Obesity Observatory: dietary surveillance and nutritional assessment in England

The National Obesity Observatory also lists some of the main sources of national data for dietary intake and nutritional status of the population in England. The data provided by each source are described and the different methodologies and their limitations are discussed.
   http://www.noo.org.uk/uploads/doc/vid_5191_Dietary_Surveillance_and_Nutritional_Assessment_in_England.pdf

National Institute for Health and Care Excellence: guidance documents on diet, nutrition and obesity

The National Institute for Health and Care Excellence publishes guidance for a range of public health subjects. These typically include recommendations for implementation and promotion of particular public health services, but also provide details of indicators and outcomes for particular types of intervention which may assist when designing and developing a programme evaluation.
   http://www.nice.org.uk/guidance/lifestyle-and-wellbeing/diet--nutrition-and-obesity

Centers for Disease Control and Prevention: evaluation tools

The US Centers for Disease Control and Prevention web site contains a list of references relevant to programme evaluation. These include generic step-by-step manuals to evaluation, in addition to more specific guides for particular aspects of evaluation.
   https://www.cdc.gov/eval/resources/index.htm

Medical Research Council: diet and physical activity measurement toolkit

The UK Medical Research Council has funded an online toolkit providing resources for evaluation of diet and physical activity interventions. Links to validated questionnaires, discussion of the most appropriate methodologies to use in different situations, as well as practical considerations are covered in this online toolkit.
   http://dapa-toolkit.mrc.ac.uk/
   Links valid 29 December 2016.

28.4 Data analysis and statistics

Without the use of suitable data analysis methodology the resources spent collecting data are wasted and, moreover, the interpretation may be misleading. It is important to consider the evaluation objectives in order to carry out the analysis and present the data in a way that addresses these most closely. Some of the issues to consider are: What is the target audience for the evaluation and, therefore, how will it be best to present and communicate the results (e.g. text, tables or graphs)? What are the limitations of the data and how does this influence the interpretation? Can the data collection be improved for future evaluations?

Statistical analysis is critical to the interpretation of quantitative data collated during the evaluation process. A p value of <0.05 is normally an appropriate limit for statistical significance. The simple statistical tests described here will be suitable for well-defined discrete interventions, but it may be advantageous to discuss the most appropriate analysis methodology with a statistician or data analysis expert, particularly where the interventions are of a more complex nature. The statistical methods most likely to be useful for evaluation of simple nutritional interventions include t-tests and McNemar's post-hoc test for paired data (e.g. same person baseline and follow-up) when analysing continuous data, and chi-squared or odds ratio testing for non-continuous data.

A useful online resource is the GraphPad Software web site (http://www.graphpad.com/data-analysis-resource-center/), which provides excellent advice on choosing the correct statistical test and interpreting the output, as well quick calculators for small datasets, while Andy Field's textbook provides a comprehensive guide to performing statistical analyses using SPSS software (Field, 2013).

28.5 Ethical issues

Service evaluation will not normally require evaluators to obtain specific ethics approval from a research ethics committee. This exemption is based on the understanding that the intervention being evaluated does not involve any change from the standard service delivery. However, it remains essential that whenever an evaluation is conducted, ethical principles be observed. These will include the following:

- *Informed consent.* Participants included in the evaluation study should be fully informed about the evaluation process, including who will have access to data and what the purpose of the evaluation is.

- *Rights to withdraw.* Participation should be free from coercion, and individuals should understand that they retain the right to withdraw without an explanation at any time and this will have no effect on their treatment in the service.
- *Do no harm.* The evaluation process must not cause participants any harm, physical or psychological.
- *Confidentiality and anonymity.* The minimum necessary personal information should be collected, and all data must remain confidential so that only the specific evaluation team have access to raw data. Under no circumstances should it be possible to identify participants from evaluation reports or associated publications.
- *No conflicts of interest.* The evaluation team should avoid including individuals with significant conflicts of interest related to the programme.
- *Dissemination of findings.* The findings of the evaluation should be disseminated irrespective of the outcome of the programme.

28.6 Recommendations

In this section we provide some recommendations based on our practical experience working in an academic and public health partnership.

- Ensure sufficient funding is available to cover the cost of the evaluation in terms of development and production of questionnaires, costs of equipment and funding for personnel to perform the evaluation, either internal or external to the organisation.
- Underlying any successful evaluation is an informed choice of outcomes. These must be measurable or testable activities and goals.
- It may be appropriate and advisable to, where possible, involve an academic institution in the design and statistical analysis of the evaluation to ensure that there is an evidence base and sound rationale for the choice of indicators used to assess change in outcomes.
- Evaluation should be integrated into the commissioning cycle of all public health programmes with plans for measurement of outcomes. Evaluation should be considered in the early stages of development of the intervention. We suggest that the criteria for evaluation should be contained within contract documents. This should include the requirements for data to be supplied from the service provider to the commissioners and evaluators, and that data sharing agreements are established to allow this transfer of data according to a defined schedule.

Box 28.2 Examples of effective evaluations

The following gives brief details of two programme evaluations conducted by academic staff in conjunction with a local authority public health department, demonstrating the benefits of this type of collaboration to achieve the best service for the community.

Increasing fruit and vegetable intake using a mobile food store

Jennings *et al.* (2012) provide an example of evaluation being a key consideration from the initial planning stage of the programme, through to follow-up evaluation of the service 2 years after implementation. Survey data were used together with postcode mapping to identify communities with low fruit and vegetables intake and high chronic disease risk. This information was used to set up a mobile food store service which travelled to these communities each week to provide cost-price fruit and vegetables. Evaluation results using a validated questionnaire showed use of the store resulted in a significant increase in fruit and vegetable intake, providing support for this type of targeted model. The evidence provided by this evaluation resulted in the continued commissioning of the scheme and development of a plan to extend the service to other areas of deprivation in the UK.

Improving healthy behaviours using the health trainer service

Jennings *et al.* (2013) describe an evaluation of a health trainer service in Great Yarmouth and Waveney with effectiveness assessed in terms of weight loss and healthy lifestyle behaviour change. Weight measurements, as well as blood pressure, fruit and vegetable intake and physical activity levels, were measured using established health trainer data recording systems. Analysis of this data demonstrated weight loss and positive changes in health-related behaviour were achieved by participants, thus providing support for this type of health-trainer-led intervention which led to further commissioning of heath trainer services in Norfolk.

- Where baseline data are to be supplied by the service provider, this should always be collected soon after the start of the programme. This is to preserve the integrity of the data and reduce the risk of data being 'altered' to produce results more favourable to continued commissioning of the service. This may be incorporated into routine data reporting and contract monitoring processes.
- The structure of electronic spreadsheets or databases used to record evaluation data also requires careful consideration. Not only does this need to be simple to avoid data entry errors, but it must also be comprehensive enough to allow for adequate data analysis and interpretation. It thus may be advantageous to develop a template, and associated guide, with all the necessary fields/variables included. Drop-down boxes with a set of defined options may be used where appropriate (e.g. for ethnicity) to avoid ambiguous or incorrect coding, and formulae can be used to automate calculations (e.g. of body mass index or differences pre- and post-intervention).
- Where possible the results of evaluations should be published in the peer-reviewed literature, as this generates the widest dissemination; please see Box 28.2 for examples.

28.7 Conclusions

Evaluation of public health improvement interventions is important to understand their effectiveness and for informing future practice and public health policy.

Despite the difficulties in performing RCTs in the field of public health, newer developments and acceptance of other study designs (such as 'realistic study designs', 'process evaluation' and 'natural experiments') will make evaluations in the public health setting more achievable (Bonell *et al.*, 2012; Craig *et al.*, 2012; Moore *et al.*, 2014).

Although there is currently a paucity of evidence for effectiveness and cost-effectiveness of public health nutrition interventions, and evaluation of public health nutrition interventions is considered an emerging field, this is a growing area of awareness. The acceptance of study designs beyond the RCT will contribute considerably to this area.

References

Bates, B., Lennox, A., Prentice, A. *et al.* (2014) *National Diet and Nutrition Survey: Results from Years 1, 2, 3 and 4 (Combined) of the Rolling Programme (2008/2009–2011/2012). A Survey Carried Out on Behalf of Public Health England and the Food Standards Agency.* Public Health England, London. https://www.gov.uk/government/uploads/system/uploads/attachment_data/file/310995/NDNS_Y1_to_4_UK_report.pdf (accessed 6 December 2016).

Bonell, C., Fletcher, A., Morton, M. *et al.* (2012) Realist randomised controlled trials: a new approach to evaluating complex public health interventions. *Social Science & Medicine*, **75**(12), 2299–2306.

Craig, P., Cooper, C., Gunnell, D. *et al.* (2012) Using natural experiments to evaluate population health interventions: new Medical Research Council guidance. *Journal of Epidemiology and Community Health*, **66**(12), 1182–1186.

Field, A. (2013) *Discovering Statistics using IBM SPSS Statistics*, 4th edn. Sage Publications.

HSCIC (2015) *Statistics on Obesity, Physical Activity and Diet: England 2015.* Health and Social Care Information Centre. http://www.hscic.gov.uk/catalogue/PUB16988/obes-phys-acti-diet-eng-2015.pdf (accessed 29 December 2016).

Jennings, A., Cassidy, A., Winters, T. *et al.* (2012) Positive effect of a targeted intervention to improve access and availability of fruit and vegetables in an area of deprivation. *Health & Place,* **18**(5), 1074–1078.

Jennings, A., Barnes, S., Okereke, U. and Welch, A. (2013) Successful weight management and health behaviour change using a health trainer model. *Perspectives in Public Health,* 2013 Jul; **133**(4), 221–226.

Moore, G., Audrey, S., Barker, M. *et al.* (2014) Process evaluation in complex public health intervention studies: the need for guidance. *Journal of Epidemiology and Community Health,* **68**(2), 101–102. Erratum: *Journal of Epidemiology and Community Health* (2014) **68**(6), 585.

Øvrum, A. and Bere, E. (2014) Evaluating free school fruit: results from a natural experiment in Norway with representative data. *Public Health Nutrition,* **17**(6), 1224–1231.

Pommier, J., Guével, M.-R. and Jourdan, D. (2010) Evaluation of health promotion in schools: a realistic evaluation approach using mixed methods. *BMC Public Health,* **10**, 43.

Rootman, I., Goodstadt, M., Hyndman, B. *et al.* (eds) (2001) *Evaluation in Health Promotion: Principles and Perspectives.* WHO Regional Publications, European Series, No. 92. World Health Organization Regional Office for Europe, Denmark. http://www.euro.who.int/__data/assets/pdf_file/0007/108934/E73455.pdf (accessed 29 December 2016).

Snow, J. (1855) *On the Mode of Communication of Cholera.* 2nd edn. John Churchill, London.

Steckler, A., Ethelbah, B., Martin, C.J. *et al.* (2003) Pathways process evaluation results: a school-based prevention trial to promote healthful diet and physical activity in American Indian third, fourth, and fifth grade students. *Preventive Medicine,* **37**(6 Pt 2), S80–S90.

Volpe, S.L., Hall, W.J., Steckler, A. *et al.* (2013) Process evaluation results from the HEALTHY nutrition intervention to modify the total school food environment. *Health Education Research,* **28**(6), 970–978.

rdWHO (2014) *Global Status Report on Noncommunicable Diseases 2014.* WHO Press, Geneva. http://apps.who.int/iris/bitstream/10665/148114/1/9789241564854_eng.pdf (accessed 29 December 2016).

29
Considerations for Evaluation of Public Health Nutrition Interventions in Diverse Communities

Basma Ellahi

Key messages

- Knowledge of ethnic groups, and in particular their food habits, is critical in evaluation.
- Nutritionists should ensure they are culturally competent to work with diverse communities.
- Evaluation of diverse groups requires consideration of language and cultural specific outcomes and literacy issues.

- Identifying the factors that support successful nutrition interventions in diverse groups is challenging without the appropriate tools and measures.

29.1 Introduction

We now live in increasingly multicultural societies with people of diverse heritage. Some are recent immigrants or transient, but others have been settled in the new society for several generations. Examples include people from the Indian subcontinent living in the UK and Europe, or Hispanics and Africans living in the USA. These cultural groups are often defined in terms of their ethnicity. In this context the use of the word ethnicity or ethnic group implies a cultural identity as well as other characteristics associated with ancestral heritage. These ethnic groups have shown a desire to be respected and acknowledged for their unique ancestry and contributions to society. Although often referred to as minority groups of the population, in certain locations they can represent a majority, and thus these culturally and linguistically diverse groups require special consideration when approaching evaluation.

Nutrition is a major modifiable behavioural risk factor in many non-communicable diseases, including obesity, undernutrition, diabetes, cardiovascular diseases and certain cancers and, therefore, is a key determinant of

health and well-being. Ethnic populations have a higher risk of developing nutrition-related non communicable diseases. For example, in the UK, ethnic minorities represent a significant group, many of whom originate in the Indian subcontinent (India, Pakistan and Bangladesh) and have among the highest rates of cardiovascular disease (Gilbert and Khokhar, 2008; Leung and Stanner, 2011) and diabetes (Leung and Stanner, 2011). The health needs of ethnic groups reflect the need for high-risk population groups to have specifically designed prevention or behavioural intervention approaches and an evidence base to demonstrate what is effective.

There is increasing need and motivation among nutritionists and dietitians working in public or community health to understand culture and ethnicity factors in order to provide appropriate programmes and services and for their evaluation. This increased motivation for improving quality, particularly for interventions for ethnic and culturally diverse populations, is attributable in part to the growing social presence of diverse cultural groups in society at large and their poor health profiles. This chapter discusses some of the key considerations for

Public Health Nutrition, Second Edition. Edited by Judith L Buttriss, Ailsa A Welch, John M Kearney and Susan A Lanham-New.
© 2018 by The Nutrition Society. Published 2018 by John Wiley & Sons, Ltd.
Companion website: www.wiley.com/go/buttriss/publichealth

evaluation of interventions with a focus on dietary change in diverse communities and on the implications for future research.

29.2 Cultural competency

Diversity literally means difference. Individual and group diversity need to be considered in order to ensure that everybody's needs and requirements are understood and responded to within nutrition intervention design and delivery. Evaluation can then address whether all ethnic groups respond to the programme or service in the same way and have achieved the same outcomes; for example, whether the factors contributing to enhancing motivation to change are similar or different, and what contributes to facilitating or enabling an action (such as making food-based change).

Nutritionists as educators should aim to become 'culturally competent' to work more effectively with diverse communities. By this, they should possess a set of competencies around knowledge and interpersonal skills that enable them to increase their understanding and appreciation of cultural differences and similarities which exist among and between groups, and to work competently and effectively in cross-cultural situations. Several authors describe fairly similar steps on the continuum of becoming culturally competent which can be applied to the nutrition professional. A number of models describe this process of largely similar steps. In general, these are summarised as: acquiring *cultural knowledge* (learning about the world view of other cultures); gaining *cultural awareness* (the process of becoming more aware of your own learned biases and prejudices toward other cultures, whilst becoming aware of the beliefs, values, practices, lifestyles and problem-solving strategies of other cultural groups); and having *cultural sensitivity* (an awareness of your own cultural beliefs, assumptions, customs and values as well as those of other groups, and recognition that similarities and differences exist without assigning values to those differences, such as right or wrong) (Contento, 2016).

Diverse communities often come with new sets of values, beliefs and cultural expectations. The issues of culture, literacy and language can have an impact on the provision of appropriate services. To be culturally competent and ensure effective practices with diverse groups nutritionists need to have knowledge and skills for multiethnic evaluation, including abilities to:

- recognise ethnic and cultural diversity;
- understand the role that culture and ethnicity play in the development of ethnic and culturally diverse populations;

- understand that socio-economic and political factors significantly impact on the development of ethnic and culturally diverse groups;
- help clients to understand/maintain/resolve their own sociocultural identity in relation to food choices for improved health;
- be advocates for communities by understanding and representing their needs as appropriate;
- empower communities to increase their degree of autonomy in order to enable them to represent their interests in a responsible and self-determined way, acting on their own authority.

These aspects are adapted from American Psychological Association (n.d.) but are very relevant to nutritionists. They are discussed within this chapter in relation to evaluation.

29.3 Ethnic and cultural diversity

Culture can be described as a set of beliefs, knowledge, traditions, values and behavioural patterns that are developed, learned and shared by members of a group. Culture has an important role in food, nutrition and health. For example, beliefs help determine which foods are edible and how to prepare these; traditions can influence what is eaten for health or for curative reasons; religion can affect approaches to fasting and feasting or restricted foods. Values are widely held beliefs that influence what is considered important for well-being. What may be considered desirable by one culture or group may not be so in another but may nevertheless have an influence on food and nutrition practices and, thus, for evaluation may result in a different outcome that needs to be captured.

Cultures do, however, constantly change; thus, with acculturation (that is, cultural modification of an individual, group or people by adapting to or borrowing traits from another culture), food habits change. But equally so, change can be resisted, so that cultural identity and boundaries are maintained. It is important for nutritionists to acknowledge that these cultural differences are reflected in the kinds of foods purchased, how they are prepared, and how and when they are eaten. How and when people shop for food, the timing of meals, the social context of meals and whose preferences at household level may dominate food choice and should also be considered. For example, in many cultures the elder male member of the family dominates food choice. Furthermore, we need to remember that everyone will interpret their own culture as individuals. A geographical move to another country can influence this, as food choices are affected by availability and access to the usual foods within a culture. This has implications for design of evaluations which need to capture an individual's starting position as well as the outcome. To ensure this information is captured, it is important to consider the evaluation strategy alongside programme development rather than leaving the design of the evaluation to the end of an intervention (which often happens), otherwise this insight can be lost. Strategies for evaluation should focus on the multitude of factors causing dietary changes, such as changes to meal patterns, meal composition and intake of different foods. This may mean using a variety of approaches to capture the data, embracing not only quantitative methods, but also a range of qualitative methods. In reality, this can prove challenging with funders and/or commissioners of projects, who often wish to see quantitative outcomes reflective of more robust evaluation designs, such as randomised controlled trials. However, in order to take account of the diversity of the community in relation to a health issue, we need to use an approach that is specific for the chosen behaviour being addressed, and the specific social and cultural context of the determinants of change for target intervention groups. Thus, we should ensure a variety of different approaches not only in the design, but also in the evaluation.

Furthermore, involving groups in the design of the evaluation is just as important as in the intervention design phase. Kong *et al.* (2014) present a systematic review on evaluation of diet and weight changes in African-American women. They suggest that studies with significant findings commonly report participant involvement during the formative phases. Involving the intended participants early on in the process would help uncover key attributes of the target group which helps understanding of the heterogeneity that exists even within ethnic groups, thus informing evaluation. Yancey *et al.* (2004) reviewed a number of interventions for ethnic-specific aspects. Ethnically sensitive studies placed greater emphasis on involving community and building coalitions from inception. However, again, there was an absence of studies that report how to create an interest in and sustain weight loss in ethnic groups.

From the literature looking at evaluation in diverse cultural groups, it is clear that few intervention studies have demonstrated sustained effectiveness in preventing or controlling weight gain and obesity through healthy living and active living approaches in ethnic groups/populations. This means that public health nutritionists do not have a strong evidence base for designing or implementing targeted approaches.

Finally, there is little consistency in how culture as a variable is defined or measured. Further work to address this for designing evaluations is necessary so that outcomes can be compared and thus provide a stronger

evidence base. Although there is a paucity of research on culturally specific evaluation in nutrition, culturally specific research as part of the design stage of an intervention is commonly found and can help identify appropriate measures, such as identifying ways of knowing about healthy eating, eating practices, barriers and preferences for intervention. Tiedje *et al.* (2014) explored this and concluded that 'cultural factors are not fixed variables that occur independently from the contexts in which they are embedded'. Encouraging a similar focus for evaluation with diverse communities will enhance the value (especially to others) of the outcomes reported.

29.4 Literacy

The importance of tailoring culturally specific messages and messengers is recognised (Yancey *et al.*, 2004). In the UK the Department of Health (2004) suggested that the need for clear, accessible and 'tailored advice' is critical if the behaviour change is to be made and sustained, and these principles still apply today. In this context, a distinction between general literacy and health literacy should be acknowledged. General literacy is a key determinant of health, and debate tends to centre on income and income distribution, employment, working conditions and social environment. Health literacy is more than the ability to read and write. Health literacy is linked with education and empowerment and is recognised as a potential barrier to the 'fully engaged' scenario whereby people are empowered to take control of their own health, which is supported in the UK as the most cost-effective route to health and wellbeing for all (Wanless and Health Trends Review Team, 2002). Health literacy enables people to make health decisions in the context of everyday life. Nutritionists, therefore, need to be mindful of the literacy and language levels of audiences when designing evaluations. They should be able to develop oral, visual and written communications appropriate to the level of understanding of the audience in order to enhance effectiveness. It can be extremely embarrassing for someone to admit that they cannot read or write, whether it is in English or their mother language, again demonstrating that cultural knowledge is vital to successful working.

Literacy levels will influence the approach used for evaluation. Simple instruments may be suitable for low-literacy groups or those not speaking the language of the host country. Assumptions should not be made in relation to translation of materials as many immigrants may not be educated beyond primary level, and efforts to produce evaluation materials in an alternative language may not increase the quality of responses received. Evaluation instruments should be non-intrusive and quick to complete, which may be useful when assessing children or large samples; however, limitations in the validity and reproducibility of such tools need to be considered. Most paper-based dietary assessment approaches require some level of literacy, except for the interview administered 24-h dietary recall. Whilst this method is useful, the analysis becomes more time consuming and may not be considered appropriate due to resource constraints. Pictures for common foods and portion sizes are useful here to overcome limitations (Lanerolle et al., 2013). New technologies using computer-assisted programmes or mobile applications have scope but also have limitations in relation to adoption and acceptability of these tools in diverse communities.

29.5 Evaluation of dietary change in diverse communities

Dietary assessment in ethnic groups is critical for national surveillance programmes and for implementing and evaluating effective interventions. For the latter, we are interested in assessing changes in the diet that may be due to the intervention. For this, an appropriate assessment tool is necessary to quantify the change. Many interventions in the obesity era focus on weight loss measures as outcomes; however, whilst this is valuable on its own, it may not represent the complete nature of the changes made by the individual or group. Capture of the changes in dietary intakes and nutrient composition of foods would be useful for nutritionists to explore and report in evaluations to give a sense of what works and why. For example, changes such as use of alternative fat sources or reduction of salt use in recipes, or those made when addressing malnutrition, would be very interesting and valuable but are often not reflected in the evaluation design. One useful example of qualitative research undertaken to address a malnutrition intervention and evaluation is reported by Burtscher and Burza (2015). However, available evidence does not explain how culturally adapted strategies specifically influence outcomes.

Very few tools validated for diverse communities are available that enable such dietary behaviour to be assessed. Dietary assessment methods such as diet recalls, food frequency questionnaires (FFQs) and unweighed food records can be used. However, because of the popularity of amorphous foods – that is, foods that take the shape of the container they are in, such as noodle and rice dishes – this makes estimating the portion size a challenge.

In the UK, Sevak et al. (2004) validated an FFQ to assess macro– and micronutrient intake among South Asians in the UK. More recently, the development of a validated FFQ for use in Ghanaian migrants in the UK was developed from an assessment of commonly eaten foods (Adinkrah, 2010). At community practice level, many evaluations design their own tools to capture food consumed, but owing to a lack of validity or time these evaluations may not make it into the published literature.

Whilst these tools are useful, they have limitations, most crucially the accurate estimation of portion sizes (Cypel et al., 1997) and the literacy levels of those expected to complete them.

With evaluation, the use of strategies to recall portion size during dietary assessment by both interviewers and respondents can potentially improve data collection. This can include approaches such as guidance on quantities, such as 'large', 'medium' and 'small' in quantitative FFQs, or using portion size estimation aids such as food models, household utensils, photographs or diagrams, in 24-h recalls, although the performance of these tools is variable (Almiron-Roig et al., 2015). Commonly used in the UK is *A Photographic Atlas of Food Portion Sizes* (Nelson et al., 1997), which includes pictorial representations of commonly eaten foods and subsequent serving sizes. However, this may be of limited value as many ethnic minorities consume composite dishes (dishes made from many ingredients) and the ingredients are not always the same, depending on season and/or availability. Thus, whilst we may get a picture of portion size, without composition data the atlas has limited use.

Another difficulty with measuring diet in ethnic groups is that recipes can differ between areas, family preferences and cultural aspects. A common recipe is not often followed: there is often a 'know-how' that guides preparation and cooking which can be passed on to subsequent generations, but this may not have been recorded. Composition data for commonly eaten ethnic foods is available in most good databases based on *McCance and Widdowson* (Finglas et al., 2015) and more tailored information collected through recipe analysis for South Asians in the UK has also been published (Kassam-Khamis et al., 2000). The latter was based on household-level observations by collecting recipe information. More recently, the publication of an atlas of Indian foods has helped with assessment of commonly consumed Indian subcontinent foods and provides information on portion tools and servings and macronutrient composition (Sudha et al., 2013). These can be of use for evaluation of dietary data for these ethnic groups in the UK but require validation.

Lastly, a further complexity is that of cultures where food is consumed directly from a shared dish (such as is commonly observed in Arab and some African countries, particularly in the north), and this makes it difficult to assess individual diet and so requires resource-intensive techniques such as direct observation. This makes evaluation of dietary change interventions in these groups challenging.

Acculturation is known to have an observable effect on food choices and dietary habits (Ludwig *et al.*, 2011). Host nation foods are becoming popular and mainstreamed into the diet of minority groups replacing more traditionally consumed foods, and thus dietary acculturation is commonly observed (Satia-Abouta *et al.*, 2002). Furthermore, food and nutrient intakes vary among different ethnic groups but also differ within ethnic groups by migrant generation status (Ngo *et al.*, 2009); thus, intergenerational aspects need to be captured as these can have an influence on evaluation outcomes. This makes any attempt to assess diet in these groups difficult as any tool has to capture the complexity of the diet, which may be a combination of ethnic foods and those commonly consumed that may be typical of the autochthonous diet. What is needed is the development and publication of ethnic-specific assessment methods including portion size that would enable dietary changes to be better assessed as part of evaluation.

In summary, our ultimate goal must be to identify the factors that support successful nutrition interventions in ethnic groups, and this in itself is challenging for nutritionists or evaluators to capture without the appropriate tools. Strategies for dietary evaluation should not only include how dietary advice is delivered, but also focus on the multitude of factors leading to dietary changes, such as changes to meal pattern, meal composition and intake of different foods.

29.6 Conclusion

Nutritionists and service providers need to consider the socio-cultural framework and the diversity of values, interactional styles and cultural expectations in a systematic fashion within evaluation. To develop effective intervention strategies, it is vital to understand not only how changes occur, but also how different factors influence dietary habits.

A number of public health nutrition projects are undertaken with the aim of influencing nutrition-related behaviour change at community level and may include a specific focus on an ethnic group or groups. There is a good body of literature exploring the cultural aspects relevant to designing interventions.

However, limited literature exists on the evaluation of nutrition interventions in diverse communities including ethnic groups. There could be a number of reasons for this, as the issue in evaluation with diverse communities is that many interventions are population-based approaches and may only recruit small numbers of ethnic minority groups, thus limiting their impact. The evaluation design used may also not be robust enough to be published in the research literature or may only be reported to the funders/

commissioners. In an increasingly diverse society we should aim to address the health needs of different ethnic groups (whether generically or within targeted programmes); a well-considered evaluation can help to assess whether we have achieved this.

To conclude, a number of considerations emerge from this chapter for future research:

- The need for development of other sensitive ethnic-specific tools for assessing diet that can be used to assess dietary change.
- The development and validation of portion size assessment methods for quantitative assessment.
- The evidence reflecting differences relating to enabling and influencing factors and barriers to change in diverse groups compared with the mainstream population for interventions.
- Efforts to standardise definitions of culture and measures used as variables linking them to outcomes will be important to enhance future evaluations.
- There is a need to obtain evidence that shows the effectiveness of culturally adapted strategies and their influence on outcomes.

References

Adinkrah, J. & Bhakta, D. (2010) First generation Ghanaian migrants in the UK; dietary intake, anthropmetric indices and nutrition intervention through black churches. *Proceedings of the Nutrition Society*, **69** (OCE1).

Almiron Roig, E., Aitken, A., Galloway, C. and Ellahi, B. (2015) Assessing portion size in ethnic minorities in the U.K.: a systematic review of existing instruments. *Proceedings of the Nutrition Society*, **74** (OCE5), E306.

American Psychological Association (n.d.) Guidelines for Providers of Psychological Services to Ethnic, Linguistic, and Culturally Diverse Populations. http://www.apa.org/pi/oema/resources/policy/provider-guidelines.aspx (accessed 30 December 2016).

Burtscher, D. and Burza, S. (2015) Health-seeking behaviour and community perceptions of childhood undernutrition and a community management of acute malnutrition (CMAM) programme in rural Bihar, India: a qualitative study. *Public Health Nutrition*, **18** (17), 3234–3243.

Contento, I.R. (2016) *Nutrition Education: Linking Research, Theory, and Practice*. Jones & Bartlett Learning, Burlington, MA.

Cypel, Y.S., Guenther, P.M. and Petot, G.J. (1997) Validity of portion-size measurement aids: a review. *Journal of the Amercan Dietetic Association*, **97** (3), 289–292.

Department of Health (2004) *Choosing Health: Making Healthy Choices Easier*. The Stationery Office, London. http://webarchive.nationalarchives.gov.uk/+/dh.gov.uk/en/publicationsandstatistics/publications/publicationspolicyandguidance/dh_4094550 (accessed 30 December 2016).

Finglas, P.M., Roe, M.A., Pinchen, H.M. *et al.* (2015) *McCance and Widdowson's The Composition of Foods*, 7th summary edn. Royal Society of Chemistry, Cambridge.

Gilbert, P.A. and Khokhar, S. (2008) Changing dietary habits of ethnic groups in Europe and implications for health. *Nutrition Reviews*, **66** (4), 203–215.

Kassam-Khamis, T., Judd, P.A. and Thomas, J.E. (2000) Frequency of consumption and nutrient composition of composite dishes commonly consumed in the UK by South Asian Muslims originating from Bangladesh, Pakistan and East Africa (Ismailis). *Journal of Human Nutrition and Dietetics*, **13** (3), 185–196.

Kong, A. Tussing-Humphreys, L.M., Odoms-Young, A.M. *et al.* (2014) Systematic review of behavioural interventions with culturally adapted strategies to improve diet and weight outcomes in African-American women. *Obesity Reviews*, **15** (Suppl 4), 62–92.

Lanerolle, P., Thoradeniya, T., and de Silva, A. (2013) Food models for portion size estimation of Asian foods. *Journal of Human Nutrition and Dietetics*, **26** (4), 380–386.

Leung, G. and Stanner, S. (2011) Diets of minority ethnic groups in the UK: influence on chronic disease risk and implications for prevention. *Nutrition Bulletin*, **36**, 161–198.

Ludwig, A.F., Cox, P. and Ellahi, B. (2011) Social and cultural construction of obesity among Pakistani Muslim women in North West England. *Public Health Nutrition*, **14** (10), 1842–1850.

Nelson, M., Atkinson, M. and Meyer, J. (1997) *A Photographic Atlas of Food Portion Sizes*. MAFF Publications, London.

Ngo, J., Gurinovic, M., Frost-Andersen, L. and Serra-Majem, L. (2009) How dietary intake methodology is adapted for use in European immigrant population groups – a review. *British Journal of Nutrition*, **101**, 86–94.

Satia-Abouta, J., Patterson, R.E., Heuhouser, M.L. and Elder, J. (2002) Dietary acculturation: applications to nutrition research and dietetics. *Journal of American Dietitic Association*, **102**, 1105–1118.

Sevak, L., Mangtani, P., McCormack, V. *et al.* (2004) Validation of a food frequency questionnaire to assess macro– and micro-nutrient intake among South Asians in the United Kingdom. *European Journal of Clinical Nutrition*, **43**, 160–168.

Sudha, V., Mohan, V., Anjana, R.M. and Krishnaswamy, K. (2013) *Dr Mohan's Atlas of Indian Foods*. Dr Mohans's Health Care Products Pvt Ltd, Chennai.

Tiedje, K., Wieland, M.L., Meiers, S.J. *et al.* (2014). A focus group study of healthy eating knowledge, practices, and barriers among adolescent immigrants and refugees in the United States. *The International Journal of Behavioral Nutrition and Physical Activity*, **11**, 63.

Wanless, D. and Health Trends Review Team (2002) *Securing our Future Health: Taking a Long-Term View. Final Report*. HM Treasury, London. http://webarchive.nationalarchives.gov.uk/20130107105354/ http://www.hm-treasury.gov.uk/consult_wanless_final.htm (accessed 30 December 2016).

Yancey, A.K., Kumanyika, S.K., Ponce, N.A. *et al.* (2004) Population-based interventions engaging communities of color in healthy eating and active living: a review. *Preventing Chronic Disease*, **1** (1), A09.

Appendix

Dietary energy and nutrient reference values have been developed in a number of countries to provide a method of estimating the adequacy of diets in the population. Key differences in terminology between countries are summarised here, together with changes in the UK in recent years.

Daily Reference Values in the UK

In the UK, the Department of Health published *Dietary Reference Values for Food Energy and Nutrients for the United Kingdom* in 1991 based on advice given by the Committee on Medical Aspects of Food and Nutrition Policy (COMA). This established a set of figures known as Dietary Reference Values (DRVs) which cover a range of intakes (Table A.1). These replaced the single values previously published as Recommended Daily Amounts (RDAs). Full details and tables are available in the COMA report (Department of Health, 1991).

The purpose of developing these values is to provide a benchmark for assessing the adequacy of diets in a population. They are not intended for use as recommendations or target intakes for individuals. DRVs are defined for different ages and sexes since nutrient requirements may differ significantly with age, sex and physiology, with differing growth patterns, nutrient absorption and functional capacity contributing to this variability. Variability in older individuals is particularly high.

DRVs are based on the distribution of nutritional requirements in the healthy population, and the values for any nutrient assume the requirements for all other nutrients are met. DRVs assume a normal distribution of requirements within the population (Figure A.1), and are typically presented as follows:

Estimated Average Requirement (EAR) Defined as the intake estimated to meet the average (median) requirements (i.e. 50%) of the population.

Reference Nutrient Intake (RNI) At this level of intake, the requirements of 97.5% of the population will be met (calculated as 2 Standard Deviations above the EAR).

Lower Reference Nutrient Intake (LRNI) At this level of intake, 2.5% of the population will meet their needs (calculated as 2 Standard Deviations below the EAR).

Safe Intake Used where there is insufficient evidence to set an EAR, RNI, or LRNI. The safe intake is the amount estimated to avoid deficiency or excess.

COMA has since been superseded by the Scientific Advisory Committee on Nutrition (SACN) that focuses on nutrients for which there is cause for concern and advances to evidence have been made, rather than reviewing all the nutrients together: https://www.gov.uk/government/groups/scientific-advisory-committee-on-nutrition).

To support the population to meet the DRVs and eat a healthy, balanced diet, Public Health England created the Eatwell Guide (https://www.gov.uk/government/publications/the-eatwell-guide) with scientific rationale provided by Scarborough *et al.* (2016). The history of the guide and the main changes and methodology used to develop the guide, have been summarised by Buttriss (2016).

Updated energy recommendations in the UK

In 2011, the Scientific Advisory Committee on Nutrition (SACN) published a report entitled *Dietary Reference Values for Energy*. This contained revised figures based on a number of factors, including improved methodology for calculating energy requirements and updated WHO/FAO recommendations for energy requirements. The approach used in this report calculated EAR as Basal

Public Health Nutrition, Second Edition. Edited by Judith L Buttriss, Ailsa A Welch, John M Kearney and Susan A Lanham-New.
© 2018 by The Nutrition Society. Published 2018 by John Wiley & Sons, Ltd.
Companion website: www.wiley.com/go/buttriss/publichealth

Table A.1 Estimated average requirements for energy and reference nutrient intakes for selected nutrients in the UK.[a]

	Children					Males				Females				Pregnant females
Age:	Under 1	1 to 3	4 to 6	7 to 10	11 to 14	15 to 18	19 to 50	50+	11 to 14	15 to 18	19 to 50	50+	16 to 50
													reference nutrient intake per person per day
Energy[b] kcal	721	1197	1630	1855	2220	2755	2550	2340	1845	2110	1940	1877	2140
Protein g	13.5	14.5	19.7	28.3	42.1	55.2	55.5	53.3	41.2	45.0	45.0	46.5	51.0
Calcium mg	525	350	450	550	1000	1000	700	700	800	800	700	700	700
Iron mg	1.7	6.9	6.1	8.7	11.3	11.3	8.7	8.7	14.8	14.8	14.8	8.7	14.8
Zinc mg	4.0	5.0	6.5	7.0	9.0	9.5	9.5	9.5	9.0	7.0	7.0	7.0	7.0
Magnesium mg	55	85	120	200	280	300	300	300	280	300	270	270	270
Sodium[c] g	0.3	0.5	0.7	1.2	1.6	1.6	1.6	1.6	1.6	1.6	1.6	1.6	1.6
Potassium g	0.8	0.8	1.1	2.0	3.1	3.5	3.5	3.5	3.1	3.5	3.5	3.5	3.5
Thiamin mg	0.2	0.5	0.7	0.7	0.9	1.1	1.0	0.9	0.7	0.8	0.8	0.8	0.9
Riboflavin mg	0.4	0.6	0.8	1.0	1.2	1.3	1.3	1.3	1.1	1.1	1.1	1.1	1.4
Niacin equivalent mg	4	8	11	12	15	18	17	16	12	14	13	12	13
Vitamin B6 mg	0.3	0.7	0.9	1.0	1.2	1.5	1.4	1.4	1.0	1.2	1.2	1.2	1.2
Vitamin B12 µg	0.3	0.5	0.8	1.0	1.2	1.5	1.5	1.5	1.2	1.5	1.5	1.5	1.5
Folate µg	50	70	100	150	200	200	200	200	200	200	200	200	300
Vitamin C mg	25	30	30	30	35	40	40	40	35	40	40	40	50
Vitamin A (retinol equivalent) µg	350	400	500	500	600	700	700	700	600	600	600	600	700

[a] Department of Health, Dietary Reference Values for Food Energy and Nutrients for the United Kingdom. HMSO, 1991.

[b] Estimated Average Requirement

[c] The RNI for sodium is the amount that is sufficient for 97 per cent of the population. In May 2003 the Scientific Advisory Committee on Nutrition made recommendations about the maximum amount of salt that people should be eating, i.e. that the average salt intake for adults should be no more than 6 grams per day, equivalent to 2.4 grams of sodium per day.

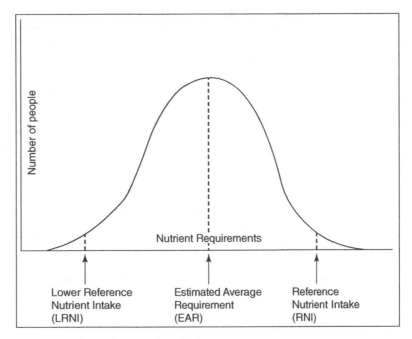

Figure A.1 Nutrient requirements for the population. *Source:* British Nutrition Foundation.

Metabolic Rate (BMR) multiplied by Physical Activity Level (PAL). The BMR values used were estimated using healthy body weights to ensure that if followed, the new energy requirements would lead to weight loss in overweight individuals and weight gain in underweight individuals. This prescriptive approach is one of the most radical changes from the previous methodology used, and was driven by the increasing percentage of the UK population with unhealthy body weights and activity levels. Further details of the SACN report can be found at (https://www.gov.uk/government/uploads/system/uploads/attachment_data/file/339317/SACN_Dietary_Reference_Values_for_Energy.pdf).

Other updates to recommendations in the UK

In 2017, SACN advised on military-specific DRVs for energy for those roles and/or activities where energy expenditures are different from the EAR for UK population groups in the *Statement on Military Dietary Reference Values for Energy* (https://www.gov.uk/government/publications/sacn-statement-on-military-dietary-reference-values-for-energy).

SACN reviewed the evidence on Vitamin D and health, and published a report with revised recommendations in July 2016 (https://www.gov.uk/government/publications/sacn-vitamin-d-and-health-report).   See chapter 20 for details.

The *SACN Carbohydrates and Health Report* (https://www.gov.uk/government/publications/sacn-carbohydrates-and-health-report) was published in July 2015 providing revised recommendations for intake of dietary fibre and free sugars. See chapter 17 for details. Public Health England published a report, *Government Dietary Recommendations: Government Recommendations for Food Energy and Nutrients for Males and Females Aged 1–18 Years and 19+ Years*, which updates guidelines in light of the SACN carbohydrate recommendations (https://www.gov.uk/government/uploads/system/uploads/attachment_data/file/547050/government__dietary_recommendations.pdf).

SACN gave an overview of the current evidence and the adequacy of dietary intakes of iodine in the UK in the *2014 Statement on Iodine and Health* (https://www.gov.uk/government/publications/sacn-statement-on-iodine-and-health-2014 on Iodine and Health). See chapter 9 for an update on current iodine status.

In February 2011, the *SACN Iron and Health Report* was published (https://www.gov.uk/government/publications/sacn-iron-and-health-report) reviewing the evidence and identifying population groups at risk of deficiency. See chapter 9 for details on the risks of iron deficiency.

The *SACN Folate and Disease Prevention Report* (https://www.gov.uk/government/publications/sacn-folate-and-disease-prevention-report) reviewed the available evidence on folate and health, particularly the need

Table A.2 Global terminology for dietary reference values.

UK	USA	European Communities	WHO/FAO	Explanation
Daily Reference Value (DRV)	Dietary Reference Intake (DRI)			Overall range of recommended intakes
Estimated Average Requirement (EAR)	EAR	Average Requirement (AR)		Meets the requirements of 50% of the population
Reference Nutrient Intake (RNI)	Recommended Dietary Allowance (RDA)	Population Reference Intake (PRI)	RNI	Meets the requirements of 97.5% of the population
Lower Reference Nutrient intake (LRNI)		Lower Threshold Intake (LTI)		Meets the requirements of 2.5% of the population
Lower end of safe intake range	Adequate Intake (AI)	Lower end of safe intake range		Lowest safe intake
Upper end of safe intake range	Tolerable Upper Intake Level (UL)	Upper end of safe intake range	Tolerable Upper Intake Level (UL)	Highest safe intake

Links to relevant data sources for each region are provided at the end of this appendix.

for adequate intakes of folate at the time of conception to reduce the risk of neural tube defect affected pregnancies.

Outside of the UK

The terminology used in other countries and regions varies, but the principle underlying the measures used are similar. However, the use of different age boundaries and different average weights within these groups means that there are minor variations between the guidelines given in each region. The USA, Europe and the World Health Organisation (WHO) and Food and Agriculture Organisation (FAO) have each developed their own reference values. These are summarised in Table A.2.

Interpretation and use

It is important to make a distinction between assessment of diet for population groups and individuals. For population groups, EFSA now recommends the use of the AR (or EAR) to estimate prevalence of inadequate intakes of micronutrients, assuming the nutrient intakes are normally distributed and independent of requirements (http://www.efsa.europa.eu/en/efsajournal/pub/1458). The PRI (or RNI/RDA) is likely to result in overestimating the proportion at risk of inadequacy and therefore should be used with caution in this situation. For macronutrients, it may be useful to determine the proportion of the group outside the lower and upper limits of the safe intake range to identify those at risk of adverse health effects. The mean intake of energy of a population group can be compared with the AR (or EAR) to determine adequacy of energy intake.

The use of DRVs for assessment of nutrient intake adequacy in individuals is limited. Intakes below the AR (or EAR) are likely to be insufficient and those below the LTI (or LRNI) are highly likely to be insufficient, while those above the UL (upper end of safe intake range) may be associated with adverse consequences.

More in-depth discussion of the use of the different dietary reference terms to describe intakes is provided elsewhere (e.g. Murphy *et al.*, 2006).

Reference intakes used in food labelling

The nutritional information provided on food labelling in the UK is controlled by the European Food Information Regulation (FIR) (see Chapter 24). Guidelines for dietary intakes of energy and key nutrients are defined by a single set of reference intakes (RIs). The RI values (Table A.3) are based on the requirements for an average female adult with no special dietary requirements and an assumed energy intake of 2000 kcal, and are intended as maximum amounts to be consumed per day.

The use of RIs replaces the previous use of guideline daily amounts (GDAs) in the UK. Food labels should

Table A.3 Food label reference intakes.

Nutrient or energy	Reference Intake (RI)
Energy	8400 kJ (2000 kcal)
Fat	70 g
Saturates	20 g
Carbohydrate	160 g
Total sugars	90 g
Protein	50 g
Salt	6 g

show the percentage of each RI provided per 100 g or 100 ml. No specific RIs are available for children.

References

UK data

Buttriss, J.L. (2016) The Eatwell Guide refreshed. *Nutrition Bulletin*, **41** (2): 135–141.

Department of Health (1991) Report on health and social subjects. Dietary Reference Values of Food Energy and Nutrients for the United Kingdom: Report of the Panel on Dietary Reference Values of the Committee on Medical Aspects of Food Policy, HMSO, **41**, 1–210, London.

Public Health England: https://www.gov.uk/government/publications/the-eatwell-guide

Scarborough *et al* (2016) http://bmjopen.bmj.com/content/6/12/e013182.full?keytype=ref&ijkey=Uo55Bu2X5HD3ukv

Scientific Advisory Committee on Nutrition (SACN): https://www.gov.uk/government/groups/scientific-advisory-committee-on-nutrition

WHO/FAO data

World Health Organisation. Worldwide dietary recommendations http://www.who.int/nutrition/topics/nutrecomm/en/

European data

European Food Safety Authority (EFSA): http://www.efsa.europa.eu/en/press/news/nda100326

Food Label Reference Intakes (Food and Drink Federation): http://www.foodlabel.org.uk/label/reference-intakes.aspx

USA data

Institute of Medicine. Dietary Reference Intakes. Washington, DC: National Academies Press.

Murphy, S.P., Guenther, P.M., Kretsch, M.J. (2006) Using the dietary reference intakes to assess intakes of groups: pitfalls to avoid. *Journal of the American Dietetic Association*, **106** (10), 1550–1553.

United States Departments of Agriculture (USDA): https://www.cnpp.usda.gov/dietary-guidelines

Index

Public Health Nutrition, Second Edition. Edited by Judith L Buttriss, Ailsa A Welch, John M Kearney and Susan A Lanham-New.
© 2018 by The Nutrition Society. Published 2018 by John Wiley & Sons, Ltd.
Companion website: www.wiley.com/go/buttriss/publichealth

Printed and bound by CPI Group (UK) Ltd, Croydon, CR0 4YY

27/10/2024

14580203-0002